T0305510

DRUG REPOSITIONING

About the Cover

Drug repositioning can be a daunting challenge, but one filled with possibility. There is a story in *The Art of Possibility* by Rosamund Stone Zander and Benjamin Zander of a man who comes upon a woman on a beach, surrounded by starfish that have washed ashore. She picks up individual starfish and throws them back into the water, in an almost "ritualistic dance." The man approaches her: "There are stranded starfish as far as the eye can see. What difference can saving a few of them possibly make?" Smiling, she bends down and once more tosses a starfish out over the water, saying serenely, "It certainly makes a difference to this one."

Like the woman, drug repositioning sifts through many compounds, particularly those "washed up," failed compounds, to find the one that makes a difference to patients.

Art of Possibility: Transforming Professional and Personal Life by Rosamund Stone Zander and Benjamin Zander. Harvard Business Press Books, 2000.

Cover image by Rachel Frail

DRUG REPOSITIONING

BRINGING NEW LIFE TO SHELVED ASSETS AND EXISTING DRUGS

Edited by

Michael J. Barratt

Donald E. Frail

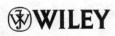

A JOHN WILEY & SONS, INC., PUBLICATION

Copyright © 2012 by John Wiley & Sons, Inc. All rights reserved

Published by John Wiley & Sons, Inc., Hoboken, New Jersey
Published simultaneously in Canada

No part of this publication may be reproduced, stored in a retrieval system, or transmitted in
any form or by any means, electronic, mechanical, photocopying, recording, scanning, or
otherwise, except as permitted under Section 107 or 108 of the 1976 United States Copyright
Act, without either the prior written permission of the Publisher, or authorization through
payment of the appropriate per-copy fee to the Copyright Clearance Center, Inc., 222
Rosewood Drive, Danvers, MA 01923, (978) 750-8400, fax (978) 750-4470, or on the web at
www.copyright.com. Requests to the Publisher for permission should be addressed to the
Permissions Department, John Wiley & Sons, Inc., 111 River Street, Hoboken, NJ 07030, (201)
748-6011, fax (201) 748-6008, or online at http://www.wiley.com/go/permissions.

Limit of Liability/Disclaimer of Warranty: While the publisher and author have used their best
efforts in preparing this book, they make no representations or warranties with respect to the
accuracy or completeness of the contents of this book and specifically disclaim any implied
warranties of merchantability or fitness for a particular purpose. No warranty may be created
or extended by sales representatives or written sales materials. The advice and strategies
contained herein may not be suitable for your situation. You should consult with a professional
where appropriate. Neither the publisher nor author shall be liable for any loss of profit or any
other commercial damages, including but not limited to special, incidental, consequential, or
other damages.

For general information on our other products and services or for technical support, please
contact our Customer Care Department within the United States at (800) 762-2974, outside the
United States at (317) 572-3993 or fax (317) 572-4002.

Wiley also publishes its books in a variety of electronic formats. Some content that appears in
print may not be available in electronic formats. For more information about Wiley products,
visit our web site at www.wiley.com.

Library of Congress Cataloging-in-Publication Data:

Drug repositioning : bringing new life to shelved assets and existing drugs / edited by
Michael J. Barratt, Donald E. Frail.
    p. ; cm.
  Includes bibliographical references and index.
  ISBN 978-0-470-87827-9 (cloth)
  I. Barratt, Michael J. II. Frail, Donald E.
  [DNLM: 1. Drug Repositioning. 2. Computational Biology–methods. 3. Drug
Industry–economics. 4. Pharmaceutical Preparations–economics. QV 55]

  338.4'76151–dc23

          2011044253

Printed in the United States of America

ISBN: 9780470878279

10 9 8 7 6 5 4 3 2 1

CONTENTS

7. **Predicting the Polypharmacology of Drugs: Identifying New Uses through Chemoinformatics, Structural Informatics, and Molecular Modeling-Based Approaches**   **163**
Li Xie, Sarah L. Kinnings, Lei Xie, and Philip E. Bourne

8. **Systematic Phenotypic Screening for Novel Synergistic Combinations: A New Paradigm for Repositioning Existing Drugs**   **207**
Margaret S. Lee

ABOUT THE EDITORS

Michael J. Barratt was a founding member and Senior Director of Pfizer's Indications Discovery Unit, where he led the Biomarker, Computational Biology, and Screening initiatives and later took on responsibility for academic alliances, a key element in the Unit's external drug repositioning efforts. Previously, Michael has held positions as Head of Molecular Pharmacology and Head of Dermatology Molecular Sciences for Pfizer in Ann Arbor, Michigan, and Skin Research Platform Leader for Unilever in New Jersey. With broad experience in drug discovery technologies and preclinical/early clinical drug development spanning multiple therapeutic, Michael has been involved in bringing more than 15 drug candidates into the clinic. In addition, he has fostered and led numerous strategic alliances in both the pharmaceutical and consumer health industries. Michael earned a degree in Biochemistry from Exeter College, Oxford University and obtained his PhD in Molecular Sciences from King's College London, where he also completed a postdoctoral fellowship.

Donald E. Frail is currently Vice President, Science, in the New Opportunities iMED at AstraZeneca, a research unit focused on identifying developing new medicines through external partnerships and drug repositioning. Prior to this, Don founded and led the Indications Discovery Unit at Pfizer, a dedicated research unit focused on drug repositioning, and was an architect of the groundbreaking partnership between Washington University School of Medicine and the Indications Discovery Unit. He has also held positions as Site Head for Pfizer's St. Louis Laboratories, Head of Biology for the St. Louis Laboratories, Head of Central Nervous Systems Research at Pharmacia, and positions at Women's Health at Wyeth and Neuroscience at Abbott. He has been involved in bringing more than 20 potential new medicines into the clinic across multiple indications. He obtained his PhD in Biochemistry from McGill University and completed a postdoctoral fellowship at Washington University School of Medicine.

■ ACKNOWLEDGMENTS

This book is dedicated to the many scientists who have worked tirelessly to produce the outstanding drug candidates that provide opportunities for drug repositioning and hope for patients. We thank all of our authors for sharing their expertise through insightful contributions. We also thank our colleagues in industry and academia, who have provided incredibly thoughtful perspectives and debates over the past few years. Our appreciation and gratitude are also extended to Lauren Frail for her expertise in indexing this first comprehensive work on this subject. Finally, none of this would have been possible without the understanding and patience of our families, to whom we are indebted for affording us the time to work on this project.

CONTRIBUTORS

Christos Andronis, Biovista Inc., Charlottesville, Virginia, USA

Makiko Aoyama, Sosei R&D Ltd., London, UK

John Arrowsmith, Thomson Reuters, London, UK

Michael J. Barratt, Washington University School of Medicine, St. Louis, Missouri, USA

Philip E. Bourne, University of California, San Diego, La Jolla, California, USA

Curtis R. Chong, Massachusetts General Hospital, Boston, Massachusetts, USA

Kuldip D. Dave, Michael J. Fox Foundation for Parkinson's Research, New York, New York, USA

Spyros Deftereos, Biovista Inc., Charlottesville, Virginia, USA

Louis DeGennaro, The Leukemia & Lymphoma Society, White Plains, New York, USA

Donald E. Frail, AstraZeneca Pharmaceuticals, Waltham, Massachusetts, USA

Scott L. Harbeson, Concert Pharmaceuticals, Lexington, Massachusetts, USA

Richard Harrison, Thomson Reuters, Philadelphia, Pennsylvania, USA

James Kasper, The Leukemia & Lymphoma Society, White Plains, New York, USA

Sarah L. Kinnings, University of California, San Diego, La Jolla, California, USA

Ourania Konstanti, Biovista Inc., Charlottesville, Virginia, USA

Margaret S. Lee, Zalicus Inc., Cambridge, Massachusetts, USA

Christopher A. Lipinski, Melior Discovery, Inc., Waterford, Connecticut, USA

Craig E. Masse, Nimbus Discovery, Inc., Cambridge, Massachusetts, USA

Richard Mazzarella, Appistry, Inc., St. Louis, Missouri, USA

John McCall, Polycystic Kidney Disease Foundation, Kansas City, Missouri, USA

Maria L. Miller, BioMed-Valley Discoveries, Inc., Kansas City, Missouri, USA

Mark A. Mitchell, Pfizer Inc., St. Louis, Missouri, USA

Akinori Mochizuki, Sosei Group Corporation, Tokyo, Japan

Adam J. Morgan, Concert Pharmaceuticals, Lexington, Massachusetts, USA

Damian O'Connell, Bayer HealthCare Pharmaceuticals, Berlin, Germany

Bhaumik A. Pandya, Concert Pharmaceuticals, Lexington, Massachusetts, USA

Jill Panetta, Polycystic Kidney Disease Foundation, Kansas City, Missouri, USA

Andreas Persidis, Biovista Inc., Charlottesville, Virginia, USA

Aris Persidis, Biovista Inc., Charlottesville, Virginia, USA

Ken Phelps, Camargo Pharmaceutical Services, LLC, Cincinnati, Ohio, USA

Andrew G. Reaume, Melior Discovery, Inc., Exton, Pennsylvania, USA

Michael S. Saporito, Melior Discovery, Inc., Exton, Pennsylvania, USA

Aaron Schimmer, Ontario Cancer Institute, Toronto, Ontario, Canada

David J. Sequeira, Upsher-Smith Laboratories, Maple Grove, Minnesota, USA

Anuj Sharma, Biovista Inc., Charlottesville, Virginia, USA

Todd B. Sherer, Michael J. Fox Foundation for Parkinson's Research, New York, New York, USA

Elizabeth T. Stark, Pfizer Inc., St. Louis, Missouri, USA

Alison Urkowitz, Michael J. Fox Foundation for Parkinson's Research, New York, New York, USA

Vassilis Virvilis, Biovista Inc., Charlottesville, Virginia, USA

Craig Webb, Van Andel Research Institute, Grand Rapids, Michigan, USA

Richard Winneker, The Leukemia & Lymphoma Society, White Plains, New York, USA

Lei Xie, University of California, San Diego, La Jolla, California, USA; and Hunter College, the City University of New York, New York, New York, USA

Li Xie, University of California, San Diego, La Jolla, California, USA

Introduction

MICHAEL J. BARRATT and DONALD E. FRAIL

Drug repositioning, also commonly referred to as drug reprofiling or repurposing, has become an increasingly important part of the drug development process for many companies in recent years. The process of identifying new indications for existing drugs, discontinued, or "shelved" assets and candidates currently under development for other conditions—activities we refer to as "indications discovery"—is an attractive way to maximize return on prior and current preclinical and clinical investment in assets that were originally designed with different patient populations in mind. It is widely appreciated that the business impetus to recoup the vast investments in pharmaceutical research and development (R&D) is enormous. As discussed by Arrowsmith and Harrison in Chapter 1, output of new medical entities (NMEs) approved by the U.S. Food and Drug Administration (FDA) has remained steady at around 25 per year over the last decade, while pharmaceutical R&D expenditure has increased over 50% in the same time frame [1, 2]. Against this backdrop of escalating costs associated with increased development timelines and requirements, along with growing regulatory and reimbursement pressures, drug repositioning has emerged as a lower cost and potentially faster approach than *de novo* drug discovery and development. The objective of Part I of this book is to examine in detail the medical and commercial drivers underpinning the repositioning industry, and to highlight the key strategic, technical, operational, and regulatory considerations for drug repositioning programs.

Among the numerous case studies that are described throughout this book, perhaps the best known example of successful implementation of drug repositioning is that of the blockbuster and first approved treatment for erectile dysfunction (ED), Viagra® (sildenafil citrate). The story of the development of this drug, which was originally being developed by Pfizer for the treatment

Drug Repositioning: Bringing New Life to Shelved Assets and Existing Drugs, First Edition.
Edited by Michael J. Barratt and Donald E. Frail.
© 2012 John Wiley & Sons, Inc. Published 2012 by John Wiley & Sons, Inc.

of angina, offers a fascinating insight into how keen observation and good science can unlock the full potential of safe biotherapeutics that are either already marketed or, as was the case for sildenafil, under development for other indications [3]. This example serves to highlight some of the essential elements that underpin the rationale behind, and opportunities that exist in, drug repositioning.

At its core, drug repositioning takes advantage of three fundamental principles. First is the reality of biological redundancy, namely that "druggable" biological targets can contribute to the etiologies of seemingly unrelated conditions, due to common underlying pathology and/or shared biological signaling networks. In the mid-1980s, the biological target of Viagra®, an enzyme called phosphodiesterase 5 (PDE5), was being studied for its involvement in regulating nitric oxide (NO) signaling in smooth muscle cells associated with coronary blood vessels. NO activates the enzyme guanylate cyclase, which results in increased levels of cyclic guanosine monophosphate (cGMP), leading to smooth muscle relaxation, increased blood flow, and the associated hemodynamic effects characteristic of nitrates. cGMP PDE enzymes such as PDE5 inactivate cGMP by converting it into guanosine monophosphate (GMP), and attenuate NO signaling. With this underlying biology in mind, sildenafil was at the time being considered as an antiangina therapy. After initial clinical trials in angina indicated modest hemodynamic effects (i.e., efficacy) but dose-limiting adverse events including erections, attention turned to ED, where the role of NO/cGMP was emerging at the time; but the role of PDE5 in the corpus cavernosum of the penis had not previously been appreciated [3]. New biology was thus uncovered and the rest, as they say, is history.

A second key driver for drug repositioning, which is also highlighted by the Viagra® story, is that the pharmaceutical drug discovery process is typically therapy area–focused and sequential, meaning that a candidate is usually designed and developed single-mindedly for one disease, regardless of whether the drug target may have roles in other diseases in different therapy areas. Because of this focus—though less frequent now than in the past—consideration of alternative therapeutic applications for a candidate may not occur until it either succeeds in the primary indication (typically in Phase III or beyond), or fails. Even then, repositioning or "indications discovery" efforts are not guaranteed and certainly rarely systematic, due to potential stigma associated with a failed asset, or risk aversion in a successful primary project team that "owns" the candidate, or simply lack of cross-therapeutic expertise/ mindset. As described in Chapter 2 of the book, one consequence of this for a pharmaceutical company's pipeline is that valuable patent life may be lost by delaying exploration of other opportunities, particularly if the candidate's safety, pharmacokinetics (PK), and pharmacology have been adequately demonstrated—often several years previously—in Phase I studies. Thus, repositioning applies not only to previously shelved candidates or marketed drugs, but increasingly to candidates that are still under clinical development in a primary indication.

Among the key elements of any repurposing program are the unique clinical, regulatory, and logistical considerations of conducting patient studies with candidates in secondary indications. The purpose of Chapter 3 is to outline some of the requirements for generating a robust data package for a second indication, as well as to highlight some of the often underappreciated challenges of repositioning candidates to different patient populations, where the safety package, route of administration, site of action, and PK/pharmacodynamic (PD) requirements can all differ. Part I concludes with a review of some unique regulatory and market exclusivity opportunities that can be applied to repositioned candidates (Chapter 4).

Fortunately, for both companies and the patients they serve, the traditional, sequential approach to drug discovery is changing. Increasingly, companies are leveraging internal expertise and external collaborators in a more cross-therapeutic manner to assess the applicability of pipeline or shelved candidates (and in some cases, external opportunities) in alternative indications that may be in noncore areas, in a more systematic and intentional way. A key component of a systematic approach to repositioning is the application of bio- and chemoinformatics-based approaches to interrogate vast amounts of internal and published preclinical/ clinical data (both on the drug candidates themselves and their cognate biological targets/pathways) to generate new hypotheses for experimental testing. Part II of this book—"Application of Technology Platforms to Uncover New Indications and Repurpose Existing Drugs"—addresses this aspect and outlines a number of computational strategies, tools, and databases that have been developed or successfully applied to repositioning studies. Authors in this section have been drawn from large pharmaceutical and biotechnology companies, as well as academia, in order to provide a wide spectrum of perspectives. Chapters in this section include descriptions and case studies using the numerous information sources that are publicly available to facilitate repositioning.

Also covered in Part II of the book is the topic of screening approaches for drug repositioning. As a complementary strategy to "hypothesis-driven" indications discovery, screening clinical candidates or marketed drugs in disease-relevant *in vitro* assays or animal models in an unbiased manner increases the probability of uncovering not only previously unknown connections between drug targets and diseases, but also the potential to reveal pharmacologically important "off-target" effects of a candidate. Off-target biology—the elicitation of useful pharmacology by a drug that was not intended or appreciated at the time of development—is a third and important driver for drug repositioning, particularly for older compounds that were less extensively profiled than present day candidates. For example, amantadine, originally developed for influenza through its ability to interfere with the viral M2 protein [4], was later found to have, among other activities, dopaminergic and noradrenergic effects and was subsequently repurposed for Parkinson's disease [5]. Another well-known example is thalidomide. Originally prescribed as sedative, it was found to have antiemetic effects leading to its use by pregnant women in the late 1950s and early 1960s with tragic teratogenic consequences for the developing fetus [6]. Despite these tragic beginnings, thalidomide has since been found to have a number of pharmacologically beneficial effects including antitumor necrosis factor (TNF) and antiangiogenic activities and has been approved for use in erythema nodosum leprosum (ENL) and multiple myeloma [7].

From the perspective of drug repositioning, phenotypic, disease-relevant *in vitro* screening assays, or animal models are unbiased with respect to "on-target" or "off-target" effects; any activity that modulates the endpoint being measured will be detected, regardless of cause. Although often more complex to prosecute and automate than conventional target-based biochemical assays used in the drug discovery process, such models provide the significant benefit of enabling an investigator to probe all the possible activities of a candidate, or cohort of candidates, across a wide therapeutic spectrum of disease models. Examples of cell-based screening approaches, including searching for novel synergistic combinations of marketed drugs, are described in the Chapter 8 by Lee, while the application of "multiplexed" *in vivo* screening platforms to identify new indications clinical candidates is described in Chapter 9 by Saporito et al.

The final chapter in Part II by Morgan et al. addresses a common strategy employed for drug repositioning or "drug salvaging," namely the development of chemically modified analogs of approved agents which are either metabolized *in vivo* into the parent drug molecule (prodrugs), or may themselves be viewed essentially as NCEs, in the case of deuterium-labeled analogs. Also covered in this chapter is the "chiral switch" approach, namely single enantiomer variants of previously approved chiral drug mixtures. Collectively, such strategies have yielded numerous clinically relevant, enhanced drug properties including increased bioavailability, improved PK profiles, more convenient dosing regimens, dramatic changes in tissue distribution, and decreased adverse events. A number of case studies are provided to illustrate these concepts.

It is noteworthy that many of the strategies covered in Part II have been driven by specialist companies that have developed and validated technology platforms to provide unique and cost-effective screening/repurposing services to the pharmaceutical/biotechnology industry. In many cases, these same companies have utilized their own platforms together with strategic alliances with large pharmaceutical companies to build internal pipelines of repurposed drugs of their own.

In Part III of the book, we turn our attention to repositioning approaches being pursued outside the industry, but often in partnership with it; specifically some of the efforts being championed in academia and by not-for-profit organizations/foundations. One of the increasingly important contributions that academic investigators and foundations provide in the field of drug discovery in general—and repositioning in particular—is their advocacy for rare or neglected diseases (sometimes collectively termed orphan diseases), which are frequently overlooked by big pharmaceutical companies due to lack of commercial return. In the United States, the Rare Disease Act of 2002 [8] defines rare disease strictly according to prevalence, specifically as "any disease or condition that affects less than 200,000 persons in the United States," or about 1 in 1500 people. A similar definition exists in Europe [9]. Neglected diseases [10] generally refer to a group of tropical infections prevalent in developing countries of Africa, Asia, and south/central America but essentially nonexistent in developed nations (e.g., parasitic trypanosomal and helminth infections, bacterial infections such as cholera, and viral episodes such as dengue fever). Chapter 11, written by Curtis Chong, describes several examples of repositioned candidates for diseases of the developing world that have been identified through open source screening campaigns such as the Johns Hopkins Clinical Compound Screening Initiative. Chapter 12 provides case studies from several different patient advocacy groups/foundations to highlight the unique work these organizations perform, as well as the tremendous potential advantages afforded by repositioning for patients suffering from rare diseases whose existing treatment options are often extremely limited. The book concludes with an overview of some of the business thinking that is currently being applied to drug repositioning within the pharmaceutical and biotechnology sectors with an emphasis on partnerships between the various stakeholders that are engaged in this sector. Chapter 13 highlights the increasing use of strategic alliances and risk-sharing partnerships as approaches to increase the industry's clinical development capacity and number of successful proof-of-concepts and recoup value on otherwise stalled assets. This chapter examines the various drivers for each party in such alliances and assesses the potential of current and future repositioning joint ventures between industry, academia, and not-for-profit organizations. Finally, Chapter 14 exemplifies some of the key considerations for drug repositioning partnerships through a case study on the Japanese biopharmaceutical company Sosei, which pioneered a unique business platform for reprofiling previously shelved drug candidates using a sophisticated shared risk partnership model.

The Appendix at the end of the book seeks to provide a compilation of valuable resources for the prospective repositioner, providing information on drug repositioning and reformulation companies, databases, relevant government resources and organizations, links to regulatory agency guidance, along with academic and nonprofit organization initiatives related to repositioning.

We hope that the book is as informative to the reader as it has been enlightening to compile.

REFERENCES

1. DiMasi, J.A., Grabowski, H.G. (2007). The cost of biopharmaceutical R&D: Is biotech different? *Managerial and Decision Economics*, *28*, 469–479.
2. DiMasi, J.A., Feldman, L., Seckler, A., Wilson, A. (2010). Trends and risks associated with new drug development: Success rates for investigational drugs. *Clinical Pharmacology and Therapeutics*, *8*, 272–277.

3. Bell, A. (2005). The Viagra Story: From Laboratory to Clinical Discovery. Medicinal and Bioorganic Chemistry Foundation Winter Conference, January 24, 2005. http://www.mbcfoundation.org/pdfs/Blockbuster%20Drug%20Symposium%20Final.pdf

4. Wang, C., Takeuchi, K., Pinto, L.H., Lamb, R.A. (1993). Ion channel activity of influenza A virus M2 protein: Characterization of the amantadine block. *Journal of Virology*, *67*(9), 5585–5594.

5. Verma, U., Sharma, R., Gupta, P., Kapoor, B., Bano, G., Sawhney, V. (2005). New uses for old drugs: Novel therapeutic options. *Indian Journal of Pharmacology*, *37*(5), 279–287.

6. Mekdeci, B. How a commonly used drug caused birth defects. http://www.birthdefects.org/research/bendectin_1.php

7. Teo, S.K., Stirling, D.I., Zeldis, J.B. (2005). Thalidomide as a novel therapeutic agent: New uses for an old product. *Drug Discovery Today*, *10*(2), 107–114.

8. Rare Disease Act of 2002. Public Law 107–280. November 6, 2002. 107th U.S. Congress. http://frwebgate.access.gpo.gov/cgi-bin/getdoc.cgi?dbname=107_cong_public_laws&docid=f:publ280.107

9. Use Information on Rare Diseases from an EU Perspective. European Commission Health & Consumer Protection Directorate General. http://ec.europa.eu/health/ph_information/documents/ev20040705_rd05_en.pdf

10. Wikipedia. Neglected diseases. http://en.wikipedia.org/wiki/Neglected_diseases

PART I

DRUG REPOSITIONING: BUSINESS CASE, STRATEGIES, AND OPERATIONAL CONSIDERATIONS

PART III

DRUG REPOSITIONING: BUSINESS
CASE, STRATEGIES, AND
OPERATIONAL CONSIDERATIONS

███████ **CHAPTER 1**

Drug Repositioning: The Business Case and Current Strategies to Repurpose Shelved Candidates and Marketed Drugs

JOHN ARROWSMITH and RICHARD HARRISON

1.1. INTRODUCTION

Drug repositioning or "repurposing" has become one of the major sources for revenue growth within the pharmaceutical industry [1]. Repurposing encompasses everything from new indications for failed compounds to line extensions for existing drugs and is expected to generate up to $20 billion in annual sales in 2012 [2]. This opportunity for revenue generation has led to an increase in companies such as Biovista, Melior, Marco Polo Pharma et al., consortia such as CTSA (http://www.ctsapharmaportal.org), and specialist units within major pharmaceutical companies that are dedicated to bringing new life to existing compounds, as well as summit meetings specifically designed on this topic [3].

It is easy to understand why repurposing drugs is so attractive since those that failed have been through much of the preclinical and some early human clinical trials and in many cases have been found to be safe. In general, drugs that have been approved for an indication have a greater likelihood of being safe in a new indication and different patient population. This increased knowledge of a drug shortens its development cycle relative to new molecular entities (NMEs[1]), bringing significant savings and lower risk to the cost of development. In addition, the continually evolving knowledge of targets and

---

[1] NME: new molecular entity, which includes new chemical entity (NCE) and new biological entity (NBE).

Drug Repositioning: Bringing New Life to Shelved Assets and Existing Drugs, First Edition.
Edited by Michael J. Barratt and Donald E. Frail.
© 2012 John Wiley & Sons, Inc. Published 2012 by John Wiley & Sons, Inc.

pathways means that developing drugs for rare diseases or stratified populations of common diseases has become a more technically viable research and
development (R&D) strategy.

This chapter will begin with a historic overview of why drugs fail and will
explore the reasons for failures at each stage in the development paradigm,
highlighting differences in success rates between therapeutic areas. Next, we
will discuss how some of these failures led to the drugs that are on the market
today. Finally, we will identify some of the common themes of repurposing
failed—or "shelved" compounds—with the goal of highlighting some of the
key learnings from these failures.

1.2. IS PHARMACEUTICAL R&D FAILING?

> The only time you don't fail is the last time you try anything—and it works
> —William Strong

Failure is a common problem in any research environment. Yet it is from these
failures that many of the greatest successes are born. When Thomas Edison's
experiments failed to produce a storage battery, he simply muttered, "I have
just found 10,000 ways that won't work." Failure is a fundamentally inherent
property in the pharmaceutical research and development process. It is due to
the difficult nature of the problems being solved that makes it so, and is not
reflective of the work that goes into the process. Despite the working of some
of the most creative scientific minds, most drug candidates fail. Statistically,
after testing up to one million potential candidates, one is picked to enter
clinical trials, and only 1 out of 20 compounds that enter into clinical trials
goes on to be a marketed product [4, 5]. Put another way, 95% of new drug
candidates entering human clinical trials fail. Furthermore, pharmaceutical
research data [6] suggest that drug candidates are failing more often. As shown
in Figure 1.1, the success rate for compounds progressing through clinical
development from Phase II to Regulatory Submission actually decreased over
the period from 2004 to 2009.

> Success is not final, failure is not the end. It is the guts to carry on that counts.
> —Winston Churchill

The pharmaceutical industry faces unprecedented challenges in its R&D productivity. Despite the continued increase in R&D investment up to 2008, with
a slight flattening in 2009–2010, the number of NMEs approved globally per
annum has fallen and cycle times for candidate development have risen [7]
(Figure 1.2). The sales figures in Figure 1.2 would at first glance suggest a fairly
optimistic future for R&D-based pharmaceutical companies; however the
growth in sales of branded drugs is more than offset by patent expiry such that
the majority of future sales growth comes from generic drugs and emerging

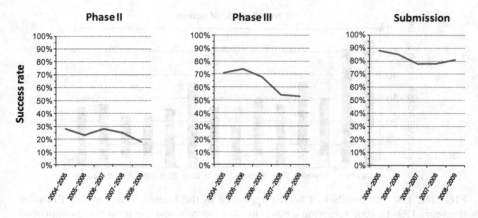

© CMR International, a Thomson Reuters business

FIGURE 1.1. Average success rates for compounds successfully advancing to the next phase of clinical trials for the years 2004 through 2009 for a cohort of 40 large and mid-sized pharmaceutical companies. *Source:* CMR International 2010 Global R&D Performance Metrics Programme. Reproduced with permission.

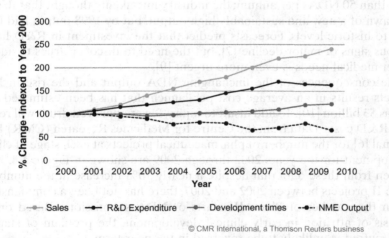

© CMR International, a Thomson Reuters business

FIGURE 1.2. The percent change in pharmaceutical investment in R&D, drug development times, and global NME output over a 10-year period indexed to 2000 for a cohort of 40 large and mid-sized pharmaceutical companies. *Source:* CMR International 2011 Pharmaceutical Fact Book [7]. Reproduced with permission.

markets. Generic sales are expected to be worth $400 billion by 2015. The shift from branded to generic drugs has a major negative impact on the profitability of traditional pharmaceutical companies [8].

Despite the steady increase in pharmaceutical R&D budgets over the last ~15 years, the number of new drug applications (NDAs) approved per annum

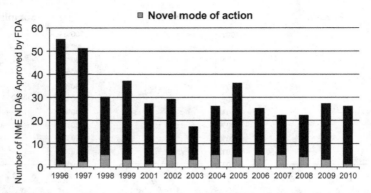

FIGURE 1.3. The number of NMEs approved in the United States by the FDA for the years 1996 to 2009 targeting a novel mode of action, and the total NMEs approved for a cohort of 40 large and mid-sized pharmaceutical companies. *Source*: Thomson Reuters Integrity database.

has remained reasonably constant (Figure 1.3). The only exception to this trend in output was in the period from 1995 to 1997 when output spiked to more than 50 NDAs per annum; the industry mistakenly thought that this was the dawn of a new and sustainably high output, but by 1998 output had fallen back to historic levels. Forecasts predict that the investment in R&D has no obvious signs of major decline [7], but the need to discover drugs to address unmet medical needs is even more urgent [9].

The consequences of the unchanging NDA output and the rise in R&D budgets results in an average cost per launch that has been estimated at as high as $3 billion [10]. To add insult to injury, fewer approved drugs will recoup their R&D costs. Data from the Centre for Medicines Research (CMR) International [6] for the number of pharmaceutical projects at each stage of clinical development for the years 2002 through 2009 are shown in Figure 1.4. It can be seen from these data that despite a nearly 70% increase in the number of Phase II projects between 2002 and 2007, there has not been a commensurate rise in the number of Phase III starts or NDA submissions. Based on this analysis of attrition in early clinical development, the problem of stagnant NME output is unlikely to be reversed in the near term.

Many explanations are offered for this productivity decline, but in reality, it results from a combination of multiple factors. From a biological standpoint, "breakthrough" drugable targets are often elusive, particularly for complex multigenic diseases such as Alzheimer's, cancer, and diabetes. There is also increased understanding of and attention to the safety risk–benefit profile of candidate therapeutics by the industry and regulatory authorities. Changes in strategic focus and cost reductions within corporate portfolios and ensuing reorganizations can halt entire therapeutic areas and delay progress in others. In addition, there is growing pressure from payers to reimburse only those new medicines that are clearly differentiated from existing standards of care,

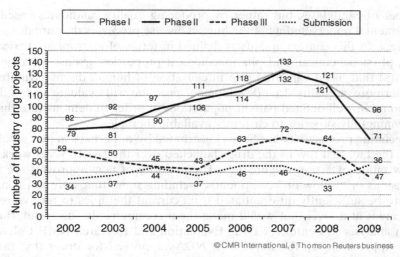

FIGURE 1.4. The number of NMEs entering each stage of clinical development from 2002 to 2009 for a cohort of 40 large and mid-sized pharmaceutical companies. *Source:* CMR International Global R&D Performance Metrics Programme. Reproduced with permission.

which themselves in many areas are increasingly dominated by lower cost generics as patents on branded medicines expire.

It is perhaps ironic that the current challenges are in part the result of past success. The pharmaceutical industry had a period of extraordinary growth in the mid-1990s, producing a far greater number of NDAs per year between 1995 and 1997 than ever before. In addition, a significant proportion of this cohort became blockbuster drugs, such as Lipitor®, Norvasc®, Zocor®, and Zoloft®. The underlying assumption at the time was that the discovery of new targets and new drugs was a "scalable commodity," and to increase drug launches one simply needed to increase the number of compounds entering clinical trials. Thus, if it required 10 first-in-human (Phase I) starts to get one blockbuster drug then, according to this logic, 20 Phase I starts would produce two launches. What followed was a major increase in R&D spending and capacity, and in addition research groups within these companies began to be incentivized to produce more drug development candidates; the number of new drug candidates became a primary goal. This flawed basis for improved productivity was built around a "shots on goal" philosophy. Since the average research and development time for a new drug is nearly 12 years, it took a while for the industry to recognize that more early clinical programs per se was not resulting in the anticipated number of late stage programs and launches. The increased attrition of candidates in development and the flat NDA approval rates was not an aberration. It became apparent that pharmaceutical R&D productivity could not be enhanced solely by increasing the number of candidates, but rather by producing quality candidates based on fundamental understanding of the human disease processes they are designed to affect. In this context, quality is defined in terms of appropriate toxicological, physicochemical, and pharmacological properties against a biological target(s) that has a validated role in causation of human disease/symptoms. Furthermore, a quality drug development program will evaluate such a drug candidate in well-defined patient populations in order to demonstrate that it is meaningfully superior to currently available therapies.

Declining productivity has been exacerbated by, or perhaps in part resulted from, the fact that few of the drugs launched over the last 10 years work via a new mode of action (Figure 1.3). The majority of new approvals are line extensions or "follow-on" compounds, including some that were not considered to be sufficiently differentiated from current therapies to receive reimbursement at a level that would make them commercially successful. Based on an analysis of Center for Drug Evaluation and Research NME Calendar Year Approvals [11], the number of NDAs approved for drugs that target unprecedented molecular mechanisms remains fairly steady at about 3–4 per annum. New regulatory hurdles now mandate that new drugs show superiority over existing therapies; the effectiveness of a drug (as measured in the United States) and the cost-effectiveness of a drug (as measured in the European Union) is the new standard for assessing drug value, further compounding the decline of drugs that are perceived to be only equal to or marginally more effective than currently available therapies. This greater need to differentiate from current therapy to enable reimbursement is driving the industry to a mantra of being "first and/or best in class" for each new drug candidate that it invests in. However in this regard, the concentration of research effort among companies working on the same mechanisms for the same or similar indications is a concern, since only a few of the drugs that come from this work will ever be approved and reimbursed. For example, according to an analysis by the authors in the Thomson Reuters Integrity database, 71 different organizations are listed as working beta-secretase as a drug target for Alzheimer's disease. It is reasonable to assume that, at best, only a very small number of these efforts will result in a medically beneficial and commercially successful product; and even this is assuming that the target turns out to be a viable therapeutic approach.

In summary, new targets for the complex diseases that remain poorly served are elusive, as are the drugs to safely and effectively modulate their activity. Biological complexity and redundancy will likely mean that in many cases a single "magic bullet" will not be found. These factors have combined to contribute to the progressive decrease in drug candidate survival in most phases of development and along with it, the probability of success to market. To make matters worse, many of the blockbuster drugs launched in the 1990s reach the end of their period of exclusivity in the period from 2005 to 2013 and there are not enough new drugs of high value to replace these revenue streams for their innovators. Even the emergence of high cost per treatment biologics is insufficient to bridge the revenue gap across the industry. The consequence of lower Pharma revenues, coupled with the higher cost of development, has led to reduction in R&D footprints, increased use of out-sourcing, and a need to refill development pipelines using strategies such as company mergers and acquisitions, in-licensing, orphan drug approaches, and repurposing.

1.3. WHY ARE DRUGS FAILING?

> Remember the two benefits of failure. First, if you do fail, you learn what isn't working and second, the failure provides you the possibility to try a new approach.
> —Roger Von Oech

Data collected by Thomson Reuters have uncovered the reasons for failure from Phase I to submission over the last 6 years for a cohort of 20 pharmaceutical companies (Figure 1.5). The data highlight the fact that the causes of failure change during the course of development. Early in the process, compounds fail primarily for safety reasons. Compounds that successfully navigate Phase I increasingly drop out due to lack of efficacy in Phase II/III. As noted previously, this decrease in pharmaceutical industry productivity (as judged by the number of products approved per money invested) appears to have no obvious signs of an immediate upward inflection. Attrition is not just increasing in early development but also in Phase III and at the approval stage [12]. Despite being the most expensive phase of development, more than half of the compounds fail to move from Phase III to approval. Table 1.1 lists some of the more notable failures of 2009.

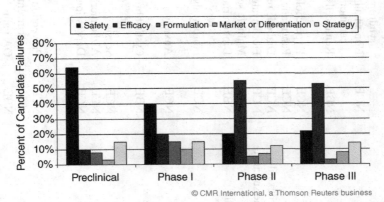

© CMR International, a Thomson Reuters business

FIGURE 1.5. A retrospective analysis of the reasons for a compound failing to advance to the next stage of clinical trials for the year 2009 as reported by a cohort of large and mid-sized pharmaceutical companies that represent approximately 70% of global R&D expenditure. *Source:* CMR International 2010 Global R&D Performance Metrics Programme. Reproduced with permission.

TABLE 1.1. Phase III Project Terminations Reported in 2009 and Reasons for Termination [12]

Product	NCE/NBE	Indication	Company	Status When Dropped	Reason
Mepolizumab	NBE	Hypereosinophilic syndrome	GSK	MAA Filed	Insufficient benefit–risk
Vandetanib	NCE	Non-small cell lung carcinoma	AstraZeneca	NDA/MAA Filed	No survival advantage
Vitespen	NBE	Renal cell carcinoma	Antigenics	MAA Filed	Negative opinion from CHMP
AVE-5530	NCE	Hypercholesterolemia	Sanofi-Aventis	Phase III	Lack of efficacy
Axitinib	NCE	Pancreatic cancer	Pfizer	Phase III	Lack of efficacy
Candesartan cilexetil	NCE	Diabetic retinopathy	Takeda	Phase III	Lack of efficacy
Desvenlafaxine succinate	NCE	Fibromyalgia	Wyeth	Phase III	Lack of efficacy
Dirucotide	NBE	Multiple sclerosis	Lilly/BioMS	Phase III	Lack of efficacy
DTP-HepB-Hib	NBE	Diphtheria tetanus, pertussis, Hep B, Hib	Sanofi-Aventis	Phase III	Reallocation of resources
Esreboxetine	NCE	Fibromyalgia	Pfizer	Phase III	Lack of superiority over existing drugs
Imagabalin	NCE	Anxiety	Pfizer	Phase III	Lack of superiority over existing drugs
Liprotamase	NBE	Cystic fibrosis	Altus	Phase III	Reprioritization of portfolio
Resatorvid	NCE	Sepsis	Takeda	Phase III	Lack of efficacy
Rosiglitazone	NCE	Alzheimer's	GSK	Phase III	Lack of efficacy
Saredutant	NCE	Depression	Sanofi-Aventis	Phase III	Negative study in combination with escitalopram
Sarpogrelate	NCE	Prevention of recurrent stroke	Mitsubishi Tanabe	Phase III	Lack of efficacy
Tanezumab	NBE	OA pain	Pfizer	Phase III	Safety—exacerbation of OA symptoms

MAA, marketing approval authorization; NBE, new biological entity; NCE, new chemical entity; NDA, new drug application; Hep B, hepatitis B; Hib, *Haemophilus influenzae* type B; OA, osteoarthritis.

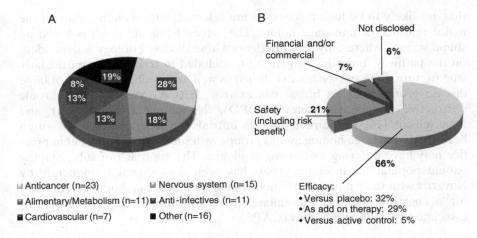

A

19%
8%
13%
13%   18%
28%

⊔ Anticancer (n=23)
▣ Alimentary/Metabolism (n=11)
▣ Cardiovascular (n=7)
▣ Nervous system (n=15)
▣ Anti-infectives (n=11)
■ Other (n=16)

B

Not disclosed
Financial and/or
commercial   6%
                  7%

Safety   21%
(including risk
benefit)

66%

Efficacy:
• Versus placebo: 32%
• As add on therapy: 29%
• Versus active control: 5%

Modified from Arrowsmith, J. (2011). Nature Reviews Drug Discovery, 10, (1), 87. *Nature Publishing Group*

FIGURE 1.6. Phase III and submission failures: 2007–2010, by therapeutic area (A) and reason for failure (B). Modified from Reference [12].

The failures at this late stage of development fall into a small number of categories, either lack of efficacy (defined as undifferentiated from current standard of care, no advantage as add-on therapies, or no advantage vs. placebo) or an unacceptable safety or risk-to-benefit ratio. The decrease in late-stage candidate survival seems to apply to both and large and small molecules and also occurs more frequently in complex, multigenic disorders such as neurodegenerative disease and cancer, where early promise in Phase II does not always translate into positive outcomes in larger Phase III trials (Figure 1.6). Another area of concern for cancer drug development is that the previously approvable endpoint of progression-free survival is being questioned for some tumor types where current therapies exist, and the higher hurdle of overall survival is now seen as the gold standard approvable clinical endpoint [13, 14]. This change in approval criteria has even impacted drugs that had previously been approved and marketed against the original endpoint of progression free survival.

To exacerbate the problem, even if a drug candidate successfully navigates its way through the R&D maze, the probability of it becoming a blockbuster drug has become increasingly difficult [15]. To maximize the potential for differentiated efficacy, it has also become increasingly important to stratify patient groups, which further compounds the challenge of producing a rapid rise in revenue after the initial launch of a new drug. Some companies have attempted to address this issue through launch of "incremental blockbusters," whereby they focus on the drug target, leverage an understanding of disease pathways that are dependent on modulating that drug target, and then target the responder groups across numerous diseases. In this way, only those patients that are likely to be high responders are selected, thus avoiding some of the major reasons for late-stage failure. The value of this approach is based on sound science where only those patients whose disease etiology is dependent on the pathway under investigation are included in trial. This is particularly true for rare diseases (see later sections) as well as for subpopulations of large disease groups such as breast cancer (e.g., BRCA1 vs. BRCA2), chronic obstructive pulmonary disease (COPD), rheumatoid arthritis (RA), and hypertension [16]. In the past, patients in trials for these diseases have often been treated as large homogeneous groups with similar symptoms but in practice may have differing underlying etiologies. The approach of sub-grouping patient populations in clinical trials has been demonstrated eloquently by Novartis with their novel IL-1β monoclonal antibody, canakinumab (Ilaris®) for a spectrum of rare autoinflammatory syndromes, termed cryopyrin-associated periodic syndromes (CAPS).

1.4. OVERCOMING FAILURES

Failure is success if we learn from it.

—Malcolm Forbes

Pharmaceutical companies have adopted a number of strategies in order to offset the issues caused by the fall in R&D productivity, price constraints, reimbursement issues, and generic intrusion. At a macro scale, companies are trying to maintain revenue streams and decrease a heavy reliance on a flow of novel drugs for the United States and Western European markets by moving more aggressively into emerging markets, building or buying generic drug capability, diversifying the business into animal health or consumer health, and focusing on rare diseases. There has been consolidation in the industry through mergers and acquisitions; there has been downward pressure on costs through staff reductions, outsourcing, and in-licensing. Many of the traditional "small molecule" companies have invested heavily in vaccines and biologics ("large molecules"). In addition, companies have increasingly extracted more value from their assets through life cycle management as seen in new indications (often related to the original indication), new formulations, combination products, and targeting new patient groups for previously approved products. Typically, this type of life cycle management used to occur as a product matured and the end of its period of exclusivity came closer, but in recent years the trend has been to advance these types of life cycle activities earlier in the period of patent protection. Clearly, life cycle management is dependent on a flow of new NMEs and so this practice will become more challenging as the flow of new products slows and exclusivity is lost. While biologics have remained relatively immune to generic intrusion, the recent introduction of legislation (U.S. Patient Protection and Affordable Care Act; European Medicines Agency guideline on similar biological medicinal products) [17, 18] will allow biosimilar production; and so this area is now under threat. Thus premium pricing that drives the value of biologics is expected to face challenges. However, the cost of entry into biosimilar development remains very high compared with small molecules, so it cannot be assumed that market share for biologic innovator drugs will be eroded as quickly as has been seen for small molecules.

Fundamentally the industry needs more strategies from which it can develop new and commercially attractive drugs at reasonable cost. Traditional life cycle management was discussed above; however, one area that still remains relatively underexploited is drug repurposing. With better understanding of drug targets and disease pathways, there are potentially significant opportunities to take existing drugs, or previously discontinued candidates, and repurpose them in new indications with high unmet medical need and so complement the usual *de novo* approach to R&D.

1.5. DRUG REPURPOSING

Failure is a back road, not a dead-end street.

—Zig Ziglar

1.5.1. The Case for Repurposing

Table 1.1 provides a summary of the Phase III program terminations in the pharmaceutical industry in 2009. Although not exhaustive, the data clearly show that compounds are failing in Phase III primarily for efficacy reasons. While the detailed causes for each of these failures are beyond this chapter, the following points are noteworthy:

- The majority of these compounds were safe at the doses administered in the Phase II and Phase III trials.
- The compounds have desirable pharmacokinetic (PK) and pharmacodynamic properties.
- It is estimated that around 2000 failed drugs are sitting on companies shelves and that this number grows at the rate of 150–200 drugs per annum [19].

The drivers for repurposing highlighted in this chapter are:

- Pharmaceutical companies need to have additional strategies that will bring new and reimbursable drugs to market quickly.
- There is much substrate available on which to build a repurposing strategy.
- The science to evaluate or re-evaluate new diseases continues to evolve so that science-led repurposing (rather than random screening) is a viable business model.

- The risk of failure is decreased.
- The cost of a repurposing program is significantly cheaper than *de novo* R&D.
- The cycle time of a repurposing program is significantly shorter than *de novo* R&D.

With repurposing strategies, companies are going back to re-examine these failed drug candidates with an eye toward new indications. Current estimates suggest that around 2000 failed drugs are sitting on companies' shelves and this number grows at the rate of 150–200 drug candidates per annum [19]. Clearly not all of these failed drugs are amenable to repositioning; some were shown to be unsafe or have poor PK properties, but there are a large number of molecules that could be considered for science-led re-evaluation.

Drug repositioning offers an attractive route to halt the declining productivity trend. An analysis of the reasons for a compound's failure—particularly where safety was not the primary cause—can be used to turn these failures into insights into how to be successful in the future. There is a growing list of examples of drugs that were initially designed for one indication and have either been discontinued or gone on to be successful after repurposing in additional indications. Some of these examples are shown in Table 1.2.

And why wouldn't the pharmaceutical industry want to build on this model? The time and cost to re-evaluate shelved drugs is less than the time and cost required to create NMEs, and can be a highly effective approach to developing new or better drugs that meet medical needs and that are also reimbursable [1, 2]. With a robust rationale in place, including confidence in the target and its relationship to the disease state in humans, a drug candidate can get a "second chance" to make it to market or extend the franchise of an existing approved drug. This second chance will benefit from the continually evolving science on targets and pathways, which not only elucidates new pathways of disease, but also enables the repositioning of drugs to them.

Understanding why a drug fails will help identify whether it can potentially be repurposed and, if so, the most likely therapeutic applications based on its known mechanism of action. Clearly when a drug has been shown to be unsafe in humans (e.g., TeGenero TGN1412, [20]) it would not be considered for repurposing. However, when a drug is dangerous in specific populations (e.g., thalidomide in women of child bearing potential) it has been demonstrated that carefully selected alternative populations can benefit from such drugs [21]. The definition of a "safe drug candidate" can therefore be indication/patient population specific. There are also drugs that express pharmacology in humans but do not translate into meaningful clinical outcomes (e.g., thromboxane synthetase inhibitors) yet may be synergistic with other pharmacologically active agents. Finally there are potential repositioning candidates among assets dropped from a company's portfolio for strategic reasons (e.g., Roflumilast, a

TABLE 1.2. Examples of Repurposed Drugs and Their Original Indications

Drug	Innovator	Mechanism	Original Indication	Repurposed Indication
Gemcitabine	Eli Lilly	Inhibition of DNA synthesis	Antiviral	Anticancer
Raloxifene	Eli Lilly	Estrogen agonist/antagonist	Breast cancer	Osteoporosis
Buproprion	GSK	Norepinephrine–dopamine reuptake inhibitor	Depression	Smoking cessation
Dapoxetine	Eli Lilly	Selective serotonin reuptake inhibitor (SSRI)	Analgesia	Premature ejaculation
Fluoxetine	Eli Lilly	SSRI	Depression	Premenstrual dysphoria
Hydroxychloroquine	Sanofi	Lysosomal alkalinization; TLR inhibitor	Antiparasitic	Antiarthritic
Doxepin	Boehringer Mannheim (Roche)	Serotonin–norepinephrine reuptake inhibitor (SNRI)	Antidepressant	Antipruritic
Bimatoprost	Allergan	Prostaglandin analog	Glaucoma	Eyelash growth

phosphodiesterase 4 [PDE4] inhibitor for COPD that was dropped by Pfizer but subsequently launched by Nycomed/Forest). Therefore, a thorough understanding of the reasons for termination provides a basis for rational decision making on future investments.

As will be discussed in greater detail in subsequent chapters of this book, a number of technologies have been employed in drug repurposing, including computational approaches [22–26], *in vitro* and *in vivo* methods [27–29], and screening for synergies among combinations of existing drugs [30]. Success stories can be found in diverse therapeutic areas such as HIV [31], cancer [21, 32], diabetes, [33] and erythema nodosum leprosum (ENL) [21] among numerous others.

1.6. EXAMPLES OF SUCCESSFUL REPURPOSING

A discussed, repurposing or repositioning is a smart way to capitalize on the cost of developing a new drug or resurrecting a shelved candidate. It has become a major driver for increased revenue within the industry [2]. Numerous small companies have been started with the sole purpose of repurposing drugs, but increasingly larger companies are building this capability into their R&D function. Successful repurposing can result in three potential outcomes: (1) new indications for shelved candidates, (2) line extension for existing drugs, and (3) new targets and new indications for existing drugs. The first category, shelved drugs, can be further subdivided into those that failed for efficacy, safety, and strategic reasons. We will examine each of these in greater detail with examples.

1.6.1. Drug Candidates That Lacked Efficacy in their Primary Indications

1.6.1.1. Sildenafil   Perhaps the most frequently cited example of drug repurposing is Viagra® (sildenafil), a phosphodiesterase 5 (PDE5) inhibitor that was under development for the treatment of angina in the 1990s. Clinical trials for the drug were suspended after it was shown that the compound had PK properties that were inconsistent with the prolonged control of angina in patients [34]. However, in these trials, researchers identified a striking side effect that helped define a new disorder—erectile dysfunction (ED). The poor PK properties that made the compound unsuitable as an antiangina treatment were ideal for a drug prescribed for ED. This case also exemplifies the point that some diseases are only considered as targets for therapeutic intervention when an efficacious drug is discovered, as was also the case for migraine prior to Imigran (sumatriptan). Subsequent to their use for ED, PDE5 inhibitors have been tested in a variety of other indications and found to be effective in pulmonary arterial hypertension (PAH) [34] for which sildenafil is now approved and marketed as REVATIO®.

1.6.1.2. Canakinumab   Another recently discontinued drug that was repurposed provides a good example of a new paradigm for drug discovery. Canakinumab, (trade name, Ilaris®) is a recombinant monoclonal antibody developed by Novartis that works by blocking an immune system protein known as interleukin-1beta (IL-1β), It was originally tested as a therapy for RA in a Phase II trial, where the drug failed to reach its clinical endpoints and was discontinued. Subsequently, a separate group of researchers at Novartis knew of a rare disease, termed Muckle–Wells syndrome, in which patients were genetically predisposed to high levels of IL-1β [35]. Although this rare and potentially life-threatening illness affects only a few thousand patients worldwide, the researchers successfully argued for additional trials. The results of these showed that Ilaris® produced rapid and sustained remission of symptoms in up to 97% of patients, with most of them responding within hours of the first injection [36]. The U.S. Food and Drug Administration (FDA) has approved and given orphan drug status to the drug for two forms of cryopyrin-associated periodic syndrome (CAPS): Muckle–Wells and familial cold auto-inflammatory syndrome. It has also received priority approval in the EU. Novartis is now conducting trials to extend the drug to other inflammatory indications such as COPD, gout, RA, ostheoarthritis (OA), and vasculitis in stratified groups of patients whose disease is highly dependent on IL-1β overproduction. The lesson here is that a clear understanding of the disease pathway is an extremely important factor in *de novo* drug discovery and is essential to unlocking the full potential of the many thousands of drugs that are available for repurposing.

1.6.1.3. Pertuzumab   Another recent example from Genentech involves pertuzumab, a first-in-class monoclonal antibody that acts as a "HER dimerization inhibitor", which was intended to be the successor to Herceptin®. In 2005, the Phase II clinical trials of pertuzumab in prostate, breast, and ovarian cancers met with limited success [37]. However, when evaluated in newly diagnosed early stage HER-2 positive breast cancer, pertuzumab used in combination with other chemotherapeutic agents caused cancers to disappear in 49% of patients, compared with 29% of patients receiving Herceptin® and chemotherapy [38].

1.6.2. Drugs That Failed for Safety Reasons in the Primary Patient Populations

1.6.2.1. Thalidomide   Thalidomide, launched by Grünenthal in 1957, was found to act as an effective tranquilizer and painkiller [21]. It was also found to be an effective antiemetic and had an inhibitory effect on morning sickness during pregnancy. Soon after launch, severe side effects began to be noticed as thousands of children were born with severe developmental abnormalities of the limbs and face (phocomelia) as a consequence of thalidomide use. The drug was withdrawn in 1962. Subsequent studies revealed the compound was an enantiomer, and only one of the two optical isomers was responsible for the teratogenic effects [39]. Unfortunately the two isomers interconvert in humans, so it is impossible to separate the risk from the benefit in women of childbearing age. However, despite the catastrophic effects on the developing fetus, thalidomide has since been used successfully in the treatment of ENL, a painful complication of leprosy, and tuberculosis [21]. Mechanistic studies have revealed that the efficacy observed may be due to its ability to inhibit tumor necrosis factor (TNF) alpha signaling. Further studies have been carried out to develop the potential for thalidomide in Kaposi's syndrome (a complication of AIDS) and multiple myeloma [21, 40]. Sales of thalidomide produced $550 million in revenue for Celgene in 2008. There is, therefore, renewed interest in thalidomide and its derivatives, and a recent literature search by these authors (Thomson Reuters Integrity database) has revealed investigation into its use in more than 30 alternative indications.

1.6.2.2. Plerixafor   Plerixafor was initially developed at the Johnson Matthey Technology Centre for potential use in the treatment of HIV because of its role in the blocking of CXCR4, a chemokine receptor that acts as a co-receptor for certain strains of HIV. Development of this indication was terminated because of poor oral bioavailability, cardiac disturbances, and its teratogenic potential. Plerixafor (Mozobil®) was subsequently repurposed as an immunostimulant used to multiply hematopoietic stem cells in cancer patients and the stem cells are subsequently transplanted back to the patient [41]. Hence the limitations that resulted in failure as an oral drug were not relevant for this innovative application.

What all of these compounds have in common is that they previously failed to meet safety and/or efficacy goals for their original indication. Additional studies brought about by keen observations of the clinical data or a deeper understanding of disease pathways led them to this innovative application.

1.6.3. Drug Candidates That Were Discontinued for Strategic Reasons

There is a category of drugs that were discontinued during clinical development for commercial or strategic reasons. These include drugs:

- In therapeutic areas that were exited by a company.
- That were "backups" or "follow-ons" to lead candidates.
- Where the likelihood of getting a return on investment was low either because the target population is small or because the development costs were very high.
- That, based on data generated or timelines, were not going to be first- or best-in-class.

TABLE 1.3. Examples of Drug Development Candidates Discontinued for Strategic Reasons

Drug	Company	Indication	Termination Reason
Roflumilast	Pfizer	Reduced exacerbation of COPD	Pfizer's Phase III efficacy endpoints not reached. This PDEi has subsequently been launched by Nycomed/Forest Daxas®/Daliresp®.
Alvespimycin hydrochloride	Kosan	Cancer	Hsp 90 inhibitor dropped due to reallocation of resources
AVE-0847	Sanofi-Aventis	Type 2 diabetes	Glitazar; reprioritization of product portfolio
INCB9471	Incyte	AIDS	Market potential; competing CCR5 antagonists already launched. Out-licensed.
TS-033	Taisho	Type 2 diabetes	Sodium-glucose transporter (SGLT) inhibitor dropped in Phase II in favor of backup compound

Drug candidates that have been discontinued during development for strategic reasons may be offered for out-licensing if a company assesses that there is no impact on their retained portfolio.

One example of a strategic discontinuation was Pfizer's Factor Xa inhibitor eribaxaban, which was shelved when a competing, but more advanced Factor Xa inhibitor, apixiban, was licensed-in from BMS.

Other examples of strategic terminations can be found in Table 1.3.

1.7. REPURPOSING EXISTING DRUGS

1.7.1. Line Extensions

A line extension is a variation of an existing product. The variation can be a new formulation of an existing product or an additional indication of an existing molecular entity [42].

It has been estimated that over half of the top 50 pharmaceutical companies expect to increase revenue by implementing some form of line extension on current products. This is clearly one of the best ways to maximize the potential of a compound, and this has not gone unnoticed by the pharmaceutical industry. One example of a drug that was extended beyond the original indication is bevacizumab, sold under the trade name Avastin®. The drug is a monoclonal antibody raised against vascular endothelial growth factor (VEGF), one of the primary mediators of blood vessel growth (angiogenesis). It was approved by the FDA in 2004 for use alongside the chemotherapeutic drug 5-fluorouracil in patients with advanced colorectal cancer and in Europe in 2005 as a first-line treatment of patients with colorectal cancer in combination with chemotherapy. Since the initial approval, Avastin® has been approved for a variety of indications both as a first-line treatment and in combination with existing therapies. Table 1.4 lists a few other examples of line extensions to expand the monopoly that these drugs gained.

The advantages of a line extension are many. Approval rates are greater for line extensions than for first-in-class molecules. While a new development project has a 10% chance of going from Phase II to approval, a line extension or repurposed candidate at the same stage (excluding reformulations or new combinations) has a 25% chance of approval (Figure 1.7). Similarly increased approval rates are also seen for compounds from Phase III to submission. Line extensions also expand patient populations and increase revenues with lower development costs than a new drug.

1.7.2. New Indications for Existing Drugs

Human pathophysiology is complex, with many interconnected signaling pathways. Unfortunately for the drug discoverer, compounds often affect more than one pathway, which can have safety implications. Conversely, the same signaling pathway can be involved in different disease states, meaning that a compound used for one indication can just as easily be applicable to other diseases. One such example is Avastin®, which as described above, is used extensively in treatment for many types of cancer, but has shown promise as a treatment for macular degeneration.

Several additional recent examples of new indication approvals for existing drugs [40] include:

- Duloxetine (Cymbalta®), a selective serotonin and norepinephrine reuptake inhibitor (SSNRI) indicated for the treatment of major depressive disorder, neuropathic pain associated with diabetic peripheral neuropathy, and generalized anxiety disorder, has been approved for treatment of chronic musculoskeletal pain.
- Onabotulinumtocin A (Botox®) is a neurotoxin complex indicated for the treatment of cervical dystonia, severe primary axillary hyperhidrosis (underarm sweating), and upper limb spasticity, and has been approved recently for the prevention of chronic migraine.
- Finasteride, a 5-alpha reductase inhibitor, expanded use from prostate cancer (Proscar®) to hair loss (Propecia®).
- Hydroxychloroquine (Plaquenil®), a compound that increases lysosomal pH and inhibits toll-like receptors (TLR), expanded use from an antiparasitic to an approved antiarthritic agent.

TABLE 1.4. Examples of Line Extensions and the Increased Years of Monopoly

Name (Marketed Since); Company	Monopoly Protection Until	Number of Monopoly Years	Second Drug (Marketed Since); Relationship to first drug	Monopoly Protection Until	Number of Monopoly Years	Additional Monopoly Gained
Citalopram (1989); Lundbeck	2002	13	Escitalopram (2002); (S)-enantiomer	2022	20	20
Omeprazole (1988); Astra Zeneca	2002	14	Esomeprazole (2000); (S)-enantiomer	2019	19	17
Risperidone (1993); Janssen Cilag	2007	14	Paliperidone (2007); active metabolite	2022	15	15
Loratadine (1988); Schering Plough	2002	14	Desloratadine (2001); active metabolite	2019	18	17
Paroxetine (1991); GSK	2003	12	Paroxetine CR (2002); controlled release	2017	15	14
Venlafaxine (1994); Wyeth/Pfizer	2006	12	Venlafaxine XR (2001); extended release	2017	16	11

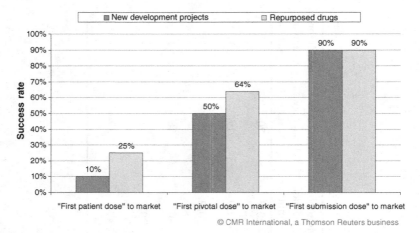

FIGURE 1.7. Probability of success to market for new development projects versus repurposed drugs for decisions made between 2004 and 2009. Repurposed drugs are defined as those drugs that have entered Phase II after the parent drug has been launched; it excludes reformulations, combinations, or same indications. *Source:* CMR International Global R&D Performance Metrics Programme. Reproduced with permission.

- Doxepin (Sinequan®, Adapin®), an SNRI, expanded use from an approved antidepressant to a topical antipruritic agent.
- Naltrexone, an opioid receptor antagonist, expanded use from an opioid addiction therapeutic to alcohol withdrawal therapy.

1.8. ORPHAN DRUGS

The focus of this chapter has been on repurposing failed drugs; some fail for safety reasons, some fail for lack of efficacy in the target indication, some fail because the patient population has not been appropriately stratified to eliminate nonresponders, and some fail because they no longer fit into a portfolio. The financial and time advantages of repurposing drugs have also been discussed. It is also appropriate to mention orphan drugs in the context of repurposing. The definition of an orphan drug in the United States is a rare disease with prevalence of less than 200,000 and/or for which drug development costs are unlikely to be recovered through sales in the United States. There are a number of incentives in the United States to encourage company involvement in orphan drug programs, including extended periods (7 years) of market exclusivity (and the potential for 10 years in EU/Japan), tax credits for 50% of development costs, R&D grants, fast track approval status with the FDA, and waived drug application fees. Similar concessions are available outside the United States. These incentives can make repurposing drugs to rare diseases particularly attractive. It is estimated that there are between 5000 and 8000 rare diseases and there is already orphan drug designation for over 1800 of these in the United States [43].

Orphan diseases make a sound platform for a repurposing drug strategy since there are excellent exclusivity and R&D incentives offered with the Orphan Drug Act and price restrictions around such drugs are lacking. In fact, companies like Genzyme (acquired by Sanofi-Aventis) and Shire (through its acquisition of Transkaryotic) have made rare disease and orphan drugs their core business. Other major companies like Pfizer and GSK are aggressively entering this opportunity space. An important note here is that 90% of approved treatments for rare diseases were not originally developed for these rare diseases. Moreover, the strong rationale for a particular mechanism in a rare disease can provide an initial lower risk and quicker path to commercialization before expanding to more prevalent diseases where the rationale may not be as strong, as in the case of Ilaris®.

1.9. CONCLUSIONS

There will never be a shortage of discontinued compounds; this is simply the cost of doing business in the pharmaceutical environment. But if we learn from these failures and apply the constantly developing understanding of biology and human disease, value can be salvaged through repurposing efforts from these failed compounds, which is important in today's R&D environment where new drugs are difficult and expensive to develop and many medical needs remain underserved. Repurposing drugs, including those that have failed in their primary indications or have been shelved for strategic reasons, is an important part of a pharmaceutical company's R&D strategy and is also a key component of the operating model for several specialist companies, as well as numerous academic and foundation initiatives. Subsequent chapters of this book will explore examples of these in more detail.

While there are numerous diverse examples of successfully repurposed drugs, a number of key themes emerge from them:

- Keen scientific observation or specific detailed knowledge of disease states created new opportunities for R&D.
- The time to market was significantly shortened since fewer preclinical studies were needed and Phase I clinical trials were often unnecessary.
- Cooperation was imperative across the entire R&D organization to move these compounds through to market.
- There is plentiful substrate within large Pharma companies, or potentially available for licensing from other companies.
- Pharmaceutical companies are increasingly willing to explore opportunities for previously shelved compounds in which much investment has already been sunk.

Some key enablers of a repurposing strategy are to have:

- Support and belief in the value of repurposing from R&D leaders.
- Resources to execute high quality preclinical/human translational validation experiments, including exposure–response relationships, and proof-of-concept experiments.
- Access to one of the high quality databases, such as Thomson Reuters Integrity, that accurately curate and record R&D success and failure activity from across all of Pharma.
- Access to a high quality database that mines and analyzes the continually emerging knowledge in systems biology to understand the underlying biology behind disease pathways (see for example http://www. GeneGo.com).

REFERENCES

1. Ashburn, T.T., Thor, K.B. (2004). Drug repositioning: Identifying and developing new uses for existing drugs. *Nature Reviews. Drug Discovery*, *3*, 673.
2. Tobinick, E.L. (2009). The value of drug repositioning in the current pharmaceutical market. *Drug News & Perspectives*, *22*, 119.
3. Campas, C. (2009). Drug repositioning summit: Finding new routes to success. *Drug News & Perspectives*, *22*, 126.
4. Kaitin, K.I., DiMasi, J.A. (2011). Pharmaceutical innovation in the 21st century: New drug approvals in the first decade, 2000–2009. *Clinical Pharmacology and Therapeutics*, *89*, 183.
5. DiMasi, J.A., Feldman, L., Seckler, A., Wilson, A. (2010). Trends in risks associated with new drug development: Success rates for investigational drugs. *Clinical Pharmacology and Therapeutics*, *87*, 272.
6. CMR International 2010 Global R&D Performance Metrics Programme. http:// cmr.thomsonreuters.com/services/programs/randd/.
7. CMR International 2011 Pharmaceutical Fact Book. http://cmr.thomsonreuters.com/.
8. IMS Institute for Healthcare Informatics (2011) The Global Use of Medicines: Outlook through 2015; May 2011.
9. EvaluatePharma World preview 2016 "Beyond the Patent Cliff" (June, 2011).
10. Munos, B. (2009). Lessons from 60 years of pharmaceutical innovation. *Nature Reviews. Drug Discovery*, *8*, 959.
11. Food and Drug Administration (FDA) Drug and Biologic Approval Reports. http://www.fda.gov/Drugs/DevelopmentApprovalProcess/ HowDrugsareDevelopedandApproved/DrugandBiologicApprovalReports/ default.htm
12. Arrowsmith, J. (2011). Trial watch phase III and submission failures: 2007–2010. *Nature Reviews. Drug Discovery*, *10*(1), 87.
13. D'Agostino, R.B. (2011). Changing end points in breast-cancer drug approval—The avastin story. *The New England journal of medicine*, *365*, e2.

14. Food and Drug Administration (FDA) Drug and Biologic Approval Reports. http://www.fda.gov/downloads/Drugs/GuidanceComplianceRegulatoryInformation/Guidances/ucm071590.pdf

15. Jack, A. (2010). Big pharma aims for reinvention. *The Financial Times*, October 2, 2010.

16. Food and Drug Administration (FDA) Drug and Biologic Approval Reports. http://www.fda.gov/downloads/Drugs/ScienceResearch/ResearchAreas/Pharmacogenetics/ucm085575.pdf

17. Food and Drug Administration (FDA) Drug and Biologic Approval Reports. http://www.fda.gov/Drugs/GuidanceComplianceRegulatoryInformation/ucm215089.htm

18. Food and Drug Administration (FDA) Drug and Biologic Approval Reports. http://www.ema.europa.eu/docs/en_GB/document_library/Scientific_guideline/2009/09/WC500003517.pdf

19. Jarvis, L. (2006). Teaching an old drug new tricks. *Chemical and Engineering News*, *84*, 52.

20. Bhattacharya, S., Coghlan, A. (2006). One drug, six men, disaster. *New scientist (1971)*, Mar 25–31;*189*(2544), 10–11.

21. Matthews, S.J., McCoy, C. (2003). Thalidomide: A review of approved and investigational uses. *Clinical Therapeutics*, *25*, 342.

22. Bernard, P., Dufresne-Favetta, C., Favetta, P., Do, Q.T., Himbert, F., Zubrzycki, S., Scior, T., Lugnier, C.P. (2008). Application of drug repositioning strategy to TOFISOPAM. *Current Medicinal Chemistry*, *15*, 3196.

23. Bisson, W.H., Cheltsov, A.V., Bruey-Sedano, N., Lin, B., Chen, J., Goldberger, N., May, L.T., Christopoulos, A., Dalton, J.T., Sexton, P.M., Zhang, X.K., Abagyan, R. (2007). Discovery of antiandrogen activity of nonsteroidal scaffolds of marketed drugs. *Proceedings of the National Academy of Sciences of the United States of America*, *104*, 11927.

24. Dubus, E., Ijjaali, I., Barberan, O., Petitet, F. (2009). Drug repositioning using in silico compound profiling. *Future Medicinal Chemistry*, *1*, 1723.

25. Ren, J.Y., Xie, L., Li, W.W., Bourne, P.E. (2010). SMAP-WS: A parallel web service for structural proteome-wide ligand-binding site comparison. *Nucleic Acids Research*, *38*, W441.

26. Subramanian, G., Sud, M. (2010). Computational modeling of kinase inhibitor selectivity. *ACS Medicinal Chemistry Letters*, *1*, 395.

27. Bhattacharya, A., Mishra, L.C., Bhasin, V.K. (2008). *In vitro* activity of artemisinin in combination with clotrimazole or heat-treated amphotericin B against *Plasmodium falciparum*. *The American Journal of Tropical Medicine and Hygiene*, *78*, 721.

28. Iorio, F., Bosotti, R., Scacheri, E., Belcastro, V., Mithbaokar, P., Ferriero, R., Murino, L., Tagliaferri, R., Brunetti-Pierri, N., Isacchi, A., Di Bernardo, D. (2010). Discovery of drug mode of action and drug repositioning from transcriptional responses. *Proceedings of the National Academy of Sciences of the United States of America*, *107*, 14621.

29. Kinnings, S.L., Liu, N., Buchmeier, N., Tonge, P.J., Xie, L., Bourne, P.E. (2009). Drug discovery using chemical systems biology: Repositioning the safe medicine Comtan to treat multi-drug and extensively drug resistant tuberculosis. *PLoS Computational Biology*, *5*, e1000423.

30. Tartaglia, L.A. (2006). Complementary new approaches enable repositioning of failed drug candidates. *Expert Opinion on Investigational Drugs*, *15*, 1295.

31. Clouser, C.L., Patterson, S.E., Mansky, L.M. (2010). Exploiting drug repositioning for discovery of a novel HIV combination therapy. *Journal of Virology*, *84*, 9301.

32. Gills, J.J., LoPiccolo, J., Dennis, P.A. (2008). Nelfinavir, a new anti-cancer drug with pleiotropic effects and many paths to autophagy. *Autophagy*, *4*, 107.

33. Saporito, M.S. et al. (2007). CINF 14-MLR-1023: A drug candidate for type II diabetes with a novel molecular target discovered by using an *in vivo* drug repositioning approach. *Abstracts of Papers of the American Chemical Society*, *234*, 14.

34. Ghofrani, H.A., Osterloh, I.H., Grimminger, F. (2006). Sildenafil: From angina to erectile dysfunction to pulmonary hypertension and beyond. *Nature Reviews. Drug Discovery*, *5*(8), 689–702.

35. U.S. National Library of Medicine. http://ghr.nlm.nih.gov/condition/muckle-wells-syndrome

36. Lachmann, H.J., Kone-Paut, I., Kuemmerle-Deschner, J.B., Leslie, K.S., Hachulla, E., Quartier, P., Gitton, X., Widmer, A., Patel, N., Hawkins, P.N.; Canakinumab in CAPS Study Group (2009). Use of canakinumab in the cryopyrin-associated periodic syndrome. *The New England Journal of Medicine*, *360*(23), 2416–2425.

37. Menendez, J.A., Lupu, R. (2007). Targeting human epidermal growth factor receptor 2: It is time to kill kinase death human epidermal growth factor receptor 3. *Journal of Clinical Oncology*, *25*(17), 2496–2498.

38. Roche. http://www.roche.com/med-cor-2010-12-10

39. Fabro, S., Smith, R.L., Williams, R.T. (1967). Toxicity and teratogenicity of optical isomers of thalidomide. *Nature*, *215*(5098), 296.

40. Ng, S.S., Brown, M., Figg, W.D. (2002). Thalidomide, an antiangiogenic agent with clinical activity in cancer. *Biomed Pharmacother*, *56*(4), 194–199.

41. DiPersio, J.F., Uy, G.L., Yasothan, U., Kirkpatrick, P. (2009). Plerixafor. *Nature Reviews. Drug Discovery*, *8*, 105.

42. Drugs.com. http://www.drugs.com/new-indications.html

43. Food and Drug Administration (FDA) Drug and Biologic Approval Reports. http://www.accessdata.fda.gov/scripts/opdlisting/oopd/index.cfm

████████ **CHAPTER 2**

Opportunities and Challenges Associated with Developing Additional Indications for Clinical Development Candidates and Marketed Drugs

DONALD E. FRAIL and MICHAEL J. BARRATT

2.1. INTRODUCTION

While drug repositioning is most often thought of as finding new uses for discontinued, or older marketed drugs, the merits of identifying additional indications for a compound or biologic that is being actively developed in a primary indication, or a patent-protected, approved drug are often stronger. More than 90% of drugs on the market are approved for additional indications beyond those for which they were originally developed and launched [1]. Furthermore, over 30% of new drugs or biologics that were approved or launched for the first time in the United States in 2009 were either drugs repositioned for new indications, reformulations, or new combinations of existing drugs [2]. Collectively, this clearly indicates a high success rate in extending franchises for those drugs that do initially make it to the market.

Conversely, most drugs fail in clinical development, as has been discussed in greater detail in the previous chapter and therefore the pursuit of additional indications in parallel with the initial indication offers a greater probability of reaching the market with maximum patent life. Much attention has been given to the performance of pharmaceutical and biotechnology research and development (R&D) organizations over the past decade and the lack of new medicines to replace the large wave of patent expirations and lost revenue (reviewed in Chapter 1). As a consequence, there has been considerable attention given recently to intentional drug repositioning strategies in order to maximize the

Drug Repositioning: Bringing New Life to Shelved Assets and Existing Drugs, First Edition.
Edited by Michael J. Barratt and Donald E. Frail.
© 2012 John Wiley & Sons, Inc. Published 2012 by John Wiley & Sons, Inc.

value of the R&D efforts. The aim of this chapter is to outline the opportunities and concomitant challenges associated with identifying and developing additional indications both for new medical entities (NMEs) that are being actively developed for a primary indication, as well as for patent-protected, approved drugs.

Since "drug repositioning" often connotes the "rescue" of a discontinued drug, we often use "indications discovery" to describe repositioning activities involving both discontinued drugs and those that are in active clinical development for a primary indication. Our perspective is based primarily on our experience in large pharmaceutical companies where extensive pipelines provide numerous repositioning opportunities, although these are usually competing with other portfolio priorities for finite resources. Despite this backdrop, many of the principles we highlight in this chapter are applicable to anyone considering a repositioning program.

2.2. THE VALUE PROPOSITION

While the value proposition for drug repositioning is highlighted in numerous ways throughout this book, there are three fundamental underlying premises. First, the biological targets that are the subject pharmaceutical development are components of complex biological pathways and networks. As a result, even the "on target" effects of many medicines modulate more than one system or disease process, which can provide both an opportunity for additional indications and a source of potential safety concerns. The enzyme phosphodiesterase 5 (PDE5), the target for the erectile dysfunction drugs sildenafil (Viagra®), tadalafil (Cialis®), and vardenafil (Levitra®), is involved in regulation of cyclic guanosine monophosphate (cGMP) and nitric oxide, mediators of endothelial function in multiple physiological contexts. Thus, PDE5 inhibitors impact overall vascular elasticity and have particularly profound effects on vascular elasticity of both the corpora cavernosa in the penis and the pulmonary vasculature due to high PDE5 concentrations in these tissues. Consequently, although sildenafil was not sufficiently effective in its first clinical studies in angina, it was highly successful in subsequent studies of erectile dysfunction (Viagra®) and pulmonary arterial hypertension (REVATIO®) and has therefore become an important example of drug repositioning [3].

Despite the success of PDE5 inhibitors, this example also highlights a second key driver for focused reprofiling efforts—the fact that in large pharmaceutical companies, drug repositioning/indications discovery has historically been the result of serendipity and, consequently, "sequential" in nature. In other words, the exploration of alternative uses for a compound or biologic often does not occur—if at all—until the primary indication has reached a pivotal decision point. The presumption that the primary studied indication is the "best" fit for a candidate may often be incorrect; moreover, with diminishing patent life, this is an inefficient strategy from a return on investment perspective, particularly once a viable candidate has been identified in Phase I/IIa studies. The time, cost, and risk involved in developing a compound that has existing toxicology and human data are significantly reduced. Repositioning a compound provides a significant shortcut to proof-of-concept (PoC) studies in humans, avoiding the time and costs involved in the discovery of a new compound, non-GLP (good laboratory practice) and GLP toxicology and safety testing, and, in some cases, Phase I human studies. Thus a significant advantage of repositioning existing drugs or advanced development candidates is the reduced risk of attrition due to toxicology or human pharmacokinetics. Importantly, however, there is no reason to believe that Phase II attrition—the initial testing of efficacy and safety in patients—will be lower for a repositioned compound. In other words, all else being equal, there is the same likelihood of *efficacy* for an NME entering Phase II in its first indication as there is for a repositioned candidate moving into Phase II for a completely new indication.

The third underlying premise for drug repositioning is that potential drugs are not necessarily selective for a single target and, as a result, multiple biological systems may be modulated due to these "off-target effects." Off-target biology—the elicitation of useful pharmacology by a drug that was not intended or appreciated at the time of development—is an important driver for drug repositioning, particularly for older compounds that were less extensively profiled than present-day candidates. For example, amantadine, originally developed for influenza through its ability to interfere with the viral M2 protein [4], was later found to have, among other activities, dopaminergic and noradrenergic effects, and was subsequently repurposed for Parkinson's disease [5]. Another well-known example of this phenomenon is thalidomide. Originally prescribed as a sedative, thalidomide was found to have antiemetic effects, leading to its use by pregnant women in the late 1950s. Tragically, its use resulted in birth defects, subsequently determined to be a result of teratogenicity in the developing fetus [6]. Despite these tragic beginnings, thalidomide has since been found to have a number of additional pharmacologically beneficial effects, including anti-TNF and anti-angiogenic activities, and has been approved for use in erythema nodosum leprosum (ENL) and multiple myeloma [7]. The additional biology elicited by "off-target" activities of a drug can further expand the opportunities for repositioning but may also lead to additional—and harder to predict—safety issues. As just one example, the analgesic effects of aspirin are complicated by a risk for gastrointestinal bleeding.

The strong value proposition for drug repositioning has led to an explosion of activity in academia and pharmaceutical companies as well as the formation of new companies that are based on a new technology or platform focused on drug repositioning, some of which are discussed in this book. Still, there are significant considerations and challenges involved in repositioning a compound and many of these are discussed next, with particular emphasis on pipeline candidates and approved drugs.

2.3. MANAGING THE RISK: ORGANIZATIONAL CHALLENGES

While generally thought to be lower than for a *de novo* drug development program, there are risks involved in repositioning a compound. These risks differ depending on whether the compound is "shelved" (i.e., no longer being pursued in another indication), if it is being pursued in another indication but not yet achieved clinical PoC, or if it is being pursued in another indication that has demonstrated PoC (Table 2.1). For compounds that are still under active development for a primary indication, there is often a concern by the project team that exploration of additional indications could uncover undesirable results that will negatively affect the development and marketing of the primary indication. Some of these concerns are based on real risks that must be considered for each compound and development program. In other cases, concerns are not based on true risks to the program but rather behavioral elements, including a strong sense of ownership of the compound by the project team. Breaking this down into discrete scenarios is instructive.

For those compounds in ongoing clinical development programs where the initial questions of efficacy and safety have already been addressed, typically Phase IIb or beyond, the chances of reaching the market are much improved. In addition, at this point there is a strong focus on the final label, including discussions and agreements with the regulatory authorities on what is required for approval. The investments at these stages are very high. Project teams whose candidates have reached Phase IIb are therefore loath to take on additional risks, and for good reasons. One less obvious risk, though, is a potential loss of focus on the primary program since any other activities will create complexity, be a distraction, and can slow timelines. A compound at this stage will likely require the full support of the primary project team and excellent communication across the teams.

For compounds that have not yet achieved PoC in their primary indications, there continues to be a high risk of attrition due to lack of suitable efficacy or safety. While all project teams believe that their project is going to be a winner, by far the majority do not make it, as the discussion in Chapter 1 highlights starkly. Yet there is often resistance by the project team to allow additional investigations for fear of jeopardizing the primary program, and often compounds in development are only pursued for additional indications after their failure (assuming not safety-related) in the primary indication. In these cases, a fundamental shift in organizational behavior and support from senior leaders is required for a successful repositioning program.

For those compounds that are not subject to ongoing clinical development programs, the organizational challenges are quite different. Since there is no longer a project team in place, a significant obstacle can be gaining access to all of the historical data and experiences with the compound or biologic. Ideally, former project team members can be engaged—if still present in the organization—to gain the best understanding of past events rather than relying solely on written documentation. Fortunately, these project team members are

TABLE 2.1. Repositioning Opportunities and Challenges Vary Depending on Status of Development in the Primary Indication

	Primary Program Ongoing: Pre-PoC	Primary Program Ongoing: Post-PoC or Approved	Primary Program Shelved/Discontinued
Opportunities	– Strong intellectual property (IP) position (NCE/NBE) – Ability to leverage primary project team resources—cost and time savings – Programs that have passed Phase I and have established proof of human pharmacology represent the "sweet spot" for indications discovery studies	– Strong intellectual property (IP) position (NCE/NBE) – PoC provides improved probability of success in second indication (assuming hypothesis is valid)	– No open IND to limit early investigation – Existing preclinical/clinical data packages can save years of work for the new indication – Existing composition-of-matter IP: value depends on filing date and assumes patent maintenance
Challenges	– Open IND; need to minimize risk of safety findings that are not relevant to the primary indication – Likelihood of attrition for efficacy is not reduced and attrition due to safety is only somewhat reduced	– Open IND/NDA; need to minimize risk of safety findings that are not relevant to the primary indication – High cost of investment post-PoC dictates even greater control of asset. Often second indications best led by primary project/brand team at this stage – Pricing and branding in different indications can be challenging	– Access to old data packages and expertise – New regulatory/safety standards may require additional toxicology or PK studies (in addition to clinical efficacy in new indication) – Loss of patent exclusivity; maybe reliant on less robust (e.g., formulation/methods patents) or shorter duration protection (regulatory exclusivity) – Organizational fatigue

often motivated to contribute in order to see the fruits of their past labors achieve success. A separate challenge, however, can be gaining the support of the organization to continue to invest in a compound that has failed in a primary indication. The justification required to gain the support to restart a failed program can often be higher than the justification required to initiate an entirely new program.

2.4. PRACTICAL CONSIDERATIONS, REAL RISKS, AND MITIGATION STRATEGIES WHEN DEVELOPING ADDITIONAL INDICATIONS FOR A CANDIDATE OR MARKETED DRUG

Organizational challenges and perceived risks aside, there are important practical considerations and real issues that must be understood for an effective drug repositioning program, particularly when the candidate is being actively developed or marketed for a primary indication. These are addressed in detail below.

2.4.1. Safety

A major source of anxiety associated with indications discovery efforts for candidates that are in clinical development for a primary indication is the potential to uncover additional safety risks that jeopardize the success or slow the progress of the primary indication. But wait—don't we want to know everything about the safety of a compound? Certainly organizations do want to know about relevant safety issues with a candidate as early as possible. However, it is possible during the pursuit of an alternate indication that safety findings that are not relevant to the primary indication's patient population can be uncovered. Consider these examples:

- The primary indication is an acute treatment and the secondary indication is chronic indication, so much longer safety studies are required for the secondary indication.
- The doses required for the repositioning indication are higher than those required for the primary indication.
- The primary indication and the repositioning program target different, non-overlapping disease populations (e.g., adults and pediatric, respectively) and therefore a safety signal could arise in the repositioning program that is not relevant to the primary indication.
- The formulation of the compound for the repositioning program differs from that used in the primary program, particularly if the route of administration differs (e.g., topical vs. oral).

In each case, the risk of discovering additional safety concerns that are not relevant to the lead indication's patient population could jeopardize the success of the primary program and most certainly slow it down.

However, there are strategies that can be implemented to mitigate the safety risks involved in the parallel assessment of additional indications for a clinical development candidate. In particular, the risks can be limited by an agreement within the organization that indications discovery/repositioning activities can proceed unencumbered as long as the repositioning program uses the compound within the existing limits defined by the safety studies submitted to the regulatory authorities. That is, the doses of the compound, the length of dosing of the compound, and dosing route, along the species in which the compound is used, are all within the scope of the existing data package. In this way, the probability of uncovering a new safety finding, particularly one that is relevant to the primary indication, in preclinical and clinical studies is low. Since any new finding that is deemed relevant to the primary indication is a reportable event to the regulatory authorities, these agreed upon limitations significantly reduce the risk of jeopardizing the success or slowing the primary project, without unnecessarily encumbering parallel exploration of additional indications.

For a candidate that has already been shelved or discontinued in its lead indication (e.g., for lack of efficacy or commercial reasons), the concern that a repositioning program could jeopardize other development efforts is obviously irrelevant. However, there are still practical considerations regarding safety. First, if the discontinued compound is older, there may be a need to upgrade the safety studies to present-day standards given the evolving guidelines (e.g., the need to assess the toxicity of metabolites or impurities if these exceed a certain level). Repeat or additional toxicity studies may be needed, for example, if the new indication requires (1) a longer dosing period than originally planned for the primary program, (2) a better definition of the maximum tolerated dose, (3) a different route of administration—for example, topical formulations may need additional local (dermal/ocular) tolerability and phototoxicity testing, or (4) the use of a different preclinical species with greater translatability for the new indication. The potential need for additional safety studies is but one of several reasons that debunk the belief that repositioning a failed compound is as simple as initiating a single clinical study in humans.

2.4.2. Preclinical Efficacy Testing

Almost all repositioning programs require at least some preclinical assessment for efficacy. As discussed in the previous chapter, a major cause of attrition is a lack of efficacy in Phase II studies, which can either be due to the hypothesis being invalid, or that the dosing regimen of the compound used was insufficient to achieve efficacy. Again, while there is a belief that a repositioning program can simply jump into a clinical trial, preclinical experiments are most likely needed to address the following:

- Enhance the *confidence that the rationale for the project is sound* through assessment in an animal model. While the utility of animal models to predict success in the human disease can be debated, these experiments are most likely needed if alternative approaches to increasing the probability of success of the program are lacking.

- The choice of *dose selection and dose duration* for the repositioning indication must be based on data and not simply assumed to be the same for the primary indication. In many cases this is determined in an animal model of the disease.

- Likewise, the *pharmacodynamic response* of the compound in the repositioning indication must also be based on data and not simply assumed to be the same for the primary indication. Again, in many cases this is determined in an animal model of the disease.

- A biomarker to assess target coverage relevant to the repositioning indication, *and the relationship between dosing, biomarker response, and disease outcome in the new indication*, must also be defined.

Such preclinical experiments can take up to a year, depending on the animal model and the extent of the biomarker work required. Without these data in hand, the repositioning program will not truly know if they have appropriately tested the compound in the indication if efficacy is not subsequently observed in the clinic.

2.4.3. Pharmaceutical Sciences Activities: Formulation, Drug Supply, and Packaging

Practical considerations regarding pharmaceutical sciences-related activities can easily be overlooked when first entering into a drug repositioning program. When the compound is also still under development in a primary indication, significant coordination is required between the respective project teams in order to avoid redundant activities, avoid any delays of the primary program, and expedite the repositioning program. Because there is already a project team in place, existing expertise and plans for formulations and drug supply ("active pharmaceutical ingredient" [API] also known as "bulk drug substance") can significantly accelerate the repositioning program and save costs if there is good cooperation between the programs. In the absence of an existing project, pharmaceutical sciences activities must be reinitiated for the new program, which is seldom trivial. In all cases, any drug repositioning program must address the following practical considerations:

- *Formulations.* If the formulation for the repositioning program differs from the primary indication, particularly if the route of administration is different, then significant formulation work is required prior to initiating a clinical study. Depending on the extent of the reformulation, additional toxicology studies and human PK studies may be required.

- *Drug Supply (Amount, Qualification, Purity).* Of course, drug supply is required for the clinical studies, but may also be required for additional toxicology and safety studies. If existing supply exists from the previous program, it may be "qualified" with acceptable stability for immediate use or it may be expired. In the latter case, it may be possible to requalify the supply. As part of this process, purity must be within the accepted range and this may have changed due to drug instability, or due to a change in regulations affecting the purity criteria. For a compound that is in development for a primary indication, excess drug supply may be available for use by the repositioning program, although this is not the norm. Instead, a new synthesis is likely required and this can take significant time.

– *Packaging.* The preferred packaging of drug supply for clinical studies can differ depending on the clinical study design and indication, and therefore new packaging may be required for the indication targeted for repositioning. Stability testing may also be required.

Such pharmaceutical sciences considerations can be vastly underappreciated at the outset of a repositioning program and the impact can be very significant given that they may take substantial time and specialist expertise to complete (e.g., a drug resupply could take up to a year) and the costs can be very high. Pharmaceutical sciences activities can often be the most time-consuming and costly activities required to initiate a clinical study for a drug repositioning program and one of the biggest challenges for drug repositioning efforts in academia and many small companies. This topic is discussed further in Chapter 3.

2.4.4. Regulatory

There are also practical regulatory considerations in pursuing a repositioning program that differ between the repositioning of a discontinued compound and one that is still under development in a primary indication. Some of these regulatory considerations are also considered in the context of the clinical study in Chapter 3. For those repositioning programs in which there is not an open investigational new drug (IND) application, the IND must be updated for the new indication, and perhaps to new standards for an older compound, and resubmitted to the appropriate regulatory division. In addition, it is not uncommon that the last active program did not archive detailed documentation of the last studies completed since the program was being terminated, and therefore additional internal diligence may be needed.

The situation is more complex for the repositioning of a compound that is also in development for a primary indication. There are several factors that create this complexity. First, an assessment of the type of regulatory filing required is needed, since the repositioned indication may be under the jurisdiction of a different division within the regulatory body (e.g., Metabolism and Endocrinology vs. Pulmonary, Allergy and Rheumatology divisions of the FDA) if the two studies are within the same country. A division may allow a study in a different indication to proceed under their jurisdiction depending on the size and complexity of the study and the comfort level of the division. More often, a new IND must be submitted to the different division, with updated sections relevant to the new indication and a cross-reference to the primary development program. Of course, a new filing is required if the studies for the new indication are to take place in a different country from that for the primary indication. In all cases, it is essential that there is excellent communication, collaboration, and coordination between the two program teams.

Perhaps the most important requirement for a repositioning program of a compound already in development is the coordination of safety reporting between the two programs and the regulatory bodies. An adverse event in one program, and the steps taken to address it, can have direct impact on the other program and a system for efficient cross-reporting and collaborative discussions between programs on how best to address must be in place. In addition, reportable adverse events in one program must be efficiently and appropriately communicated to the regulatory bodies of all programs. This can be particularly complex with an "independent investigator research" study where an academic investigator holds the IND and executes a clinical trial while the same compound is in development within a company for another use. Mechanisms must be established whereby the investigator-initiated study design, compliance, and safety reporting is aligned with the primary (internal) clinical study, which could include protocol review, oversight above what may normally be established, and a collaborative adverse event reporting and evaluation process.

As in any drug development program, the type of regulatory filing must be considered, from a full IND package to an exploratory IND. Many drug repositioning programs have full toxicology data packages and even Phase I studies completed, and therefore IND strategies like exploratory INDs are less likely to apply. However, a less recognized regulatory path in the United States, the use of a 502(b)(2) filing, may be applicable to certain repositioning programs and this is described in detail in Chapter 4.

2.4.5. Exclusivity Protection

Drug development is a high risk and expensive activity and therefore a term of market exclusivity sufficient to obtain a return on investment commensurate with the high risks is required. There are two means to achieve this. The first is through a patent and the second is through regulatory exclusivity.

Patents are the standard means of obtaining marketing exclusivity. In return for disclosing an invention, one is granted an exclusivity period that prevents others from practicing the invention. Many marketed compounds are covered by issued patents on the structures themselves ("Composition of Matter" patents), and therefore the generics are prevented from entering the market until the patent on the compound expires (20 years from original filing in the United States). Additional patent protection can be gained through other means, for example, from new methods of use or novel formulations. Since repositioning programs typically utilize compounds that are in development or launched, and patents are typically sought well before entry into development, a major challenge for repositioning programs can be that there is not sufficient patent life remaining to achieve a sufficient return on investment. In addition, the costs of maintaining patents are not insignificant and therefore patents on discontinued programs may have already been abandoned. In fact, there may be many potentially useful medicines that will never be developed because there is insufficient patent life remaining on the compound.

As stated previously, there are potential paths for new patents on older compounds. A "Method of Use" patent may be submitted for the new use of the older compound if this truly is a novel finding that has not been disclosed previously or obvious from existing disclosed data. However, one challenge is that many composition of matter compound patents claim a very large number of uses for the compound, even indications well beyond those initially demonstrated by the data, and therefore the "new" indication may be previously disclosed in the compound patent simply by referencing them as possibilities. Still, there are examples of methods of use patents for repositioning of compounds, including the use of thalidomide [7, 8] and the use of lyn kinase inhibitors for diabetes, as described in detail in Chapter 9.

Formulation patents have also been successfully used to provide market exclusivity. For example, the immunosuppressant drug cyclosporine, which has poor water solubility, has been developed in a topical emulsion for treating inflammation caused by keratoconjunctivitis sicca (dry eye syndrome) and marketed under the trade name Restasis® (0.05%) [9]. Numerous formulation companies have engaged in repurposing efforts, although technically these are often to extend the range of use (see Appendix).

A less well-recognized means of obtaining marketing exclusivity is to obtain regulatory exclusivity. Regulatory exclusivity was implemented by regulators to provide a means of market exclusivity for the developer of the first use of a compound and therefore a return on investment may be possible. It is important to note that regulatory exclusivity is completely independent from patent protection and thus provides an opportunity for even an off-patent drug to have a period of market exclusivity. For example, when generic drugs are developed, the generic company references data in the original innovator filing to support their regulatory filing, including efficacy and safety data. Regulatory exclusivity provides a defined period, independent of, but concurrent with any remaining patent protection, in which a generic developer cannot reference the initial filing. Until this period of exclusivity is over, the generic company could only gain approval if they completed the prohibitively long and expensive studies for a complete data package. In the United States, this period

TABLE 2.2. Marketing Exclusivity Periods for NCEs, NBEs, and New Indications

Territory	NCE	NBE	New Indication	Orphan Indication
U.S. [10, 13]	5 years	12 years	3 years	7 years
EU [10, 13]	8 years data + 2 additional years marketing[b]	NCE and NBE harmonized	1 year	10 years[a]
Japan [16]	6 years	Not distinguished	4 years	10 years

[a] 12 years for an orphan drug for children.
[b] A generic can reference but not file for these 2 years.

of exclusivity for new chemical entities (NCEs) is 5 years for the first use of a compound and 3 years for a new indication. In Europe, these periods are up to 10 years and 1 year, respectively (Table 2.2) [10]. While this does provide a path to market exclusivity, it can be a challenge to obtain a return on investment commensurate with the risk within five years (or less) of approval for two reasons. First, Phase III trials are typically the most costly phase of drug development by far and these are not avoided in a typical repositioning program. Second, the uptake of a new drug by physicians and patients is incremental and full acceptance, and maximal annual sales, can take five years (or more), just when the market exclusivity period is ending. Therefore, regulatory exclusivity may be an acceptable path when the total Phase III investment is on the lower end, which typically means shorter trials and fewer patients, and the unmet need is high so acceptance is much quicker than the norm. This strategy has not been used often, but there are examples. Both Taxol® (Paclitaxel) for use in cancers and Eprex® (Epeotin Alpha) for use in anemia were supported by regulatory exclusivity provisions that exceeded the remaining patent life [11]. One example that gained attention in 2009 was the approval of the use of colchicine for the treatment of gout, this despite the availability of generic colchicine for over a century and its common use in gout by the medical community despite the lack of U.S. Food and Drug Administration (FDA) approval. The generic colchicine, although not FDA approved for any use, was available prior to the 1938 Food, Drug, and Cosmetic Act and was thus allowed to remain on the market (see Chapter 4 for more details). UCL Pharma completed both pharmacokinetic (PK) and efficacy studies in gout patients and gained FDA approval based on these data. Because it was a new approved indication, it was granted 3 years of exclusivity. At the same time, UCL Pharma also gained approval for the treatment of familial Mediterranean fever (FMF) and was granted 7 years of exclusivity based on this orphan disease. Following approval, UCL Pharma sought to remove all other versions of colchicine from the market and raised the price by a factor of 50. This particular use of the regulatory exclusivity provisions captured the attention of the *New England Journal of Medicine* [12].

Only recently have regulatory authorities defined regulatory exclusivity periods for new biologic entities (NBEs). In contrast to the 5-year period provided to NCEs, the period provided to NBEs is 12 years in the United States, while in Europe NCE and NBE exclusivity has been harmonized at 10 years (plus an additional year for a new indication) [13].

Approvals for orphan disease indications are an exception to the standard NCE regulatory exclusivity period. In the United States, orphan indications are defined as those in which there are fewer than 200,000 patients in the United States [14]. The European Union (EU) definition of an orphan condition is broader than that of the United States, in that it also covers some tropical diseases that are primarily found in developing countries [15]. In order to stimulate the development of new drugs for orphan diseases, governments provided additional incentives. Among several incentives implemented in the United States with the 1983 Orphan Drug Act (ODA), which may include tax credits for a portion of the development costs, R&D grants, fast track approval status, and waived drug application fees, is a longer marketing exclusivity period of 7 years. The EU legislation, Regulation (EC) No. 141/200 [15], provides for 10 years of marketing exclusivity, but no tax incentives because there is no centralized EU taxation system. Japan also provides for up to 10 years of marketing exclusivity [16].

One must first seek orphan disease designation from the regulators, which is typically done at some point in the discovery or development phase, and there is a common European Medicines Agency/(EMEA)/FDA application available online. The application requires, among other things, a description of the drug and a discussion of the scientific rationale for the use of the drug for the rare disease or condition, including all relevant supporting data from nonclinical laboratory studies, clinical investigations, and other evidence that is available to the sponsor, whether positive, negative, or inconclusive. Also required is documentation that demonstrates that the number of people afflicted by the disease meets the respective statutory prevalence threshold, and a summary of prior regulatory submissions for the drug [17]. The FDA publishes those programs that have been granted orphan disease status [18] and the European Medicines Agency maintains a similar database [19]. The number of programs that have obtained orphan disease status has increased substantially since implementation of these incentives—there are now over 1800 designations in the FDA database—suggesting that the longer data exclusivity period is indeed stimulating the development of new drugs for orphan disease.

In summary, one potential challenge with repositioning a drug is limited patent life. Regulatory exclusivity is an alternative means to market exclusivity, although the standard 5-year term for NCEs in the United States is often not sufficient to stimulate investment. However, the longer terms provided by various orphan drug regulations clearly have stimulated investment in this category, given the number of records now in the FDA's Orphan Drug Database [18]. It is likely that additional drug repositioning efforts, particularly of the thousands of NCEs with limited patent life, would be strongly stimulated by a change of the U.S. data exclusivity terms for NCEs from the current 5 years up to the 10 years afforded orphan indications (and NCEs in Europe) or even the 12 years now provided to NBEs in the United States [13].

2.4.6. Parallel Development Programs

There are real risks and complexities that need to be considered when the compound of interest for a drug repositioning program is also being actively developed for another indication. The potential risks to the primary program fall into two categories—the risk of generating data that raises concerns and the risk of lack of focus and time delays.

Data can be generated in the drug repositioning program that unnecessarily jeopardize the primary program, including additional toxicology findings that are not relevant to the primary program, as previously described in the safety section. In addition, a poorly designed clinical study, including the choice of the patient population for the repositioning clinical study, and a poorly monitored clinical study can also provide results that unnecessarily jeopardize the primary program. Each of these factors into the considerations to reduce the risks, as previously described in the regulatory section.

There is also the potential that a drug repositioning program can have a real impact on the timelines set for the primary program, while at the same time a primary program can accelerate the timelines for the repositioning program. Some examples include:

- The need for the repositioning program to engage and coordinate with the primary program, creating a distraction for the primary program and potentially delays.
- The production of drug supply for a clinical study is typically done as synthetic "campaigns" that require advanced planning and months to complete. It is ideal for a drug repositioning if they can simply increase the production target of a campaign project if the program can be simply increased. However, this requires perfect timing in the design and finalizing of the repositioning clinical study or a delay in the campaign to complete the clinical study design. While the latter may create a short time delay to the primary program, it would typically save a significant amount of time, up to a year or more, that would be needed to schedule an entirely separate campaign. Exactly how the decision is made regarding the drug supply planning options, particularly one that would cause a short delay to a primary program to greatly accelerate the repositioning program, can be contentious.
- Also highlighted previously is the need to closely coordinate the adverse event assessment and reporting between the two project teams, which creates additional complexity.

2.4.7. Pricing, Reimbursement, and Prescribing Practices

There are significant issues that must be considered regarding both pricing and marketing for any program, some unique to repositioning. There are various scenarios that differ depending on the status of marketed competitor molecules that are targeting either the same mechanism or a different mechanism for the same indication. Marketing exclusivity does not guarantee that the new drug will be reimbursed by government programs and private insurers, which are a major segment of the market. Some of the various scenarios and considerations are outlined below.

2.4.7.1. Scenario: A New Use for a Compound That Is the Only NCE/NBE in the Mechanistic Class on the Market   This is the best-case scenario. This is the case for the lyn kinase repositioning program being pursued by Melior Discovery (described in Chapter 9). This old drug failed in Phase III clinical development many years ago as a treatment for gastric ulcers [20]. Using its *theraTRACE®* screening platform, Melior discovered that the compound had anti-diabetic effects in multiple animal models of type 2 diabetes, and subsequently defined the molecular target as lyn kinase. They have filed methods of use patents for the compound—named MLR-1023—and for lyn kinase inhibitors in general [21]. Based on these new findings, an IND was granted by the FDA [22]. If Melior is granted the methods of use patents and successfully reaches the market with a lyn kinase inhibitor, in addition to patent exclusivity, they will also have pricing flexibility since there is not a competing lyn kinase molecule on the market. Clearly, though, like all new products, it will need to be priced appropriately relative to competing anti-diabetic agents that target different mechanisms.

2.4.7.2. Scenario: A New Use for a Compound in the Same Mechanistic Class as Other Proprietary Compounds That Are on the Market for Other Indications   With any new drug development program, pricing of the new drug must be carefully considered and is heavily influenced by both regulatory authorities and those in the distribution chain. In certain countries, the regulatory authorities consider the value (or cost-effectiveness) of the new medicine in their approval process, value being roughly defined as the amount of medical impact of the new medicine relative to the currently available treatments divided by the costs. In addition to regulatory considerations, national health plans may consider the value of the new medicine and only add to the national health formulary if they deem the value to be sufficiently high. In these cases, regulatory approval is only the first step to obtaining formulary status, while reimbursement by the national health plans, which typically cover a relatively high percentage of total patients, is nearly essential for commercial success. A subset of examples illustrates various situations below.

- The National Institute for Health and Clinical Excellence (NICE) has powers in the UK to deny reimbursement of drugs through the National

Health Service that are not deemed to be cost-effective. Notable examples include the breast cancer drug Herceptin®, and treatments for macular degeneration, Macugen® and Lucentis®. While these powers will be rescinded in 2014, in part as a result of public pressure, they are being replaced with a value-based pricing system in which the UK government will negotiate with pharmaceutical companies to agree a price, based on a drug's effectiveness [23]. While applicable to all market entrants, including repositioned drugs, this clearly raises the bar for reimbursement of new medicines reaching the market in the UK and is indicative of a growing global trend to combat rising healthcare costs.

• The case study of Avastin® and Lucentis® illustrates how the commercial success of a molecule for a new indication can be affected by the existence of a marketed compound against the same biological target (in this case vascular endothelial growth factor [VEGF]) for a different indication. Avastin®, an oral drug, is on the market for oncology indications while Lucentis®, a drug delivered by injection into the eye, is on the market for age-related macular degeneration. The price of Lucentis® for macular degeneration was set around $2000 per injection in the United States while equivalent doses resulting from "splitting" Avastin® vials between multiple patients costs around $50 [24]. Although Avastin® was not approved for macular degeneration, physicians have the prerogative to use Avastin® off-label and have shown it to be effective. This puts considerable pressure on the developer to justify the high price of Lucentis® when a lower cost option is potentially available. It is noteworthy in this case, however, that the risks of off-label use have recently been highlighted by reports of a number of patients contracting serious eye infections and in some cases losing their sight, after unapproved off-label use of Avastin® [24].

It is also important to note that a second potential hurdle is the practice of "prescription switching." In the United States, there is flexibility that allows the switching of the physician-prescribed drug to an alternative, including generics, in a number of states. Typically, at least in the United States, the profit margins to those in the distribution chain, from wholesalers to retailers to payers, for generic drugs are higher than for branded drugs and therefore those in the distribution chain have a large incentive to encourage the switching of branded prescriptions to generics. Often the patient's co-pay is less for generic drugs and therefore the patients also have an incentive to switch to a generic. One complication is that reimbursements for a drug for non-approved indications can be complex and vary among the many payers. Regardless, if there is a potential alternative choice, there will be significant pressure on the developer to justify pricing and therefore truly innovative medicines are the surest path to commercial success.

Although not a repositioning example per se, the prescription switching scenario is illustrated well by the multiple statins that have revolutionized the treatment of hyperlipidemia. Certain statins are now at, or nearing their end of patent life and therefore available as generics. With the availability of generic Zocor® at a lower price than the branded super statins, sales of Lipitor® and Crestor® began to be negatively impacted in part due to both the prescribing of generic Zocor® and the switching of Lipitor® and Crestor® prescriptions to generic Zocor®. Similarly, it is speculated that the availability of generic Lipitor® will have a further negative effect on the sales of branded Crestor®. While this example is not for a repositioned drug, it still applies equally to a repositioned asset. If a generic is available with the same biological mechanism as the repositioned drug, it is likely that the use of the repositioned drug will be competing with the generic due to prescribing and reimbursement practices; moreover, the availability of a method-of-use patent on the repositioned drug may not prevent these practices from occurring. Consider the case for repositioning a statin. While there have been numerous publications regarding the use of statins for a variety of indications, there is little incentive from a purely commercial perspective to invest in the clinical trials needed to demonstrate medical utility, even if a method-of-use patent is obtained.

In summary, there are pricing, reimbursement, and prescribing practice considerations for any drug development program, with some nuances and complexities specific for drug repositioning programs. Earlier, a method-of-use patent was discussed as a means to obtaining market exclusivity. However, the value of a method-of-use patent for a new indication requires analysis and debate in cases when the same compound is generic for use in another indication, or when a generic compound in the same class is available, regardless of indication.

2.5. CONCLUSION

Although many of the considerations involved in a successful drug repositioning program are similar to all drug development programs, some are unique to drug repositioning. The advantages of having significantly more data, which can include human data, for a repositioning program must be balanced with the challenges of parallel progression of several indications (for compounds or biologics still under clinical development for their primary indication) or the possibility of limited patent life and market exclusivity (for discontinued compounds and marketed drugs). A common theme highlighted by the various nonprofit foundations in Chapter 12 is that a major barrier to developing promising repositioned molecules is the lack of suitable patent life required to provide the incentives for industry to invest in their costly development, particularly Phase III, which is beyond the means of the foundations. A consequence is that many potential new drugs will never be developed unless alternative incentive mechanisms, such as regulatory exclusivity, are developed or enhanced.

REFERENCES

1. Gelijns, A.C., Rosenberg, N., Moskowitz, A.J. (1998). Capturing the unexpected benefits of medical benefits. *The New England Journal of Medicine, 339*, 693–698.
2. Graul, A.I., Sorbera, L., Pina, P., Tell, M., Cruces, E., Rosa, E., Stringer, M., Castañer, R., Revel, L. (2010). The year's new drugs & biologics—2009. *Drug News Perspect, 23*(1), 7–36.
3. Bell, A. *The Viagra® Story: From Laboratory to Clinical Discovery.* http://www.mbcfoundation.org/pdfs/Blockbuster%20Drug%20Symposium%20Final.pdf.
4. Wang, C., Takeuchi, K., Pinto, L.H., Lamb, R.A. (1993). Ion channel activity of influenza A virus M2 protein: Characterization of the amantadine block. *Journal of Virology, 67*(9), 5585–5594.
5. Verma, U., Sharma, R., Gupta, P., Kapoor, B., Bano, G., Sawhney, V. (2005). New uses for old drugs: Novel therapeutic options. *Indian Journal of Pharmacology, 37*(5), 279–287.
6. Mekdeci, B. How a Commonly Used Drug Caused Birth Defects. http://www.birthdefects.org/research/bendectin_1.php.
7. Teo, S.K., Stirling, D.I., Zeldis, J.B. (2005). Thalidomide as a novel therapeutic agent: New uses for an old product. *Drug Discovery Today, 10*(2), 107–114.
8. Celgene Corporation. http://www.thalomid.com/thalomid_history.aspx
9. Allergan, Inc. http://www.restasis.com/default.htm?x=Restasis
10. Hathaway, C., Manthei, J., Scherer, C. (2009). Exclusivity strategies in the United States and European Union. *Update (Loma Linda University. Ethics Center), 3*(May–June), 34–39.
11. Pugatch, M.P. (2004). Intellectual Property and Pharmaceutical Data Exclusivity in the Context of Innovation and Market Access. http://www.iprsonline.org/unctadictsd/bellagio/docs/Pugatch_Bellagio3.pdf
12. Kesselheim, A.S., Solomon, D.H. (2010). Incentives for drug development—The curious case of colchicine. *The New England Journal of Medicine, 362*, 2045–2047.
13. Grabowski, H., Long, G., Mortimer, R. (2011). Data exclusivity for biologics. *Nature Reviews. Drug Discovery, 10*, 15–16.
14. Wikipedia. http://en.wikipedia.org/wiki/Orphan_drug
15. Official Journal of the European Communities (1999). http://ec.europa.eu/health/files/eudralex/vol-1/reg_2000_141/reg_2000_141_en.pdf
16. Masuda, S. (2008). The market exclusivity period for new drugs in Japan: Overview of intellectual property protection and related regulations. *Journal of Generic Medicines, 5*(2), 121–130.
17. U.S. Food and Drug Administration (1992). How to Apply for Designation as an Orphan Product. http://www.fda.gov/ForIndustry/DevelopingProductsforRareDiseasesConditions/HowtoapplyforOrphanProductDesignation/ucm135122.htm
18. U.S. Food and Drug Administration. Search Orphan Drug Designations and Approvals. http://www.accessdata.fda.gov/scripts/opdlisting/oopd/index.cfm
19. European Medicines Agency. Rare Disease (Orphan) Designations. http://www.ema.europa.eu/ema/index.jsp?curl=pages/medicines/landing/orphan_search.jsp&murl=menus/medicines/medicines.jsp&mid=WC0b01ac058001d12b

20. Lipinski, C.A., et al. (1980). Bronchodilator and antiulcer phenoxypyrimidinones. *Journal of Medicinal Chemistry*, *23*, 1026–1031.

21. Reaume, A., Saporito, M.S. Methods and formulation for modulating lyn kinase activity and treating related disorders, USPTO, Patent Number: 7,776,870 2010.

22. Melior Discovery Press Release (2009). http://www.meliordiscovery.com. Melior Discovery Announces IND Approval for Novel Diabetes Drug MLR1023. Press release.

23. Department of Health, Medicines, Pharmacy & Industry Group, United Kingdom (2011). A New Value-Based Approach to the Pricing of Branded Medicines. http://www.dh.gov.uk/prod_consum_dh/groups/dh_digitalassets/documents/digitalasset/dh_128404.pdf

24. Jack, A. (2001). Setback for off-label use of Roche drug. *Financial Times*, http://www.ft.com/cms/s/0/82afcb50-d536-11e0-bd7e-00144feab49a.html?ftcamp=rss#axzz1X70hNSuP. Sept. 2 2011.

CHAPTER 3

Clinical and Operational Considerations in Repositioning Marketed Drugs and Drug Candidates

DAMIAN O'CONNELL, DAVID J. SEQUEIRA, and MARIA L. MILLER

3.1. INTRODUCTION

One of the most attractive aspects of drug repositioning is the reduced time to clinically test the hypothesis compared with a *de novo* drug discovery program. In many cases, shorter routes to the clinic are possible because *in vitro* and *in vivo* screening, chemical optimization, toxicology, bulk manufacturing, formulation development, and even early clinical development have already been completed and can therefore often be bypassed in a repositioning program. In this chapter we will aim to provide the reader with an appreciation of the clinical considerations and operational complexities that are unique to a repositioning program. In many cases, the clinical validation strategy is influenced both by the existing data and by the ability to take advantage of factors that could shave several years, along with substantial risk and cost, from the pathway to the market.

The reduced risk offered by an existing favorable safety and pharmacokinetic profile of a repositioning candidate can be offset if the asset has not established proof-of-mechanism (PoM, or alternatively referred to as proof of pharmacology) in the clinic. Furthermore, toxicology or pharmacokinetics (PK) that were collected for the candidate in the original indication might now be inadequate due to the changes in regulatory standards. However, pioneering efforts can pay off handsomely: for example, achieving first-in-class status can allow for a significant head start on the competition, as exemplified by the first-mover advantage of about 5 years that Pfizer's sildenafil (Viagra®) had on Lilly and ICOS's tadalafil (Cialis®) and GlaxoSmithKline and Bayer's

Drug Repositioning: Bringing New Life to Shelved Assets and Existing Drugs, First Edition.
Edited by Michael J. Barratt and Donald E. Frail.
© 2012 John Wiley & Sons, Inc. Published 2012 by John Wiley & Sons, Inc.

vardenafil (Levitra®). Brand awareness built during the first years of sales played a key part in maintaining Viagra's® position in the market despite strong competition.

3.2. CHALLENGES AND OPPORTUNITIES IN ESTABLISHING A DRUG REPOSITIONING PORTFOLIO: MARKETED DRUG, LEAD CANDIDATE, OR BACKUP?

A portfolio of drug repositioning candidates can be comprised of marketed compounds and/or new chemical/biological entities (NCE/NBE). The amount of development risk and resource needed for clinical validation will vary depending on how far the candidate has progressed in its primary indication. If the candidate is a marketed drug, the extent of any remaining patent coverage and the potential for generic or off-label competition from drugs of the same mechanistic class will be key considerations. On the other hand, if the repositioning candidate is an NCE/NBE with recently granted patent protection, then the stage of development and amount of clinical and preclinical toxicological data will be the primary drivers. Another consideration when repositioning an NCE is that the lead candidate may have a clinical data package, whereas a "backup" candidate of the same class might only have preclinical data. Thus, the additional risk and time needed to establish clinical validation will be a factor for the latter.

Figure 3.1 captures the advantages and disadvantages of drug repositioning when there is a choice between selecting an NCE that is progressing in its primary indication versus a "backup" candidate of the same class that is less advanced. The development of a single NCE in two indications will increase the probability of the NCE reaching the market and maximizing return on investment. However, there are other factors requiring careful consideration. If the severity of the disease and co-morbidities across both patient populations are considerably different, there is a risk that nonrelevant label warnings will be "carried over" into the healthier patient indication label (e.g., risk for black box warning). Also pricing flexibility will be limited due to the potential for off-label use despite branding efforts, as discussed in Chapter 2. The commercial impact of these factors could be huge and therefore play a key role in the selection of a "backup" NCE for the second indication, despite the efficiency advantages that result from parallel development of the alternate indications with the "lead" candidate.

3.2.1. Proof-of-Concept (PoC) Trial Design

As previously mentioned, the repositioning of a drug candidate can provide many benefits that will vary depending on the stage of development at the time of repositioning. Many candidates will have extensive or complete Phase I clinical data packages while others may have Phase II or even Phase III data. Marketed compounds will have abundant clinical and safety data from

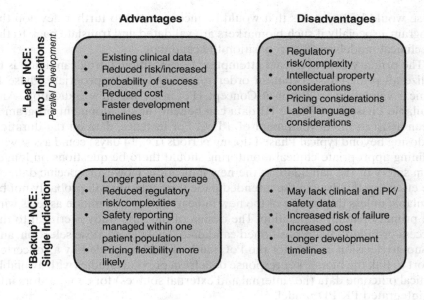

FIGURE 3.1. Advantages and disadvantages of using a "lead" NCE versus a "backup" NCE when repositioning an active development candidate or marketed drug.

numerous Phase III and Phase IV clinical programs. This can be both a positive and a negative depending on the history of the clinical program and the overall value of the drug to the company if it is currently on the market. Additionally, how close the drug is to its patent expiry will impact the potential return on investment for a new indication.

The principal value of a legacy Phase I program for developers of a candidate in a new indication comes from the pharmacokinetic and pharmacodynamic (PK/PD) data package generated in these prior studies. Critical dosing information will be available along with exposure limits and general safety of the compound in healthy subjects. The existing data can be used to develop appropriate PK/PD models to assist with dose range projections for the new indication or aid in development of additional preclinical work if warranted. However, dosing and PK/PD for the new indication should be determined empirically, as they may differ from the first indication. If the data package has areas requiring clarification or missing information, additional Phase I clinical evaluations should be performed as appropriate to support the development plan. For example, these may include drug–drug interaction (DDI) studies, bioavailability/bioequivalence studies for new formulations, studies in a special population such as the elderly, and/or other safety studies that would apply specifically to the second indication (e.g., tolerability for local administration). If there are biomarker data, or other specialized methodology such as imaging studies that are beneficial to the proposed new indication, then these would be key items that would be incorporated to further develop the program, especially if such biomarkers are validated and translate back to the preclinical models used to reposition the candidate.

The primary goal of a team attempting to reposition a drug candidate is to utilize all prior Phase I data in order to proceed into appropriate Phase II clinical validation or Proof-of-Concept (PoC) for the new indication. Any available Phase II or Phase III data can benefit the development program if it can assist in the development of a PoC. For instance, data on the duration of dosing beyond typical Phase I dosing periods (i.e., 14 days) could assist with defining appropriate clinical monitoring should there be questions on longer term safety of the candidate in the new indication. However, specific data on the effects of the drug in the intended patient population will probably not be available unless the disease of the new indication shares common aspects with the primary patient population. The design of the PoC study is critical to the success or failure of a repositioned candidate. Trial design, dose selection, and go-no-go decision criteria for the PoC study should be guided by a concerted effort to link the biomarker response data from previous studies with available clinical outcome data (i.e., internal and external sources) for comparators into an integrated PK/PD model.

If the PoC design is sound, as assessed for example by peer review or an appropriate scientific advisory committee, the PK/PD is well understood, and the results are compelling once completed, then the candidate can often proceed directly into Phase III testing. This can lead to more rapid commercialization for the candidate; however, it must be noted that additional complementary data may also be required for gaining approval depending on the indication under evaluation (e.g., acute vs. chronic disease). There are some scenarios where Phase IIb or Phase IIb/III adaptive design studies will be needed. For example, such studies will be required to support an alternative route of administration or when there is a large uncertainty in the estimates of efficacious dose.

When designing a PoC study it is important that repositioning teams bring in relevant therapeutic expertise and, wherever possible, retain access to the primary indication team's knowledge of the asset to assist in the development of the candidate for its new indication. Within big pharmaceutical companies, where this latter scenario is most likely to apply, this is a consideration that should not be underestimated due to the organizational challenges often faced when working across multiple therapeutic areas. Very often the expertise in the new therapeutic area may not reside inside the company or division repositioning the candidate, especially if the approach used to generate the repositioning hypothesis was unbiased (e.g., broad phenotypic screening or computational mining). Use of an academic research organization (ARO) is one way to access the requisite expertise since the research physicians are often well versed in both industry development and treatment of the patient population under study. For example, in the cardiovascular space, the Thrombolysis In Myocardial Infarction (TIMI) Study Group of Brigham and Women's

Hospital and Harvard Medical School is an excellent resource. Interactions with groups such as these can help to ensure the best possible PoC trial design is taken forward. It is also important to ensure that both the statistical and regulatory support available to the repositioning team is well versed in trial designs for the specific therapeutic area/indication in question (e.g., oncology, neuroscience, and infectious disease). The amount of resource required to perform a PoC can vary depending on the size of the intended PoC trial and nature of the repositioning trial sponsor. Large companies will probably be able to attain most of the required resource internally, whereas small companies or biotechs will often need to rely on outsourcing. However, even large companies are increasingly taking advantage of opportunities to outsource or partner in this space.

3.3. PROOF-OF-MECHANISM (PoM) FOR REPOSITIONED COMPOUNDS AND THE USE OF CLINICAL PROBES

The primary aim of drug repositioning studies is to characterize the pharmacodynamic effects of the candidate that could be used to treat other as yet untested condition(s). By using the appropriate study population (healthy volunteers vs. specific patient subgroup) and methodology, efficacy and safety/toleration profiles can be determined in these new indications. Use of these drugs as pharmacological probes can facilitate the discovery of new drug targets. Doing so with a readily available internal candidate or a marketed/licensed drug that has a well-characterized safety profile, albeit perhaps in different populations, enables safe testing in new indications, minimizing the risk to patients or healthy volunteers.

If a drug repositioning study is conducted with a well-characterized compound (e.g., marketed/licensed drug or a drug candidate that is in Phase IIb/III clinical testing) with pharmacokinetic and safety profiles appropriate for the new indication, this can serve as a PoM study. PoM is a key concept that underpins the conduct of indications discovery studies. It entails demonstration that the drug binds and modulates its intended target at a safe dose (acceptable therapeutic index) in humans. The required degree of target modulation (enzyme inhibition, receptor occupancy, etc.) should be defined prior to the PoM study based on preclinical data or clinical data from compounds with a similar mechanism. PoM is usually demonstrated in Phase I in healthy volunteers using a target or mechanism biomarker or in a Phase Ib/IIa study in a target population (e.g., antigen challenge study in asthma patients, fluorodeoxyglucose [FDG] positron emission tomography [PET] signal in cancer patients, etc.) if target or mechanism biomarkers are not feasible in healthy subjects. A clear demonstration of PoM reduces the risk that an unprecedented or novel mechanism is unsafe in humans and helps define the effective dose range to evaluate in Phase II to fully test the drug target. PoM also increases the chance of program success and means additional indications for which there exists strong confidence in rationale (CIR) can also be tested with greater likelihood of clinical success.

The following is an example of such a study. Phosphodiesterase 5 (PDE5) is a widely expressed enzyme. There is evidence that PDE5 inhibition can be useful in treating a number of conditions, including a range of cardiovascular diseases. Sildenafil, a PDE5 inhibitor approved for use in male erectile dysfunction, has been tested in studies in both systemic and pulmonary arterial hypertension (PAH). Results from these relatively small clinical target validation (CTV)/PoM studies in the appropriate patient populations suggested acceptable efficacy/target modulation at well-tolerated doses. The potential for its use in these additional indications was subsequently evaluated in larger confirmatory patient trials, which ultimately led to sildenafil being approved for PAH under the trade name REVATIO®.

When a marketed drug is used "off-label" in a drug repositioning study, the sponsor may have no intention of developing it for the new indication, but use the data from such a clinical pharmacology study to guide the discovery of another compound with the appropriate efficacy, safety, pharmacokinetic profile along with patent protection that would enable the development of a "best-in-class" drug. When using another marketed drug, a sponsor can use publicly available data such as the Summary of Product Characteristics or the European Public Assessment Reports (EPAR) for preclinical and clinical safety data to ensure that the drug can be used safely as a pharmacological tool. Subject safety should be the paramount consideration and the "off label" use of licensed drugs should be carefully considered to ensure that the program is conducted according to International Conference on Harmonization (ICH) principles.

3.4. IMPLICATIONS OF DRUG REPOSITIONING FOR CLINICAL PLANNING AND OPERATIONS

As already discussed, candidates for drug repositioning include both marketed compounds and NCE/NBEs. Each candidate presents unique operational challenges for the repositioning development plan before initiation of any clinical validation can proceed. One of the most frequent questions to arise once a drug candidate has been identified for repositioning is: "What do we need to do to get it into the clinic?" If the compound was originally developed "in-house," then compilation of the various data components (e.g., clinical protocols and study reports, preclinical data, clinical databases, and regulatory documents) should be relatively straightforward. It should be noted, however, that internal constraints (sharing of clinical supplies, timing of Investigator's Brochure updates, etc.) could exist if the compound is also involved in another development program, being co-developed, or is a marketed agent. On the other hand, if the compound was brought in from the outside, or had development activities spread across one or more companies, then bringing together a cohesive package can be challenging. Teams must ensure that the original data package meets current regulatory standards if it is to be utilized to support the new indication. It is prudent for a repositioning team to include appropriate commercial and legal representation to ensure the best path forward for development as competitive landscape, intellectual property, and patent issues can make the development path complex.

The discussion below will focus on clinical and operational planning considerations when repositioning NCEs. There will be some differences, including regulatory pathway and manufacturing complexity, which will need to be considered for NBEs.

3.4.1. NCE/NBE

In order to test an NCE/NBE in a new indication, the sponsor will need to have access or ability to cross-reference all preclinical and clinical safety data and chemical, manufacturing, and controls (CMC) information. From an operational perspective, the drug supply plan will play a key role on the development timeline and budget. Drug substance and drug product manufacturing may be rate-limiting for the start of supportive toxicology or clinical studies. Critical information for estimating total drug supply requirements includes having the outline of the clinical protocol(s) with projected number of patients, route of administration, proposed doses, dosing period, and study design (i.e., placebo control and/or use of a blind comparator, parallel vs. cross-over design) including an estimate of the number of sites and countries, which will all be required to draft the overall plan. If the route of administration is different from that used in the existing toxicology package, then additional preclinical toxicology studies along with formulation development will be needed. For example, if an oral drug is being repositioned for a topical indication, a new formulation will need to be developed and new local tolerability preclinical studies will be required prior to human testing. If there is a strong rationale in support of abbreviated preclinical studies, then the sponsor should plan for a pre-investigational new drug (IND) with the U.S. Food and Drug Administration (FDA) meeting prior to triggering long and costly preclinical toxicology studies.

When a new formulation or drug product strength is required for the new indication, the repositioning team might need to trigger a bioavailability/bioequivalence study prior to the PoC study in patients. The need for these additional studies is determined by the formulation type or biopharmaceutical properties of the drug substance (permeability, solubility, etc.).

A repositioning program will also need to assess if the duration of the existing preclinical toxicology package will be adequate to support the proposed clinical dosing period. In general, the dosing period of the preclinical toxicology package needs to be of equal or larger duration than the proposed dosing period of the clinical study. If deemed insufficient, this could have a considerable impact on the development timeline and budget for the start of the new study. A particularly costly scenario would be if a longer good laboratory practice (GLP) toxicology study is needed for the new indication and the compound is relatively safe. In this situation, not only would the duration of the study impact program timelines, but also large amounts of drug substance would be needed due to both the duration and the high doses required to obtain adequate understanding of margins. On the other hand, for anti-cancer Phase I oncology studies, treatment of patients can continue beyond the dosing period of the preclinical toxicological package as long as the patient is responding. Refer to the International Conference on Harmonisation of Technical Requirements for Registration of Pharmaceuticals for Human Use (ICH) S9 guidelines [1, 2] for different preclinical toxicology schedules based on examples of proposed oncology study designs and durations.

Once the drug supply needs are drafted, an assessment of the existing drug substance and drug product technology including inventory will need to be conducted. The best scenario will be that the supplies are available along with adequate storage stability and expiry dates. For compounds that are no longer in active development, that is, those that were previously discontinued, the inventory of available supplies will likely need requalification, depending on how long they have been in storage. When drug substance has been stored for longer periods than the assigned expiry date (based on previously collected stability data), it will need to be retested and subjected to further stability work to ensure acceptability prior to use in additional clinical studies. Drug substance expiry dates and usability are generally longer than the final drug product at early premarket stages, for example, due to higher risks for potential interactions with excipients in the latter. If drug substance is available, it may therefore be possible to use this existing material to manufacture a new drug product for clinical use. In addition, these supplies will need to have been stored under good manufacturing practice (GMP) conditions to maintain the chain of custody and GMP status. Analytical assays will also need to meet current regulatory standards. If not, assay development and validation work should be factored into the cost and timeline for the project.

In the case where no supplies are available or the stored material is deemed unsuitable for human studies, a new manufacturing campaign will be needed. Complexity of drug substance synthesis and quantities required will directly affect resources and time required for the manufacture of supplies. In order for a new lot to be released for clinical use, the levels of any impurities will need to be comparable to, or lower than those in the lot(s) used in the preclinical toxicology studies. For example, for a maximum NCE daily dose of ≤2 g/day, if a new impurity reaches a threshold of 0.10% or 1 mg/day intake (whichever is lower), the impurity will need to be qualified by conducting additional impurities/safety assessment studies per the FDA Q3A Guideline document [3]. In some cases, data might be available in the scientific literature (paper assessment) to support the qualification of the impurity without the need to conduct new *in vivo* qualification studies.

In parallel to the supply plan, the regulatory strategy to support the activities through PoC will need to be developed. A flow chart to assist with the investigational medicinal product dossier planning for new indications is shown in Figure 3.2. The project team should start building the dossier using the Common Technical Document (CTD) format and then edit specific sections (i.e., CMC) to satisfy different country requirements, if needed. However, if the paper format filed previously is acceptable to the regulatory authority, then any updates (i.e., justification for the new indication) can take place in paper version. In the meantime, plans to convert the paper version into a CTD format should take place in parallel with the ongoing clinical studies in the new indication to expedite future regulatory submissions.

In addition, key to the dossier preparation will be the status of the regulatory application for the original indication. For example, in the United States, if the sponsor has an existing open IND in another indication/division, the sponsor will be able to cross-reference sections from the open IND. For an inactivated IND, reactivation may occur with submission of new clinical study protocol, updated manufacturing information, and so on. The submission will be subject to a 30-day review clock. An IND enters in an inactive status when there has been no activity for a period of 2 years or more, or if all studies under the IND remain on clinical hold for 1 year or more. However, withdrawn (sponsor requests to end IND) and terminated (FDA orders sponsor to end all clinical activity) INDs cannot be cross-referenced and therefore a new IND submission will be required.

The operational aspects regarding drug safety, drug substance, drug product, and clinical supplies availability are summarized in Figure 3.3. The specific timelines to compile the dossier for submission will depend on the extent of any additional CMC and safety package requirements.

3.4.2. Approved Drugs

For an approved drug, using the same flow chart and considerations shown in Figures 3.2 and 3.3 will provide a good start in the planning process. From a regulatory perspective, if the drug is already approved, the sponsor is not required to own the data or have the right to reference from the original applicant. The application will include external published data and the FDA's previous findings of safety and effectiveness. In the United States, this may be done using the 505(b)(2) new drug application (NDA) application process (see Chapter 4 of this book).

With a good understanding of the compound's safety and pharmacokinetic properties, fewer clinical and/or toxicological studies will be required to support the IND application for the secondary indication. In the event of a positive PoC study, progressing the program using the 505(b)(2) NDA application process is likely to be completed faster and at a lower cost than a traditional 505(b)(1).

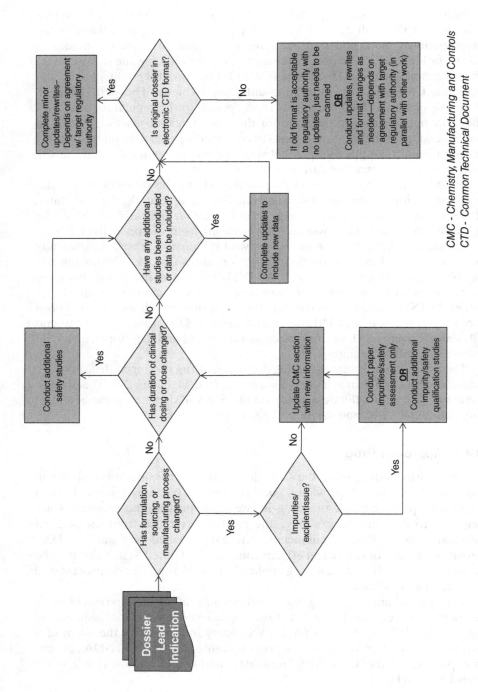

FIGURE 3.2. Dossier flow chart: Considerations when repositioning drug candidates.

CMC - Chemistry, Manufacturing and Controls
CTD - Common Technical Document

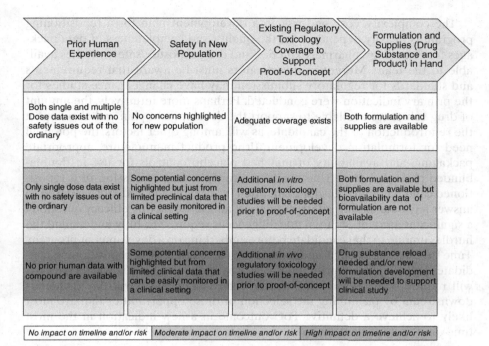

Prior Human Experience	Safety in New Population	Existing Regulatory Toxicology Coverage to Support Proof-of-Concept	Formulation and Supplies (Drug Substance and Product) in Hand
Both single and multiple Dose data exist with no safety issues out of the ordinary	No concerns highlighted for new population	Adequate coverage exists	Both formulation and supplies are available
Only single dose data exist with no safety issues out of the ordinary	Some potential concerns highlighted but just from limited preclinical data that can be easily monitored in a clinical setting	Additional *in vitro* regulatory toxicology studies will be needed prior to proof-of-concept	Both formulation and supplies are available but bioavailability data of formulation are not available
No prior human data with compound are available	Some potential concerns highlighted but from limited clinical data that can be easily monitored in a clinical setting	Additional *in vivo* regulatory toxicology studies will be needed prior to proof-of-concept	Drug substance reload needed and/or new formulation development will be needed to support clinical study

No impact on timeline and/or risk	Moderate impact on timeline and/or risk	High impact on timeline and/or risk

FIGURE 3.3. Impact of availability of key data on clinical timelines/risk for repositioning drug candidates.

3.5. CONCLUSION

The repositioning of drugs to new indications can help companies increase the depth and value of their research portfolios, and importantly, provide opportunities to accelerate the delivery of new treatment options in areas of unmet medical need. Current trends of increased time-to-market approval, higher regulatory hurdles, and consolidation of industry research programs in recent years have created an environment where drug repositioning programs provide an attractive means to offset these challenges. Clinical validation of the candidate NCE, NBE, or marketed drug in a new indication is pivotal to this process. Development plans based upon existing preclinical and clinical data, CMC packages, and drug substrate provide significant leverage and give the repositioned candidate a head start to achieving PoM and/or PoC in the clinic. Overall, the risks and development costs associated with repositioning drug candidates are generally lower than those for NCEs being developed from "lead" status for a first indication. Importantly, however, as has been highlighted in this chapter and also that which preceded it, a repositioning team must be careful not to overlook critical operational, regulatory, and strategic considerations at the outset of the clinical program.

The complexity, cost, and risk in a development plan for a repositioning program is heavily dependent on the quality and completeness of data packages for toxicology, pharmacokinetics, and drug exposure/safety profiles available to the team. Moreover, investigators must be aware that requirements and standards for regulatory submission may have changed since studies for the primary indication were conducted. Perhaps more intuitively, the amount of drug substance available to support the development plan will also impact the reintroduction of the candidate, as will, among other factors, the potential need for formulation development, drug product manufacture, appropriate packaging, and availability of matched placebo controls for use in double-blinded patient studies. Thus, while in principle the progression of a repositioned candidate into the clinic can often be streamlined and more focused to answer any outstanding safety, regulatory, and subsequently efficacy questions, a significant amount of initial due diligence is required to fully understand the hurdles unique to that candidate before embarking on a development program. Time invested upfront to understand the current status of repositioning candidates and all relevant prior data, as well as to define what a new data package will require—and hence what needs to be in the plan—will pay dividends downstream by facilitating the selection of those opportunities that are most likely to achieve a definitive PoC outcome in a new indication in the most time- and cost-efficient manner.

ACKNOWLEDGMENTS

The authors would like to thank Mary Sommer, Neil Duncan, and Heather Dowty for their contributions to Figure 3.2, and Denise Pretzer for her helpful comments.

REFERENCES

1. U.S. Department of Health and Human Services Food and Drug Administration. http://www.fda.gov/downloads/RegulatoryInformation/Guidances/UCM129110.pdf
2. European Medicines Agency. http://www.ema.europa.eu/docs/en_GB/document_library/Scientific_guideline/2009/09/WC500002867.pdf
3. U.S. Department of Health and Human Services Food and Drug Administration. http://www.fda.gov/downloads/RegulatoryInformation/Guidances/ucm127984.pdf

CHAPTER 4

Regulatory Considerations and Strategies for Drug Repositioning

KEN PHELPS

4.1. INTRODUCTION

This chapter focuses on regulatory strategies available in the United States for drug repositioning, with particular reference to the 505(b)(2) approach. Although this approach is less well known than the 505(b)(1) route (in which the sponsor owns the data or has right of reference), 505(b)(2) may be applied to certain drug repositioning and drug repurposing programs to reduce the time and cost involved for approval. Similar approaches exist in other countries, notably the hybrid application in Europe, which is based on Article 10 of Directive 2001/83/EC, which covers a generic, hybrid, or similar biological application [1].

Historically, most new drug applications (NDAs) have arisen from the creation of new molecules that were studied for their toxicity and putative efficacy in preclinical models and then advanced through clinical studies to demonstrate safety and efficacy. The duration of these studies consumes patent life, and although some of this can be recovered in the United States by patent term extension under the Hatch–Waxman provision of the Food, Drug, and Cosmetic (FDC) Act, the net result is a shortened time on the market to recoup the substantial development costs and provide profits to support further research efforts. After patent protection and any additional marketing exclusivity (see later section in chapter) has expired, many companies are poised to erode the branded market with generic copies that are approved via an abbreviated new drug application (ANDA) in the United States. An ANDA contains data that when submitted to the U.S. Food Drug Administration (FDA)'s Center for Drug Evaluation and Research (CDER), Office of Generic

Drug Repositioning: Bringing New Life to Shelved Assets and Existing Drugs, First Edition. Edited by Michael J. Barratt and Donald E. Frail.
© 2012 John Wiley & Sons, Inc. Published 2012 by John Wiley & Sons, Inc.

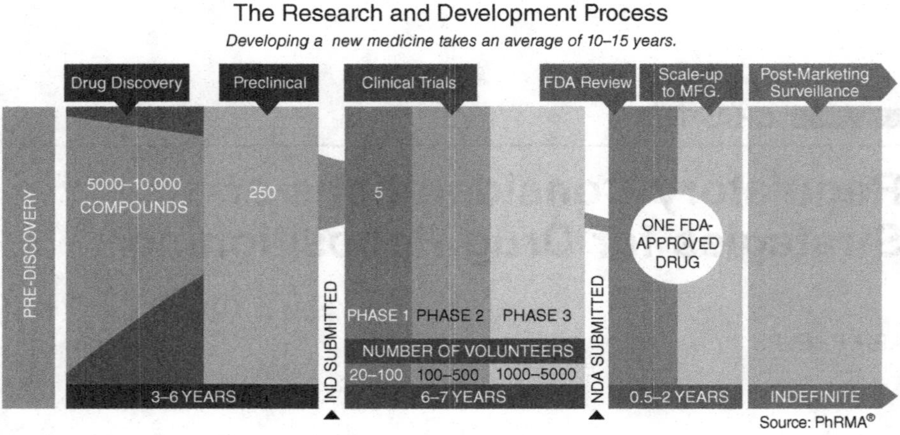

The Research and Development Process
Developing a new medicine takes an average of 10–15 years.

FIGURE 4.1. The pharmaceutical research and development process (reproduced with permission from PhRMA).

Drugs, provides for the review and ultimate approval of a generic drug product. Once approved, an applicant may manufacture and market the generic drug product to provide a safe, effective, low cost alternative [2].

The pharmaceutical industry trade organization, PhRMA, has estimated that of 5000–10,000 compounds that come from drug discovery, only one is likely to be approved for market (Figure 4.1) [3]. Due to the substantial cost of research and development (R&D) and this failure rate, which is described in detail in Chapter 1, it is understandable that the pharmaceutical industry is examining ways in which failures can be mitigated and the market for approved drugs can be expanded. This has spurred the development of numerous techniques, collectively referred to as repurposing or repositioning, which may be aimed at improving a drug's properties or adding additional therapeutic indications, in order to maximize return on investment in the asset.

From a U.S. regulatory perspective, the development of changes to an existing or pipeline drug candidate falls within the scope of an NDA for a small molecule [4], or a biologic license application (BLA) for biologics [5, 6]. Thus, changes to a company's marketed drug are usually handled via a supplement to its existing NDA or BLA. Changes to a drug that is in the R&D pipeline are similarly handled via the investigational new drug (IND) and NDA processes. Another company can make changes to the originator's drug substance or product and is required to obtain approval under the current NDA or BLA standards, which may differ from those when the originator drug was approved. For example, drugs approved decades ago lack the modern toxicology programs that are required under current NDA standards.

A sponsoring pharmaceutical company has two choices when deciding how to meet an NDA approval requirement: either obtain the information by conducting the studies itself through its own funding, or reference the information that has arisen from the work conducted by others. Most practitioners understand how to design and conduct the studies that are necessary to obtain an initial NDA approval of a drug product, but typically lack an understanding of what is required for NDA approval that involves modifications to an existing drug. For instance, what studies are needed to support approval of an oral extended release dosage of an existing parenteral?

The goal of this chapter is to aid the practitioner in understanding some of the regulatory considerations that arise from making drug or drug product modifications and facilitate the repositioning of an existing drug substance or product. To meet this goal, this chapter will focus on the regulatory background and examples of drug modifications that rely on a mixture of sponsor studies and public information to obtain NDA approval of small molecules.

4.2. HISTORY/BIRTH OF THE 505(b)(2)

In 1938, Congress passed the FDC Act [7], which included the definition of requirements for the approval of a new drug, thereby ushering in the modern era of drug development regulation. For the first time, the Act required that a new drug application contain evidence that the drug could be safely used before putting it on the market.

Although amendments were added that addressed chemicals in food and cosmetics, the next big change in U.S. drug regulation did not occur until 1962 with the passage of the Kefauver–Harris Amendment, which was introduced in response to the birth of thousands of deformed infants in Europe whose mothers had taken the sedative thalidomide [8]. Passed unanimously by Congress, the Drug Amendments of 1962 [9] tightened control over prescription drugs, new drugs, and investigational drugs, acknowledging that no drug can be considered safe unless it is also proven effective in its intended use. The Act also required that evidence of effectiveness be established by the manufacturer prior to marketing—a significant change in the development process [10].

4.2.1. An Era of Increased Scrutiny

To address previously approved but unproven drugs then on the market, the FDA's Drug Efficacy Study Implementation program (DESI) was established in the 1960s [10]. Under DESI the FDA began to evaluate the efficacy of all drug products marketed and approved based on the grounds of safety alone between 1938 and 1962. Although these DESI-reviewed drugs may continue to be marketed until the administrative proceedings evaluating their effectiveness are concluded, the FDA may intervene in the process and conclude that further marketing presents safety or efficacy problems; continued marketing is then permitted only if an NDA is approved for such drugs. Currently, the

FDA is pursuing an Unapproved Drug Initiative against as many as 3000 drugs still on the market without approval. While DESI has had significant negative consequences for many manufacturers, it does offer opportunities for savvy, progressive companies, as illustrated by the following example.

In March 2009, the FDA sent warning letters to seven manufacturers of morphine sulfate (oral solution, 20 mg/mL), after judging that the high concentration of morphine posed a safety hazard and gave them 6 months to stop shipping the drug. While most simply shut down production and destroyed their inventory, Roxane Laboratories saw the warning as an opportunity. They submitted what is known as a 505(b)(2) application, which is discussed in more detail below, and in January 2010 received FDA approval, giving them limited marketing exclusivity while their competitors are subject to seizure and injunction if they ship additional drug product. These competitors must now seek ANDA approval to re-enter the market.

4.2.2. The Birth of 505(b)(2)

For some time after the 1962 FDC Amendment, the FDA had an informal policy to review and approve NDAs based solely on the literature. These "paper NDAs" were also used for copies of approved drugs, called generics, which lacked formal approval requirements. That changed in 1984 when Congress passed the Drug Price Competition and Patent Term Restoration Act (known as the Hatch–Waxman Amendments). This Act sets forth the process by which marketers of generic drugs can file ANDAs and legally formalized the "paper NDA" under 505(b)(2) [4].

A 505(b)(2) application is one for which one or more of the investigations relied upon by the applicant for approval "were not conducted by or for the applicant and for which the applicant has not obtained a right of reference or use from the person by or for whom the investigations were conducted" (21 U.S.C. 355(b)(2)).

In the Act, an ANDA was defined to be "the same as" a drug product previously approved as an NDA, whereas 505(b)(1) is the standard procedure for a new drug product that had *not* been previously approved by the FDA. What, then, was the intended purpose of 505(b)(2)?

4.2.3. Defining 505(b)(2)

In 1987, long-time FDA Director Paul Douglas Parkman, co-discoverer of the rubella virus and vaccine, issued a letter defining what he thought was covered under 505(b)(2) [11]. Among other conclusions, Dr. Parkman asserted that 505(b)(2) addressed modifications to an approved drug that require submission of clinical data. Industry, even FDA staff, did not agree, however, and in 1989, the FDA issued proposed revisions to the regulations. In 1992, these regulations were published under 21 CFR 314.54.

Some confusion regarding, for example, what products were covered and how to reference investigations contained in the public domain still lingered. In 1999, the FDA issued a draft guidance document entitled "Applications Covered by Section 505(b)(2)" [12]. Although many practitioners are misled by some of the statements provided in the guidance, this author is unaware of any effort to update it. Some pharmaceutical companies did not accept the legality of the regulations [13]. A series of citizen petitions challenged submissions under 505(b)(2) as a violation of their rights under the Fourth Amendment to the U.S. Constitution, arguing that a 505(b)(2) application referencing their NDA constituted an illegal taking of property. These legal actions had a chilling effect on potential 505(b)(2) sponsors and only a handful of applications were received prior to 2003.

In October 2003, Dr. Janet Woodcock, Director of the CDER, issued a consolidated response, denying all of the Citizen Petitions. In her denial letter [14], Dr. Woodcock essentially said that Industry had given up the privacy rights in the exchange for patent life extensions in the 1984 Drug Price Competition and Patent Term Restoration Act. Dr. Woodcock's letter removed the legal barrier to the development of 505(b)(2) drug products and cleared the way for the surge of 505(b)(2) drugs in development.

4.2.4. ANDA Suitability Petition Versus 505(b)(2)

Among other provisions, the Hatch–Waxman Amendments allowed an ANDA to cover small changes from the innovator drug. Called a suitability petition, a sponsor could petition the FDA to make a change as defined in the regulations:

- A different active ingredient in a combination product in which the other active ingredients match those of the Reference Listed Drug (RLD).
- A different route of administration.
- A different dosage form.
- A different strength.

Although at first glance these would appear to be the same product differences addressed in 505(b)(2), the distinction between the two is that the *ANDA can contain only those differences that do not need clinical evidence for efficacy and safety*. Indeed, because the FDA requires clinical studies for the majority of changes, there are very few approved ANDA suitability petitions.

The ANDA suitability petition is a very public process, requiring the applicant to file the petition in a public docket and to seek public input in addition to review by the FDA Office of Generic Drugs and the CDER. Only after the decision has been published and the petition approved can an ANDA be filed. For this reason—and because once a suitability petition is approved—anyone can use the approval to file for the same change—many pharmaceutical companies use consultants or their legal firms to file to avoid publicity.

It is important to note that approval of the suitability petition does not necessarily mean that the FDA will approve the ANDA when filed, and the reasons for denial are many:

- Changes to the active pharmaceutical ingredient (API) in a single-ingredient product.
- The petition does not offer proof to show that the different active ingredient of the drug product is of the same pharmacological or therapeutic class as the ingredient of the RLD.
- The different active ingredient is not an active ingredient in a listed drug.
- The remaining active ingredients are not identical to those of the listed combination drug.
- Any of the proposed changes from the listed drug would jeopardize the safe or effective use of the product so as to necessitate significant labeling changes to address the newly introduced safety or effectiveness problem.
- The FDA has determined that the RLD has been withdrawn from sale for safety or effectiveness reasons.

4.2.5. The Pediatric Rule

ANDA suitability petitions were popular in the late 1980s and 1990s because the FDA determined that many changes did not require additional clinical studies. In 1999, however, Congress passed the Pediatric Rule [15], which states in part:

> . . . each application for a new active ingredient, new indication, new dosage form, new dosing regimen, or new route of administration shall contain data that are adequate to assess the safety and effectiveness of the drug product for the claimed indications in all relevant pediatric subpopulations. 21 CFR 314.55(a)

If there was any question that this applied to ANDA Suitability Petitions, the FDA covered it: ". . . if a petition is submitted for a change that would require a pediatric study under this rule, the petition may be denied." 63 Fed. Reg. at 66641 (FDA response to Comment 10).

The Pediatric Research Equity Act (PREA) of 2003, renewed and extended by Title IV of 2007 FDAAA [16], stipulated that an assessment was required for all applications submitted after April 1999 that contain a new active ingredient, indication, dosage form, dosing regimen, or new route of administration for pediatric populations. Indeed, in early 2007, PREA caused the FDA to rescind approval of scores of suitability petitions on this basis. Today, the ANDA Suitability Petition is limited to drug products for which there is clearly no use in pediatrics and will not require clinical studies.

4.3. SOURCES OF INFORMATION CITED IN 505(b)(2) SUBMISSIONS

By definition, the 505(b)(2) application must contain information to which the applicant does not have right of reference, but it may also—and often will—contain information generated by the sponsor in support of the application. "Information" in this case is that which is considered necessary for approval of an NDA, generally, animal studies or human clinical trials contained in modules 4 and 5 of the NDA application.

4.3.1. Standards of Acceptability for Referenced Information

Regardless of the regulatory pathway that is chosen for approval of an NDA (505(b)(1) or 505(b)(2)), the FDA standards for the demonstration of efficacy and safety are the same; it is only the *source* of information that differs between the two paths. The requirements for acceptance of the data are the same regardless of approval pathway. Nonetheless, many potential 505(b)(2) developers have difficulty understanding how a reference to a publication can substitute for data packages, statistical outputs, and so on, found in sponsored studies. Indeed, the issue of what constitutes sufficient evidence is still being debated within the Agency, by the scientific community and within the industry. Guidance documents from International Conference on Harmonisation (ICH) and the FDA can help shed light on the requirements for preclinical and clinical study report contents. For example, FDA's *Guidance for Industry: Providing Clinical Evidence of Effectiveness for Human Drug and Biological Products* is one of the most useful tools for understanding information requirements for clinical studies [17]. Some of the pertinent concepts contained in this *Guidance* are described below.

4.3.2. Defining "Substantial Evidence" of Efficacy

The 1962 Drug Amendments, as adopted by Congress, include a provision requiring manufacturers of drug products to establish a drug's effectiveness by "substantial evidence."

> Substantial evidence is defined in section 505(d) of the Act [18] as "evidence consisting of adequate and well-controlled investigations, including clinical investigations, by experts qualified by scientific training and experience to evaluate the effectiveness of the drug involved, on the basis of which it could fairly and responsibly be concluded by such experts that the drug will have the effect it purports or is represented to have under the conditions of use prescribed, recommended, or suggested in the labeling or proposed labeling thereof."

Although it has been FDA's position that Congress generally intended to require at least two adequate and well-controlled studies—each convincing on its own—to establish effectiveness, the Agency has broadened the interpretation of the Congressional requirements, where the data on a particular drug were convincing. In section 115(a) of the Food and Drug Administration Modernization Act of 1997 (FDAMA), Congress amended section 505(d) to make it clear that the Agency may consider "data from one adequate and well-controlled clinical investigation and confirmatory evidence" to constitute *substantial evidence* if such data and evidence are determined sufficient to establish effectiveness. However, a single clinical finding of efficacy, regardless of size, design, or scope, unsupported by other independent evidence, is not generally considered adequate scientific support.

4.3.3. The Quantity of Evidence Required

There are three possible scenarios to consider: (1) situations in which effectiveness of a new use may be extrapolated entirely from existing efficacy and safety studies; (2) situations in which a single study of a specific new use can be supported by information from related studies, and (3) situations in which a single multicenter study, without supporting information from other studies, may provide evidence of efficacy and/or safety.

4.3.3.1. Extrapolation from Existing Studies When other types of data provide a way to apply the known effectiveness to a new population or to a different dose, regimen, or dosage form, the effectiveness of a new product may be adequately demonstrated without additional clinical efficacy trials. Situations in which effectiveness and/or safety might be extrapolated from efficacy and safety data for another claim or product include:

- *Pediatric.* The Agency must conclude that the course of the disease and the effects of the drug are sufficiently similar to permit extrapolation from adult efficacy data to pediatric patients. Evidence may include common pathophysiology of the disease; common drug metabolism; and experience with other drugs in its therapeutic class.
- *Bioequivalence.* Alternative formulations and new dosage strengths may be assessed on the basis of evidence of bioequivalence.
- *Modified Release Dosage Forms.* In some cases, modified release dosage forms may be approved on the basis of pharmacokinetic data linking the new dosage form to an approved immediate-release dosage form.
- *Different Doses, Regimens, or Dosage Forms.* Where blood levels and exposure are not very different, it may be possible to conclude that a new dose, regimen, or dosage form is effective on the basis of pharmacokinetic data alone.

4.3.3.2. Demonstration of Effectiveness by a Single Study and Related Data A single study for a new use, when combined with independent substantiation from study data in related uses, can often provide evidence of effectiveness:

- Different doses, regimens, or dosage forms.
- Studies in other phases of the disease.
- Studies in other populations.
- Studies in combination or as monotherapy.
- Studies in a closely related disease.
- Studies in less closely related diseases, but where the general purpose of therapy is similar.
- Studies of different clinical endpoints.
- Pharmacologic/pathophysiologic endpoints.

4.3.3.3. Evidence of Effectiveness Based Solely on a Single Multi-center Study   The nature of clinical trials has changed substantially since the effectiveness requirement was implemented in 1962. At the time, the standard efficacy study consisted of a single institution with a single investigator conducting a relatively small trial. Relatively little attention was paid to blinding procedures, prospective study design, identification of outcomes, and analyses.

Today, however, major clinical efficacy studies are typically multicentered, with clear, prospectively determined clinical and statistical analytic criteria. These studies are less vulnerable to bias, can be more easily generalized, expand the safety database, and can often be evaluated for internal consistency across different subgroups, centers, and endpoints. Because of the added rigor and size of modern clinical trials, a single adequate and well-controlled study, without independent substantiation from another controlled trial, may be sufficient for approval. The characteristics that follow, although not determinative, can contribute to a conclusion that a single study would be adequate to support an effectiveness claim:

- A large multicenter study in which no single study site provides an unusually large fraction of the patients and no single investigator is disproportionately responsible for the favorable effect.
- Consistency across key patient subsets to address concerns about generalizability of findings to various populations.
- Multiple *studies* in a single program to provide separate demonstrations of activity of a drug as monotherapy, and in combination with another drug
- Multiple prospectively identified primary or secondary endpoints, in which each demonstrates a different but beneficial effect.
- Statistically persuasive findings with a very low P-value, and overall consistency of results across multiple centers.

4.3.4. Documenting the Quality of Evidence Supporting an Effectiveness Claim

In addition to documenting the data in support of an application, sponsors must show evidence that the studies were adequately designed and conducted, including documentation of trial planning, protocols, conduct, and data, as well as detailed patient records. The FDA accepts different levels of documentation of data quality, as long as the adequacy of the scientific evidence can be assured [19].

4.3.5. Reliance on Published Reports of Studies

The FDA can accept studies for which it has less than usual access to data or detailed study reports, to partially or entirely support an effectiveness claim. To increase the likelihood that a published report will in fact support an effectiveness claim, the Agency recommends having:

- The protocol used for the study, as well as any important protocol amendments that were implemented during the study, and their relation to study accrual or randomization.
- The prospective statistical analysis plan and any changes from the original plan that occurred during or after the study, with particular note of which analyses were performed pre- and post-unblinding.
- Randomization codes and documented study entry dates for the subjects.
- Full accounting of all study subjects, including identification of any subjects with on-treatment data who have been omitted from analysis and the reasons for omissions, and an analysis of results using all subjects with on-study data.
- Electronic or paper record of each subject's data for critical variables and pertinent baseline characteristics. Where individual subject responses are a critical variable (e.g., objective responses in cancer patients, clinical cures and microbial eradications in infectious disease patients, death from a particular cause), detailed bases for the assessment, such as the case report, hospital records, and narratives, should be provided when possible.
- Where safety is a major issue, complete information for all deaths and drop-outs due to toxicity.

4.3.6. Submission of Published Literature Reports Alone

A 505(b)(2) application may be made based solely on peer-reviewed articles and other published literature reports, as evidenced by the approval of secretin for evaluation of pancreatic function [20]. However, this is not an easy path, and literature most likely to support approval of a new product or new use will require at least some of the following elements:

- Consistent results from multiple studies conducted by different investigators.
- A significant level of detail, including descriptions of statistical plans, analytic methods, and study endpoints, as well as a full accounting of all enrolled patients.

- Clearly appropriate endpoints that can be objectively assessed.
- Persuasive results achieved by protocol-specified analyses yielding a conclusion of efficacy without post hoc analysis of subsets of subjects.
- Studies conducted by groups with a demonstrated history of utilizing properly documented operating procedures.

4.3.7. Reliance on Studies with Limited Monitoring

On-site and central monitoring and auditing procedures to assure data quality may vary depending on where, when, and by whom a study was conducted. According to an ICH guideline on good clinical practice [21], the extent of monitoring in a trial should be based on the design, complexity, size, and type of study outcome measures. Different studies can accommodate different degrees of on-site monitoring. Many valuable studies with important mortality outcomes had little on-site monitoring, but addressed quality control through close control and review of documentation, and extensive guidance and planning efforts with investigators.

Factors that positively influence whether studies with limited or no monitoring may be relied on include the following:

- A prospective plan to assure data quality.
- Features that make the study inherently less susceptible to bias, such as those with relatively simple procedures and readily assessed outcomes.
- An ability to sample critical data and make comparisons to supporting information such as hospital records.
- Study conducted by groups with a demonstrated history of utilizing properly documented operating procedures.

4.3.8. FDA Labeling and Summary Basis of Approval (SBA)

When a drug product under development is based on a drug currently or previously approved by the FDA[1], information that is germane to the proposed 505(b)(2) candidate may be obtained from the currently approved labeling of the RLD (see Figure 4.2).

---

[1] An NDA may make reference to a drug previously approved in the United States. Generally, the NDA cannot reference this drug unless it was withdrawn for reasons other than safety or efficacy. The FDA makes these determinations and publish in the Federal Register (e.g., http://www.scribd.com/doc/2823882/Notice-Human-drugsDrug-products-withdrawn-from-sale-for-reasons-other-than-safety-or-effectiveness8212-PEPTAVLON-Pentagastrin-for-subcutaneous). Generally, these determinations are the basis for the submission of an ANDA, but the same holds for a 505(b)(2). However, if the purpose of the 505(b)(2) project is to remove the reasons for withdrawal or otherwise is unrelated to the safety or efficacy reason, then this determination is moot.

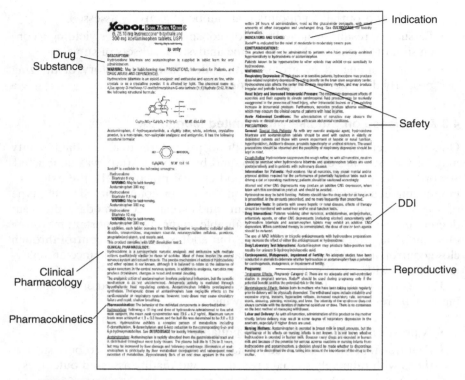

FIGURE 4.2. Approved product labeling. (DDI = drug-drug interaction)

FDA Approval Packages (formerly and still popularly called the Summary Basis of Approval or SBA) contain the FDA reviewers' summaries of the studies and information contained in the NDA of the reference drug. With care, some of this information can be referenced for the candidate 505(b)(2) drug product, bearing in mind that the reviewers' summaries, opinions, and conclusions are not binding and can be overridden by supervision. If there is basic consistency between the SBA and the approved labeling, it may be safe to use the specific SBA information.

4.4. WHERE TO FIND THE PUBLIC INFORMATION NEEDED FOR 505(b)(2) SUBMISSIONS

4.4.1. Publications

Academic and industry-sponsored studies are published in a wide variety of journals. The quality of the studies and the published reports require careful evaluation to determine their usefulness in providing pivotal information required for 505(b)(2) NDA approval. Generally, the strongest evidence comes from well-known, reputable, peer-reviewed publications. Reports of industry or government-sponsored studies are often more usable than academic studies because the former tend to follow study designs compatible with FDA approval standards.

A peer-reviewed article is published in a journal only after it has been subjected to multiple critiques by scholars in that field. Peer-reviewed journals follow this procedure to make sure that published articles reflect solid scholarship and advance the state of knowledge in a discipline. The upside is that peer-reviewed articles present the best and most authoritative information that disciplines have to offer. The downside is that these articles may not appear for years after the study was conducted.

4.4.2. Databases

A variety of companies, organizations, and consortia provide central databases of drug information that can be useful in support of a 505(b)(2) application. They often contain information on facets of drugs that were not available at the time of approval.

Key publicly accessible databases of information include the following:

4.4.2.1. *Cochrane Reviews*   http://www.cochrane.org/cochrane-reviews

The Cochrane Collaboration was established in 1993 and includes an international network of professionals preparing and updating Cochrane Reviews, which are systematic reviews of primary research in human healthcare and health policy. The Reviews investigate the effects of interventions for prevention, treatment, and rehabilitation, and assess the accuracy of a diagnostic test for a given condition in a specific patient group and setting. There are over 4500 Reviews published online.

4.4.2.2. *TOXNET*   http://toxnet.nlm.nih.gov/

TOXNET is a part of the U.S. National Library of Medicine and includes a cluster of databases covering toxicology, hazardous chemicals, environmental health, and related areas. Among the valuable databases that can be accessed are:

> *Hazardous Substances Data Bank.* A factual database focusing on the toxicology of over 5000 potentially hazardous chemicals.
>
> *Integrated Risk Information System.* A database from the U.S. Environmental Protection Agency (EPA) containing carcinogenic and noncarcinogenic health risk information on over 500 chemicals.
>
> *International Toxicity Estimates for Risk.* A database that is compiled by Toxicology Excellence for Risk Assessment (TERA) and contains over 650 chemical records.

Chemical Carcinogenesis Research Information System. Developed and maintained by the National Cancer Institute; contains over 9000 chemical records with carcinogenicity, mutagenicity, tumor promotion, and tumor inhibition test results.

GENE-TOX (Genetic Toxicology). Created by the EPA; contains genetic toxicology test results on over 3200 chemicals.

LactMed (Drugs and Lactation). A database of drugs and other chemicals to which breastfeeding mothers may be exposed.

Carcinogenic Potency Database. Provides standardized analyses of the results of 6540 chronic, long-term animal cancer tests that have been conducted since the 1950s.

Comparative Toxicogenomics Database. Describes cross-species chemical and gene–protein interactions, as well as chemical and gene disease relationships.

4.4.2.3. Adverse Event Reporting System (AERS)   http://www.fda.gov/ Drugs/GuidanceComplianceRegulatoryInformation/Surveillance/Adverse DrugEffects/default.htm

AERS is a computerized information database designed to facilitate the FDA's post-marketing safety surveillance program for all approved drug and therapeutic biologic products. The system accepts adverse event reports from healthcare professionals, as well as consumers. Reports in AERS are evaluated by clinical reviewers in the CDER and the Center for Biologics Evaluation and Research (CBER) to monitor the safety of products after they are approved by FDA.

4.4.2.4. World Health Organization Global Health Observatory   http:// www.who.int/research/en/

The Global Health Observatory (GHO) is the World Health Organization's (WHO's) online portal to data and analyses for monitoring the global health situation. The GHO data repository provides access to over 50 datasets on priority health topics, including mortality and burden of diseases, the Millennium Development Goals (child nutrition, child health, maternal and reproductive health, immunization, HIV/AIDS, tuberculosis, malaria, neglected diseases, water, and sanitation), noncommunicable diseases and risk factors, epidemic-prone diseases, health systems, environmental health, violence, and injuries, among others. The site also provides access to World Health Statistics reports, a variety of category health reports, and other valuable information.

4.5. INTELLECTUAL PROPERTY AND DATA EXCLUSIVITY

One significant advantage an NDA (either 505 (b)(1) or 505(b)(2)) enjoys over a standard 505(j) ANDA is that the former may be eligible for up to 7 years of market exclusivity—a potentially breakaway marketing advantage. The

TABLE 4.1. Requirements and Years of US Marketing/Data Exclusivity

Years of Marketing/ Data Exclusivity	Requirements
0	Only bioavailability/bioequivalence studies needed for NDA approval
3	One or more clinical investigations essential for approval of the application (e.g., new indication for existing approved drug) 21 CFR 314.50(j); 314.108(b)(4) and (5)
5	New chemical entity—in whatever indication(s) sought in original NDA 21 CFR 314.50(j); 314.108(b)(2)
7	Orphan Drug 21 CFR 314.20-316.36

provision of market exclusivity arose from the concerns of industry in the discussions leading up to the passage of the 1985 Hatch–Waxman Amendments (formally entitled Drug Price Competition and Patent Term Restoration Act). At issue were the lengthy NDA review process and the lack of remaining patent life to market a drug. Congress decided to grant a period of marketing exclusivity based loosely on the amount of investment that a company made in the product development. This market exclusivity enables investments in some products that have short patent protection or even those that lack any patent protection. For example, the latter category could cover a change from an immediate-release to extended-release oral product, or a combination product containing drugs from two innovators where composition of matter patents have expired. Table 4.1 provides a summary of the years of marketing/data exclusivity and their requirements available under Hatch–Waxman.

A major difference between a 505(b)(1) and 505(b)(2) is that patent certification may be required of a 505(b)(2). If the 505(b)(2) NDA application references a listed drug, then the sponsor must supply a patent certification statement. A patent certification statement in an NDA declares the sponsor's view of the potential patent infringement of its product versus the patent(s) of the listed drug. 505(b)(2) patent certification statements are similar to those in an ANDA submission. There are four types of certifications, referred to as Paragraphs, as shown in Table 4.2.

Thus, approval of a 505(b)(2) may be delayed because of patent and exclusivity rights that apply to the listed drug (21 CFR 314.50(i), 314.107, and 314.108 and section 505A of the Act).

4.6. 505(b)(2) CASE STUDIES

The following case studies are presented to illustrate the range of public information and sponsor-led studies that are required for 505(b)(2) approval. These

TABLE 4.2. Types of Patent Certification

Type	Patent Status	Potential FDA Action
Paragraph I	Required patent information has not been filed	FDA may approve 505(b)(2) immediately
Paragraph II	Patent has expired	FDA may approve 505(b)(2) immediately
Paragraph III	Patent has not expired but will expire on a certain date	FDA may approve 505(b)(2) effective on patent expiry date
Paragraph IV	Patent is invalid or non-infringed by applicant	Applicant provides notice to NDA holder; approval may or may not occur

examples illustrate that a 505(b)(2) can require anything from few, if any, studies to almost a full development program.

4.6.1. NovoLog®—Approval for a New Route for Insulin Administration, Based on a Single Clinical Study

Another use of the SBA is to provide access to an RLD that can be used as a comparator drug in trials for a candidate 505(b)(2) drug product. For instance, Novo Nordisk obtained a supplemental new drug application (sNDA) approval in 2008 to supplement its NDA, to add the administration of insulin aspart (NovoLog®) in children by continuous subcutaneous insulin infusion (CSII). The basis for the approval was a single Phase III study comparing the administration by CSII of insulin aspart with Lilly's insulin lispro (Humalog®). The study demonstrated that administration of insulin aspart by CSII was comparable (by standard measurements for glycemic control) to the control in children and adolescents aged 4 to 18 years.

To turn the tables, Lilly could now add this route of administration to Humalog® by submitting a 505(b)(2) NDA referencing the NovoLog SBA, product labeling, and the published study [22].

4.6.2. Makena®—Use of a Publicly Funded Study

The use of a publicly funded single study is illustrated by the approval of KV Pharmaceutical's Makena®. Makena® (17α-Alpha hydroxyprogesterone caproate or 17P) is the first FDA-approved drug intended to reduce the risk of preterm birth in women who have a history of singleton spontaneous preterm birth. The NDA was approved under Subpart H regulation 21 CFR 314.510—also referred to as accelerated approval—based on a single pivotal study [23].

In 2003, an article in the *New England Journal of Medicine* reported on results of a clinical trial that was sponsored by the National Institute for Child Health and Human Development and conducted by the Maternal–Fetal

Medicine Units Network. The double-blind, placebo-controlled trial examined the potential of 17P to prevent recurrent preterm birth [24]. Adeza Biomedical Corporation discussed with the FDA's Division of Reproductive and Urologic Products (DRUP) the possibility of basing an NDA on this report, and subsequently submitted an NDA in April 2006 with the proposed trade name Gestiva®. The initial NDA relied on the single study and a follow-up safety study of the offspring exposed to 17P in the previous study; the NDA was based solely on published literature.

The NDA was the subject of an August 2006 meeting of the Advisory Committee for Reproductive Health Drugs. Since these studies were not designed to meet FDA requirements for pivotal studies for NDA approval, FDA had a number of concerns and issued an Approvable Letter (meaning there are deficiencies that prevent immediate approval of the drug) in October 2006. Adeza was acquired in April 2007 by Cytyc Corporation, which in turn was acquired by Hologic, Inc. in October 2007. Hologic provided the first response on January 2009 under the newly proposed trade name Makena®. In the same month, the FDA sent another letter identifying clinical deficiencies. The second response to address these issues was submitted by Hologic on July 12, 2010, and the drug product was ultimately approved on February 3, 2011.

In this example, the original study was not designed to meet FDA standards for drug approval. It lacked follow-up data and an assurance that the product used in the trial was the to-be-marketed drug product. In addition, efficacy endpoints—a reduction in the incidence of preterm births prior to 37, 35, and 32 weeks gestation—were surrogates, not clinical [25].

The FDA's Statistical Review and Evaluation of 17P [26] cites the following among the reasons for *not recommending* approval of the drug based on a single trial:

- The optimal time to start study drug was not identified.
- There was inadequate randomization of study site and gestational age.
- One center accounted for 44% of subjects enrolled at 18 weeks of gestation or earlier.
- Some centers had a deficit of subjects enrolled at 18 weeks of gestation or earlier.
- Fetal and neonatal deaths among women treated with 17P occurred earlier than among women treated with placebo.
- One center accounted for a relatively large proportion of all subjects enrolled.

The rules for Accelerated approval require a second confirmatory clinical study. However, in addition to the first trial, a post-approval commitment [23] illustrates the FDA's willingness to consider published literature for an approval. An edited excerpt of the Agency's position or basis for approval follows:

Submission of an <u>academic publication</u> of pharmacokinetic data on hydroxyprogesterone caproate and its metabolites in plasma and urine of pregnant women throughout different stages of gestation. If the publication listed in this postmarketing commitment is not submitted by December 31, 2011 or if the results from the publication do not include all the relevant findings (e.g., urinary metabolites), you will conduct the following clinical trial:

A non-randomized clinical pharmacokinetic trial of hydroxyprogesterone caproate and its metabolites in pregnant women. This trial will provide data characterizing the pharmacokinetics of hydroxyprogesterone caproate and its metabolites in plasma and urine throughout the different gestational stages.

This approval also shows how the medical division handles approval in spite of reviewers' dissent. In the Statistical Review and Evaluation of Makena®, reviewers identified significant concerns with the quality of the proof of efficacy and made stringent recommendations about limitations on label claims. Yet in the end the FDA recommended approval for <37 weeks endpoint, by "recognizing an important public health need for the commercialization of this drug product" [27].

4.6.3. TRIESENCE®—An NDA with Minimal New Studies

The power of the 505(b)(2) process is most apparent when the sponsor has to conduct few, if any, studies to get their drug product approved. For many drugs, there is a wealth of data in the public domain. The challenge is in locating and preparing it for the FDA in such a way that the reviewers will understand how it applies to a company's product formulation. The following is an example of a sponsor gaining approval for a reformulation of a previously approved drug with minimal additional studies.

Alcon received approval in November 2007 for Triamcinolone Acetonide Injectable Suspension via 505(b)(2) for use in sympathetic ophthalmia, temporal arteritis, uveitis, ocular inflammatory conditions unresponsive to topical corticosteroids, and visualization of the vitreous during vitrectomy. The drug had been in systemic use for many years as KENALOG® from Bristol Myers Squibb, which was approved in 1965 under DESI. Despite containing benzyl alcohol as a preservative, and being known to cause sterile endophthalmitis when injected into the vitreous, KENALOG® has been used off-label with more than a 40-year history in ophthalmic settings, and there exists a large body of safety and efficacy information on such uses [28]. The FDA Medical Officer readily accepted this history in lieu of studies. Alcon took advantage of this data.

Under the brand name TRIESENCE®, Alcon reformulated the solution to remove benzyl alcohol and packaged it in a sterile, single-use vial. They conducted no Phase I or Phase II studies, and, in fact, could have received approval for all but the last of the aforementioned indications without any clinical studies. The safety and efficacy of the product was based on 299 publications, a meta-analysis, and a single clinical trial conducted by Alcon [29] to demonstrate safety and efficacy in visualization of the vitreous during vitrectomy (interestingly, although this is a device indication, it is considered a drug indication when coupled with the other drug indications). The indication of visualization of the vitreous during vitrectomy had never been approved by the FDA and thus the Agency required a clinical study for approval; the other indications were approved for KENALOG® and no studies were required since the only formulation difference between TRIESENCE® and KENALOG® was the benzyl alcohol.

This case study illustrates how 505(b)(2) can be especially beneficial for off-label uses that are backed by solid pharmacokinetic and/or clinical studies. However, it is of critical importance to have sufficient product differences (formulation, package, etc.) to distinguish a new product of this sort from the generics.

4.6.4. COLCRYS®—A Drug Marketed for Centuries without Proper Use and Understanding, Finally Approved Under 505(b)(2)

The drug colchicine has been used since ancient times for the treatment of gout. Products containing colchicine have been marketed for centuries in the United States without FDA approval. After 50 reports of adverse events associated with intravenous colchicine use—including 23 deaths—the drug for the treatment of gout in adults and Familial Mediterranean Fever (FMF) was taken off the market by the FDA in February 2008 [30]. According to the FDA news release, three of the intravenous colchicine-related deaths that occurred were the result of preparation errors that increased drug potency by a factor of 8 [30]. In October of that same year, Mutual Pharmaceutical sought an NDA under 505(b)(2) for colchicine tablets on the strength of a single Phase III study of low-dose colchicine in patients with gout flares, and literature describing a separate drug-drug interaction study examining the effect of clarithromycin on the pharmacokinetic profile of colchicine in healthy adults [31]. An NDA for COLCRYS® tablets was approved in July 2009.

4.6.5. Ulesfia™—A Common Cosmetic Excipient Given New Molecular Entity Status Under 505(b)(2)

Until recently, head lice infestation in children was treated with unapproved insecticides, with only marginal success because the eggs were not killed. The Sciele Pharma division of Shionogi, Inc. determined that a 5% benzyl alcohol lotion had a unique mode of action to achieve high levels of effectiveness in killing both the louse and its eggs [32].

Although a widely used chemical in the cosmetics industry, benzyl alcohol had never been approved as an active ingredient and a 505(b)(2) application was therefore made as a new molecular entity (NME). Sciele carried out an *in vitro* study that utilized a scanning electron microscope to demonstrate how the breathing spiracles of the louse are occluded and become nonfunctional after treatment with benzyl alcohol, in effect asphyxiating the lice [32]. Because the formulation was determined to be non-neurotoxic with no observable systemic side effects, it is appropriate for children as young as 6 months.

The development program for benzyl alcohol [33] under the 505(b)(2) application consisted of:

Nonclinical Studies

- Literature for repeat dose and genetic toxicology.
- Literature for *in vitro* studies demonstrating mechanism of action.
- 2-year toxicology and carcinogenesis studies from the National Toxicology Program.

Clinical Pharmacology

- Pharmacokinetic (PK) study.

Efficacy

- Two Phase III trials, totaling 615 subjects, with 240 on treatment. Study findings included no live lice observed in 76.2% of patients (vs. 4.8% for vehicle) in Study 1 and 75% (vs. 26.2% for vehicle) in Study 2.

Safety

- Relied on its database of eight studies including two Phase III, three Phase II, two Phase I, and one special safety study.
- Extensive publication review.

When the FDA granted an NDA in April 2009, it also granted the sponsor 5 years of data exclusivity because it was an NME.

4.6.6. CAFCIT®—An Example of a Common Commodity Approved Under 505(b)(2) as a New Molecular Entity and Given Orphan Status

In premature babies, the part of the central nervous system that controls breathing is not yet fully developed, causing a condition called apnea of prematurity (AOP) [34]. The condition causes large bursts of breath followed by periods of shallow breathing or breathing that stops entirely for 15–20 seconds. Primarily affecting babies born at less than 35 weeks gestation, AOP also causes bradycardia or a slowing of the heart rate, which may cause babies to appear pale or bluish. Although a fairly common condition, it is frightening to observe; fortunately most babies outgrow it as they mature [35].

In this example of the use of 505(b)(2), a clinical trial was conducted to evaluate the efficacy of caffeine citrate in apnea. Eighty-five infants, 28–32 weeks post-conception and 24 hours or more after birth who had six or more apnea episodes within 24 hours were enrolled in a multicenter, parallel, randomized, double-blind, placebo-controlled trial by the Department of Pediatrics, University of Arizona Health Sciences Center. The study data showed that caffeine citrate was significantly more effective than placebo in reducing apnea episodes by at least 50% in 6 days and approached statistical significance in 3 days; it was significantly better than placebo in eliminating apnea in 5 days and approached significance in 2 days [36].

In addition to this single clinical trial, the 505(b)(2) application for this drug included literature from 19 human PK studies and 71 articles supporting drug–drug interaction aspects of the NDA. No human PK studies were conducted; plasma caffeine levels from subjects in the study and special software were used to perform a population PK analysis. CAFCIT®, the brand name of caffeine citrate, was approved as an NME and granted orphan drug status and 7 years data exclusivity as well as expedited review.

4.7. PRODRUGS

An increasing number of prodrugs are being developed. Prodrugs are drugs that are designed to release an active moiety after administration; the prodrug itself is inactive or, at least, much less active than the active moiety. The regulatory concerns for this class can be with the intact prodrug, the active moiety, and the balance of the prodrug that remains unconverted. To determine the regulatory pathway—505(b)(1) or 505(b)(2)—it is sufficient to know where the prodrug is converted into the active moiety [37] (Table 4.3).

Type IA will always require a full development program (505(b)(1)) because there is no useful available public information on the active moiety to reference in a 505(b)(2). A Type IB can be either a 505(b)(1) or a 505(b)(2) depending on the residence time of the prodrug in the systemic circulation—longer time means greater exposure to the prodrug. Type IB as, Type IA, are almost always NMEs. Type II A or B are always 505(b)(2) candidates when the active

TABLE 4.3. Prodrug Conversion Location [37]

Class	Conversion Site	Subclass	Location of Conversion	Examples
I	Intracellular	I A	Therapeutic target tissues or cells	Zidovudine 5-flurouracil
		I B	Metabolic tissues (e.g., liver, lung)	Captopril Cyclophosphamide
II	Extracellular	II A	Gastrointestinal fluid	Sulfasalazine Loperamide oxide
		II B	Systemic circulation	Fosphenytoin Bambuterol

moiety has been previously known and public data are available to support some pivotal aspect of NDA approval.

4.7.1. Case Study: Valacyclovir—An Example of a Type IB Prodrug

Valacyclovir is an antiviral prodrug used in the management of herpes simplex and herpes zoster (shingles) [38]. It is administered in an inactive form that is metabolized in the body into an active metabolite through a process termed bioactivation. Prodrugs are usually designed to improve oral bioavailability. In this case, an esterized version of acyclovir is converted by esterases to the active drug acyclovir, as well as the amino acid valine, via first-pass hepatic metabolism. The result is significantly greater bioavailability—about 55%—as compared with acyclovir, which is 10–20% [39].

The 505(b)(2) NDA sought to establish valacyclovir as an NME, using acyclovir as the RLD. This allowed the sponsor to rely on some acyclovir nonclinical and clinical data; however, the NDA required nonclinical studies for the NME, a full Phase I PK program, a Phase II dose-ranging trial, and a controlled Phase III study. For this relatively small amount of additional clinical research, however, the sponsor was granted 5 years of marketing exclusivity [40].

4.8. SUMMARY

The 505(b)(2) pathway is used to obtain FDA approval of changes to existing drugs. These drugs may be under development by innovator companies, approved drugs in the United States or other regulatory bodies, drugs marketed based on historical reasons, or repurposed chemicals. The case studies presented in this chapter highlight a broad range of improvements that can be made to the existing drug under 505(b)(2) as well as the scope of development requirements that can range from simple bioavailability or bioequivalence studies, to more complete Phase II/Phase III clinical programs. Ultimately, the true test of a successful development program is improvement in the lives of patients. The visionaries in 1984 who provided the 505(b)(2) pathway would be pleased to see how improved drugs have enhanced the health and welfare of patients.

REFERENCES

1. Camargo Pharmaceutical Services, LLC. http://www.camargoblog.com/index.php/2009/11/04/does-europe-have-a-pathway-for-approval-of-drugs-analogous-to-the-fdas-505b2-pathway/
2. U.S. Department of Health & Human Services. http://www.fda.gov/drugs/developmentapprovalprocess/howdrugsaredevelopedandapproved/approvalapplications/abbreviatednewdrugapplicationandagenerics/default.htm

3. Pharmaceutical Research and Manufacturers of America. http://www.phrma.org/sites/default/files/159/phrma_chart_pack.pdf, p. 18.

4. Applications for FDA Approval to Market a New Drug. 21 CFR 314.

5. Biological Products: General. 21 CFR 600.

6. U.S. Department of Health & Human Services. http://www.fda.gov/BiologicsBloodVaccines/DevelopmentApprovalProcess/BiologicsLicenseApplicationsBLAProcess/default.htm

7. United States of America. Public Law No. 75-717 available at: http://constitution.org/uslaw/sal/052_statutes_at_large.pdf

8. U.S. Department of Health & Human Services. http://www.fda.gov/AboutFDA/WhatWeDo/History/ProductRegulation/PromotingSafeandEffectiveDrugsfor100Years/default.htm

9. United States of America. Public Law No. 87-781 available at: http://constitution.org/uslaw/sal/076_statutes_at_large.pdf

10. U.S. Department of Health & Human Services. http://www.fda.gov/ICECI/ComplianceManuals/CompliancePolicyGuidanceManual/ucm074382.htm

11. U.S. Department of Health & Human Services. http://www.fda.gov/ohrms/dockets/dailys/03/oct03/102303/01p-0323-pdn0001-vol1.pdf, p. 36.

12. U.S. Department of Health & Human Services. http://www.fda.gov/downloads/Drugs/GuidanceComplianceRegulatoryInformation/Guidances/ucm079345.pdf

13. U.S. Department of Health & Human Services. http://www.fda.gov/ohrms/dockets/dailys/03/Sept03/090303/03p-0408-cp00001-08-Tab-G-vol3.pdf

14. U.S. Department of Health & Human Services. http://www.fda.gov/ohrms/dockets/dailys/03/oct03/102303/01p-0323-pdn0001-vol1.pdf

15. Pediatric Use Information. 21 CFR 314.55(a).

16. U.S. Department of Health & Human Services. http://www.fda.gov/Drugs/DevelopmentApprovalProcess/DevelopmentResources/ucm049867.htm

17. U.S. Department of Health & Human Services. http://www.fda.gov/downloads/Drugs/GuidanceComplianceRegulatoryInformation/Guidances/UCM078749.pdf

18. U.S. Department of Health & Human Services. http://www.fda.gov/RegulatoryInformation/Legislation/FederalFoodDrugandCosmeticActFDCAct/FDCActChapterVDrugsandDevices/ucm108125.htm

19. U.S. Department of Health & Human Services. http://www.fda.gov/downloads/Drugs/GuidanceComplianceRegulatoryInformation/Guidances/UCM072008.pdf

20. U.S. Department of Health & Human Services. http://www.accessdata.fda.gov/drugsatfda_docs/appletter/2004/21256ltr.pdf

21. U.S. Department of Health & Human Services. http://www.fda.gov/downloads/Drugs/GuidanceComplianceRegulatoryInformation/Guidances/UCM073122.pdf

22. Weinzimer, S.A., Ternand, C., Howard, C., Chang, C.T., Becker, D.J., Laffel, L.M. (2008). A randomized trial comparing continuous subcutaneous insulin infusion of insulin aspart versus insulin lispro in children and adolescents with type 1 diabetes. *Diabetes Care*, *31*(2), 210–215.

23. U.S. Department of Health & Human Services. http://www.accessdata.fda.gov/drugsatfda_docs/appletter/2011/021945s000ltr.pdf

24. Meis, P.J., Klebanoff, M., Thom, E., Dombrowski, M.P., Sibai, B., Moawad, A.H., Spong, C.Y., Hauth, J.C., Miodovnik, M., Varner, M.W., Leveno, K.J., Caritis, S.N., Iams, J.D., Wapner, R.J., Conway, D., O'Sullivan, M.J., Carpenter, M., Mercer, B., Ramin, S.M., Thorp, J.M., Peaceman, A.M. (2003). Prevention of recurrent preterm delivery by 17 alpha-hydroxyprogesterone caproate. *The New England Journal of Medicine, 348*, 2379–2385.

25. U.S. Department of Health & Human Services. http://www.fda.gov/downloads/Drugs/DevelopmentApprovalProcess/DevelopmentResources/UCM252976.pdf

26. U.S. Department of Health & Human Services. http://www.fda.gov/downloads/Drugs/DevelopmentApprovalProcess/DevelopmentResources/UCM252978.pdf

27. U.S. Department of Health & Human Services. http://www.fda.gov/downloads/Drugs/DevelopmentApprovalProcess/DevelopmentResources/UCM252976.pdf

28. U.S. Department of Health & Human Services. http://www.accessdata.fda.gov/drugsatfda_docs/nda/2007/022048s000_022223s000_MedR.pdf, p. 25.

29. U.S. Department of Health & Human Services. http://www.accessdata.fda.gov/drugsatfda_docs/nda/2007/022048s000_022223s000_MedR.pdf, p. 30.

30. U.S. Department of Health & Human Services. http://www.fda.gov/NewsEvents/Newsroom/PressAnnouncements/2008/ucm116853.htm

31. U.S. Department of Health & Human Services. http://www.accessdata.fda.gov/drugsatfda_docs/nda/2009/022352s000_SumR.pdf

32. U.S. Department of Health & Human Services. http://www.accessdata.fda.gov/drugsatfda_docs/nda/2009/022129s000_MedR.pdf

33. U.S. Department of Health & Human Services. http://www.accessdata.fda.gov/drugsatfda_docs/nda/2009/022129s000TOC.cfm

34. U.S. National Library of Medicine National Institutes of Health. http://www.ncbi.nlm.nih.gov/pubmedhealth/PMH0004488/

35. Nemours. http://kidshealth.org/parent/medical/lungs/aop.html

36. Erenberg, A., Leff, R.D., Haack, D.G., Mosdell, K.W., Hicks, G.M., Wynne, B.A. (2000). Caffeine citrate for the treatment of apnea of prematurity: A double-blind, placebo-controlled study. *Pharmacotherapy, 20*(6), 644–652.

37. Wu, K.M., Farrelly, J.G. (2007). Regulatory perspectives of Type II prodrug development and time-dependent toxicity management: Nonclinical Pharm/Tox analysis and the role of comparative toxicology. *Toxicology, 236*, 1–6.

38. Wikipedia. http://en.wikipedia.org/wiki/Valacyclovir

39. U.S. National Library of Medicine National Institutes of Health. http://www.ncbi.nlm.nih.gov/pubmed/8275615

40. U.S. National Library of Medicine National Institutes of Health. http://www.ncbi.nlm.nih.gov/pubmed/7979285

APPLICATION OF TECHNOLOGY PLATFORMS TO UNCOVER NEW INDICATIONS AND REPURPOSE EXISTING DRUGS

PART II

APPLICATION OF TECHNOLOGY PLATFORMS TO UNCOVER NEW INDICATIONS AND REPURPOSE EXISTING DRUGS

███████ **CHAPTER 5**

Computational and Bioinformatic Strategies for Drug Repositioning

RICHARD MAZZARELLA and CRAIG WEBB

5.1. INTRODUCTION

The information age has transformed the drug discovery process, yielding extensive volumes of data that have provided the basis for our increased understanding of the molecular mechanisms of human disease. Despite clear advances in the post-genomic era, we remain challenged in our ability to identify, retrieve, and analyze all of the pertinent data on any human pathological state in an efficient and comprehensive fashion. This challenge requires the appropriate use of bioinformatic and computational strategies to retrieve relevant information among terabytes of disparate data, to integrate data mining and knowledge management methodologies in a coherent and human-browsable manner, and to effectively analyze the information to formulate testable hypotheses with clinical relevance. This chapter describes various bioinformatic techniques and computational strategies used to compile and mine this information effectively to postulate new drug indications hypotheses.

The complete sequencing of the human genome near the end of the 20th century has revolutionized the landscape of drug discovery. Enormous volumes of genetic, transcriptomic, proteomic, metabolomic, and pharmacologic information is now scattered in various databases widely accessible through the World Wide Web. In addition, there has been an explosion in the number of publications in the scientific literature concomitant with the development of sophisticated protein and pathway databases that collectively provide a representation of our current knowledge of disease mechanisms. These disparate resources have demanded the development of bioinformatic and computational techniques in order to collect, analyze, and interpret the data.

Drug Repositioning: Bringing New Life to Shelved Assets and Existing Drugs, First Edition.
Edited by Michael J. Barratt and Donald E. Frail.
© 2012 John Wiley & Sons, Inc. Published 2012 by John Wiley & Sons, Inc.

Furthermore, these strategies when coupled with prediction algorithms have resulted in the formulation of new hypotheses aligning diseases to experimental or marketed drugs. Most of these techniques can be employed to postulate new hypotheses both for drug discovery and for drug repositioning. This review will highlight those approaches that can be used for the discovery of new indications, as well as new mechanisms and drug targets when applicable. Many of the databases and tools described are publically available and, as such, web addresses along with pertinent references will be provided where possible.

A current survey of available resources reveals that there are 1230 databases spanning various disciplines within molecular and cell biology [1]. In May 2009, there were approximately 18 million PubMed abstracts with about 55% of them describing human data [2]. This vast collection of data and knowledge provides an invaluable resource to use as starting point for hypothesis generation in drug repositioning but is too immense for any person to effectively review in even one disease area. Previous reviews are primarily focused on analysis of compound library data or bioinformatic approaches toward data management, simplification, and visualization [3, 4]. In addition to these important areas, this review discusses some specific algorithms for hypothesis generation of new disease indications for biopharmaceuticals that are applicable regardless of whether these are already marketed drugs, were previously terminated for reasons other than safety, or subject to ongoing clinical or preclinical development programs.

The first part of this chapter illustrates some of the computational approaches that have been previously applied within a pharmaceutical setting, as exemplified by Pfizer's Indications Discovery Unit [5]. This section is divided into four major areas: knowledge and data integration, the Connectivity Map algorithm and related strategies, sequence and genetic analysis methods, and pathway and network-based approaches. The second section of this chapter will utilize an illustrative example of the application of computational methods to align drugs to disease, in the area of personalized oncology. In this section, we will describe how the real-time application of specific bioinformatic approaches is beginning to be used to predict efficacy of existing non-oncology drugs for the treatment of cancer. In this application, molecular-based hypotheses of drug efficacy are aligned with knowledge mining to provide oncologists with information in support of medical decision making.

5.2. KNOWLEDGE MINING AND INTEGRATION STRATEGIES

The complexity of the problem that confronts computational biologists challenged with extracting and assimilating the most relevant data from various sources for the purpose of hypothesis generation has given rise to a plethora of strategies. At a high level, the primary differences between these various approaches usually relate to the identification and appropriate weighting of the key data sources. Therefore, the formation of a drug repositioning opportunity combines both a significant informatics effort along with a biological (and often commercial) assessment of the viability of an asset for the new drug indication. In its most systematic form, the informatics strategy for new indications hypothesis generation is usually a supervised automated approach, coupled with input from biologists or disease area experts to evaluate the proposed diseases, rank the most promising prospects, and formulate experimental study designs to test the most compelling hypotheses.

One such knowledge integration strategy used by Pfizer involves the assembly of drug-to-target and target-to-disease indication information [6]. This drug-centric informatics system involves the incorporation of various public and commercial pharmacologic databases to discern the drug's mechanism of action (MOA). In addition, various competitive intelligence databases (Prous Integrity, TrialScape, BioPharm Insight) are mined to determine current disease indications for each drug MOA. This information can be extremely useful for indications discovery methods to reposition other drug targets in the same pathway to drugs with known efficacy against the disease. Also, the collation of all known information regarding an MOA can directly implicate the drug target in additional disease indications based on either a small number of publications or on genetic knockout or association data.

This drug-centric informatic strategy takes advantage of the ever increasing number of bioavailable agents and information about the drug target. In their approach, Harland and Gaulton [6] have identified more than 20 commercial and public sources of drug target information from which drug MOAs can be attained. After the identification of the target information for each drug has been collected, all of this information is incorporated into a target-centric knowledgebase called TargetBook. This database unifies Pfizer internal results regarding the drug's properties and screening data with competitor intelligence information, text mining of patent and literature databases and data from external bioactivity databases. This method also requires the development of complex target ontologies for each drug of interest since the drug may have potent activity against multiple targets and the target may have multiple splice and post-translational forms. In addition, the target may be part of a protein complex or multiple protein complexes with differential roles or activities in different biological contexts. Once established, this type of data structure forms the backbone for other strategies, which lead to the formulation of new indication opportunities in drug discovery.

A target-based informatics approach can be coupled to high-throughput data mining strategies in order to incorporate known disease relevant data [7]. Target biology includes information on function, biological pathway, tissue expression, polymorphisms, and knockout phenotype as well as disease genetic linkage and association knowledge. There are more than 1000 publicly available databases that can be used as *in silico* resources for indications drug discovery efforts and this does not include numerous commercial sources. Therefore, part of the computational challenge is not just what information to extract or what algorithms to use, but more fundamentally, which high quality databases with rich content data should be leveraged for hypothesis generation. Loging et al. [7] describe about 30 key resources that include the Investigational Drugs Database, the Prous Integrity database, and the Ingenuity Pathway Analysis, which provide fervent material for electronic biology drug repositioning methods.

One vital component to any new disease indication strategy is the final prioritization or ranking of the disparate pieces of information in order to appropriately weight the evidence for each disease supposition. In addition, an absolute scoring system also enables one disease hypothesis to be evaluated against another. For premarket drug candidates/MOAs, efficacy data from Phase II/III clinical trials provides the highest level of evidence for the association of a biological target with a new indication, whereas an ongoing trial without published data (e.g., mined from Clinicaltrials.gov) would suggest that preclinical data have been generated, even if not published, and thus provides a somewhat lower level of confidence. Genetic evidence from either functional polymorphism or human disease association studies and mouse knockout data would be the third level of evidence for involvement of the target in a new indication. Finally, new indication hypotheses can be generated from sophisticated text mining methods using MEDLINE® [8]. In this approach, co-occurrences of disease and biological target terminologies in a title are scored more highly than abstract sentence co-occurrences, which in turn are stronger than co-occurrences anywhere in an abstract. The number of unique abstract hits is also tallied and contributes to the disease ranking system.

Challenges with this data extraction and scoring system result from the fact that there are a large number of resources to mine (e.g., currently about 20 million MEDLINE® abstracts), which exist in different formats, and frequently with different target and disease synonyms used by different authors. Therefore, different scripts need to be written to effectively extract the correct information from each database. In addition, a lot of "manual" work is required in compiling target and disease synonyms—that are of interest to the investigator—which are not degenerate to minimize the number of false positives recovered (which in turn requires disease area expert input). Finally, integration of the huge amount of data that results from such an approach remains a formidable challenge and it also needs to be constantly refreshed given the ever expanding public knowledgebase. If implemented correctly, however, this approach can lead to the development of a large number of high quality hypotheses, which serve as substrate for additional approaches to aid prioritization prior to experimental validation.

In an attempt to solve the problem of obtaining both an overview and specific evidence of drug-to-target-to-disease landscape, a data integration and visualization method called target opportunity universe (TOU), has been developed [9]. This tool provides a visualization of all the drug-to-target-to-disease data including druggability, competitor intelligence, genetic and disease association results, and the text mining hierarchy. Each disease is plotted with

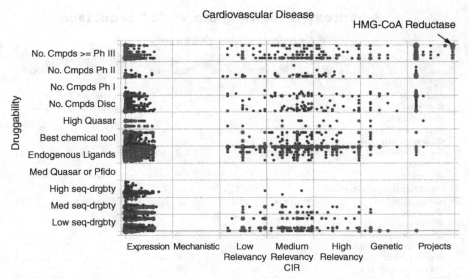

FIGURE 5.1. Target Opportunity Universe (TOU) plot for all genes that show evidence for a role in cardiovascular disease. The target's position on the graph is calculated from the body of evidence supporting both its biological role for the disease state and available chemical data. Increasing values in the y-axis indicate higher confidence in target chemical doability and increasing values in the x-axis denote growing confidence-in-rationale (CIR) in the target's role in the disease pathology. Low, medium, and high relevancy buckets on the plot are calculated from the type of the abstract co-occurrences between the disease and target terms. Larger dots denote multiple targets occupying the same position on the graph. The target 3-hydroxy-3-methylglutaryl-CoA reductase (HMG-CoA reductase) is represented by the highest x- and y- coordinates dot on the graph since it is a marketed compound target for cardiovascular disease. Selecting this target reveals the evidence summary shown in Figure 5.2.

drug targets in two dimensions, with a precedented duggability y-axis (availability of chemical matter at various stages of development) and increasing evidence of linkage of a biological target with the disease (confidence in biological rationale) plotted on the x-axis (Figure 5.1). Thus, each graph corresponds to a particular disease of interest with each point on the graph corresponding to a biological target. The point with the greatest x- and y-coordinate values is the disease target with the highest level of confidence for a role in the disease state. When a point is double-clicked on the graph all of the hyperlinked summarized underlying evidence can be seen, and clicking each piece of evidence takes one directly to the database result or the abstract from which the disease connection was garnered. The ability to quickly appraise entire disease landscape is extremely powerful, especially since the original data can be found rapidly within a few mouse clicks (Figure 5.2).

3-hydroxy-3-methylglutaryl-CoA reductase

Cardiovascular Disease

Summary of Evidence			
CIR			
Data domain	Evidence		CIR context
ⓘ Expression	3	⊕ View	cardiovascular disease
ⓘ Mechanistic			
ⓘ Low Relevancy			
ⓘ Medium Relevancy			
ⓘ High Relevancy	15	⊕ View	cardiovascular disease
ⓘ Genetic			
ⓘ Projects	5	⊕ View	cardiovascular disease
Target Chemical Doability			
Realm	Evidence		
ⓘ Low seq-drgbty			
ⓘ Med seq-drgbty			
ⓘ High seq-drgbty	1.84	⊕ View	
ⓘ Med Quasar or Pfido	6	⊕ View	
ⓘ Endogenous Ligands	6	⊕ View	
ⓘ Best chemical tool	30	⊕ View	
ⓘ High Quasar			
ⓘ No. Cmpds Disc	235	⊕ View	
ⓘ No. Cmpds Ph I	8	⊕ View	
ⓘ No. Cmpds Ph II	10	⊕ View	
ⓘ No. Cmpds >= Ph III	20	⊕ View	
Enablers			
Realm	Evidence		
ⓘ Mouse KO	2	⊕ View	
ⓘ Reviews	283	⊕ View	
ⓘ Crystal structures	4	⊕ View	
ⓘ Struct info	26	⊕ View	

FIGURE 5.2. Summary of evidence for HMG-CoA reductase from the TOU analysis. Shown are all of the supporting data from both the target compound chemical doability (y-axis) and confidence-in-rationale (CIR) for the target's involvement in the disease condition (x-axis). Additional enabler information not utilized for the calculation of the x- and y-coordinates for the target is also shown. Detailed underlying information for each category can be examined by clicking the View button.

For drug repurposing objectives, where a viable development compound/biologic or marketed drug is known to be available, the y-axis can be eliminated since late stage compounds have already addressed issues of solubility, bioavailability, and safety, and so by definition have high target chemistry values. This enables the biological rationale values to be moved to the y-axis and different disease states can now be plotted along the x-axis. This altered visualization method enables one to plot only one drug target on the graph and then survey all diseases for that target (Figure 5.3). Consequently, the drug landscape is easily assessed since the best diseases for the drug's repositioning have the highest y values. Targets with biological rationale will be revealed by this approach and are by definition the most precedented or

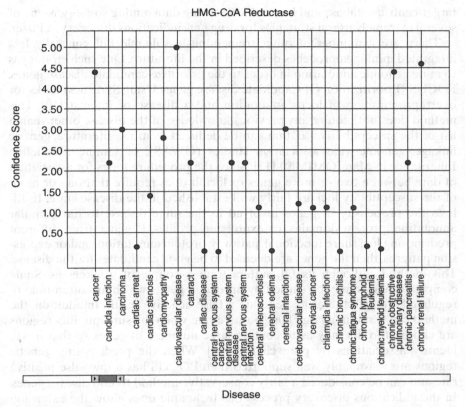

FIGURE 5.3. Drug target versus disease universe plot. This example shows the amount of information for each disease indication in the range of the sliding window for the target, HMG-CoA reductase. The confidence score is hierarchical value system where target-disease abstract co-occurrences are plotted from 0 to <1, sentences co-occurrences from 1 to <2, and the title co-occurrence is found in the range from 2 to <3. Diseases with genetic evidence for the target are plotted from 3 to <4 while clinical trials for the indication are found between 4 and <5 and are scored according to phase. A value of 5 is given if a drug for the target was approved for that indication. Intermediate values in the range are based on the total number of supporting data sources. This graph not only demonstrates that inhibitors of HMG-CoA reductase have been approved to treat cardiovascular disease but also that clinical trials targeting the enzyme for cancer, chronic obstructive pulmonary disease, and chronic renal failure have been or are being pursued. This analysis also suggests several novel disease indications.

obvious opportunities and therefore may lack commercial attractiveness. For most drug repositioning cases, the "sweet spot" in these plots lies in areas where high confidence co-occurrence or genetic evidence exists but additional work is likely required to make the targets viable opportunities. In other words, it is a balance between strength of confidence-in-rationale (CIR) and commercial opportunity. Therefore, this visualization tool, which overlays the target-centric database and hierarchical scoring data mining strategy, is one of several extremely useful strategies for drug new indications discovery at Pfizer.

There are a number of other tremendously valuable but generally less integrated mining approaches described in the literature. One such strategy is to mine genomic annotation in order to the prioritize candidate disease genes. POCUS (Prioritization Of Candidate disease genes Using Statistics) looks for overrepresentation of locus annotation and a disease of interest [10]. This method does not require any previous knowledge of the disease other than a list of the susceptibility loci that can be deduced from the literature, genetic linkage, genome-wide association studies (GWAS), or Online Mendelian Inheritance in Man (OMIM®) [11]. Since the procedure looks for association of data between two or more genes or loci, it does require that one or more of the susceptibility loci are fairly well established in the disease state. It utilizes the propensity of genes involved in the same disease to have similar annotation, protein domains, or expression profiles. If genes from different predisposing loci share functional, pathway, protein annotation, and/or expression patterns, then the genes are deemed to be good candidates for the disease. This method, although useful, suffers from a couple of weaknesses. Some complex diseases may be caused by unrelated genes which are often not co-regulated and will therefore generate a false negative result. In addition, the method can result in a large false positive rate when the susceptibility regions are chosen too liberally as to contain large numbers of genes so that it will identify associations by pure chance [10]. When the predisposing genetic regions are reasonably well supported then POCUS has a low false positive rate and can be considered a fairly conservative method to find disease genes. In the indications discovery process this technique does allow the extension of known disease loci to other suspected loci in the drug portfolio.

An important tool to the indications discovery process is the investigation of the pairwise association of biomedical concepts. The association of a gene or biological pathway with a translatable disease model or human disease pathology is central to the drug repositioning process. For example, an investigator can determine which drugs have been used for a given disease or what genes have been described to be involved in that disease. Simple well-known text mining search engines of utility for hypothesis formation include PubMed [12] and HubMed [13]. iHOP is a sophisticated is gene-centric literature navigation tool [14, 15]. This program extends the literature search through genetic and protein interaction networks such that gene function, disease phenotypes, and pathologies can be explored. The sentences displaying the interaction from the literature abstracts are extracted so that the investigator can determine the validity of the association. In the result, each interaction gene and associating verb is highlighted for quick survey of the association information and this approach can detect relatively distant relationships in comparatively few intermediate gene interactions. This analysis can then construct a graph of the shortest path between any two genes that on average are only four connections away from one another. The effective mining of pathway and network information by this strategy enables investigators to discover novel associations for known drug targets in new disease indications.

FACTA is another web-based text mining search engine that enables the investigator to formulate these types of queries [16]. This program allows one to explore the pairwise relationship of any terms in MEDLINE® and then examine six categories of relevant concepts, which include gene or protein, disease, symptom, drug, enzyme, and compound. An advantage of FACTA over other text mining tools is that the results are generated in real time. It is able to dynamically query pre-indexed words and concepts and then rapidly compute the association statistics.

EBIMed is a web-based text mining program that can also be used to investigate pairwise relationships between biomedical terms and concepts. It merges the document retrieval process with a co-occurrence analysis of MEDLINE® abstracts [17]. The user inputs a PubMed-style query and then the program examines the matched abstracts to find gene and protein names, Gene Ontology (GO) cellular component, GO biological process, GO molecular function, drug names, and species information. EBIMed uses an extensive list of synonyms for gene, protein and drug names in order to increase its sensitivity. All of the frequently occurring concepts appear in a summary table and one can then directly examine the sentence associations for each concept through the use of a hyperlink. The same group also developed the web server program MedEvi to provide supplementary textual evidence [18]. This tool enforces a positional restriction on top of the co-occurrence of terms in order to effectively resolve multiple-term queries. It also allows the use of BOOLEAN operators and differs from other search engines by directly analyzing text fragments to determine if semantic relationships exist between the queried terms.

PolySearch is an improved web-based text mining program that can determine relationships between genes, proteins, drugs, diseases, single-nucleotide polymorphisms (SNPs), pathways, tissues, subcellular localization, and metabolites [19]. It not only mines literature data from PubMed like other tools but also searches text from a number of additional databases including DrugBank, SwissProt, Human Gene Mutation Database (HGMD), Human Metabolome Database (HMDB), Human Protein Reference Database (HPRD), and Genetic Association Database (GAD). Queries result in a summary display that ranks key sentences from the matched text and contains links to the information in the external databases. This ranking system is based on the type of co-occurrence of query terms, association words, and database terms, and a rules-based pattern recognition algorithm. The program then calculates an overall Relevancy Score based on both the frequency and type of co-occurrence of term associations (Figure 5.4). PolySearch's principal limitation is that it only provides a simple dictionary method to find biomedical associations and does not extract context or meaning from identified sentences.

SciMiner is a web-accessed tool that uses functional enrichment analysis for target identification [20]. It automatically collects MEDLINE® abstracts

Z Score	Relevancy Score	Gene/Protein Name	Synonyms	PubMed Hits
12.7	1282 (4,9,10,90)	IL23R	IL 23R; IL23R; Interleukin 23 receptor; Interleukin 23 receptor isoform 1; Interleukin 23 receptor isoform 2 F1; Interleukin 23 receptor isoform 2 F2; Interleukin 23 receptor isoform 3 F1; Interleukin 23 receptor isoform 3 F3...	15 (1,2,3,27)
8.5	872 (3,11,23,220)	tumor necrosis factor alpha	Cachectin; DIF; TNF; TNF alpha; TNF a; TNFA; TNFSF 2; TNFSF2...	104 (3,11,23,192)
7.1	731 (1,6,7,147)	NOD2	ACUG; BLAU; CARD15; CD; Caspase recruitment domain containing protein 15; IBD 1; IBD1; Inflammatory bowel disease protein 1...	34 (1,5,6,71)
6.8	706 (6,11,12,63)	Toll like receptor 4	CD284; CD284 antigen; TLR 4; TLR4; TOLL; Toll like receptor 4; Toll like receptor 4 precursor; hToll...	20 (6,11,12,61)
6.7	692 (6,7,8,53)	P glycoprotein	ABC20; MDR1; ABCB 1; ABCB1; ATP binding cassette sub family B member 1; CD243; CD243 antigen; CLCS...	7 (6,7,8,22)
6.1	640 (0,1,14,48)	IBD1	Aldose 1 epimerase; IBD1; BLOCK 25; BLOCK25 protein; GALM; Galactose mutarotase; Galactose mutarotase (aldose 1	–

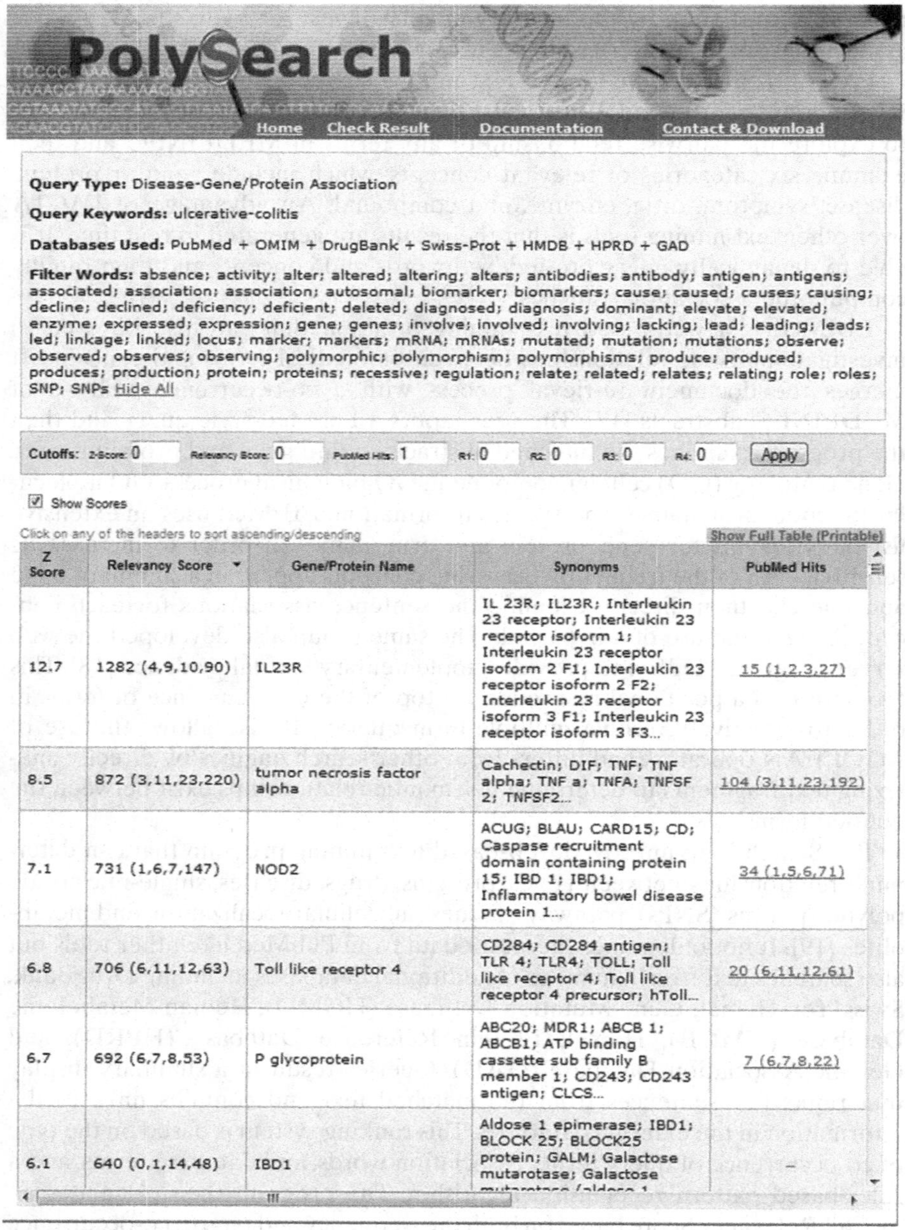

FIGURE 5.4. PolySearch example output. Displayed are the top ranked genes that are associated with the disease query "ulcerative colitis." Reproduced from the PolySearch website with the permission of Craig Knox and David Wishart of the University of Alberta.

and publically available full-text articles. It can also be downloaded and run locally to include institutional subscriptions to additional journals. In addition, this program allows users to edit the search results and carry out comparisons of the results between multiple queries. Identified targets are extracted from the articles and are ranked by hit number. The genes are then further analyzed for their enrichment in protein–protein interaction pathways, GO pathways and terms, and Medical Subject Heading terms. The Fisher's exact test [21] is then applied to identify statistically overrepresented targets, terms, and pathways to discover possible important biological processes.

PathText is an integrated tool that merges literature text mining information with biological pathway visualization [22]. It achieves this goal in part by leveraging the unique strengths of three text mining programs, FACTA [16], KLEIO [23], and MEDIE [24]. As previously discussed, FACTA has the unique ability to perform real-time co-occurrence searches. KLEIO is a program that provides semantic search functions to named entity recognition results. KLEIO uses Lucene, an open-source search and indexing tool, to generate a gene, protein, metabolite and medical term concepts. Then KLEIO utilizes its ability to link entities to acronyms via a recognition and disambiguation process in order to maximize the sensitivity and selectivity of the subsequent literature searches. MEDIE is an intelligent search engine that uses a deep syntactic analysis of individual sentences in order to retrieve biomedical knowledge from large text databases. Since MEDIE can perform the analysis of syntactic and semantic relationships, complex queries describing precise relational concepts can be formulated to identify instances in the literature. PathText integrates knowledge from three disparate data sources: external databases such as SwissProt, MGD, Flybase, and Entrez Gene; text databases such as MEDLINE and publisher journals; and pathway information, which is organized as statements of biological interactions. PathText's primary shortcoming is that it has a separate process for each of the three text mining tools and it is the responsibility of the user to determine the concurrence and inconsistencies of the results between the three different outputs. Other noteworthy text mining programs, which are variations on the previous themes, include XplorMed [25, 26], MedlineR [27], LitMiner [28], AliBaba [29], and Anni [30].

Recent development of a Disease–Drug Correlation Ontology (DDCO) has created a framework capable of interconnecting drug mechanisms and disease biology [31]. This new ontology system is the result of evolution in the development of the Semantic Web [32] and Ontology Web Language (OWL). This application of Semantic Web technology enables data integration and knowledge representation. DDCO is able to extract pharmacological and biological knowledge from diverse databases comprised of unique ontologies and database schemes. In the end, this new ontology creates efficient and robust environment to mine drug MOA and disease pathology associations. This knowledge base has been constructed to integrate with DrugBank, EntrezGene, GO, OMIM, KEGG, BioCarta, Reatome, UMLS, and the Gene Expression Omnibus (GEO) [33]. The chief weakness of this method, like many other high quality informatic efforts, is that it requires the manual curation and integration of many of the external database information. All of this knowledge is semantically assembled as a pharmacome–diseasome structure, which can be visualized by a graphical web network representation. Once constructed, graphics-based approaches using betweenness and closeness centrality algorithms can be applied to determine the rank order of the best drug candidates for a particular disease condition. Using this strategy the authors were able to repurpose tamoxifen as candidate drug for the treatment of systemic lupus erythematosus (SLE) [31]. This hypothesis is the result of estrogen receptor 1 and androgen receptor ranking highest in both closeness and betweenness centrality measures. Subsequent manual mining of the literature confirmed that both of these receptors appear to be involved in SLE disease pathology.

5.2.1. Genetic Analysis Methods

One fertile approach for providing new drug indication hypotheses is the analysis of genetic data. This information can be particularly enlightening especially when corroborated by independent data such as clinical expression analyses or preclinical studies. Depending of the type and source of the genetic data, this strategy can yield a number of high quality drug repositioning hypotheses. The success of this approach has led to the development of many sequence, expression, and phenotype-based genetic analysis methods.

Perhaps one of the most well-known tools used for mining the association of genes to genetically inherited diseases is G2D—Genes to (2) Disease [34–36]. The method has been used successfully to identify asthma [37] as well as type 2 diabetes (T2D) and obesity candidate genes [38]. The publicly available web server tool merges classical genetic methods with a computational data mining approach. G2D selects candidate genes genetically linked or in regions associated with the disease condition. It uses three different algorithms that differ based on the type of prioritization strategy used to produce the resulting rank-ordered candidate gene list for the disease based on fuzzy set theory. To identify and score relationships between terms Perez-Iratxeta et al. [34] defined two different fuzzy relations to measure the degree of association between medical and chemical controlled vocabularies. Identified susceptibility genes have functions related to the disease phenotype as defined by literature, genetic, or protein databases. The main assumption of the original prioritization algorithm (phenotype method) is that for any particular disease with unknown contributory gene X, there exists a phenotypically similar disease with identified associated gene Y, and genes X and Y are functionally related and relevant to the disease phenotype [35]. Therefore, G2D makes candidate predictions by scoring a number of BLASTX matches of unknown disease genes versus known disease genes. The final ordered list of predicted disease genes ultimately depends on the gene's annotation. Later, two additional prioritization algorithms based on different principles were developed [36]. The second algorithm (known genes method) uses the knowledge of genes already identified or suspected to be involved in a similar disease or disease variant but existing in a genomic location other than the one under consideration. This assumes that the gene involved in the disease of interest will have a function similar to the phenotypically related disease with known causal gene(s). The final algorithm (protein–protein interactions method) requires another locus in addition to the one under examination that is well established as contributing to the disease phenotype. The assumption is that some of the genes that exist in both loci will be involved in the same protein complex or pathway. The method will then prioritize candidates according to whether or not functional interactions are detected between proteins from both loci.

The phenotype and known-genes methods show a similar performance and will, on average, identify the causal gene in the top 25% of all prioritized genes under consideration. In contrast, the protein–protein interactions method is fairly insensitive as it produces results only about 25% of time, but when successful the disease contributing gene is generally found in the top 10% of the prioritized genes. The performance of the G2D phenotype method can be enhanced through the use of an R-score [38]. This is a relative score of the gene sequence according to the distribution of annotation scores of all the genes under consideration as contributing to the disease phenotype. R-scores near zero suggest a strong likelihood that the gene is associated with the disease. This additional score also allows for the direct comparison of candidates from different genomic regions.

GeneSeeker is a public tool that extracts and combines information from a series of open access genetic databases to generate a list of disease candidate genes [39]. It mines several sources to compile information about the cytogenetic localization, the human and mouse gene associated phenotypes, the function, and the available tissue expression of disease gene candidates. The program is also able to resolve gene name nomenclature differences among databases. The query form allows the user to specify genetic location and tissue expression while permitting the exclusion of housekeeping genes and certain databases. The query interrogates all the genetic databases in parallel and returns data exactly matching the user parameters, possible genes of interest that exhibit the appropriate expression patterns but map outside the candidate region, and genes that map to the region but are not expressed in the target tissues.

A sequence-based strategy to identify genes in Mendelian and multigenic diseases is utilized by the PROSPECTR (Priorization by Sequence and Phylogenetic Extent of Candidate Regions) program [40]. Traditional linkage studies as well as GWAS can identify genomic disease regions implicating tens to hundreds of candidate genes. Identification of the most probable disease-causing candidates becomes crucial to the drug repositioning process. One approach is to attempt to match the gene's functional annotation to the disease phenotype. This is unlikely to be successful in many instances since it depends on knowledge of involvement of the gene in some known pathogenesis. This strategy suffers from the fact that many genes in the genome lack functional annotation and available information is strongly biased by well-characterized genes. One theory is that most human diseases share genes that have common sequence features such as gene structural elements or functional protein features. PROSPECTR uses a machine learning algorithm to identify common sequence feature patterns among the candidate genes to recommend the likely most disease-causing targets. After testing a variety of algorithms, the alternating decision tree algorithm [41] was chosen because the classification rules that it produces can be easily understood and the results are just as predictive as other methods. An assessment of PROSPECTR performance demonstrated that it correctly identifies disease genes with about 70% accuracy, although it has an approximately 40% false positive rate. This same group developed a subsequent program called SUSPECTS to analyze the relationships between the functional annotation and expression profiles of disease candidate genes [42]. This tool attempts to resolve a potential problem with their previous sequence-based method since it prioritizes genes based on shared characteristics with disease genes but not necessarily the particular disease of interest to the investigator. It complements their previous approach using the hypothesis that genes involved in the same disease process will also tend to share either functional annotation or expression patterns that ultimately reflect their common participation in a biological pathway. In this method, the entire set of candidate genes are first identified by PROSPECTR for common sequence features. Second, the list of candidates is analyzed for correlations of co-expression based on the Genomics Institute of the Novartis Research Foundation (GNF) Gene Atlas expression data [43]. Third, the genes are analyzed for occurrences of rare Interpro domains. Finally, the list is assessed by the extent of semantic similarity among GO terms [44]. Each analysis generates an independent score and then the four scores are weighted by the amount of evidence, combined, and ranked by the final score. This approach identifies the correct disease gene in the top 5% of candidates with 56% accuracy. Both PROSPECTR and SUSPECTS can be run from a publicly available web interface.

Another group has designed an approach similar to PROSPECTR, called Disease Gene Prediction (DGP), which builds a decision tree-based model constructed from the similar features of disease-causing proteins [45]. This strategy is founded on the assumption that human disease genes have distinct properties that make them more susceptible to mutations causing pathological states. Therefore, their computational model is assembled from a sequence analysis of known disease proteins to detect their common sequence features. Disease proteins appear to contain more amino acids that are expressed in more phylogenetic groups and have a greater degree of sequence conservation among paralogs than their nondisease-causing counterpart proteins. To represent each protein's properties, this method computes two scores in addition to the length measure. To capture the degree of phylogenetic expression, they calculate a Z-score, and for the degree of paralog conservation, they compute a conservation score. They then utilize the Kolmogorov–Smirnov statistic to test the distribution between the conservation scores of disease proteins and all known human proteins to derive a P-value. This technique is also applied to the length distributions. Using a jack-knife test with 75% of 1567 known disease proteins to build the model, they demonstrate that they accurately predict 70% of the known disease genes in the remaining 25% test set of disease data. Furthermore, they describe the top 20 scoring putative disease genes not yet proven to be involved in human pathology, although several of them are implicated by other methods.

GWAS data are becoming useful for elucidating the genetic basis for the susceptibility to many human diseases. A tool called GWAS Analyzer integrates both phenotypic and genotypic data from many public GWAS resources [46]. The program compiles statistical information from association studies, HapMap data, microRNA results from miRBase, differential splice site knowledge, and microarray expression experiments. The web interface allows researchers to browse and analyze the available data and to quickly identify SNPs from candidate gene regions that satisfy the search query for further investigation. Using the tool, genomic regions surrounding the candidate SNPs can be subsequently examined for potential structural variants that may be contributing to the disease phenotype.

The creation of the Semantic Web has enabled a strategy that utilizes mouse and human genomic and phenomic knowledge to identify disease genes associated with orthologous phenotypes [47]. To accomplish this task, OWL and Resource Description Framework are used to integrate genomic and phenomic annotation knowledge from a variety of public data sources. Genomic information is garnered from GO, KEGG, BioCarta, BioCyc, and Reactome, while phenomic knowledge is obtained from MGI, OMIM, and the Multiple Congenital Anomaly/Mental Retardation Syndrome database. Analysis of a gene candidate list results in a directed acyclic graph. Degree centrality analysis is applied to the graph to determine the relative importance of each node and thus score each gene by its comparative significance to the network. Therefore, the gene score is inferred from both its functional significance from genomic data and its preclinical and clinical phenomic knowledge. The measure of centrality is based on the Semantic Web adapted version of the Kleinberg algorithm [48] similar to the method used by Google to determine page ranks. This gene prioritization scheme was used to rank 216 differentially expressed genes in idiopathic dilated cardiomyopathy. The top ranked and fifth ranked genes, *DMD* and *CRYAB*, had firmly established roles in the disease pathology. Two additional candidates in the top 10, *GJA1* and *RYR2*, had strong evidence for their involvement in cardiac function. This group later developed a public server called PhenoHM to enable investigators to perform this type of comparative analysis [49].

Another group of investigators has developed a similar approach to identify human disease genes based on the phenotypic appearance from an arbitrary disease query [50]. Their algorithm is based on the assumption that phenotypically similar diseases are caused by related molecular mechanisms. Their method clusters diseases with similar clinical features to an unknown query disorder and then computationally identifies the known causal genes of well-characterized disorders. Best scoring candidate genes for the disease query are proposed on the basis on their functional similarity to their corresponding known disease genes. This method relies on the analysis of GO annotations of disease gene clusters. The scoring algorithm estimates the degree of association between the candidate gene and the disease query as long as at least one known disease cluster appears to be similar. Thus, if no known disease cluster is detected as similar to the query disease, then the method fails and no disease candidate gene can be scored although different similarity thresholds can be attempted.

TOM (Transcriptomics of OMIM) is an algorithm that utilizes genetic mapping, expression, and functional information from public resources to predict candidate disease genes [51]. The approach requires at least one known disease gene and the genetic area of association or else at least two disease genetic areas of association. Given a list of disease candidates, TOM will identify the mostly likely causal gene based on common transcriptional co-regulation and functional role in cellular pathways. The strategy consists of a three-step filtering algorithm to identify the candidate genes for a particular disease. The first step is to compile a list of possible causal genes based on sequence information from the genetically associated areas. Step two is to use transcriptional data from either public or private databases to determine which gene sets have related expression profiles by calculating correlation coefficient values. Bonferroni statistics are used to correct for multiple sampling given the high number of correlation tests. Finally, candidate genes are further filtered on their related functional roles by GO annotation using hypergeometric distribution. This method has been successfully validated to identity the known disease genes for polycystic kidney disease and familial breast cancer. In addition, this approach has postulated candidate genes for the predisposition to thyroid cancer although these require further verification.

A *tour de force* approach to identify T2D and obesity candidate genes using a concert of algorithms has been described [38]. Metabolic syndromes are excellent case studies to evaluate different bioinformatic approaches since there are extensive clinical phenotypic information, genetic studies, and biomedical literature in these disease areas. This strategy utilizes seven different methods and takes a consensus approach to find genes that are identified by five or more procedures. These methods include GeneSeeker, eVOC analysis, (DGP), PROSPECTR, SUSPECTS, G2D, and POCUS. All of these strategies, with the exception of eVOC system analysis, have been previously discussed. The eVOC system is a controlled vocabulary developed to unify different types of gene expression data [52]. The subsequent eVOC analysis is the frequency of association of an eVOC anatomy term with a disease name in PubMed abstracts [53]. Using this approach, POCUS was by far the most selective while the eVOC analysis was the most nonspecific. GeneSeeker, SUSPECTS, and G2D leveraged the greatest amount of available information and the latter two are relatively complementary in approach to GeneSeeker in the formulation of the consensus view. Using a starting set of 9556 candidate genes, six of seven methods selected nine genes as potential T2D candidates and five genes as potential obesity candidates. Two of these genes, *LPL* and *BCKDHA*, overlap between the two diseases. Five of seven algorithms identify 94 candidates for T2D and 116 candidates for obesity with 58 genes in common. Although most of these candidates are implicated in these disorders by their involvement in oxidative metabolic pathways, insulin responsiveness, inflammatory pathways, and lipid and fatty acid metabolism, very few of these genes are actually validated for their role in the disease state. Therefore, it is difficult to assess the sensitivity and selectivity of this consensus algorithm approach although the underlying methods are based on diverse strategies and so it would seem unlikely that a gene would have a candidate co-occurrence on five or more methods by chance. This group later refined this strategy to include additional criteria in an effort to further improve the candidate gene selection procedure [54]. In addition, the method Endeavour was substituted for the POCUS algorithm. Endeavour ranks candidate genes utilizing Entrez Gene and GO annotation, InterPro and Bind interaction data, KEGG pathway information, expression data, and TFBS *cis*-regulatory modules [55, 56]. In this subsequent method, a supplementary analysis of the disease phenotypes and the relative frequency of the disorder symptoms in several populations were calculated [54]. With this additional filter, candidate genes from the multiple computational approaches were given a clinically relevant score based on the disease phenotypes and their frequency of occurrence in the disorder. In contrast to the previous study, Tiffin et al. [54] analyzed the disease phenotypes of metabolic syndrome in populations that are distinct but overlap with those of T2D and obesity. Fifty-four genes were selected for all five metabolic syndrome phenotypes by every one of the methods utilized, although when using phenotype frequency weightings for different populations only 19 genes were in common with both candidate datasets. These remaining genes were found to be most commonly represented in the pathways involving lipid and lipoprotein metabolism and in transmembrane signaling and signal transduction. Eight of the genes were previously implicated in metabolic syndrome although only one gene was previously described to contribute to all five phenotypes. Three of the genes had no prior connection to any of the metabolic syndrome phenotypes and represent truly novel candidate genes [54].

5.2.2. Connectivity Map Strategy

Perhaps the most innovative approach for the discovery of new indications in the drug repositioning process is the concept of the Connectivity Map [57, 58]. This is a computational approach for the generation of new disease indications hypotheses from microarray-based transcriptional profiling data, although the approach can be readily extended to other "omics" platforms. This method theoretically can connect small molecule compounds to their MOA as well as to novel diseases based on their respective gene expression "signatures." For application to drug repositioning, this strategy uses gene signatures primarily from human disease tissue to find inverse correlations with fingerprints constructed from drug-treated human cell lines. In theory, the better the correlation of disease signature to the inverse drug profile, the more likely the drug will be effective in reversing the disease genotype/phenotype—so-called disease modification.

In connectivity mapping, reference transcriptional profiles generated using microarrays are assembled by calculating the differential expression of a cell line treated with a series of compounds, relative to untreated controls. A rank order of this differential expression for each compound is then constructed. Disease query signatures can be generated from a variety of sources including disease microarrays (for example, GEO) or known information from the literature. Up-regulated and down-regulated genes from the disease queries are calculated for either positive or negative connectivity to the reference compound profiles [57]. Strong positive connectivity means that there is a good match between the up-regulated and down-regulated genes of both fingerprints, whereas strong negative connectivity means that there is an excellent correlation between the up-regulated genes of disease query and the down-regulated genes of the compound signature and vice versa. Therefore, the ideal drug will provide the precise inverse signature relative to the disease state, that is, restore the normal phenotype. This method has the advantage that it is independent of platform for the compound reference profiles and source of the disease signatures. Since it is a computational approach, large numbers of possible direct and inverse relationships within a myriad of disease states can be determined in a matter of seconds. This method has been applied to identify new drug indications in several areas. Five antiviral drugs with broad spectrum anti-influenza activity were identified and validated by their inhibition of the new pandemic H1N1 even though the virus was not used to generate the infection-mediated gene expression signature [59]. This demonstrates that this strategy can be utilized to discover antiviral agents through their effects on cellular gene expression. Phenoxybenzamine was predicted by the Connectivity Map and experimentally validated to be a potent analgesic in the rat Complete Freund's Adjuvant (CFA) osteoarthritic pain model [60]. MT7, a novel molecule from a combinatorial compound library, was indicated by the Connectivity Map to be a tubulin inhibitor by the similarity of its drug-treated expression profile to other known tubulin inhibitors [61]. Further characterization of the compound demonstrated that MT7 did inhibit tubulin polymerization even though it did not bind to purified tubulin. Cellular assays showed that the compound disrupted mitotic spindle formation and arrested cells at mitosis indicating that it may be useful as a novel anticancer [61].

The Connectivity Map method is based on the Kolmogorov–Smirnov statistic [62] using a nonparametric, rank-based, pattern-matching strategy called the Gene Set Enrichment Analysis (GSEA) [63]. In this approach, the disease query signature is comprised of a nonrank ordered list of genes correlated with the disease state, along with a sign indicating whether the gene is up- or down-regulated. The compound reference gene expression profiles are also represented in a nonparametric manner, but instead each gene is rank-ordered by its degree of differential expression relative to untreated controls. Each gene in the disease query signature is then compared against the rank-ordered list of each compound reference signature, and the strength of its positive or negative connectivity yields a score ranging from +1 to −1 for each compound signature (Figure 5.5). A connectivity score near 1 indicates a strong positive connectivity between the query and compound signatures whereas a score near −1 designates strong negative or inverse connectivity. As discussed above, for drug repositioning purposes a strong inverse connectivity is desired such that the compound restores the equilibrium disrupted by the disease condition. Since there is frequently variability in the compound profiling data, it is usually more accurate to have multiple instances of the drug-treated cell lines (Figure 5.6).

While innovative and potentially very powerful, the Connectivity Map strategy has a few limitations in its implementation as described in the original paper [57]. First, the disease query signatures are basically snapshots of the condition at or near a relatively steady state in time. In contrast, the compound reference signatures are relatively dynamic and are only snapshots of a fairly short (typically 6 hours) drug exposure. Profiles for longer exposures yield data with a different rank-ordered expression (unpublished observations). Therefore, there is a potential need for temporal optimization such that it may be possible to obtain more accurate connectivity scores from longer term drug treatments. Second, in the method as currently described, drug treatments are carried out at standard concentrations, usually 1 and 10 µM, and therefore they are independent of the compound's IC_{50} or IC_{90} (compound concentration at which 50% or 90% inhibition of the biological response is observed, respectively). Thus, in many cases the drug treatment is performed at suprapharmacological levels and the resulting compound signature may represent a combination of "on-" and "off-" target activities. Therefore, obtaining compound reference signatures at its IC_{90} may more accurately reflect the drug's primary biological activity. Finally, the Connectivity Map has implemented one algorithm to represent the degree of connectiveness between the disease query and the compound signature. Although this computational framework appears to be particularly useful in a number of cases, it is not readily apparent that the algorithm is the most productive representation of connectivity. For example, it may be naïve to assume that better connectivity between the drug and disease state is generated by requiring the gene signature to match at the extremes of the rank order profile. Therefore, a number of investigators have

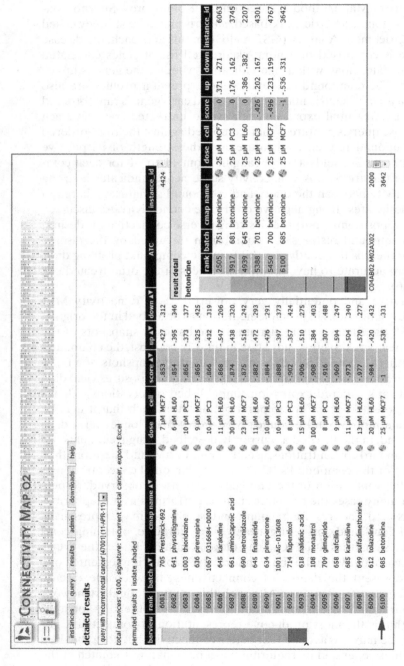

FIGURE 5.5. Connectivity Map results per instance. Shown are the instance results ranked from highest positive connectivity to best negative connectivity for a 30-gene signature for recurrent colon cancer [101]. The most negatively (inversely) connected compound treatment (betonicine) instance is shown at the bottom. Closer examination of all instances (shown at right insert) reveals that only the bottom three of six experiments are inversely connected to the signature. In addition, an identical experiment to the most negatively connected instance (shown at right insert at top) is positively connected to the up- and down-regulated query genes. Therefore, a permuted perturbation result frequently gives a more accurate view of the compound profile as seen in Figure 5.6. Reproduced from the Connectivity Map website with the permission of Justin Lamb of the Broad Institute.

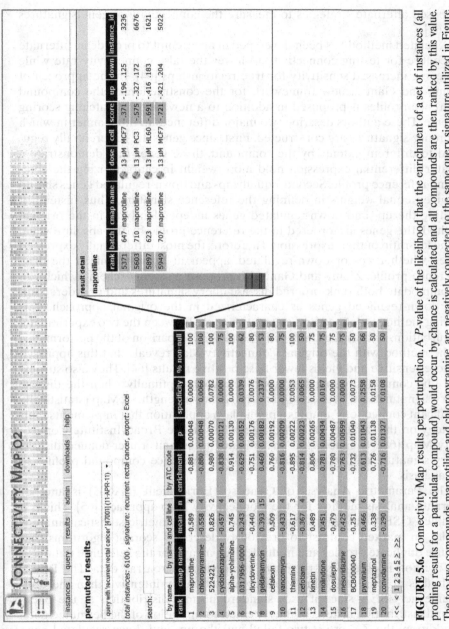

FIGURE 5.6. Connectivity Map results per perturbation. A *P*-value of the likelihood that the enrichment of a set of instances (all profiling results for a particular compound) would occur by chance is calculated and all compounds are then ranked by this value. The top two compounds, maprotiline and chloropyramine, are negatively connected to the same query signature utilized in Figure 5.5. The right side of the figure shows that all instances of maprotiline are inversely connected to the gene signature. While maprotiline has been used to treat depression and bipolar disorder, this result suggests that it might be effective in the management of recurrent rectal cancer. Reproduced from the Connectivity Map website with the permission of Justin Lamb of the Broad Institute.

proposed alternate strategies to measure the connectivity of gene signatures [64–67].

A related method has been developed in an attempt to provide an alternate procedure for testing connectivity to lower the false connectivity rate while achieving increased sensitivity for true relationships [64]. In the approach of Zhang and Gant, a new framework for the construction of the compound reference profiles is proposed in addition to a new pattern matching scoring scheme. These authors describe two major differences in the manner in which reference signatures are constructed. First, since genes are differentially regulated to different extents by the compound, those genes that demonstrate a greater differential expression hold more weight in characterizing the compound reference profile. Second, equally up- and down-regulated genes should be given equal weights in defining the reference signature. Thus, instead of treating the up- and down-regulated genes independently as in the original method, the genes are ordered in the reference profile by the absolute value of the log-ratio of their expression. Therefore, the most differentially expressed genes, whether up- or down-regulated, appear at highest rank in the drug reference profile. Zhang and Gant also propose a scoring scheme which can accommodate both rank-ordered disease query signatures and unordered up- and down-regulated genes as characterized in the original approach. This scoring method is defined by a connection score between the two experimental perturbations in the range between -1 and $+1$. Comparison of the performance of the method with the original Connectivity Map reveals that this approach is more sensitive and yields fewer false positive results [64]. They also suggest that this connectivity mapping approach works optimally when the disease query signatures are between 10 and 100 genes in length. sscMap (statistically significant connections' map) is a public Java application that implements their strategy on the current state of drug profiles in the Broad Institute Connectivity Map [68]. It enables the investigator to submit a user-defined disease query signature and to also include custom reference compound profiles in the analysis.

The Parametric Analysis of Gene set Enrichment (PAGE) is another alternate analysis method for the Connectivity Map approach [65]. This is a modified GSEA procedure that is based on a parametric statistical analysis model. In marked contrast to previously described scoring algorithms that require duplicate profiles and multiple drug arrays for the reference database, this method is able to score singlet compound microarray data. The PAGE method is at least 1000 times less computationally intensive than the non-parametric GSEA since it uses standard normal distribution as the background distribution instead of the repeated computation of the permuted data. In addition, the Z-score is two-tailed and the up- and down-regulated gene sets can be calculated in one analysis, whereas one-tailed statistical inference programs must be calculated in each direction separately. PAGE P-values are significantly lower than corresponding GSEA values and result in a larger number of significant gene sets that impart PAGE with greater sensitivity.

The method also appears to be relatively insensitive to different probe levels and microarray platforms since comparison of analyses with these variables yields the same outcomes. A web-based gene set analysis program called Gazer (gene set analyzer) uses both distribution-based and distribution-free models [69]. The tool detects significantly differentially expressed gene sets using the z-statistic, gene permutation, and multiple testing statistical analysis algorithms.

Geneva (GENE Vector Analysis) is a vector-based method that relies on the magnitude of differential expression of both the query and the reference database [66]. To quantify the increase or decrease in the differential expression of each gene, Tanner and Agarwal used the cyber-T statistic, which captures both direction and confidence. This statistical program also has a web-accessed interface and contains computational methods for estimating false positive and false negatives in microarray data using P-value distribution modeling [70]. After the cyber-T statistic is computed for all reference compound datasets, an all versus all vector query is performed. The resulting P-value represents the significance of a particular correlation relative to all correlations in the database. This technique requires replicate datasets although far fewer than the GSEA or Zhang and Gant methods, and it has the advantage that background distributions can be pre-computed. Geneva appears to be more accurate than other permutation-based models.

In a modified application of the Connectivity Map approach, one group has developed a Bayesian method to use public disease signatures to construct an automated diagnosis database and to establish new drug-to-disease relationships [67]. This strategy leverages the tremendous amount of disease information contained within the GEO database, which captures both quantitative differential expression data and complex phenotypic knowledge. Implementation of the method requires both standardization of the expression profiles to eliminate platform and experimental differences and the transformation of the associated disease information into a standardized language format using the Unified Medical Language System (UMLS). Analysis of the arrays is performed by ranking the expression values and by taking the logarithm of the expression values, resulting in a log-rank-ratio termed the standardized profile. Two microarrays can then be compared for their similarity by Pearson correlation. The Bayesian framework for automated disease diagnosis is a hierarchical classification approach where query profiles are placed into one or more disease classes using the UMLS hierarchy. Application of this method in a Connectivity Map approach identifies many known drug side effects and discovers a large number of novel disease–drug associations. In addition, numerous links between obesity and anticancer drugs were identified due to the global similarity of their expression patterns [67].

In addition to the previously discussed reference compound database biases due to temporal sampling and fixed compound concentrations, circadian rhythm [71] and food intake status [72] can potentially affect the disease query expression signatures. Diurnal variation significantly impacted expression of at least 25% of genes in adipose tissue from mildly obese people [71]. The affected genes were a subset of the circadian rhythm expression signature and principally involved in energy metabolism and antiapoptotic pathways. Inhibitors of growth factor pathways appear to be inversely related to the diurnal signature by the Connectivity Map algorithm and publicly available database. Additional studies suggest that food intake status affects the blood expression signatures of obesity-associated genes [72]. These results suggest that a pair of expression profiles, one from each of the fasted and fed states, is required to accurately reflect an individual's two distinct metabolic states. Further analysis by this group using the Granger causality test [73] has identified *PER1*, a circadian rhythm gene, as a top causal gene in both the diurnal variation and food intake status networks [74]. This suggests that care must be taken in the interpretation of the results of the Connectivity Map results due to possible confounders of the disease data, and it may be necessary to compare and contrast multiple disease datasets that encompass this biological variance.

5.2.3. Network Analysis Methods

The analysis of the complexity of the biological systems and the diversity of different types of data representing a disease state is greatly facilitated by network analysis methods. These approaches have the ability to both mathematically and graphically represent the diverse protein interactions found in higher organisms. These methods generally focus on motifs that are overrepresented in nodes and edges in the global biological network structure. This analysis can be extended to network hubs that appear to be critical proteins in the interaction networks of many hub proteins. The identification of these hubs can be particularly useful as key intervention points in a particular disease condition and thus are important protein therapeutic targets.

A network analysis method of differential expression data has been developed to identify the causal genes from particular disease linkage and association regions [75]. Most gene prioritization methods require previous knowledge about the disease processes to identity putative drug targets. In these previously described approaches, a variety of data sources are mined and then candidate genes are ranked by the amount of evidence to determine their "guilt by association." This method replaces this precondition of disease knowledge with the differential comparison of expression between healthy and disease states. Many gain of function disease defects are readily observed since they are overexpressed in the syndrome. Since many diseases arise from loss of function mutations or increased protein activity, the gene itself does not need to show increased expression to be implicated in the disorder in this strategy. Instead a functional biologic approach is taken to determine the relative enrichment of differentially expressed genes in a canonical pathway or deduced network relative to the normal state to focus on important gene sets. This enables one to look at the genes downstream to a possible defective protein and therefore using this method, one can deduce defective point in the network and therefore the candidate gene target. To accomplish this end, Nitsch et al. [75] constructed a distance network constructed from a variety of data types including genomic proximity, differential expression and co-expression data. They evaluated their strategy on four disease datasets with known causal genes: fragile X syndrome, Marfan syndrome, cystic fibrosis, and Becker muscular dystrophy. In all of these disease test cases, the known gene responsible for the syndrome was ranked in the top seven candidate genes. They also used their approach to deduce the possible causal genes for Stein–Levental syndrome, which results in obesity, hyperandrogenism, and chronic anovulation in women. They determined follistatin (*FST*), fibrillin 3 (*FBN3*), and DEAD box 4 among the best scoring genes responsible for the disease phenotype.

One network approach to establish disease-specific drug–protein relationships from molecular interaction information and PubMed abstracts based on the principle of the connectivity map has been developed [76]. This computational method uses known molecular interaction networks and established text mining techniques to determine particular disease, drug, and protein connectivity maps. The strategy not only has the capability of compiling disease-related drug information but also has the potential to uncover novel uses of marketed drugs. Thus, this approach is ideal for drug repositioning research since it can reveal new disease applications for old compounds. The framework strategy consists of three essential parts in order to construct the disease analysis: network construction, text mining and information extraction, and molecular connectivity mapping. This approach was applied to Alzheimer's disease (AD) to evaluate its effectiveness and to identify new drugs for the treatment of the disorder [76]. Li, Zhu, and Chen identified likely 22 AD candidate drugs for a list of 2019 compounds and 222,609 AD-associated PubMed abstracts. Seventeen of the candidates were used for the treatment of the disease; seven were approved for use according to DrugBank [77]. Three drugs that are known to treat cardiovascular disease were identified as possible therapies for AD. Diltiazem, prazosin, and quinidine had very similar drug–protein connectivity profiles. Another cardiovascular drug, Valsartan, has been demonstrated to reduce AD symptoms in a mouse model. Further investigation showed Prazosin is currently under investigation for the treatment of aggression in AD patients. This suggests the remaining two drugs may be potential AD therapeutics. In another application, Li et al. [76] tested the performance of the method against six types of cancer and determined that both the specificity and sensitivity of the approach were generally affected by the amount of characterization of the disease. Thus, the better studied cancers showed more favorable performance using this strategy than those cancers that were less characterized.

Another connectivity map-based method to build human disease–drug, disease–disease, and drug–drug networks using GEO expression profiles has been described [78]. The main hypothesis of this strategy is that drug and disease expression profiles can be correlated to one another in both direct and indirect relationships. This assumption is the basis of all connectivity map-related approaches. This group utilizes the cyber-T statistic which was employed by the same group in the previously described GENEVA strategy. Profile similarities are determined by calculating the Pearson correlation of the cyber-T statistic by two gene expression profiles. Gene enrichment is then established by generating a signature from one profile and then using connectivity map algorithm to assess the nonrandom distribution of the signature in the comparison profile. This enrichment procedure is essential for the construction of the drug–disease network to determine the global relationships from the public data. Among the new indications suggested by this approach is the use of tamoxifen for atopy and antimalarial drugs to treat Crohn's disease [78].

An online network analysis tool called MANTRA (Mode of Action by Network Analysis) is also inspired by the connectivity map approach [79]. This method is also based on the change in transcriptional expression of cell lines in response to drug treatment. The program is designed to discover a drug's MOA if unknown and find its off-target effects. The relatedness of two drugs is founded on the degree of commonality of their differential gene signatures. In this application of the technique, a consensus expression signature of the drug response on multiple cells lines and at different compound concentrations was constructed. A network was constructed containing 1302 drug nodes containing more the 41,000 edges relating the similarities between drug pairs. In an analysis of this network, Iorio et al. [79] were able to discover MOAs of many uncharacterized compounds and that these pathways fit well into the drug's known indication. In addition, unreported MOAs presumably due to off-target effects of well-known drugs or unknown connections between biological pathways were also ascertained and formed the basis of new indication hypotheses. One such drug is fasudil, a well-established rho-kinase inhibitor. Examination of the network showed the drug was closely connected to thapsigargin, trifluoperazine, and gossypol, known inducers of autophagy. Subsequent *in vitro* validation of fasudil treatment of human fibroblasts and HeLa cells confirmed its effect on autophagy activation. These data suggest that fasudil might be able to be repositioned as a treatment for neurodegenerative disorders [79].

Another web-based program that leverages the principle of the connectivity map is GEM-TREND (Gene Expression data Mining Toward Relevant Network Discovery) [80]. This tool enables researchers to search the public GEO database using gene expression signatures from drug data to identify diseases matching the query (Figure 5.7). It also facilitates the search of the database using keyword text queries. A co-expression network from this public database is also generated in order to discover genes which share similar regulation patterns using Pearson correlation coefficients and K-means clustering. Correlated genes are assembled in clusters based on the Pearson coefficients and subsequently into sub-networks, which interconnected the global network based on a Euclidean distance measure. Closely clustered diseases should share similar treatments and therefore a therapy utilized for one disease might

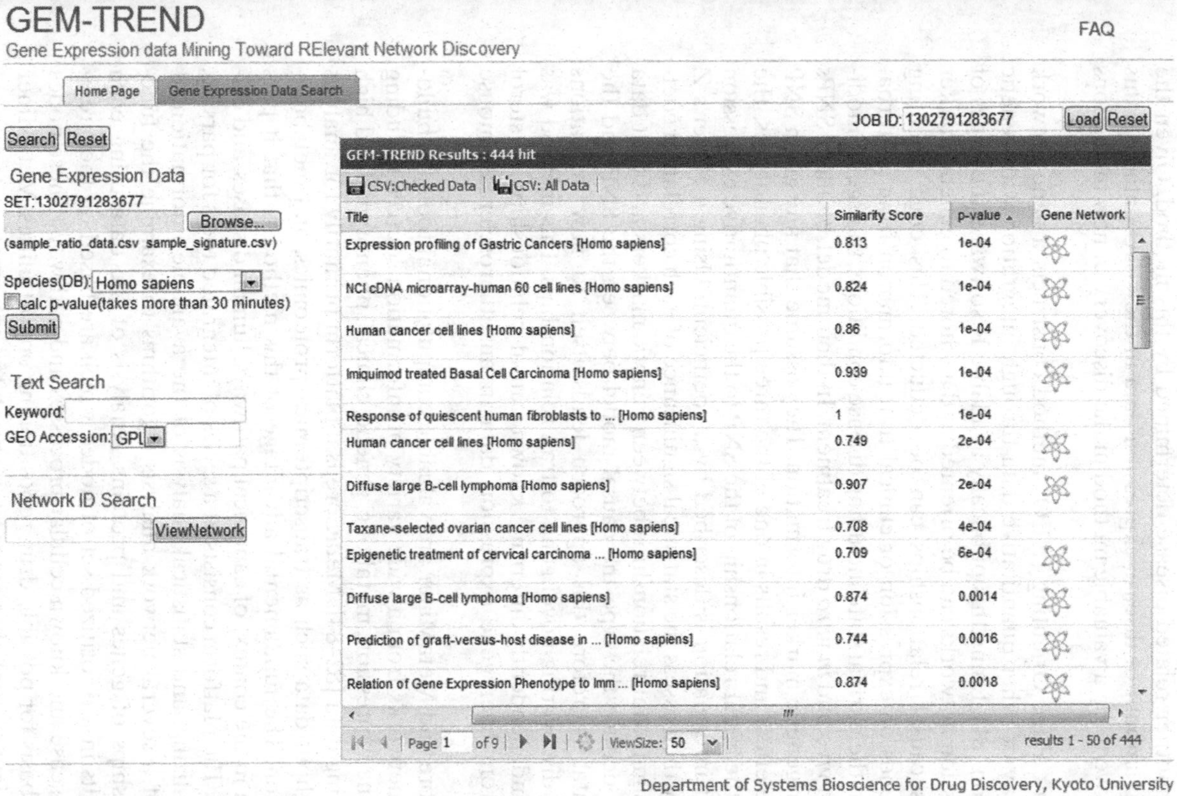

FIGURE 5.7. GEM-TREND example output. Shown are the GEO expression profiles identified by using the inverse of the histone deacetylase (HDAC) inhibitor gene signature [102]. Since GEM-TREND only detects transcription profiles that display positive connectivity, the inverse compound signature can discover novel disease indications. In this example, the inverse HDAC signature identifies many cancer profiles. Although HDAC inhibitors have been marketed mood stabilizers and antiepileptics, a number of drug trials are currently underway to investigate its use to treat a wide variety of cancers. Reproduced from the GEM-TREND website with the permission of Yasushi Okuno of Kyoto University.

117

be useful for another related disease determined by this method. Given the ever increasing amount of disease expression data in the GEO database, this tool should prove to be a valuable method in the discovery of new indications hypotheses.

The Network Edge Orienting (NEO) method constructs a gene network from microarray or other quantitative data through integration with genetic trait information [81]. Using this publically available R software, the edges of gene co-expression networks can be oriented and anchored to genetic marker data and thus causal relationships can be deducted. This edge orienting approach depends on expression or clinical trait information from perturbations relative to the normal state including disease conditions, transgenic modifications, and *in vivo* and *in vitro* drug treatment. In their model, bi-allelic SNPs are utilized for genetic marker information. They assume that any given SNP has an additive effect and results in one of the three possible phenotypes. The correlation of the linear relationship of the SNP to the quantitative expression or clinical trait information is described by a coefficient. Using a Fisher's Z transform, they then assess the statistical significance of each correlation coefficient. These significant relationships between genetic markers and trait data allow them to deduce the type the causal model between the SNP and the phenotypic data. Therefore this approach lends itself to new indications hypotheses by discovering novel gene to trait relationships. This method was validated by independently inferring known causal relationships in sterol homeostasis from liver gene expression data in an atherosclerosis mouse model [81].

The MetaCore and MetaMiner are valuable computational tools for building biological networks from a wide variety of information sources including protein and gene expression, metabolic, genetic, clinical, phenotypic, and high content screening data [82–84]. MetaCore is a platform primarily for analysis of high throughput data such as transcriptomics, proteomics, and metabolomics information. The fundamental advantage of this method is that it puts molecular data in the context of canonical pathways, human diseases, and cellular processes. The platform consists of a series of integrated tools for parsing, querying, visualizing, and statistical analysis of the available information. It also consists of a several network analysis algorithms to examine the functional relationships of genes and proteins. Analysis of the data using each algorithm results in a prioritized set of nodes, which are based on their relevance to the disease and known cellular processes and pathways. These nodes then form the basis for possible drug repositioning opportunities. MetaMiner is a disease-oriented tool that integrates annotated information for gene–disease associations, known compounds that are utilized to treat disorder- and disease-specific networks and pathways. This method has been applied to cystic fibrosis and is an effort to assemble all of the known data and information regarding the disease into one central disease repository [84]. The goal of the approach is to do a comprehensive analysis of all available knowledge using the network analysis tools to suggest alternate therapies for management of the disorder. This MetaMiner strategy has been recently extended to the analysis of chronic obstructive pulmonary disease (COPD), asthma, diabetes, and oncology [84].

A novel computational approach to identify disease genes is to determine their topological statistical significance in biological networks [85]. This method scores network nodes that are constructed from experimentally determined differential transcriptional and/or protein expression information. The scoring algorithm is based on the connectivity relationship of genes or protein nodes to the global disease expression network. In contrast to other methods, this strategy is independent of the node's centrality and thus not dependent on the node's degree of physical connections. The goal is to enhance significant nodes in the prioritization scheme while greatly reducing the network scores of nodes that have chance connectivity. The output of the analysis is a prioritized list of network nodes that show significant connectivity with the disease state and provides the researcher with possible drug targets to reverse the disease condition. If a safe marketed drug exists for the identified node, then this provides an immediately testable hypothesis for pursuit using preexisting therapeutic resources. In the next section, we will briefly describe how disease network modeling, in conjunction with some of the other approaches described in this chapter, is beginning to be used to identify possible therapeutic interventions for cancer patients based on the molecular profile of their tumor.

5.3. CASE STUDY: APPLICATION OF COMPUTATIONAL DRUG REPOSITIONING APPROACHES IN THE VAN ANDEL RESEARCH INSTITUTE PERSONALIZED MEDICINE INITIATIVE

A number of the methodologies used to identify new indications hypotheses that have been outlined in this chapter also have logical utility in the area of personalized or precision therapeutics. Personalized therapeutics refers to the utilization of molecular information obtained from an individual patient or their disease to identify agents with optimal therapeutic index. While the prediction of drug efficacy remains the common objective for both indications discovery and personalized therapeutics, the latter requires special consideration of practical restraints associated with support of clinical decision making. First, samples and data must be processed in real time; in the setting of relapse/ refractory cancer patients, we have set an upper limit of a 10 business day turnaround from patient enrollment to final report to be compatible with the needs of the treating physician. Second, sample processing must be performed in a CLIA (Clinical Laboratory Improvement Amendments) certified laboratory, which, in itself, requires finalized standard operating procedures and introduction of the necessary quality control and quality assurance measures to ensure assay performance and reproducibility. Third, and arguably the most demanding requirement, the information provided back to the treating physician must be in an actionable and readily interpretable format to support its practical use in therapeutic decision making. In this section, we will briefly describe our recent efforts to treat relapse/refractory cancer patients on the basis of molecular profiling of their tumors. While other disease states are certainly eligible for this individualized approach, the molecular heterogeneity of cancer coupled with the vast number of oncology drugs currently in clinical development, the high failure rates of these agents in Phase III trials, the projected healthcare costs associated with treating cancer over the coming decades, and the sheer incidence and toll of this disease on society mean that oncology is leading the revolution in personalized healthcare [86].

Per U.S. Food and Drug Administration (FDA), a biomarker is defined as a biological feature that can be objectively measured and used to predict or detect the progression of disease or the effects of treatment [87]. In the field of pharmacogenomics, biomarkers associated with differential drug efficacy or toxicity are investigated with the goal of identifying patient subsets most likely to achieve benefit from intervention. At the time of this writing, a simple PubMed search on the terms "biomarker," "cancer," and "drug" yields 60,189 hits that collectively represent a snapshot of peer-reviewed knowledge on the general topic. However, despite the unprecedented rate of pharmacogenomic biomarker discovery in the post-genomic era, few of these discoveries ultimately convert into useful clinical tools. This translational gap is widely recognized as a major bottleneck in translational research and requires the careful consideration of a long-term informatics strategy that aligns the disciplines, infrastructure, and tools of bioinformatics and medical informatics into an integrated scheme permitting the exchange of data, information, and knowledge between clinical application and discovery research [86, 88].

Despite limited progress in the clinical application of pharmacogenomics, a number of specific drug–disease–target (so-called theranostic) examples do exist that have collectively provided the proof-of-concept for personalized therapeutics. The hypothesis that the alignment of a drug's MOA with the causative driver of a disease process will result in enhanced drug efficacy and improve patient outcomes was illustratively tested in chronic myeloid leukemia (CML), which frequently harbors the *BCR-ABL* fusion gene product encoded by the Philadelphia chromosome; this is the result of a t(9:22) (q34;q11) translocation that drives the disease process (reviewed in [89]). Imatinib, a potent inhibitor of the *ABL* tyrosine kinase, was subsequently developed and shown to dramatically inhibit the proliferation of CML and improve patient outcomes. In an analogous example, trastuzumab, a monoclonal antibody that targets the *ERBB2* (*HER2*) protein, was approved on the basis of its efficacy in a subset of breast tumors expressing *ERBB2* [90]. Similarly, targeting metastatic melanoma's harboring an oncogenic B-Raf kinase mutation with a targeted Raf-kinase inhibitor (PLX4032) has shown early efficacy [91], while targeting activating *EGFR* mutations or *ALK* rearrangements frequently present in non-small cell lung carcinomas with corresponding inhibitors have also shown promise in clinical trials (reviewed by [92]). Collectively, these and an increasing number of other studies have demonstrated that drugs targeting the molecular drivers of the malignant phenotype of the tumor cell can exhibit robust clinical responses. However, these biomarkers are currently being developed in a drug–disease–target-specific fashion, which, ultimately, given the number of drugs, diseases, and targets available for this approach, is likely not sustainable from a healthcare economics vantage point. At some point in the near future the treating physician will become inundated with all possible theranostic tests, each with its own price point and turnaround time contributing to increased costs and delays in patient care. In addition, the complexity of the cancer genome and its ability to rapidly evolve has naturally resulted in the acquisition of resistance to single agent therapies, dictating the need to develop approaches to identify the optimal combinational treatments that target the collective Achilles' heel of the cancer cell and its microenvironment [93]. The fundamental challenge in the area of targeted cancer treatment therefore remains how to identify optimal therapeutic strategies for heterogeneous tumors that are highly adaptive and exhibit significant inter- and intra-patient variation [94–96]. This calls for a more general, scalable, and systematic genome-pharmacopeia–phenome-wide approach to align optimal combinations of drugs to disease through the use of biomarkers and consolidated informatics strategies.

Given the above challenges, we have begun to develop the processes and technologies required to process a patients tumor in real time, predict drug(s) efficacy on the basis of the analysis of molecular information extracted from the tumor, and align molecular-based hypotheses of drug efficacy with clinically relevant evidence supporting the use of the predicted agents in the context of the patient's disease. To support the community oncologist, we have focused our initial efforts on agents already approved by the FDA for any disease indication (i.e., not necessarily cancer specific) and experimental agents in developmental trials. Our initial efforts have been focused on utilizing array-based transcriptional profiling technology due to the abundance of public domain datasets available, the ability to standardize the standard operating procedures and obtain CLIA certification, and the immediate compatibility with some of the algorithmic approaches we currently use. It should be noted that we are currently modifying our approaches to also include next-generation sequencing and phosphoproteomic technologies to provide a more broadened characterization of the tumor's molecular profile. However, in this chapter we will summarize our experience to date with gene expression profiling toward the goal of real-time personalized therapeutics.

At the onset, our long-term objective was to determine which, if any, of the multitude of methodologies available for predicting drug efficacy on the basis of molecular profiling are the most accurate, while simultaneously providing potentially useful information to treating physicians in a real-time fashion for consideration in the design of a treatment plan. In consultation with physicians faced with the somewhat arbitrary selection of therapy for relapse/refractory patients who have exhausted the standard-of-care options, it was felt that any information/knowledge that could assist them in drug selection was beneficial, even if the underlying approach had not yet been proven in the clinical setting. It is important to note that having established feasibility and safety of the approach as summarized briefly below, we are currently designing efficacy trials in which molecularly guided therapies will be compared directly with "physician choice" using current approaches to drug selection. However, our initial trials were focused on testing the hypothesis that it is feasible and safe to process a patient's tumor in real time within a CLIA-certified laboratory, and generate an actionable report for consideration in 10 business days.

In our initial 50-patient trial, 14 pediatric patients and 36 adult patients with a variety of relapse/refractory cancers were enrolled in the study. In this pivotal study, we assessed the feasibility of sampling tumors through different sites/procedures (e.g., surgical material, biopsies, ascites, and pleural effusions). We showed that viable tumor material with suitable tumor content yielding high quality RNA was obtainable from surgical resections and 28 gauge (or larger) biopsies, but not from ascites or pleural effusion fluid that required extensive processing and yielded low RNA yield of poor quality. Sampled tumor was qualified by clinical pathology to ensure a greater than 50% viable tumor content (by nuclei count to estimate RNA signal contribution), prior to further processing on the Affymetrix GeneChip® platform using established and CLIA-certified standard operating procedures. After normalization and quality control assessment of the raw Affymetrix U133 2.0 plus intensity data, data are further processed using the general workflow illustrated in Figure 5.8. Tumor derived data is first compared with a reference set of samples ranging from a set of normal tissues representing the tumor's origin, a collection of heterogeneous normal samples across the human body, and/or a collection of heterogeneous tumor samples. While beyond the scope of this chapter, the selection of the appropriate reference set against which transcript abundance in the patient's tumor is compared represents a critical step in the process, and we typically run the analysis against multiple reference sets to identify agents predicted independent of reference type. During this preprocessing step, the normalized intensity of each probe set is converted to a representative Z-score, reflecting the number of standard deviations from the mean intensity within the reference sample set. At this point, subsets of over- or underexpressed genes are processed by a variety of predictive methodologies, each with its own scientific rationale, and set of drugs that could be predicted by the respective method. The pool of drugs covered by each is not identical; in general, signature-based methods (connectivity map, parametric gene set enrichment analysis) cover many of the standard chemotherapeutic (nontargeted) agents, while target-based methods (rules and network-based methods) are naturally primed to identify drug targets and the corresponding drug(s) based on the latter's MOA. The current methodologies under investigation are:

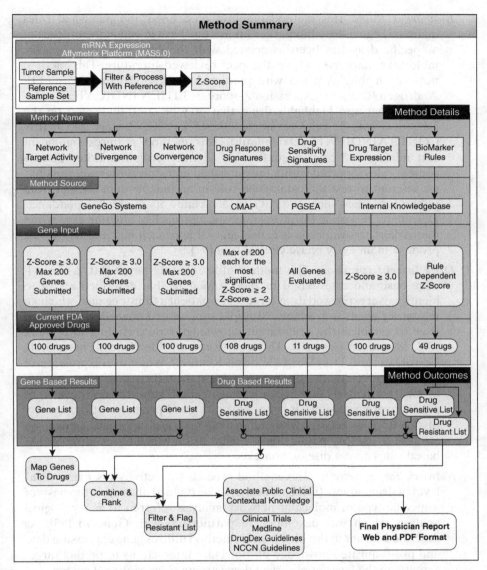

FIGURE 5.8. General work flow schema for processing tumor-derived gene expression data through a variety of methods to predict drug efficacy. Following prediction of drug efficacy by multiple methods on the basis of differential gene expression in the patient's tumor relative to a reference sample set, evidence supporting the use of the predicted agent in the context of the patient's specific disease is identified through knowledge mining of trusted sources (e.g., PubMed, clinicaltrials.gov, NCCN guidelines, and DrugDex). The end result is an interactive report summarizing information pertaining to the predicted agents and supporting evidence for consideration by the treating physician (see Figure 5.9).

Biomarker Rules. This method employs predefined and published rules maintained in a drug-biomarker knowledge base in which the efficacy of a specific drug has been associated with the expression of a specific molecular marker(s) within the peer-reviewed literature. This method not only highlights drugs with predicted sensitivity (example rule: IF Androgen Receptor Expression Z-score ≥+3 THEN INDICATE Bicalutamide), but also highlights drugs that may be contraindicated on the basis of resistance rules (example rule: IF ERCC1 Z-score ≥+3 THEN CONTRAINDICATE Oxaliplatin). This method requires significant text mining and human curation to identify drug-biomarker–disease context rules reported within the published literature. Wherever possible, we attempt to test the catalogued rule in an independent dataset from public resources such as GEO to determine its context dependence. Despite representing the most simplistic approach of aligning expression biomarkers to drug response, this general approach has recently shown promise in an early phase clinical trial [97].

Drug Target Expression. This method utilizes a drug-target (MOA) knowledge base and rules-based method similar to that described above to identify overexpressed drug targets in a patient's tumor against which an inhibitory agent is available. Multiple sources of knowledge have been used to establish the drug-target knowledge base including DrugBank [77], MetaCore (GeneGo-Thomson Reuters), MedTrack, PharmGKB, UpToDate, and DrugDex (Thomson Reuters). While overexpression of a drug target can represent a means to predict efficacy of some targeted agents (particularly biologics, e.g., trastuzumab indicated on the basis of *HER2* overexpression), it is not always a good predictor of the activity of the drug target. As with the biomarker rules approach above, we attempt to identify public domain datasets on which to test drug MOA-based rules across disease contexts.

Network Target Activity. This method predicts the activity (vs. expression) level of drug targets (same targets as those defined above) on the basis of a specific type of molecular network analysis referred to as topological analysis which was developed in partnership with GeneGo [85]. As described earlier in this chapter, this method utilizes gene expression data and pre-requisite knowledge of molecular interactions to predict target activity on the basis of observed downstream transcriptional events.

Drug Response Signatures. This method reproduces the Connectivity Map concept initially developed by the Broad Institute [57] in which the genomic consequence of drug exposure is used to connect drug effect to disease signatures. As discussed earlier, the hypothesis underlying this method is that drugs that reverse the disease genotype (gene expression profile) toward normalcy have the potential to reverse the disease phenotype. Up to 500 of the most over- and underexpressed genes in the patient's tumor are submitted to this method. Rank-based statistics are used to identify drugs with a significant inverse connectivity to the disease genotype.

Drug Sensitivity Signatures. This method reproduces the published implementation of the Parametric Gene Set Enrichment Analysis (PGSEA) method using the NCI-60 cell line sensitivity signatures [98, 99]. Pretreatment gene expression signatures associated with differential response to specific drugs on the basis of an *in vitro* drug screen are compared with the tumor-derived gene expression signature. This approach is consistent with well-published methods for inferring drug sensitivity utilizing the NCI-60 cell line dataset [98, 99].

Upon execution of the different analytical methodologies, a compiled report is generated (see Figure 5.9). The report is highly interactive, allowing the physician to quickly navigate to the underlying knowledge and evidence at multiple levels to attain more information on the specific drug, drug target, available clinical trials, and supporting literature. The report conveys the predicted efficacy (or lack of efficacy in the case of biomarker resistance rules) of the drugs identified by each of the methods and also shows any evidence that may support the use of the predicted drug in the context of the patient's specific disease state. The supporting evidence comes from a variety of sources including PubMed, clinicaltrials.gov, the FDA label, and DrugDex. Through this approach, this decision support tool not only provides molecular-based hypotheses pertaining to agent efficacy (frequently a new indication for the predicted agent), but also provides the supporting evidence and information required to efficiently practice medicine (e.g., reimbursement evidence and active clinical trials).

In our initial 50 patient trial, we demonstrated that it was feasible to enroll patients, collect and pathologically qualify suitable tumor tissue, process the tumor within a CLIA-certified environment using the Affymetrix GeneChip technology, process the molecular data through our informatics pipeline, and generate and deliver an interactive report to the treating physician in 10 business days. We also tracked utilization of the delivered information and found that, in about 50% of the cases, physicians altered their treatment plan based on the provided information. The latter was assessed through pre- and post-report questionnaire documenting planned versus actual treatments administered. While the primary objective of the trial was demonstration of feasibility, some potential responses were observed and have provided the impetus to develop proof-of-efficacy trials. Subsequent to this first study, we have completed a five-patient multisite feasibility (nontreatment) trial in pediatric neuroblastoma, and recently received FDA-Investigational Device Exemption (IDE) approval to proceed to a 14-patient treatment trial in the same indication. In parallel, we are now designing larger efficacy trials in which our molecularly informed approach to therapy selection will be compared directly with current approaches (so-called physician choice) using progression-free survival, tumor response, and/or overall survival as outcome measures. Despite

Results Summary

RANK	DRUG	METHOD	SUPPORTING INDUSTRY EVIDENCE	
			REIMBURSEMENT	OTHER
1	calcitriol	⬛ Biomarker-Based Rules – Sensitive (1 target)	1/15	46/405
2	phentolamine	⬛ Drug Target Expression (1 target)	0/15	3/405
2	trazodone	⬛ Drug Target Expression (1 target)	0/15	3/405
2	yohimbine	⬛ Drug Target Expression (1 target)	0/15	4/405
5	vorinostat	▷ Network Convergence (1 target) ⬛ Drug Target Expression (1 target)	0/15	21/405
6	phenelzine	⬛ Drug Target Expression (1 target)	0/15	2/405
6	tranylcypromine	⬛ Drug Target Expression (1 target)	0/15	2/405
8	epirubicin	⬛ Drug Target Expression (1 target)	2/15	40/405
8	etoposide	⬛ Drug Target Expression (1 target)	1/15	95/405
8	mitoxantrone	⬛ Drug Target Expression (1 target)	0/15	28/405
11	disulfiram	⬛ Drug Response Signatures (1 target)	0/15	10/405
12	topotecan	⬛ Biomarker-Based Rules – Sensitive (1 target)	1/15	22/405
13	drotrecogin alfa	⬛ Drug Target Expression (1 target)	0/15	2/405
14	dasatinib	⬛ Biomarker-Based Rules – Sensitive (1 target)	0/15	6/405
15	carmustine	⬛ Drug Sensitivity Signatures (1 target)	10/15	121/405

FIGURE 5.9. An example of a page of an informational report provided to physicians during our personalized therapeutics feasibility trials conveying a rank-ordered list of agents with predicted efficacy, and evidence supporting the use of the predicted agent in the patient's disease context (in this example, colon cancer). While impossible to ascertain from this static image, multiple aspects of the report are interactive permitting a deeper exploration of relevant information pertaining to drugs, biomarkers, methods, and supporting evidence by the physician. The pediatric column indicates agents for which there is defined pediatric dosing available in support of our ongoing pediatric oncology trials. This report format was provided by Intervention Insights (www.interventioninsights.com), who are now offering this service to oncologists [103].

the logic of aligning the mechanisms of disease and drugs, and the early promise and proof-of-feasibility, a significant amount of work lay ahead to demonstrate that this molecularly guided approach to therapy selection, on the basis of the prediction of drug efficacy, significantly impacts patient outcome.

5.4. SUMMARY AND FUTURE DIRECTIONS

There exists a wide variety of bioinformatics and computational biology tools to aid the investigator in indications discovery research. The majority of these strategies do not vary significantly between early discovery and indications discovery researchers although drug repositioning investigators are severely limited by the number of drug targets available to them. Knowledge mining and integration strategies are well-established methods and are extremely useful in the distillation of significant information from large data resources. These approaches depend, at least in part, on the co-occurrence of important terms in the knowledge bases and the computational ranking of this information is generally founded on contextual relationships. The Connectivity Map is a potentially exciting approach for drug repositioning as it qualitatively matches inversely disease and drug profiles. In theory it should be able to identify the best available compounds to reverse the disease state although this concept still requires definitive new indications discovery examples. Genetic methods can be valuable in the identification of repositioning opportunities, but application of this technique requires high quality information. This strategy assumes that a phenotypically similar disease is caused by a similarly functioning gene to a known disease gene. Therefore, the method will necessarily exclude any gene with unknown or poorly understood function, although these are generally not current drug targets. Network analysis approaches are extremely promising and many of them build on the concept of the Connectivity Map. The utility of these methods remain to be proven although there are several examples from the area of personalized medicine.

With respect to our ongoing efforts in personalized therapeutics, our past efforts have focused heavily on the utilization of gene expression data toward prediction of agent efficacy. Given the limitations of the mRNA analyte and 3′ expression arrays, we are currently adapting our approach to incorporate next-generation sequencing (NGS) (whole genome, exome, and transcriptome) to provide a much expanded view of the molecular makeup of individual patient tumors. Although some aspects of the informatics pipeline are well defined and immediately compatible with our current approaches (namely RNA-Seq), the challenge of completing the analysis in a cost- and time-effective fashion remains considerable. In addition, it will be critical to develop a necessary knowledge base that captures the association between increasingly complex molecular aberrations, the context of an individual's disease, and drug efficacy, allowing for the generation of an actionable report in support of clinical decision making [100]. Despite these barriers, it is clear that the sequencing of the cancer genome using rapidly evolving NGS technologies and informatics approaches represents a major component of the future of personalized cancer treatment.

Databases containing medically relevant information useful to the indications discovery process are expanding at near exponential rates. Therefore, the need for computational methods to crawl through and recognize important information in these databases will continue to be essential to drug repositioning strategies. Presently, there is no unsupervised substitute of a human being for quality assessment of data summaries generated by any computational or bioinformatics method. Further development of more sophisticated techniques that can address the shortcomings of current computational and bioinformatics approaches will be required to efficiently process the ever increasing volume and complexity of biological data. These issues include the need for strategies that can integrate data from a wide variety of disparate sources, for better unsupervised methods with lower false positive and false negative rates, and for approaches that can postulate unified hypotheses from several independent algorithms. Given the inaccuracy of current computational strategies, a new indication hypothesis by any method needs to be confirmed by multiple techniques and then validated by an animal model or a small clinical trial before it is a truly viable drug repositioning opportunity.

REFERENCES

1. Cochrane, G.R., Galperin, M.Y. (2010). The 2010 Nucleic Acids Research Database Issue and Online Database Collection: A community of data resources. *Nucleic Acids Res.*, *38*(Database issue), D1–D4. http://www.oxfordjournals.org/nar/database/a.
2. Tiffin, N., Andrade-Navarro, M.A., Perez-Iratxeta, C. (2009). Linking genes to diseases: It's all in the data. *Genome Med.*, *1*, 77.
3. Chen, Y.P., Chen, F. (2008). Using bioinformatics techniques for gene identification in drug discovery and development. *Curr. Drug Metab.*, *9*, 567–573.
4. Ivanenkov, Y.A., Savchuk, N.P., Ekins, S., Balakin, K.V. (2009). Computational mapping tools for drug discovery. *Drug Discov. Today*, *14*, 767–775.
5. Barratt, M.J., Frail, D.F. (2010). Integration of indications discovery efforts at Pfizer. *Int. Drug Discov.*, *5*, 72–75.
6. Harland, L., Gaulton, A. (2009). Drug target central. *Expert Opin. Drug Discov.*, *4*, 857–872.
7. Loging, W., Harland, L., Williams-Jones, B. (2007). High-throughput electronic biology: Mining information for drug discovery. *Nat. Rev. Drug Discov.*, *6*, 220–230.
8. Notter, L.E. (1972). MEDLINE—Newest service in the medical information network. *Nurs. Res.*, *21*, 101. http://www.ncbi.nlm.nih.gov/pubmed.
9. Campbell, S.J., Gaulton, A., Marshall, J., Bichko, D., Martin, S., Brouwer, C., Harland, L. (2010). Visualizing the drug target landscape. *Drug Discov. Today*, *15*, 3–15.

10. Turner, F.S., Clutterbuck, D.R., Semple, C.A. (2003). POCUS: Mining genomic sequence annotation to predict disease genes. *Genome Biol.*, *4*, R75.

11. McKusick, V.A. (1998). *Mendelian Inheritance in Man. A Catalog of Human Genes and Genetic Disorders*, 12th ed. Baltimore, MD: Johns Hopkins University Press. http://www.ncbi.nlm.nih.gov/omim/.

12. McEntyre, J., Lipman, D. (2001). PubMed: Bridging the information gap. *CMAJ*, *164*, 1317–1319. http://www.ncbi.nlm.nih.gov/pubmed.

13. Eaton, A.D. (2006). HubMed: A web-based biomedical literature search interface. *Nucleic Acids Res.*, *34*(Suppl 2), W745–W747. http://www.hubmed.org/.

14. Hoffmann, R., Valencia, A. (2004). A gene network for navigating the literature. *Nat. Genet.*, *36*, 664. http://www.ihop-net.org/UniPub/iHOP/.

15. Hoffmann, R., Valencia, A. (2005). Implementing the iHOP concept for navigation of biomedical literature. *Bioinformatics*, *21*(Suppl 2), ii252–ii258.

16. Tsuruoka, Y., Tsujii, J., Ananiadou, S. (2008). FACTA: A text search engine for finding associated biomedical concepts. *Bioinformatics*, *24*, 2559–2560. http://www.nactem.ac.uk/software/facta/.

17. Rebholz-Schuhmann, D., Kirsch, H., Arregui, M., Gaudan, S., Riethoven, M., Stoehr, P. (2007). EBIMed—Text crunching to gather facts for proteins from MEDLINE. *Bioinformatics*, *23*, e237–e244. http://www.ebi.ac.uk/Rebholz-srv/ebimed.

18. Kim, J.J., Pezik, P., Rebholz-Schuhmann, D. (2008). MedEvi: Retrieving textual evidence of relations between biomedical concepts from MEDLINE. *Bioinformatics*, *24*, 1410–1412. http://www.ebi.ac.uk/tc-test/textmining/medevi/.

19. Cheng, D., Knox, C., Young, N., Stothard, P., Damaraju, S., Wishart, D.S. (2008). PolySearch: A web-based text mining system for extracting relationships between human diseases, genes, mutations, drugs and metabolites. *Nucleic Acids Res.*, *36*(Web Server issue), W399–W405. http://wishart.biology.ualberta.ca/polysearch.

20. Hur, J., Schuyler, A.D., States, D.J., Feldman, E.L. (2009). SciMiner: Web-based literature mining tool for target identification and functional enrichment analysis. *Bioinformatics*, *25*, 838–840. http://jdrf.neurology.med.umich.edu/SciMiner/.

21. Fisher, R.A. (1922). On the interpretation of $\chi2$ from contingency tables, and the calculation of P. *J. R. Stat. Soc.*, *85*, 87–94.

22. Kemper, B., Matsuzaki, T., Matsuoka, Y., Tsuruoka, Y., Kitano, H., Ananiadou, S., Tsujii, J. (2010). PathText: A text mining integrator for biological pathway visualizations. *Bioinformatics*, *15*, i374–i381. http://www.pathtext.org.

23. Nobata, C., Cotter, P., Okazaki, N., Rea, B., Sasaki, Y., Tsuruoka, Y., Tsujii, J., Ananiadou, S. (2008). Kleio: A knowledge-enriched information retrieval system for biology. *Proceedings of the 31st Annual International ACM SIGIR Conference on Research and Development in Information Retrieval. Singapore.* ACM, Singapore, pp. 787–788. http://www.nactem.ac.uk/software/kleio/.

24. Miyao, Y., Tomoko, O., Katsuya, M., Yoshimasa, T., Kazuhiro, Y., Takashi, N., Jun'ichi, T. (2006). Semantic retrieval for the accurate identification of relational concepts in massive textbases. *In the Proceedings of COLING-ACL 2006. Sydney*, pp. 1017–1024. http://www-tsujii.is.s.u-tokyo.ac.jp/medie/search.cgi.

25. Perez-Iratxeta, C., Bork, P., Andrade, M.A. (2001). XplorMed: A tool for exploring MEDLINE abstracts. *Trends Biochem. Sci.*, *26*, 573–575. http://www.ogic.ca/projects/xplormed/.

26. Perez-Iratxeta, C., Keer, H.S., Bork, P., Andrade, M.A. (2002). Computing fuzzy associations for the analysis of biological literature. *Biotechniques*, *32*, 1380–1385.

27. Lin, S.M., McConnell, P., Johnson, K.F., Shoemaker, J. (2004). MedlineR: An open source library in R for Medline literature data mining. *Bioinformatics*, *20*, 3659–3661.

28. Maier, H., Döhr, S., Grote, K., O'Keeffe, S., Werner, T., Hrabé De Angelis, M., Schneider, R. (2005). LitMiner and WikiGene: Identifying problem-related key players of gene regulation using publication abstracts. *Nucleic Acids Res.*, *33*(Web Server issue), W779–W782. http://andromeda.gsf.de/litminer.

29. Plake, C., Schiemann, T., Pankalla, M., Hakenberg, J., Leser, U. (2006). AliBaba: PubMed as a graph. *Bioinformatics*, *22*, 2444–2445. http://alibaba.informatik.hu-berlin.de/.

30. Jelier, R., Schuemie, M.J., Veldhoven, A., Dorssers, L.C., Jenster, G., Kors, J.A. (2008). Anni 2.0: A multipurpose text-mining tool for the life sciences. *Genome Biol.*, *9*, R96. http://biosemantics.org/anni/.

31. Qu, X.A., Gudivada, R.C., Jegga, A.G., Neumann, E.K., Aronow, B.J. (2009). Inferring novel disease indications drug action and disease mechanism relationships. *BMC Bioinformatics*, *10*(Suppl 5), S4.

32. Berners-Lee, T., Hendler, J., Lassila, O. (2001). The semantic web. *Sci. Am. Mag.*, *284*, 29–37.

33. Edgar, R., Domrachev, M., Lash, A.E. (2002). Gene Expression Omnibus: NCBI gene expression and hybridization array data repository. *Nucleic Acids Res.*, *30*, 207–210. http://www.ncbi.nlm.nih.gov/geo/.

34. Perez-Iratxeta, C., Bork, P., Andrade, M.A. (2002). Association of genes to genetically inherited diseases using data mining. *Nat. Genet.*, *31*, 316–319.

35. Perez-Iratxeta, C., Wjst, M., Bork, P., Andrade, M.A. (2005). G2D: A tool for mining genes associated with disease. *BMC Genet.*, *6*, 45.

36. Perez-Iratxeta, C., Bork, P., Andrade-Navarro, M.A. (2007). Update of the G2D tool for prioritization of gene candidates to inherited diseases. *Nucleic Acids Res.*, *35*(Web Server issue), W212–W216. http://www.ogic.ca/projects/g2d_2.

37. Tremblay, K., Lemire, M., Potvin, C., Tremblay, A., Hunninghake, G.M., Raby, B.A., Hudson, T.J., Perez-Iratxeta, C., Andrade-Navarro, M.A., Lapris, C. (2008). Genes to diseases (G2D) computational method to identify asthma candidate genes. *PLoS ONE*, *3*, e2907.

38. Tiffin, N., Adie, E., Turner, F., Brunner, H.G., van Driel, M.A., Oti, M., Lopez-Bigas, N., Ouzounis, C., Perez-Iratxeta, C., Andrade-Navarro, M.A., Adeyemo, A., Patti, M.E., Semple, C.A., Hide, W. (2006). Computational disease gene identification: A concert of methods prioritizes type 2 diabetes and obesity candidate genes. *Nucleic Acids Res.*, *34*, 3067–3081.

39. van Driel, M.A., Cuelenare, K., Kemmeren, P.P.C.W., Leunissen, J.A.M., Brunner, H.G., Vriend, G. (2005). GeneSeeker: Extraction and integration of human disease-related information from web-based genetic databases. *Nucleic Acids Res.*, *33*, W758–W761. http://www.cmbi.kun.nl/GeneSeeker/.

40. Adie, E.A., Adams, R.R., Evans, K.L., Porteous, D.J., Pickard, B.S. (2005). Speeding disease gene discovery by sequence based candidate prioritization. *BMC Bioinformatics*, *6*, 55. http://www.genetics.med.ed.ac.uk/prospectr/.

41. Freund, Y., Mason, L. (1999). The alternating decision tree algorithm. *Proceedings of the 16th International Conference on Machine Learning*, pp. 124–133.

42. Adie, E.A., Adams, R.R., Evans, K.L., Porteous, D.J., Pickard, B.S. (2006). SUSPECTS: Enabling fast and effective prioritization of positional candidates. *Bioinformatics*, *22*, 773–774. http://www.genetics.med.ed.ac.uk/suspects/.

43. Su, A.I., Cooke, M.P., Ching, K.A., Hakak, Y., Walker, J.R., Wiltshire, T., Orth, A.P., Vega, R.G., Sapinoso, L.M., Moqrich, A., Patapoutian, A., Hampton, G.M., Schultz, P.G., Hogenesch, J.B. (2002). Large-scale analysis of the human and mouse transcriptomes. *Proc. Natl. Acad. Sci. U.S.A.*, *99*, 4465–4470.

44. Lord, P.W., Stevens, R.D., Brass, A., Goble, C.A. (2003). Investigating semantic similarity measures across the Gene Ontology: The relationship between sequence and annotation. *Bioinformatics*, *19*, 1275–1283.

45. López-Bigas, N., Ouzounis, C.A. (2004). Genome-wide identification of genes likely to be involved in human genetic disease. *Nucleic Acids Res.*, *32*, 3108–3114.

46. Fong, C., Ko, D.C., Wasnick, M., Radey, M., Miller, S.I., Brittnacher, M. (2010). GWAS analyzer: Integrating genotype, phenotype and public annotation data for genome-wide association study analysis. *Bioinformatics*, *26*, 560–564. http://www.nwrce.org/gwas-analyzer.

47. Gudivada, R.C., Qu, X.A., Chen, J., Jegga, A.G., Neumann, E.K., Aronow, B.J. (2008). Identifying disease-causal genes using Semantic Web-based representation of integrated genomic and phenomic knowledge. *J. Biomed. Inform.*, *41*, 717–729.

48. Kleinberg, J.M. (1999). Authoritative sources in a hyperlinked environment. *J. ACM*, *46*, 604–632.

49. Sardana, D., Vasa, S., Vepachedu, N., Chen, J., Gudivada, R.C., Aronow, B.J., Jegga, A.G. (2010). PhenoHM: Human-mouse comparative phenome-genome server. *Nucleic Acids Res.*, *38*(Web Server issue), W165–W174. http://phenome.cchmc.org.

50. Freudenberg, J., Propping, P. (2002). A similarity-based method for genome-wide prediction of disease-relevant human genes. *Bioinformatics*, *18*(Suppl 2), S110–S115.

51. Rossi, S., Masotti, D., Nardini, C., Bonora, E., Romeo, G., Macii, E., Benini, L., Volinia, S. (2006). TOM: A web-based integrated approach for identification of candidate disease genes. *Nucleic Acids Res.*, *34*(Web Server issue), W285–W292.

52. Kelso, J., Visagie, J., Theiler, G., Christoffels, A., Bardien, S., Smedley, D., Otgaar, D., Greyling, G., Jongeneel, C.V., McCarthy, M.I., Hide, T., Hide, W. (2003). eVOC: A controlled vocabulary for unifying gene expression data. *Genome Res.*, *13*, 1222–1230.

53. Tiffin, N., Kelso, J.F., Powell, A.R., Pan, H., Bajic, V.B., Hide, W.A. (2005). Integration of text- and data-mining using ontologies successfully selects disease gene candidates. *Nucleic Acids Res.*, *33*, 1544–1552.

54. Tiffin, N., Okpechi, I., Perez-Iratxeta, C., Andrade-Navarro, M.A., Ramesar, R. (2008). Prioritization of candidate disease genes for metabolic syndrome by computational analysis of its defining phenotypes. *Physiol. Genomics*, *35*, 55–64.

55. Aerts, S., Lambrechts, D., Maity, S., Van Loo, P., Coessens, B., De Smet, F., Tranchevent, L.C., De Moor, B., Marynen, P., Hassan, B., Carmeliet, P., Moreau, Y. (2006). Gene prioritization through genomic data fusion. *Nat. Biotechnol.*, *24*, 537–544.

56. Tranchevent, L.C., Barriot, R., Yu, S., Van Vooren, S., Van Loo, P., Coessens, B., De Moor, B., Aerts, S., Moreau, Y. (2008). ENDEAVOUR update: A web resource for gene prioritization in multiple species. *Nucleic Acids Res.*, *36*(Web Server issue), W377–W384. http://www.esat.kuleuven.be/endeavourweb.

57. Lamb, J., Crawford, E.D., Peck, D., Modell, J.W., Blat, I.C., Wrobel, M.J., Lerner, J., Brunet, J.P., Subramanian, A., Ross, K.N., Reich, M., Hieronymus, H., Wei, G., Armstrong, S.A., Haggarty, S.J., Clemons, P.A., Wei, R., Carr, S.A., Lander, E.S., Golub, T.R. (2006). The Connectivity Map: Using gene-expression signatures to connect small molecules, genes, and disease. *Science*, *313*, 1929–1935. http://www.broadinstitute.org/cmap/.

58. Lamb, J. (2007). The Connectivity Map: A new tool for biomedical research. *Nat. Rev. Cancer*, *7*, 54–60.

59. Josset, L., Textoris, J., Loriod, B., Ferraris, O., Moules, V., Lina, B., N'guyen, C., Diaz, J.J., Rosa-Calatrava, M. (2010). Gene expression signature-based screening identifies new broadly effective influenza a antivirals. *PLoS ONE*, *5*, e13169.

60. Chang, M., Smith, S., Thorpe, A., Barratt, M.J., Karim, F. (2010). Evaluation of phenoxybenzamine in the CFA model of pain following gene expression studies and connectivity mapping. *Mol. Pain*, *6*, 56.

61. Zhang, Z., Meng, T., He, J., Li, M., Tong, L.J., Xiong, B., Lin, L., Shen, J., Miao, Z.H., Ding, J. (2010). MT7, a novel compound from a combinatorial library, arrests mitosis via inhibiting the polymerization of microtubules. *Invest. New Drugs*, *28*, 715–728.

62. Hollander, M., Wolfe, D. (1999). *Nonparametric Statistical Methods*, 2nd ed., 178–185. New York: Wiley.

63. Subramanian, A., Tamayo, P., Mootha, V.K., Mukherjee, S., Ebert, B.L., Gillette, M.A., Paulovich, A., Pomeroy, S.L., Golub, T.R., Lander, E.S., Mesirov, J.P. (2005). Gene set enrichment analysis: A knowledge-based approach for interpreting genome-wide expression profiles. *Proc. Natl. Acad. Sci. U.S.A.*, *102*, 15545–15550.

64. Zhang, S.D., Gant, T.W. (2008). A simple and robust method for connecting small-molecule drugs using gene-expression signatures. *BMC Bioinformatics*, *9*, 258.

65. Kim, S.Y., Volsky, D.J. (2005). PAGE: Parametric analysis of gene set enrichment. *BMC Bioinformatics*, *6*, 144.

66. Tanner, S.W., Agarwal, P. (2008). Gene Vector Analysis (Geneva): A unified method to detect differentially-regulated gene sets and similar microarray experiments. *BMC Bioinformatics*, *9*, 348.

67. Huang, H., Liu, C.C., Zhou, X.J. (2010). Bayesian approach to transforming public gene expression repositories into disease diagnosis databases. *Proc. Natl. Acad. Sci. U.S.A.*, *107*, 6823–6828.

68. Zhang, S.D., Gant, T.W. (2009). sscMap: An extensible Java application for connecting small-molecule drugs using gene-expression signatures. *BMC Bioinformatics*, *10*, 236. http://purl.oclc.org/NET/sscMap.

69. Kim, S.B., Yang, S., Kim, S.K., Kim, S.C., Woo, H.G., Volsky, D.J., Kim, S.Y., Chu, I.S. (2007). GAzer: Gene set analyzer. *Bioinformatics*, *23*, 1697–1699.

70. Long, A.D., Mangalam, H.J., Chan, B.Y., Tolleri, L., Hatfield, G.W., Baldi, P. (2001). Improved statistical inference from DNA microarray data using analysis of variance and a Bayesian statistical framework. Analysis of global gene expression in Escherichia coli K12. *J. Biol. Chem.*, *276*, 19937–19944. http://cybert.ics.uci.edu/.

71. Loboda, A., Kraft, W.K., Fine, B., Joseph, J., Nebozhyn, M., Zhang, C., He, Y., Yang, X., Wright, C., Morris, M., Chalikonda, I., Ferguson, M., Emilsson, V., Leonardson, A., Lamb, J., Dai, H., Schadt, E., Greenberg, H.E., Lum, P.Y. (2009). Diurnal variation of the human adipose transcriptome and the link to metabolic disease. *BMC Med. Genomics*, *2*, 7.

72. Leonardson, A.S., Zhu, J., Chen, Y., Wang, K., Lamb, J.R., Reitman, M., Emilsson, V., Schadt, E.E. (2010). The effect of food intake on gene expression in human peripheral blood. *Hum. Mol. Genet.*, *19*, 159–169.

73. Granger, C.W.J. (1969). Investigating causal relationships by econometric models and cross-spectral methods. *Econometrica*, *37*, 424–438.

74. Zhu, J., Chen, Y., Leonardson, A.S., Wang, K., Lamb, J.R., Emilsson, V., Schadt, E.E. (2010). Characterizing dynamic changes in the human blood transcriptional network. *PLoS Comput. Biol.*, *6*, e1000671.

75. Nitsch, D., Trancheven, L.C., Thienpont, B., Thorrez, L., Van Esch, H., Devriendt, K., Moreau, Y. (2009). Network analysis of differential expression for the identification of disease-causing genes. *PLoS ONE*, *4*, e5526.

76. Li, J., Zhu, X., Chen, J.Y. (2009). Building disease-specific drug-protein connectivity maps from molecular interaction networks and PubMed abstracts. *PLoS Comput. Biol.*, *7*, e1000450.

77. Knox, C., Law, V., Jewison, T., Liu, P., Ly, S., Frolkis, A., Pon, A., Banco, K., Mak, C., Neveu, V., Djoumbou, Y., Eisner, R., Guo, A.C., Wishart, D.S. (2011). DrugBank 3.0: A comprehensive resource for "omics" research on drugs. *Nucleic Acids Res.*, *39*(Database issue), D1035–D1041.

78. Hu, G., Agarwal, P. (2009). Human disease-drug network based on genomic expression profiles. *PLoS ONE*, *4*, e6536.

79. Iorio, F., Bosotti, R., Scacheri, E., Belcastro, V., Mithbaokar, P., Ferriero, R., Murino, L., Tagliaferri, R., Brunetti-Pierri, N., Isacchi, A., Di Bernardo, D. (2010). Discovery of drug mode of action and drug repositioning from transcriptional responses. *Proc. Natl. Acad. Sci. U.S.A.*, *107*, 14621–14626. http://mantra.tigem.it.

80. Feng, C., Araki, M., Kunimoto, R., Tamon, A., Makiguchi, H., Niijima, S., Tsujimoto, G., Okuno, Y. (2009). GEM-TREND: A web tool for gene expression data mining toward relevant network discovery. *BMC Genomics*, *10*, 411. http://cgs.pharm.kyoto-u.ac.jp/services/network/.

81. Aten, J.E., Fuller, T.F., Lusis, A.J., Horvath, S. (2008). Using genetic markers to orient the edges in quantitative trait networks: The NEO software. *BMC Syst. Biol.*, *2*, 34.

82. Ekins, S., Bugrim, A., Brovold, L., Kirillov, E., Nikolsky, Y., Rakhmatulin, E., Sorokina, S., Ryabov, A., Serebryiskaya, T., Melnikov, A., Metz, J., Nikolskaya, T. (2006). Algorithms for network analysis in systems-ADME/Tox using the MetaCore and MetaDrug platforms. *Xenobiotica*, *36*, 877–901.

83. Ekins, S., Nikolsky, Y., Bugrim, A., Kirillov, E., Nikolskaya, T. (2007). Pathway mapping tools for analysis of high content data. *Methods Mol. Biol.*, *356*, 319–350.

84. Wright, J.M., Nikolsky, Y., Serebryiskaya, T., Wetmore, D.R. (2009). MetaMiner (CF): A disease-oriented bioinformatics analysis environment. *Methods Mol. Biol.*, *563*, 353–367.

85. Dezso, Z., Nikolsky, Y., Nikolskaya, T., Miller, J., Cherba, D., Webb, C., Bugrim, A. (2009). Identifying disease-specific genes based on their topological significance in protein networks. *BMC Syst. Biol.*, *3*, 36.

86. Webb, C.P. (2009). Personalized medicine: The need for system integration in the design of targeted therapies. In *Computational and Systems Biology: Applications and Methods*, eds. Mazzarella, R., Head, R., 177–195. Kerala, India: Research Signpost.

87. Katz, R. (2004). Biomarkers and surrogate markers: An FDA perspective. *NeuroRx*, *1*, 189–195.

88. Webb, C.P., Pass, H. (2004). Translational research: From accurate diagnosis to appropriate treatment. *J. Transl. Med.*, *2*, 35–47.

89. Bumbea, H., Vladareanu, A.M., Cisleanu, D., Barsan, L., Onisai, M., Voican, I. (2010). Chronic myeloid leukemia therapy in the era of tyrosine kinase inhibitors. The first molecular targeted treatment. *J. Med. Life*, *3*, 162–166.

90. Vogel, C.L., Cobleigh, M.A., Tripathy, D., et al. (2002). Efficacy and safety of trastuzumab as a single agent in first-line treatment of HER2-overexpressing metastatic breast cancer. *J. Clin. Oncol.*, *20*, 719–726.

91. Bollag, G., Hirth, P., Tsai, J. et al. (2010). Clinical efficacy of a RAF inhibitor needs broad target blockade in BRAF-mutant melanoma. *Nature*, *467*, 596–599.

92. Dienstmann, R., Martinez, P., Felip, E. (2011). Personalizing therapy with targeted agents in non-small cell lung cancer. *Oncotarget*, *2*, 165–177.

93. Hanahan, D., Weinberg, R.A. (2011). Hallmarks of cancer: The next generation. *Cell*, *144*, 646–674.

94. Sjoblom, T., Jones, S., Wood, L.D., et al. (2006). The consensus coding sequences of human breast and colorectal cancers. *Science*, *314*, 268–274.

95. Balakrishnan, A., Bleeker, F.E., Lamba, S., et al. (2007). Novel somatic and germline mutations in cancer candidate genes in glioblastoma, melanoma, and pancreatic carcinoma. *Cancer Res.*, *67*, 3545–3550.

96. Heng, H.H. (2009). The genome-centric concept: Resynthesis of evolutionary theory. *Bioessays*, *31*, 512–525.

97. Von Hoff, D.D., Stephenson, J.J. Jr, Rosen, P., et al. (2010). Pilot study using molecular profiling of patients' tumors to find potential targets and select treatments for their refractory cancers. *J. Clin. Oncol.*, *28*, 4869–4871.

98. Staunton, J.E., Slonim, D.K., Coller, H.A., et al. (2001). Chemosensitivity prediction by transcriptional profiling. *Proc. Natl. Acad. Sci. U.S.A.*, *98*, 10787–10792.

99. Lee, J.K., Havaleshko, D.M., Cho, H., Weinstein, J.N., Kaldjian, E.P., Karpovich, J., Grimshaw, A., Theodorescu, D. (2007). A strategy for predicting the chemosensitivity of human cancers and its application to drug discovery. *Proc. Natl. Acad. Sci. U.S.A.*, *104*, 13086–13091.

100. Mousses, S., Kiefer, J., Von Hoff, D., Trent, J. (2008). Using biointelligence to search the cancer genome: An epistemological perspective on knowledge recovery strategies to enable precision medical genomics. *Oncogene 27* (Suppl 2), S58–S66.

101. Kalady, M.F., Dejulius, K., Church, J.M., Lavery, I.C., Fazio, V.W., Ishwaran, H. (2010). Gene signature is associated with early stage rectal cancer recurrence. *J. Am. Coll. Surg.*, *211*, 187–195.

102. Glaser, K.B., Staver, M.J., Waring, J.F., Stender, J., Ulrich, R.G., Davidsen, S.K. (2003). Gene expression profiling of multiple histone deacetylase (HDAC) inhibitors: Defining a common gene set produced by HDAC inhibition in T24 and MDA carcinoma cell lines. *Mol. Cancer Ther.*, *2*, 151–163.

103. Garber, K. (2010). Ready or not: Personalized tumor profiling tests take off. *J. Natl. Cancer Inst.*, *103*, 84–86.

Mining Scientific and Clinical Databases to Identify Novel Uses for Existing Drugs

CHRISTOS ANDRONIS, ANUJ SHARMA, SPYROS DEFTEREOS, VASSILIS VIRVILIS, OURANIA KONSTANTI, ANDREAS PERSIDIS, and ARIS PERSIDIS

6.1. INTRODUCTION

The business case for drug repurposing (or drug repositioning) has already been emphasized in earlier chapters of this book. The present chapter attempts to provide a compendium of data types and associated data sources being exploited for the purposes of drug repositioning. Selected cases will be presented in more detail by adding example usage scenarios for the purposes of drug discovery and drug repositioning.

Serendipitous drug repositioning (i.e., based on clinical observations) has been part of the regular drug discovery process since the very first days of the pharmaceutical industry. The success stories of sildenafil and thalidomide as repositioned drugs, together with the dearth of approval of new chemical entities (NCEs) by the U.S. Food and Drug Administration and the "patent-cliff" facing many of the currently approved drugs is pushing many groups in the pharmaceutical industry to pursue directed strategies toward drug repositioning.

Another factor related to the renewed interest in drug repositioning stems from the fact that the sequencing of the human genome has not yet resulted, as many had initially expected, in an associated proliferation of the druggable target space [1, 2], limiting our ability to generate novel biological hypotheses based on newly characterized drug targets. From the above, it becomes clear that a new way of looking at the existing drug target space is needed, based on the fact that many drug targets are ultimately shared by more than one

Drug Repositioning: Bringing New Life to Shelved Assets and Existing Drugs, First Edition.
Edited by Michael J. Barratt and Donald E. Frail.
© 2012 John Wiley & Sons, Inc. Published 2012 by John Wiley & Sons, Inc.

physiological process, that is, more than one function/phenotypic effect. Such a paradigm shift is enhanced by the increasing awareness that many drugs may have more than one biological target ([3–5] and see Chapter 7 of this book on polypharmacology), as is the case for a number of psychiatric drugs [5]. This drug "promiscuity" has led several groups to pursue rational drug repositioning with promising results [4, 6–9].

Although human genome sequencing has not led to the massive discovery of novel drug targets, it has provided an improved insight into the genomic diversity of existing targets and associated pathways as well as the molecular mechanisms that modulate health and disease. Such a deep understanding of the biological mechanism connecting drug targets and human diseases is central for any successful drug repositioning project.

In recent years, rational approaches to drug repositioning have emerged both from academia and industry where the focus is on the discovery of pharmacological mechanisms of action that have not yet been described for a known molecule. The term "systematic serendipity" [10, 11] has been coined to describe these approaches where the focus is on the "systematic" and targeted innovation rather than on serendipity itself. This review will continue on the theme of the previous chapter, focusing on the data sources available for systematic drug repositioning and on some exemplary cases using these resources to infer novel associations between drugs and their targets and human diseases.

6.2. DATA SOURCES

By nature, the *in silico* element of drug repositioning relies mostly on (1) already executed laboratory experiments and studies (*in vitro*, preclinical, and clinical) with data deposited in online databases and (2) on the actual "history" of a drug as it is captured in the scientific literature either in the form of scientific articles (e.g., in PubMed) or in other sources, such as a product sheet or a patent. In addition, information regarding a drug target might be obtained by profiling the target across many genomic, expression, and literature databases and then associating these profiles with ones from multiple diseases. These data sources and associated technologies, together with the necessary domain expertise in pharmacology, usually define repurposing business strategies.

Perhaps not surprisingly, drug repositioning incorporates a core set of methodologies that are common with other *in silico* platforms linked to drug discovery. This applies to both the data sources used and the data mining techniques employed. In order to search for repurposing opportunities, one needs to be aware of the pool of candidate compounds (including discontinued and generic compounds available in countries outside the United States), as well as have readily available all the components (genes, proteins, signaling pathways, safety data) needed to reconstruct novel mechanisms of action

(MoAs) supporting a drug repositioning proposal. All in all, it becomes clear that a systematic approach to repositioning requires a comprehensive knowledge management approach that can incorporate extensive data mining (including text mining) and subsequent targeted analysis.

A selection of data sources found to be useful in our hands or used commonly in various drug repositioning projects is described below. Table 6.1 lists the URLs and the coverage of each of these databases. The emphasis is given to publicly available resources that can be downloaded and mined locally and that are being used extensively by *in silico* discovery programs, having thus become industry standards in their respective fields of coverage. Other common characteristics of these data sources is that they are either first-in-class in their field covering a niche area (e.g., DrugBank) or are mature products that have evolved over the years and overshadow other contenders due to their quality, breadth of information, and high interconnectivity with other resources (e.g., the National Center for Biotechnology Information [NCBI] databases). Key aspects relevant to *in silico* drug discovery and drug repositioning are highlighted next.

6.2.1. Bioinformatics-Related Resources

6.2.1.1. Genomic Repositories   The NCBI provides an extremely diverse set of databases ranging from genomic and transcriptomic data to compounds and bioassay datasets, to PubMed—a service that provides access to over 19 million citations from MEDLINE and additional life sciences journals.

6.2.1.2. NCBI/Entrez Gene   The Entrez Gene Database [12] is a comprehensive repository of genomic data. The information provided is gene-based and around it key connections related to chromosome map, sequence, expression, structure, function, citation, and homology data have been implemented. Unique identifiers, used throughout NCBI's databases, are assigned to genes. Apart from the unique identifiers, Entrez Gene contains official gene symbols, descriptions, and common synonyms for all genes; links to expression data; protein domain information; and so on. Being the major integrator of gene nomenclature, Entrez Gene is a key resource in data mining/text mining projects relevant to drug repositioning.

6.2.1.3. The Universal Protein Resource (UniProt)   UniProt [13] is a comprehensive resource for protein sequence and annotation data provided by the European Bioinformatics Institute (EBI), the Swiss Institute of Bioinformatics (SIB), and the Protein Information Resource (PIR). An essential part of UniProt is the UniProt Knowledgebase (UniprotKB), which consists of two sections, "Swiss-Prot" and "TrEMBL". The latter contains protein sequences, usually derived from large-scale functional characterization projects whose functional annotation has been computationally generated and in turn not reviewed by human curators. On the other hand, Swiss-Prot

TABLE 6.1. Data Sources for Drug Repositioning Featured in This Review. The Coverage Column Contains an August 2011 Snapshot of the Statistics for Each Resource

Bioinformatics Resources	Coverage	Website
Entrez Gene	8,050,454 genes belonging to 7705 taxa	http://www.ncbi.nlm.nih.gov/sites/entrez?db=gene
Swiss-Prot	531,473 sequence entries	http://www.uniprot.org/
PDB	75,694 protein structures	http://www.pdb.org/pdb/home/home.do
GEO	24,892 series; 618,783 samples	http://www.ncbi.nlm.nih.gov/geo
KEGG	409 reference pathway maps	http://www.genome.jp/kegg/pathway.html
REACTOME	1153 human pathways	http://www.reactome.org/
GO	21,330 biological process; 2,896 cellular component; 9,062 molecular function	http://www.geneontology.org/
Cheminformatics resources		
PubChem	>30 million compounds; >500,000 bioassays	http://pubchem.ncbi.nlm.nih.gov/
ChEMBL	>1 million distinct compounds	http://www.ebi.ac.uk/chembl/
Drug–target space		
DrugBank	6662 drugs; 4134 distinct drug targets	http://www.drugbank.ca/
Drugs and disease resources		
Drugs@FDA	6118 brand names; 2313 active ingredients (includes combinations)	http://www.accessdata.fda.gov/scripts/cder/drugsatfda/index.cfm
DailyMed	28,380 drug labels	http://dailymed.nlm.nih.gov/dailymed/about.cfm
AERS	2,838,106 adverse events; 12365 adverse reactions	http://www.fda.gov/Drugs/GuidanceComplianceRegulatoryInformation/Surveillance/AdverseDrugEffects/default.htm
Ontologies		
MeSH	26,142 descriptors; 190,000 headings called Supplementary Concept Records	http://www.nlm.nih.gov/mesh/meshhome.html
UMLS	1,850,214 Concept Unique Identifiers; 4,234,081 concept names[a]	http://www.nlm.nih.gov/research/umls/licensedcontent/umlsknowledgesources.html

[a] These numbers correspond to the English language Knowledge sources in the default UMLS Metamorphosis set.

contains manually annotated records with information extracted from the literature and curator-evaluated computational analysis. As such, Swiss-Prot may enhance the gene/protein nomenclature available from Entrez Gene with additional synonyms, and manually assigned keywords for each protein.

6.2.1.4. The Protein Data Bank (PDB)   PDB [14] is a database containing three-dimensional (3D) structures of large biological molecules, including proteins and nucleic acids. PDB contains over 62,000 structures from a variety of organisms and is regularly used to retrieve structures for docking studies [6, 15].

6.2.2. Microarray Repositories

6.2.2.1. Gene Expression Omnibus (GEO)   GEO [16] is a public functional genomics data repository that archives and distributes microarray and other high-throughput functional genomic data submitted by the scientific community. These data include single and dual channel microarray-based experiments measuring mRNA, miRNA, genomic DNA (including Array-comparative genomic hybridization [Array-CGH], Chromatin Immunoprecipitation-chip [ChIP-chip], and single-nucleotide polymorphism [SNP]), and protein abundance, as well as nonarray techniques such as serial analysis of gene expression (SAGE), and various types of next-generation sequence data. Two important features in the GEO database are the GEO DataSets and the GEO Profiles; the former are higher level, manually curated collections of biologically and statistically comparable GEO Samples, whereas the latter consist of the expression measurements for an individual gene across all samples in a dataset. Importantly, GEO supports the MIAME data format, which has emerged as the de facto standard for the description of microarray experiments. Collectively, GEO DataSets and Profiles can be used for profiling drug targets for gene and disease co-regulation against multiple diseases.

6.2.3. Pathway Databases

Biochemical and signaling pathways are mostly defined by the group of proteins they contain rather than a specific name or nucleotide sequence. In most cases signaling pathways are entities without well-defined ends and not always universally accepted (protein) members. This ambiguity in what constitutes a pathway is reflected to the actual naming: there is no such thing as an "official pathway name" (in analogy to an official gene symbol) and pathways may have titles taken from a ligand, for example, the "tumor necrosis factor (TNF)-pathway," a prototypical receptor representing a whole class of proteins, for example, the "Notch pathway," a major signaling component, for example, the "mammalian target of rapamycin (mTOR) pathway," or even a disease. Despite these difficulties, a few public and proprietary databases have taken upon themselves the task of trying to better define the set of proteins participating in a pathway and provide a common set of terms describing molecular networks/signaling pathways. With the exception of GO, the databases described below contain a mix of metabolic, cell signaling, and disease pathways, giving emphasis to both protein–protein and protein–small molecule interactions.

6.2.3.1. Kyoto Encyclopedia of Genes and Genomes (KEGG)   KEGG provides an extensive array of metabolic and signal transduction data, as well as human disease data, manually created and organized into a collection of pathways and pathway maps [17]. As of August 2011, KEGG contains references to 409 pathways. KEGG has been widely used as a reference knowledge base for biological interpretation of large-scale datasets generated by sequencing and other high-throughput experimental technologies.

The value of KEGG lies in the fact that it provides the molecular interactions together with the components of each pathway, cross-referenced to all organisms known to utilize each pathway.

6.2.3.2. Reactome   Reactome [18] is a free curated pathway database encompassing many areas of human biology. Information is authored by expert biological researchers, maintained by the Reactome editorial staff, and cross-referenced to a wide range of standard biological databases. The curated human data are used to infer orthologous events in 20 nonhuman species including the major animal models, *Caenorhabditis elegans*, budding and fission yeasts, two plants, and *Escherichia coli*. As of August 2011, Reactome contains 1153 human pathways, corresponding to over 4700 proteins. Reactome is a joint effort between the EBI, the Ontario Institute for Cancer Research, and Cold Spring Harbor Laboratory, and is one of the most active efforts toward a complete pathway database based on open-source standards.

6.2.3.3. Gene Ontology (GO)   GO [19] is a collection of three ontologies (Biological Process, Molecular Function, and Cellular Component) providing a controlled vocabulary of terms for describing gene products and gene product annotation data. GO is the most prominent bioinformatics initiative addressing the need of standardizing the representation of gene and gene product attributes across species and databases. Although the "Biological Process" ontology has not been constructed with the aim of being used as a signaling pathway database per se, owing to its breadth of terms and its widespread usage in grouping gene products to some high-level term related to a pathway (e.g., glucose catabolism), it has been commonly utilized as a pathway database. As of August 2011 "Biological Process" contains over 21,330 terms making it the biggest publicly accessible data resource of its kind.

6.2.3.4. Other Pathway Databases   A number of commercially available pathway databases such as TransPath® (from BioBase Inc.), MetaBase™

(from GeneGo Inc.), and Ingenuity Pathways Analysis® (IPA®; Ingenuity Systems Inc.) provide notable numbers of molecular pathways and have been regularly used in drug discovery projects.

The Nature Signaling Gateway [20] is a collaborative project between the University of California San Diego (UCSD) and Nature Publishing Group. The information provided is web-based and revolves around "Molecules," that is, proteins. Each Molecule Page provides a concise review on a single protein, the post-translational modifications it can acquire (its states), transitions that link pairs of states together, and the molecular functions the protein has (e.g., is a kinase, a receptor). Currently there are over 4000 Molecule Pages published. Nature Signaling Gateway data are freely available, providing a valuable resource, complementary to the other pathway data resources.

6.2.4. Cheminformatics-Related Resources

The primary application of cheminformatics is the storage of information relating to chemical compounds into chemical databases and the retrieval and analysis of this information [21–23]. As such, cheminformatics has become an essential part of the drug discovery decision-making process and is increasingly used for *in silico* profiling of small molecule bioactivities against arrays of drug targets [24].

6.2.4.1. PubChem PubChem [25] provides information on the biological activities of small molecules. It comprises three very comprehensive databases, BioAssay, Compound, and Substance, which are all part of NCBI's Entrez system. Being part of the NCBI infrastructure, PubChem is highly interconnected with PubMed, NCBI/Entrez Gene, and NCBI's protein 3D structure resource. Among the three databases, PubChem Compound comprises a nonredundant set of standardized and validated chemical structures, along with an extensive set of properties for each compound, including links to bioassay and toxicology data whenever these are available.

6.2.4.2. ChEMBL ChEMBL [26] is a public, freely available database containing structure activity relationship (SAR) data for over 690,000 medicinal chemistry compounds, aiming to impact the prioritization and lead discovery of drug-like molecules for use as innovative therapies. ChEMBL is a relatively new repository of bioactivity and drug data, but its wealth of information around small molecule compounds and their bioactivity has already resulted in its use in several drug discovery and drug repositioning efforts (see reference [4] for an example).

6.2.4.3. Chemistry Development Kit (CDK) and OpenBabel Although they are not data resources, Chemistry Development Kit (CDK) and Open-Babel are two open-source Cheminformatics libraries used very often in drug discovery and have been employed in various drug repositioning projects [9, 27].

CDK [28] is an open-source JAVA library that can be integrated into various environments to make its functionality available. It provides methods for common tasks in molecular informatics, including 2D and 3D rendering of chemical structures, input/output (I/O) routines, simplified molecular-input line-entry specification (SMILES) parsing and generation, ring searches, isomorphism checking, and structure diagram generation. CDK is commonly used to calculate chemical hashed fingerprints and 2D chemical similarity scores. Campillos et al. [9] used the Chemistry Development Kit to calculate 2D chemical similarity scores of existing drugs in combination with side effect similarity of otherwise unrelated drugs to predict novel targets for these drugs.

OpenBabel [29] is free software for converting between chemical file formats. It exists both as ready-to-use programs and also as a set of libraries in C++ and other languages (e.g., Perl, JAVA, Ruby) for general chemical software development.

6.2.5. Drug Target Space

Since the advent of the human genome sequencing, the pharmaceutical industry has repeatedly attempted to expand on the known space of proteins that have traditionally been used as small molecule targets for disease therapies [2, 30]. Databases describing the drug target space such as DrugBank, Super-Target, and Matador have recently emerged. The most widely used among these resources is DrugBank.

6.2.5.1. DrugBank   DrugBank [31] is a database created at the University of Alberta, Canada, linking drugs (mostly small molecule drugs) with their drug targets. As such, DrugBank sits at the interface of Bioinformatics and Cheminformatics resources. At the time of writing, DrugBank included over 1437 FDA-approved small molecule drugs, and 134 FDA-approved biotech (protein/peptide) drugs. Additionally, more than 4100 nonredundant protein (i.e., drug target) sequences are linked to these FDA-approved drug entries. DrugBank has been one of the first data sources to capture the direct link between a drug and its target in a comprehensive manner, and has thus become a widely used resource by many drug repositioning efforts that have appeared to date [6, 7, 15, 27, 32]. For example, Cockell et al. [27] constructed a graph of 120,000 concepts with 570,000 relationships between drugs, proteins, and diseases by combining data from various sources, including DrugBank, UniProt, KEGG, Pfam, SynAtlas, G-sesame, OpenBabel, and BLAST and then used this graph to infer novel drug–disease relationships.

6.2.6. Drug and Disease Data Sources

6.2.6.1. Drugs@FDA   The US Food and Drug Administration (FDA) maintains some of the most important databases related to drugs and their actions. First and foremost is the compendium of currently FDA-approved drugs (both small molecules and biologics), stored in the Drugs@FDA database [33]. Apart from active ingredients and brand names of the FDA-approved drugs, this database contains indications the drugs are approved for, marketing status, dosage, route of administration, strength, and so on. Drugs@FDA also allows viewing the approval history of a drug. Understandably, Drugs@FDA is commonly the starting point for systematic drug repositioning projects. Much of the information in Drugs@FDA originates from the "Orange Book" (Approved Drug Products with Therapeutic Equivalence Evaluations).

6.2.6.2. DailyMed   DailyMed [34] is a database maintained by the National Library of Medicine (NLM) containing drug labels for an increasing number of FDA-approved drugs (28,380 drugs as of August 2011). As such, DailyMed is complementary to Drugs@FDA. What makes DailyMed unique is that product labels for each drug are in a structured XML format (SPL format), making it amenable for text mining using standard scripting languages (Perl, Python, etc.).

6.2.6.3. Adverse Event Reporting System (AERS)   The Adverse Event Reporting System [35] is a database designed to support the FDA's post-marketing safety surveillance program for all approved drug and therapeutic biologic products. The FDA uses AERS to monitor for new adverse events and medication errors that might occur with these marketed products. FDA receives adverse event and medication error reports directly from healthcare professionals (such as physicians, pharmacists, and nurses) and consumers. AERS data are available quarterly from the FDA site and include drug information from the case reports, adverse drug reaction information from the reports and patient outcomes. Interestingly, the list of drugs also includes nutritional supplements, a class of products not regulated by the FDA. Adverse events in AERS are coded to terms in the Medical Dictionary for Regulatory Activities terminology (MedDRA) and thus can be linked to other medical conditions via the Unified Medical Language System (UMLS; see below). AERS is the successor to FDA's Spontaneous Reporting System (SRS).

6.3. ONTOLOGIES

In the context of knowledge management, ontologies hold a central role. Ontologies are used to describe a knowledge domain, describe the concepts in the domain, the relationships between them, and their properties. At a basic level, they are used as simple hierarchies that organize taxonomically a domain or provide a dictionary of certain types of concepts. Although this is not their only intended function, some of the major ontologies in the field, for example, GO, MeSH, and UMLS, are routinely used this way. However, traversal of multiple ontologies as a mechanism toward inferring novel associations between known drugs and human diseases has also been reported [7].

6.3.1. The Medical Subject Headings (MeSH) Thesaurus

The MeSH thesaurus [36] is a controlled vocabulary for biomedical terms produced by the NLM. It includes a vast array of term types, ranging from drugs, compounds, and diseases, to human physiology and anatomy, to publication types and named groups. The latest (August 2011) edition of MeSH contains 26,142 descriptors. There are also over 172,000 entry terms that assist in finding the most appropriate MeSH Heading and more than 190,000 entries called Supplementary Concept Records. Although it contains a wealth of biomedical information, there are other specialized data sources that even surpass MeSH in sheer numbers of terms in their own specialized field (e.g., SnomedCT for medical conditions). However, there are several reasons that make MeSH unique, including the fact that, being an ontology, it permits searching and traversal at various levels of specificity, many synonyms, near-synonyms, and closely related concepts are included as entry terms and most importantly, the fact that MeSH is heavily tied to PubMed/MEDLINE. Every single article in PubMed is indexed based on MeSH headings, enabling the extraction of biomedical terms contained in an article as a first step in a drug repositioning effort [7, 37]. Baker and Hemminger [37] used MeSH annotations in MEDLINE abstracts to build a repository of chemicals associated with biological activities and diseases and then used this repository (called ChemoText) to generate a list of chemicals linked implicitly to particular diseases through the literature.

6.3.2. UMLS

Unified Medical Language System is a unique compendium of controlled vocabularies in the Biomedical domain. It unifies over 100 different health and clinical vocabularies, including MeSH, SnomedCT, NCI, COSTART, ICD-10, MedDRA, OMIM, and GO. The principal component of UMLS is the Metathesaurus, which contains a collection of concepts from the various vocabularies, and their relationships. Each individual concept in the Metathesaurus is represented by a "Concept Unique Identifier" (CUI). The 2010 version of the Metathesaurus (2010AA) contains over 1.8 million CUIs, which correspond to over 4.2 million concept names from over 100 controlled vocabularies (English-language sources only). This unifying notion of UMLS allows for the creation of customized word lists containing concepts from many different UMLS vocabularies, and thus highly enriched in synonyms.

UMLS is also important because it deals directly with the modern "Tower of Babel" imposed by the various formats used by the controlled vocabularies, demonstrating that it is possible to efficiently link various terminologies spanning the entire translational spectrum. Although not in the scope of this review, the issue of data standards and differing formats impacts heavily on the transmission and linkage of data across multiple biomedical data sources [38].

6.4. LITERATURE CORPORA AND MINING

6.4.1. Information Extraction

Lately, literature mining has emerged as another important data mining strategy to infer associations between biomedical entities [38–40]. One of the earliest applications of literature mining to drug discovery was the combination of seemingly disparate bibliographic information into new knowledge as proposed by Don Swanson in the 1980s [41, 42]. These literature-based discoveries were based on the premise that two phenomena A and B, not-previously reported to bear any connection to each other, could be directly connected if there is a third phenomenon C, which is directly associated with A and B in separate instances.

In more recent years, with the advent of Natural Language Processing (NLP) techniques originating from the field of computational linguistics, literature mining has found an ever-increasing field of applications in the form of Information Extraction (IE) from scientific publications. In a first step called Entity Recognition (ER), biomedical entities (genes, diseases, drugs, etc.) are extracted (i.e., identified) from abstracts (typically MEDLINE abstracts) and then associated to each other either by simple co-citation or by contextual directed relationships via specific action terms (i.e., inhibits, antagonizes, activates, etc.). This approach has been extensively applied to the identification of physical protein-protein interactions, in an effort to reconstruct signaling pathways and protein complexes [43–45]. Methods of associations range from simple co-occurrence [46, 47] to advanced context-based NLP approaches [43, 48, 49].

6.4.2. Publicly Available Literature Mining Corpora

6.4.2.1. PubMed/MEDLINE   As discussed in an earlier chapter, PubMed is a database of citations and abstracts for biomedical literature from MEDLINE and other life science journals. At the time of writing, PubMed contains over 20 million abstracts. Each article in PubMed is indexed using MeSH. Being freely available to researchers worldwide, PubMed has emerged as the major corpus for biomedical literature mining in the last decade or so. For some of the publications in PubMed, the full-text is also available. These publications form the PubMed Central database. Part of PubMed Central—the PMC Open Access Subset—is freely available under a Creative Commons license and is therefore, suitable for downloading and use in text mining projects. Although, the number of articles in the PMC Open Access Subset is still small, it holds a great potential for literature mining in the near future.

6.4.2.2. Patent Databases   The U.S. Patent Office (USPTO), the European Patent Office (EPO), and the World Intellectual Property Organization (WIPO) all provide online public free access to the full-text of patents (granted and patent applications). The full text of patents could provide a significant resource for literature mining. However, obtaining the full text of the patents in bulk is not readily available and is not free, hampering the full potential of this resource for data mining and discovery purposes. For the time being, researchers may download small numbers of full-text patents from the USPTO for selected classes and date ranges.

6.4.2.3. Press Releases   Press releases from resources such as PR Newswire [50] could provide a significant resource for finding links among drugs, their targets and diseases. Newswire resources have been extensively used in the past for other data mining applications, such as for Business Intelligence purposes. However, given that they resemble scientific abstracts in that they describe relations between biomedical entities in a concise form, they could become a significant resource for biomedical discovery.

6.4.2.4. Scientific Conferences   Published proceedings from scientific conferences can be a complementary resource to MEDLINE abstracts in the effort to uncover indirect links between drugs and diseases. Many societies, such as the American Society of Clinical Oncology (ASCO) and the American Academy of Neurology (AAN) publish and distribute freely all the abstracts presented during their yearly events. These proceedings usually contain the results of many clinical trials which, even by themselves, can be a significant resource for new discoveries.

Table 6.2 lists a selection of additional data resources that have been used in various drug repositioning publications. A short description of the data resource as well as the corresponding URL is also provided.

6.5. STRATEGIES TO INFER NOVEL ASSOCIATIONS BETWEEN DRUGS, DRUG TARGETS, AND HUMAN DISEASES: CASE STUDIES

Several of the strategies toward *in silico* drug repositioning rely on commonly used machine learning techniques. Machine learning approaches for natural language processing (NLP), classification, clustering, and graph theory have found extensive use in analyzing medical and chemical data. In the following sections, we discuss various strategies to *in silico* drug repositioning with examples taken from the scientific literature. These strategies have been segregated into five broad categories that are driven primarily by the data types used to infer novel associations rather than the machine learning approach employed.

6.5.1. Graph and Machine Learning Approaches Integrating Chemical Data

Machine learning approaches have been widely applied to mining rich data sources currently available in the field of cheminformatics. Several papers can

TABLE 6.2. Other Data Sources Used in Drug Repositioning Publications

Data Source	Comments	Website
MetaCyc	Metabolic pathways database	http://www.metacyc.org/
BioGRID	Manually curated protein and genetic interactions database	http://thebiogrid.org/
STRING	Database of known and predicted protein interactions	http://string-db.org/
ArrayExpress	Gene expression database	http://www.ebi.ac.uk/microarray-as/ae/
OMIM	Compendium of human genes (>12,000) and genetic phenotypes	http://www.ncbi.nlm.nih.gov/omim
OPHID	Interologous Interaction Database (I2D) database: known, experimental, and predicted protein–protein interactions for five model organisms and human	http://ophid.utoronto.ca/ophidv2.201/index.jsp
Comparative Toxicogenomics Database (CTD)	Chemical–gene/protein interactions and chemical–and gene–disease interaction database	http://ctd.mdibl.org/
CTCAE Adverse reactions	Common terminology criteria for adverse events. Adverse events terminology from National Cancer Institute (NCI)	http://evs.nci.nih.gov/ftp1/CTCAE/About.html
Anatomical Therapeutic Classifications (ATC)	World Health Organization database that divides drugs into different groups according to the organ or system on which they act and their therapeutic, pharmacological, and chemical properties	http://www.whocc.no/atc_ddd_index/

(Continued)

149

TABLE 6.2. (*Continued*)

Data Source	Comments	Website
WOMBAT	Proprietary small molecule chemogenomics database	http://www.sunsetmolecular.com/
KEGG Ligand	KEGG composite database consisting of COMPOUND, GLYCAN, REACTION, RPAIR, RCLASS, and ENZYME databases	http://www.genome.jp/kegg/ligand.html
Chemical Entities of Biological Interest (ChEBI)	Dictionary of molecular entities focused on "small" chemical compounds; published by EBI	http://www.ebi.ac.uk/chebi/
ChemBank	Information about small molecules and small-molecule screens; stores cell measurements derived from cell lines treated with small molecules. Used to retrieve drug–target information	http://chembank.broadinstitute.org/
SuperTarget	Drug–target database	http://bioinf-tomcat.charite.de/supertarget/
Matador	Contains direct and indirect drug–target interactions	http://matador.embl.de/
Psychoactive Drug Screening Program (PDSP) Ki database	*In vitro* binding affinities for small molecule psychoactive compounds	http://pdsp.med.unc.edu/pdsp.php
BindingDB	*In vitro* binding affinities for small molecule compounds	http://www.bindingdb.org/bind/index.jsp
STITCH	Known and predicted interactions of chemicals and proteins	http://stitch.embl.de/

be found discussing the application of machine learning techniques working on chemical and structural data with the purpose of discovering novel associations. Typically these approaches consist of processing certain types of data for building interaction graphs, which may then be visualized or queried to find novel associations.

A methodology to predict pharmacological effects from the chemical structure of the compound and infer the drug–target interactions based on the similarity in pharmacological effect using bipartite graph inference is presented in Reference [51]. Chemical, genomic, and pharmacological data gathered from KEGG Drug, KEGG Ligand databases, JAPIC, KEGG Genes database, KEGG BRITE, BRENDA, SuperTarget, and DrugBank databases are used for demonstrating the working of the proposed methodology.

A statistical cheminformatics approach to detect novel targets for known drugs using the similarity of the ligands that bind to these targets is developed in [4]. The drug collection was extracted from the MDL Comprehensive Medical Chemistry database and the ligands associated with each drug were extracted from the MDL Drug Data Report, the WOMBAT, and the StARlite database. The associations were represented as drug–target networks.

In [9] a workflow based on target side-effect similarity of drugs is developed for repositioning purposes. Scoring of drug pairs is performed by generating two-dimensional (2D) vectors associating each drug pair, where the two dimensions consist of side-effect similarity and chemical similarity. The data used were extracted from UMLS, Matador, DrugBank, and PDSP.

In Reference [52] the authors developed drug retargeting as a viable strategy for finding new uses for existing drugs through a series of case studies. This is one of the first studies that talked about the utility and feasibility of drug repositioning and provides a good overview of the problem and how drug repositioning tackles it. The workflow described suggests screening of approved drugs with other targets to identify new candidates for clinical trials.

A network-based methodology for identifying novel uses for existing drug is described in Reference [8]. The network associations are built from a knowledge base extracted from the FDA's DRUGDEX system and UMLS. Evidence of a stable methodology is established via novel drug suggestions, a high percentage of which map to diseases in clinical trials.

Network-based approaches for drug repositioning have also been exploited by a number of commercial entities. e-Therapeutics create networks of interconnected nodes (proteins) associated with a disease state and then calculate which would be the most synergetic set of nodes to affect, using a process called "combinatorial impact analysis." After establishing these complex disease signatures, they seek molecules that have an appropriate pattern of interaction with proteins associated with the studied "disease state." These interactions can be exerted through direct binding affinity, effects on protein expression, altering specific protein functional states (for example phosphorylation), or indirect network-mediated effects—typically by affecting a near topological neighbor of a key protein for the disease [53].

As discussed in some detail in the previous chapter, scientists at Pfizer have constructed a ligand–drug target matrix in an effort to explore the global relationships between chemical structure and biological targets [24]. This matrix represents a polypharmacology interaction network where each compound may target more than one protein and may enable the rational design of selective compounds against panels of genetically or functionally unrelated drug targets.

6.5.2. Gene Expression Profiling and Machine Learning

Another area where machine learning approaches have been extensively applied is on gene expression data. Typically methods falling in this category work by constructing a connectivity map between a set of genes, diseases, and drugs. The manner in which the map is constructed varies in terms of the source data and similarity detection metric.

In a seminal paper appearing in 2006 [54], researchers from the Broad Institute presented the construction of a Connectivity Map linking drugs, genes, and diseases using genomic signatures. The Connectivity Map is built from genome-wide mRNA expression data for 164 distinct bioactive small molecules. Application of nonparametric, rank-based pattern matching (GSEA) overcomes the shortcomings of the more commonly used hierarchical clustering approach. This approach is discussed in detail in Chapter 5 of this book by Webb and Mazzarella.

A strategy for constructing a drug-associated network is presented in Reference [55]. An association is created if there is similarity in the transcription effect of the drugs across multiple treatments with varying parameters. The authors also created a web-based tool called MANTRA for querying the network (this is a static network generated for the purpose of the work presented in that article). Testing of the drug network construction algorithm was performed on data retrieved from DrugBank and ChemBank.

GEO datasets have been exploited by a group of scientists at GlaxoSmithKline to generate a large-scale disease–drug network for drug repositioning as well as drug target/pathway identification [56]. The network constructed includes 645 disease–disease, 5008 disease–drug, and 164,374 drug–drug relationships. A significant part of these links were found to be novel, such as the relation of some antimalaria drugs to Crohn's disease, and a variety of existing drugs to Huntington's disease.

Gene expression data have also been used by Compugen, in conjunction with protein interaction networks to predict associations between genes and pathologies, integrated in a computational biology platform called MED [57].

6.5.3. Structural Data and Machine Learning

Attempts have also been made to repurpose drugs to new diseases by attempting to use the structural information of the targets and the drugs [6, 58]. Given the structural data of a drug and a set of targets, it is theoretically possible to identify what targets it is likely and what targets the drug is not likely to dock with. Methods falling in this category typically attempt to reduce the problem of drug repositioning to an optimization problem that attempts to find the most suitable docking sites for a ligand, but are heavily dependent on the availability of structural data for all targets that can be studied.

The applicability of the Monte Carlo global optimization technique to finding new targets for existing drugs has been demonstrated by Bisson et al. [58]. The optimization is applied to finding the lowest energy conformation for receptors, mandating the availability of structural data for the gene of interest, allowing the determination of the appropriate ligand that can form a complex with it. Using this approach, Bisson et al. [58] identified nonsteroidal antagonists of the human androgen receptor (AR). Using a docking procedure, they selected 11 compounds with the best docking score and then tested those *in vitro* for receptor binding and AR antagonism. These initial selection steps identified the antipsychotic drugs acetophenazine, fluphenazine, and periciazine as weak AR antagonists. Further computational optimization of these phenothiazines led to the identification of a nonsteroidal antiandrogen with improved AR antagonism and marked reduction in affinity for dopaminergic and serotonergic receptors. This compound might be useful in cases where one would want inhibition of the AR, such as in prostate cancer [59].

Another workflow for starting with the 3D structure of a protein and extracting the most likely binding sites as possible pockets for small molecules is developed in Reference [6]. Using the Monte Carlo searching approach, pockets where a small molecule might dock can be identified. Data sources used for the work presented include DrugBank and PDB.

6.5.4. Text Mining

Literature analysis in the form of text mining has been extensively applied either alone or in conjunction with other methodologies and data types for the purpose of establishing novel scientific hypotheses and identifying repositioning opportunities. Text mining includes the application of machine learning techniques to extract information from data in a supervised or unsupervised manner. Several machine learning techniques have been applied to mine biomedical data and recently also with the purpose of drug retargeting.

A literature-based target discovery system is described in Reference [60]. The proposed method combines n-Grams of concepts derived from UMLS and systematic analysis based on NLP for parsing PubMed abstracts. The proposed system works at a sentence level whereby sentences are extracted from the abstracts and then co-occurrence of concepts is used to support the discovery process.

Korbel et al. [61] describe an unsupervised approach to mining MEDLINE for associations between genes and phenotypic characteristics. Using principal component analysis (PCA), the authors demonstrated that the feature sets extracted from MEDLINE abstracts can be used to identify novel genotype–phenotype relations. The key feature of the results presented is that the approach used is systematic and requires no manual curation.

A number of companies previously engaged in providing software and services based, among other data types, on the analysis of the scientific literature have recently entered the field of drug repositioning. Companies like Ingenuity, GeneGo, and Ariadne Genomics have all been providing pathway-based solutions to the pharmaceutical industry and have recently started aiming their tools toward drug repositioning. Both GeneGo and Ariadne Genomics are integrating a variety of bioinformatics and cheminformatics resources with literature analysis to identify novel drug targets for a given drug.

Given a compound to be repurposed, GeneGo combines chemical structural analysis tools with molecular interaction and pathway analysis data to produce a list of putative new indications. GeneGo associates compounds to drug targets (known and predicted through structural similarity searches), which are then analyzed for their participation in disease-related pathways. On the other hand, Ariadne Genomics have recently presented data repurposing fulvestrant to glioblastoma using an approach based on publicly available microarray data combined with their own suite of pathway analysis tools [32].

Biovista capitalizes extensively on the use of advanced literature analysis methodologies to infer novel relationships between existing drugs and new indications. Central to Biovista's efforts is its Clinical Outcome Search Space™ (COSS™) computational platform, a system incorporating text mining, cheminformatics, and data analysis and visualizations tools. COSS™ capitalizes on a proprietary database of relations among biomedical entities, which utilizes custom technological solutions to achieve high-performance access to the underlying data. It allows Biovista to repurpose drugs and drug targets, and assess their benefit/risk clinical outcome potential against the universe of all medical conditions listed in the various UMLS Knowledge sources.

The COSS™ platform consists of multidimensional profiles of biomedical terms belonging in >20 biomedical categories (diseases, adverse events, drugs, compounds, genes, pathways, etc.) and correlation tools needed to analyze the interrelations of these profiles (Figure 6.1).

The multidimensional profiles are used to generate information regarding the putative mode of action of drugs in previously unknown alternative indications but also to deliver information regarding potential adverse drug reactions. The process is strengthened by the integration of cheminformatics tools and related data sources.

This technology is currently driving the development of Biovista's pipeline in areas that include central nervous system (CNS), oncology, and autoimmune diseases. Two of the first drugs that have been announced as a result of a systematic drug repositioning effort were generated through the COSS™ platform and are BVA-101 (Dimebon) and BVA-201 (Pirlindol) for the treatment of multiple sclerosis [62]. In addition, Biovista's technology is being used by the FDA's Office of Clinical Pharmacology (OCP) in its assessment of the

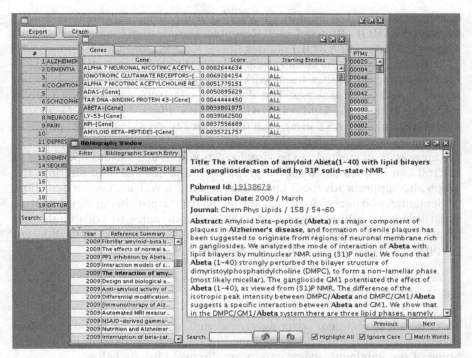

FIGURE 6.1. Example screenshot of the analysis module of the Biovista COSS™ platform. A gene-centric profile of a drug was used to generate a list of putative new indications for the drug. The profile of one of the indications (i.e., medical conditions) together with the underlying literature supporting the link is also shown.

adverse event profiles of major drug classes and drugs being evaluated by OCP/FDA.

6.5.5. Ontology-Based Approaches

A popular approach taken to the task is that of building large-scale ontologies wherein various diseases and drugs can be classified and then their interactions studied or discovered. Ontology-based approaches typically require curating data from various sources into a uniform format (or representation), allowing meaningful queries to be run and discoveries made. Also gaining popularity are techniques for visualizing the ontology data (or parts of it) using graphs to make it easier to identify "unexpected" relationships.

In Reference [7], the authors build a disease drug correlation ontology (DDCO) through manual curation for combining several existing sources of information on such interactions including DrugBank, Entrez Gene, GO, OMIM, KEGG, BioCarta, Reactome, UMLS, and GEO. The ontology is tested on finding drugs for the disease systemic lupus erythematosus (SLE). The association network is built as an ontology using Jena, allowing data mining through SPARQL Protocol and Resource Description Framework (RDF) Query Language (SPARQL) queries.

In Reference [27], the authors built a graph of 120,000 concepts with 570,000 relations using the Ondex framework. The graph shows associations between drugs, proteins, and diseases. The dataset is constructed from data sources including DrugBank, UniProt, HRPD, KEGG, Pfam, SynAtlas, G-sesame, OpenBabel, and BLAST using each data source to provide different pieces of information required to build the association graph. Using the Ondex platform, the mega-dataset created can be visualized as graphs and various operations of interest can be preformed on the graph such as expansion and filtering. The graph also supports advanced operations to allow novel association detection.

Semantic web technologies based on RDF are also being developed to assist scientists within large pharmaceutical companies to collaborate and identify internal compounds, which might have been created for a different purpose many years ago, with a utility in a new indication [63].

6.6. FURTHER READING

More detailed treatment covering various initiatives can be found in several review papers that have been published in the field over the last few years. Some of the imminent review papers are discussed briefly below.

A review of several methodologies that have successfully been applied to determining drug–target relationships through the use of chemical structures and chemical–chemical similarity between known and new targets can be found in Reference [64]. Various database resources with publicly available cheminformatics data and a comprehensive review of methodologies used for mining such data are presented in Reference [23]. Graphical methods described include "rule of five" selection schemes based on functional group filtering and chemistry space-based similarity. Also described is a range of machine learning methods applied to chemically extracted data about the drug molecule and the target structures. Dudley et al. [65] present an overview of both pattern-based and network-based approaches to *in silico* drug repositioning, such as the concept of the Connectivity Map [54] and the drug–drug networks constructed by Keiser et al. [4] and Chiang and Butte [8]. Recent publications dealing with the use of network pharmacology for the prediction of adverse events are also highlighted (References [66] and [67] as examples).

6.7. CLOSING REMARKS

Since about 2009, interest in drug repurposing has been growing to the extent that several conferences and industry reports are now wholly dedicated to this branch of drug discovery. In the present review we presented a selection of data types and accompanied data sources that have been extensively employed in various drug repositioning projects. Working examples of the usage of these data sources were also described. We believe that the information highlighted herein will provide a good starting point for someone entering the field of drug repositioning.

REFERENCES

1. Mestres, J., Gregori-Puigjané, E., Valverde, S., Solé, R.V. (2008). Data completeness—The Achilles heel of drug-target networks. *Nature Biotechnology*, 26(9), 983–984.

2. Hopkins, A.L., Groom, C.R. (2002). The druggable genome. *Nature Reviews. Drug Discovery*, 1(9), 727–730.

3. Nobeli, I., Favia, A.D., Thornton, J.M. (2009). Protein promiscuity and its implications for biotechnology. *Nature Biotechnology*, 27(2), 157–167.

4. Keiser, M.J., Setola, V., Irwin, J.J., Laggner, C., Abbas, A.I., Hufeisen, S.J., Jensen, N.H., Kuijer, M.B., Matos, R.C., Tran, T.B., Whaley, R., Glennon, R.A., Hert, J., Thomas, K.L., Edwards, D.D., Shoichet, B.K., Roth, B.L. (2009). Predicting new molecular targets for known drugs. *Nature*, 462(7270), 175–181.

5. Roth, B.L., Sheffler, D.J., Kroeze, W.K. (2004). Magic shotguns versus magic bullets: Selectively non-selective drugs for mood disorders and schizophrenia. *Nature Reviews. Drug Discovery*, 3(4), 353–359.

6. Li, Y.Y., An, J., Jones, S.J. (2006). A large-scale computational approach to drug repositioning. *Genome Informatics*, 17(2), 239–247.

7. Qu, X.A., Gudivada, R.C., Jegga, A.G., Neumann, E.K., Aronow, B.J. (2009). Inferring novel disease indications for known drugs by semantically linking drug action and disease mechanism relationships. *BMC Bioinformatics*, 6(10 Suppl 5), S4.

8. Chiang, A.P., Butte, A.J. (2009). Systematic evaluation of drug-disease relationships to identify leads for novel drug uses. *Clinical Pharmacology and Therapeutics*, 86(5), 507–510.

9. Campillos, M., Kuhn, M., Gavin, A.C., Jensen, L.J., Bork, P. (2008). Drug target identification using side-effect similarity. *Science*, 321(5886), 263–266.

10. Mucke, H.A.M. (2010) *Drug repositioning: Extracting added value from prior R&D investments*, Insight Pharma Reports. July 2010.

11. Datamonitor (2008) *Drug repositioning strategies: Serendipity by design*. DMHC2400. May 2008.

12. NCBI Gene. http://www.ncbi.nlm.nih.gov/sites/entrez?db=gene

13. UniProt Consortium (2010). The Universal Protein Resource (UniProt) in 2010. *Nucleic Acids Research*, 38(Database issue), D142–D148. http://www.uniprot.org/.

14. Berman, H.M., Westbrook, J., Feng, Z., Gilliland, G., Bhat, T.N., Weissig, H., Shindyalov, I.N., Bourne, P.E. (2000). The Protein Data Bank. *Nucleic Acids Research*, 28(1), 235–242. http://www.pdb.org.

15. Kinnings, S.L., Liu, N., Buchmeier, N., Tonge, P.J., Xie, L., Bourne, P.E. (2009). Drug discovery using chemical systems biology: Repositioning the safe medicine Comtan

to treat multi-drug and extensively drug resistant tuberculosis. *PLoS Computational Biology*, 5(7), e1000423.

16. Barrett, T., Troup, D.B., Wilhite, S.E., Ledoux, P., Rudnev, D., Evangelista, C., Kim, I.F., Soboleva, A., Tomashevsky, M., Marshall, K.A., Phillippy, K.H., Sherman, P.M., Muertter, R.N., Edgar, R. (2009). NCBI GEO: Archive for high-throughput functional genomic data. *Nucleic Acids Research*, 37(Database issue), D885–D890. http://www.ncbi.nlm.nih.gov/geo/.

17. Kanehisa, M., Goto, S., Furumichi, M., Tanabe, M., Hirakawa, M. (2010). KEGG for representation and analysis of molecular networks involving diseases and drugs. *Nucleic Acids Research*, 38(Database issue), D355–D360. http://www.genome.jp/kegg/.

18. Matthews, L., Gopinath, G., Gillespie, M., Caudy, M., Croft, D., de Bono, B., Garapati, P., Hemish, J., Hermjakob, H., Jassal, B., Kanapin, A., Lewis, S., Mahajan, S., May, B., Schmidt, E., Vastrik, I., Wu, G., Birney, E., Stein, L., D'Eustachio, P. (2009). Reactome knowledgebase of human biological pathways and processes. *Nucleic Acids Research*, 37(Database issue), D619–D622. http://www.genomeknowledge.org/cgi-bin/frontpage?DB=gk_current.

19. Ashburner, M., Ball, C.A., Blake, J.A., Botstein, D., Butler, H., Cherry, J.M., Davis, A.P., Dolinski, K., Dwight, S.S., Eppig, J.T., Harris, M.A., Hill, D.P., Issel-Tarver, L., Kasarskis, A., Lewis, S., Matese, J.C., Richardson, J.E., Ringwald, M., Rubin, G.M., Sherlock, G. (2000). Gene ontology: Tool for the unification of biology. The Gene Ontology Consortium. *Nature Genetics*, 25(1), 25–29. http://geneontology.org/.

20. Saunders, B., Lyon, S., Day, M., Riley, B., Chenette, E., Subramaniam, S., Vadivelu, I. (2008). The Molecule Pages database. *Nucleic Acids Research*, 36(Database issue), D700–D706. http://www.signaling-gateway.org/.

21. Olsson, T., Oprea, T.I. (2001). Cheminformatics: A tool for decision-makers in drug discovery. *Current Opinion in drug discovery & development*, 4(3), 308–313.

22. Brown, F. (2005). Editorial opinion: Chemoinformatics—A ten year update. *Current Opinion in Drug Discovery & Development*, 8(3), 298–302.

23. Jónsdóttir, S.O., Jørgensen, F.S., Brunak, S. (2005). Prediction methods and databases within chemoinformatics: Emphasis on drugs and drug candidates. *Bioinformatics*, 21(10), 2145–2160.

24. Paolini, G.V., Shapland, R.H., van Hoorn, W.P., Mason, J.S., Hopkins, A.L. (2006). Global mapping of pharmacological space. *Nature Biotechnology*, 24(7), 805–815.

25. Wang, Y., Xiao, J., Suzek, T.O., Zhang, J., Wang, J., Bryant, S.H. (2009). PubChem: A public information system for analyzing bioactivities of small molecules. *Nucleic Acids Research*, 37(Web Server issue), W623–W633. http://pubchem.ncbi.nlm.nih.gov/.

26. EMBL-EBI-ChEMBL. http://www.ebi.ac.uk/chembl/

27. Cockell, S.J., Weile, J., Lord, P., Wipat, C., Andriychenko, D., Pocock, M., Wilkinson, D., Young, M., Wipat, A. (2010). An integrated dataset for *in silico* drug discovery. *Journal of Integrative Bioinformatics*, 7(3), 116.

28. Steinbeck, C., Hoppe, C., Kuhn, S., Floris, M., Guha, R., Willighagen, E.L. (2006). Recent developments of the chemistry development kit (CDK)—An open-source java library for chemo- and bioinformatics. *Current Pharmaceutical Design*, 12(17), 2111–2120. http://sourceforge.net/apps/mediawiki/cdk/index.php?title=Main_Page.

29. Guha, R., Howard, M.T., Hutchison, G.R., Murray-Rust, P., Rzepa, H., Steinbeck, C., Wegner, J., Willighagen, E.L. (2006). The Blue Obelisk-interoperability in chemical informatics. *Journal of Chemical Information and Modeling, 46*(3), 991–998. http://openbabel.org/wiki/Main_Page.

30. Russ, A.P., Lampel, S. (2005). The druggable genome: An update. *Drug Discovery Today, 10*(23–24), 1607–1610.

31. Wishart, D.S., Knox, C., Guo, A.C., Cheng, D., Shrivastava, S., Tzur, D., Gautam, B., Hassanali, M. (2008). DrugBank: A knowledgebase for drugs, drug actions and drug targets. *Nucleic Acids Research, 36*(Database issue), D901–D906. http://www.drugbank.ca/.

32. Kotelnikova, E., Yuryev, A., Mazo, I., Daraselia, N. (2010). Computational approaches for drug repositioning and combination therapy design. *Journal of Bioinformatics and Computational Biology, 8*(3), 593–606.

33. Drugs@FDA. http://www.accessdata.fda.gov/scripts/cder/drugsatfda/

34. DailyMed. http://dailymed.nlm.nih.gov/dailymed/about.cfm

35. FDA AERS. http://www.fda.gov/Drugs/GuidanceComplianceRegulatoryInformation/Surveillance/AdverseDrugEffects/default.htm

36. NLM MeSH. http://www.nlm.nih.gov/mesh/meshrels.html and http://www.nlm.nih.gov/mesh/meshhome.html

37. Baker, N.C., Hemminger, B.M. (2010). Mining connections between chemicals, proteins, and diseases extracted from Medline annotations. *Journal of Biomedical Informatics, 43*(4), 510–519.

38. Sarkar, I.N. (2010). Biomedical informatics and translational medicine. *Journal of Translational Medicine, 8*, 22.

39. Jensen, L.J., Saric, J., Bork, P. (2006). Literature mining for the biologist: From information retrieval to biological discovery. *Nature Reviews. Genetics, 7*(2), 119–129.

40. Weeber, M., Kors, J.A., Mons, B. (2005). Online tools to support literature-based discovery in the life sciences. *Briefings in Bioinformatics, 6*(3), 277–286.

41. Swanson, D.R. (1986). Fish oil, Raynaud's syndrome, and undiscovered public knowledge. *Perspectives in Biology and Medicine, 30*(1), 7–18.

42. Swanson, D.R. (1988). Migraine and magnesium: Eleven neglected connections. *Perspectives in Biology and Medicine, 31*(4), 526–557.

43. Temkin, J.M., Gilder, M.R. (2003). Extraction of protein interaction information from unstructured text using a context-free grammar. *Bioinformatics, 19*(16), 2046–2053.

44. Ramani, A.K., Bunescu, R.C., Mooney, R.J., Marcotte, E.M. (2005). Consolidating the set of known human protein-protein interactions in preparation for large-scale mapping of the human interactome. *Genome Biology, 6*(5), R40.

45. Thomas, J., Milward, D., Ouzounis, C., Pulman, S., Carroll, M. (2000). Automatic extraction of protein interactions from scientific abstracts. *Pacific Symposium on Biocomputing*, 541–552.

46. Jenssen, T.K., Laegreid, A., Komorowski, J., Hovig, E. (2001). A literature network of human genes for high-throughput analysis of gene expression. *Nature Genetics, 28*(1), 21–28.

47. Stephens, M., Palakal, M., Mukhopadhyay, S., Raje, R., Mostafa, J. (2001). Detecting gene relations from Medline abstracts. *Pacific Symposium on Biocomputing*, 483–495.

48. Saric, J., Jensen, L.J., Ouzounova, R., Rojas, I., Bork, P. (2006). Extraction of regulatory gene/protein networks from Medline. *Bioinformatics*, *22*(6), 645–650.

49. Rzhetsky, A., Iossifov, I., Koike, T., Krauthammer, M., Kra, P., Morris, M., Yu, H., Duboué, P.A., Weng, W., Wilbur, W.J., Hatzivassiloglou, V., Friedman, C. (2004). GeneWays: A system for extracting, analyzing, visualizing, and integrating molecular pathway data. *Journal of Biomedical Informatics*, *37*(1), 43–53.

50. PR Newswire. http://www.prnewswire.com/

51. Yamanishi, Y., Kotera, M., Kanehisa, M., Goto, S. (2010). Drug-target interaction prediction from chemical, genomic and pharmacological data in an integrated framework. *Bioinformatics*, *26*(12), i246–i254.

52. O'Connor, K.A., Roth, B.L. (2005). Finding new tricks for old drugs: An efficient route for public-sector drug discovery. *Nature Reviews. Drug Discovery*, *4*(12), 1005–1014.

53. Zimmer, S., Young, M.P. (2009). From low productivity to efficient network-based drug discovery. *Innovation in Pharmaceutical Technology*, *18*, 38–41.

54. Lamb, J., Crawford, E.D., Peck, D., Modell, J.W., Blat, I.C., Wrobel, M.J., Lerner, J., Brunet, J.P., Subramanian, A., Ross, K.N., Reich, M., Hieronymus, H., Wei, G., Armstrong, S.A., Haggarty, S.J., Clemons, P.A., Wei, R., Carr, S.A., Lander, E.S., Golub, T.R. (2006). The Connectivity Map: Using gene-expression signatures to connect small molecules, genes, and disease. *Science*, *313*(5795), 1929–1935.

55. Iorio, F., Bosotti, R., Scacheri, E., Belcastro, V., Mithbaokar, P., Ferriero, R., Murino, L., Tagliaferri, R., Brunetti-Pierri, N., Isacchi, A., Di Bernardo, D. (2010). Discovery of drug mode of action and drug repositioning from transcriptional responses. *Proc. Natl. Acad. Sci. U.S.A.*, *107*(33), 14621–14626.

56. Hu, G., Agarwal, P. (2009). Human disease-drug network based on genomic expression profiles. *PLoS ONE*, *4*(8), e6536.

57. Compugen Press Release. http://www.cgen.com/Content.aspx?Page=press_releases&NewsId=229

58. Bisson, W.H., Cheltsov, A.V., Bruey-Sedano, N., Lin, B., Chen, J., Goldberger, N., May, L.T., Christopoulos, A., Dalton, J.T., Sexton, P.M., Zhang, X.K., Abagyan, R. (2007). Discovery of antiandrogen activity of nonsteroidal scaffolds of marketed drugs. *Proc. Natl. Acad. Sci. U.S.A.*, *104*(29), 11927–11932.

59. Vasaitis, T.S., Njar, V.C. (2010). Novel, potent anti-androgens of therapeutic potential: Recent advances and promising developments. *Future Medicinal Chemistry*, *2*(4), 667–680.

60. Weeber, M., Klein, H., de Jong-Van Den Berg, L.T.W., Vos, R. (2001). Using concepts in literature-based discovery: Simulating Swanson's Raynaud-Fish oil and migraine-magnesium discoveries. *Journal of the American Society for Information Science and Technology*, *52*(7), 548–557.

61. Korbel, J.O., Doerks, T., Jensen, L.J., Perez-Iratxeta, C., Kaczanowski, S., Hooper, S.D., Andrade, M.A., Bork, P. (2005). Systematic association of genes to phenotypes by genome and literature mining. *PLoS Biology*, *3*(5), e134.

62. Lekka, E., Deftereos, S.N., Persidis, A., Persidis, A., Andronis, C. (2011). Literature analysis for systematic drug repurposing: A case study from Biovista. *Drug Discovery Today: Therapeutic Strategies*, in press.

63. W3C: Semantic Web Use Cases and Case Studies. http://www.w3.org/2001/sw/sweo/public/UseCases/Pfizer/

64. Kuhn, M., Campillos, M., González, P., Jensen, L.J., Bork, P. (2008). Large-scale prediction of drug-target relationships. *FEBS Letters*, *582*(8), 1283–1290.

65. Dudley, J.T., Schadt, E., Sirota, M., Butte, A.J., Ashley, E. (2010). Drug discovery in a multidimensional world: Systems, patterns, and networks. *Journal of Cardiovascular Translational Research*, *3*(5), 438–447.

66. Xie, L., Li, J., Xie, L., Bourne, P.E. (2009). Drug discovery using chemical systems biology: Identification of the protein-ligand binding network to explain the side effects of CETP inhibitors. *PLoS Computational Biology*, *5*(5), e1000387.

67. Berger, S.I., Ma'ayan, A., Iyengar, R. (2010). Systems pharmacology of arrhythmias. *Science Signaling*, *3*, ra30.

■■■■■■ **CHAPTER 7**

Predicting the Polypharmacology of Drugs: Identifying New Uses through Chemoinformatics, Structural Informatics, and Molecular Modeling-Based Approaches

LI XIE, SARAH L. KINNINGS, LEI XIE, and PHILIP E. BOURNE

7.1. INTRODUCTION

Over the past two decades, rational drug design has proceeded by identifying a single disease-associated target and discovering exquisitely selective drugs for that target. Unfortunately, this approach has yielded few successes due to the lack of both drug efficacy and clinical safety. Hence, both the cost to launch a new drug and the attrition rates during the late stages of drug development are increasing. To overcome the failure of the current approach, polypharmacology has emerged as a new paradigm in drug discovery. Polypharmacology focuses on searching for multitarget drugs or multiple drugs that bind to different targets within a network, to perturb a disease-causing network, instead of designing selective ligands to target individual proteins. The proposed use of multi-target drugs has been suggested by the systems-level observations regarding the robustness and resilience of parasitic diseases, as well as the success of serendipitously discovered therapies. The rational design of poly-pharmacological drugs relies on an understanding of drug–target interactions on a proteome-wide scale. An increasing number of computational tools have been developed to detect such broad-based drug–target relationships. In this chapter, we present an overview of the computational approaches to predict polypharmacology, and their applications in drug repositioning. The methods

Drug Repositioning: Bringing New Life to Shelved Assets and Existing Drugs, First Edition.
Edited by Michael J. Barratt and Donald E. Frail.
© 2012 John Wiley & Sons, Inc. Published 2012 by John Wiley & Sons, Inc.

discussed include ligand similarity-based, binding site similarity-based, and phenotype-based approaches.

7.2. THE CONCEPT OF POLYPHARMACOLOGY AND ITS RELATIONSHIP TO DRUG RESISTANCE, SIDE EFFECTS, AND DRUG REPOSITIONING

For the past two decades, the paradigm of drug discovery has been to develop highly selective ligands that interact with specific binding sites on individual target proteins—the so-called "one gene, one drug, one disease" approach. The rationale behind this strategy is that it is possible to develop safer, more effective drugs through the minimization of undesirable side effects caused by secondary target (also known as "off-target") interactions [1, 2]. However, it is now becoming increasingly apparent that there are major issues with the key assumptions framing this reductionism-based approach to drug discovery [3]. Indeed, this strategy is only appropriate for those diseases that can be treated using a single target intervention, that is, Ehrlich's "magic bullet." It is well known that effective therapy for many multigenic, complex diseases requires the simultaneous inhibition or activation of multiple targets in order to effectively rebalance the regulatory network processes that are perturbed in the disease state, and to achieve optimal therapeutic benefit [4–6]. For instance, since the induction of most cancers has been shown to require several independent mutations, it follows that multiple interventions will be necessary in order to counter the process of oncogenesis [6]. In fact, many existing multitarget antibacterial, antiviral, and anticancer therapeutics are actually developed through drug combination (so-called "cocktails") [6]. Although drug combination is perhaps the most obvious way of designing specific pharmacology, its success is highly dependent on the optimization of dosage ranging, the understanding of drug–drug interactions, and the systematic evaluation of safety profiles. Indeed, while two drugs may be safe individually, this does not necessarily mean that they will be safe in combination. This complexity significantly raises the cost of developing combination therapies. Conversely, if the multitarget agent is a single molecule, issues in drug development, such as the prediction of absorption, distribution, metabolism, and excretion (ADME)/ toxicity (Tox) properties, are substantially less complex [2]. Therefore, the development of a single drug that is able to mediate its effects through the inhibition of multiple targets is highly desirable.

Thus, in contrast with the conventional "one gene, one drug, one disease" drug design philosophy, polypharmacology considers one drug binding to multiple targets or combination therapies of multiple drugs. In recent years it has been discovered that ligand promiscuity is actually essential for the efficacy of many approved drugs from a wide range of different therapeutic areas. For example, a number of different protein kinase inhibitors actually mediate their anti-cancer effects through the modulation of several different targets simultaneously, even though they were originally designed for a single specific target [1, 2, 7]. Sorafenib and sunitinib have been shown to bind a number of different protein kinases, thereby affecting both tumor proliferation and tumor angiogenesis pathways. Similarly, imatinib, which was originally developed as a highly selective inhibitor of c-Abl for the treatment of chronic myeloid leukemia, has since been shown to exhibit significant activity against several other protein kinases, such as c-Kit, leading to the expansion of its clinical use [8]. Microarray transcription profiles have shown that the combined synergistic effects that result from a drug acting on more than one protein kinase can be greater than the additive effects of targeting those protein kinases individually [2]. There are many other reported examples of where therapeutic efficacy is enhanced through synergistic relationships between multiple targets [9–11]. Many anti-psychotic drugs, such as clozapine, are known to mediate their effects through binding entire families of serotonin and dopamine receptors [2]. In fact, it has been proposed that the clinical failures of many anti-psychotics can be attributed to them being too selective in nature [2]. Besides the aforementioned drugs, the success of many serendipitously discovered antibiotics can be attributed to their inhibition of multiple protein targets simultaneously. Current drug discovery methods based on the assumption of single-target essentiality would have simply failed to systematically discover such therapeutics [3]. Thus, research into drug polypharmacology can make a critical contribution toward studies concerning drug resistance, side effects, and drug repositioning.

Multitarget drugs can reduce drug resistance by interacting with other targets in the same pathway or with other targets with similar functions. For example, many factors can cause drug resistance to inhibitors of individual kinases in tumor cells, such as mutation of the primary target, activation of substitute kinases, and modulation of pathway components. One compound designed through targeted polypharmacology, PP121, overrides resistance in chronic myelogenous leukemia (CML) by redundantly targeting both oncogenic tyrosine kinases and phosphatidylinositol-3-OH kinases [12]. Another example is the drug resistance of anti-infective drugs. A single amino acid substitution in the target protein is often sufficient to render a pathogen resistant to a single-target anti-infective therapeutic [3]. In principle, multitarget anti-infective drugs not only exhibit greater efficacy, but are also less vulnerable to drug resistance by impacting multiple nodes at the system level [13]. By using a single drug to inhibit two or more essential targets, it is possible to prevent the emergence of drug resistance. Indeed, while pathogens are able to rapidly acquire resistance to single-target agents through mutations in the target protein, it is much more difficult to acquire resistance to multitarget agents, since a mutation in one of the target proteins would not confer any selective advantage over the wild type. The success of the previous generation of anti-infective drugs, combined with the current failure of genome-based strategies, highlights the need to employ polypharmacology-based strategies in order to produce successful anti-infective therapies in the future. Recently,

Kinnings et al. applied a ligand binding site comparison method for an all-against-all comparison across the *Mycobacterium tuberculosis* structural genome in an effort to construct a genome-scale protein–ligand interaction network [14]. Their study revealed that a number of different proteins share similar ligand binding sites, therefore highlighting the potential for developing drugs that are able to inhibit multiple proteins within the organism, and presenting new opportunities to combat drug resistance.

An alternative strategy to counter the emergence of drug resistance is to develop anti-infective therapeutics that inhibit both an essential target and a nonessential "co-target" simultaneously. Co-targets are proteins that reside in pathways that are involved in drug resistance. Recently, Raman and Chandra [15] constructed a genome-wide protein–protein interaction (PPI) network for *M. tuberculosis*, which they then used to identify the most plausible pathways for the emergence of a number of different drug resistance mechanisms. As a result, they were able to suggest a number of important co-targets, which, when simultaneously inhibited along with the intended targets, would prevent the emergence of resistance to a given drug. In future, a detailed analysis of the binding sites of drug targets, as well as the genes that are responsible for drug resistance, will undoubtedly provide invaluable clues for the design of drugs that inhibit not only essential genes but also co-targets that are not necessarily essential for bacterial survival, but which mediate drug resistance. Even in an initial small-scale study, one such protein was identified, cytochrome P450 121, which showed significant binding site similarity to a number of potential drug targets. In order to develop antibacterial therapies that are less liable to drug resistance, we hypothesized that the inhibitor should be designed to retain binding to the primary targets while reducing binding to co-targets such as cytochrome P450 [14].

Side effect prediction requires the identification of multiple drug targets. Currently, the biggest hurdle in drug development is toxicity, which results in numerous lead compounds, especially those that are more promiscuous in nature, failing late stage clinical trials or being recalled from the market. Early characterization of toxicity is particularly important considering the emergence of polypharmacology as the new paradigm in drug discovery. As modern attitudes toward animal welfare put increasing pressure on pharmaceutical companies to minimize animal testing, the *in silico* prediction of adverse side effects is growing in popularity. Since many failures in drug design due to unacceptable side effects are often caused by drug off-target binding or binding to therapeutic targets in non-target tissue [16], the pharmaceutical industry is now putting considerable effort into the computational screening of potential off-targets, with the intention of identifying any potential problems at an early stage in the drug discovery process [17]. Indeed, by identifying and subsequently fine-tuning the binding profile of a particular compound it is possible to select for clinical development those compounds whose profiles maximally modulate a disease network while causing minimal side effects [3]. In order to predict the toxicity profile of a compound *in silico*, it is necessary to understand

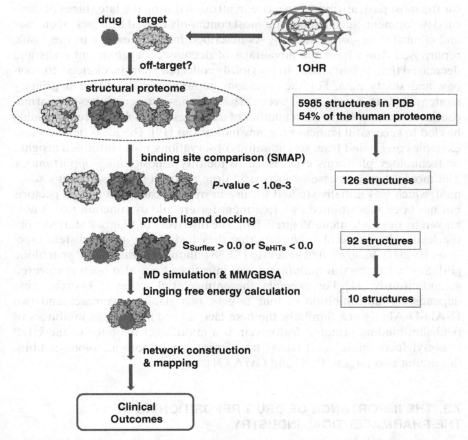

drug   target

off-target?

1OHR

structural proteome

5985 structures in PDB
54% of the human proteome

binding site comparison (SMAP)

P-value < 1.0e-3

126 structures

protein ligand docking

$S_{Surflex}$ > 0.0 or S_{eHiTs} < 0.0

92 structures

MD simulation & MM/GBSA
binging free energy calculation

10 structures

network construction
& mapping

Clinical
Outcomes

FIGURE 7.1. A structural proteome-wide off-target pipeline taken from Reference [18]. It integrates ligand binding site characterization and comparison, protein–ligand docking, molecular dynamics (MD) simulation, molecular mechanics/generalized born surface area (MM/GBSA) energy calculations, and biological network analysis. PDB, Protein Data Bank.

its cross-reactivity across the whole proteome, which requires the identification of off-targets across the whole proteome using a pipeline like the one shown in Figure 7.1 [18].

The most straightforward application of drug polypharmacology is to discover novel uses of existing drugs, that is, drug repositioning, since drugs interacting with the same targets are likely to have similar functions. Drug repositioning is the process of developing novel indications for existing drugs or clinical candidates previously withdrawn for reasons other than safety. *De novo* drug discovery has failed to efficiently supply pharmaceutical company pipelines. The decline in productivity of the pharmaceutical industry can be, for the most part, attributed to a rise in attrition during the late stages of clinical development. Such failures are most commonly caused by a lack of efficacy and clinical safety or toxicology. As described in detail earlier in this book, repurposed drugs have the advantage of decreased development costs and decreased time to launch due to previously collected pharmacokinetic, toxicology, and safety data. For these reasons, repurposing should be a primary strategy in drug discovery for every broadly focused, research-based pharmaceutical company. There are a number of examples in which drug repositioning has led to successful launches for new indications [19]. The ideas behind these examples originated from serendipitous observations, novel informed insights, or technology platforms established to identify repositioning opportunities. The most prominent case of successful drug repositioning was Pfizer's sildenafil, which was initially studied for use in hypertension and angina pectoris but has been repositioned as a treatment for erectile dysfunction and is now known by the trade name Viagra® [20]. The discovery of Viagra® started from the feedback of several volunteers that they had strong and persistent erections. By 2003, Viagra® had generated $1.88 billion for Pfizer in that year alone [19]. Several successful multitarget anti-infectives have also been discovered serendipitously [21]. For example, the antibacterial action of D-cycloserine depends on the inhibition of four targets: two alanine racemases and two D-Ala-D-Ala ligases. Similarly, the beta-lactams are multitarget inhibitors of penicillin-binding proteins; fosfomycin is a multitarget inhibitor of the UDP N-acetylglucosamine enolpyruvyl transferases, and fluoroquinolone antibiotics inhibit two targets, ParC and GyrA [21].

7.3. THE IMPORTANCE OF DRUG REPOSITIONING IN THE PHARMACEUTICAL INDUSTRY

As has been discussed in detail earlier in this book, there has been increasing interest in drug repositioning due to the sustained high failure rates and costs involved in attempts to bring new drugs to market. Despite major advances in human genomics and pharmacology, sales growth of the pharmaceutical industry is at a historic low globally [22]. Indeed the U.S. Food and Drug Administration (FDA) approved just 24 new drugs in 2008, compared with a high of 53 in 1996 [23]. Although the U.S. National Institutes of Health (NIH) doubled its research spending to $27 billion in 2003, the number of new FDA-approved drugs has remained fairly constant at around 20–30 new compounds per year [24]. At the same time, the cost of developing a new drug increases every year [25]. According to a 2009 report by Bain Capital, pharmaceutical companies spent an average of $1.1 billion on the development and launch of a new drug during the late 1990s. By 2009, the required investment had more than doubled to $2.2 billion, and the return on invested capital for new drug development had dropped from 9% in 1995–2000 to 4% in 2009. In addition, due to regulatory requirements regarding safety, efficacy, and quality, the time required for the *de novo* development of a new drug is much longer than before. With the expiration of patents on currently available drugs, and the lack of new drugs to replace them, from 2010 onward, pharmaceutical companies experienced their first decrease in revenue in four decades [3].

Current drug discovery methods are poorly equipped in the battle against drug-resistant pathogens, rapidly emerging diseases such as avian flu, and diseases with small financial markets [24]. The soaring costs associated with the high failure rate of *de novo* drug discovery, combined with the recent revelations about drug promiscuity, have renewed a keen interest in drug repositioning [26]. Drug repositioning provides a promising solution to reducing both the time and costs associated with drug development [17]. Indeed, since the drugs have already been approved for human use, it may be possible to bypass toxicological and pharmacokinetic assessment, assuming that the dose, site of action, and route of administration for the secondary indication is the same as that used for the initial use. Newly identified drug indications can be evaluated relatively quickly in Phase II clinical trials, which on average may be completed in 2 years and cost around $17 million [24, 25].

Besides the reduction in the time and costs associated with drug discovery, drug repositioning also enables drugs that are no longer covered by patents to be used to treat neglected diseases in developing countries [17, 24]. This is highly beneficial because not only is there a huge unmet need for new drugs to treat these diseases, but these countries neither have the finances nor the healthcare infrastructure to monitor the post-marketing safety of drugs in Phase IV clinical trials. A number of existing drugs have successfully been repositioned in this way, including miltefosine, which was repurposed to treat visceral leishmaniasis, a sandfly-transmitted parasite that kills around half a million people every year. Miltefosine was originally developed to treat breast cancer, but it was never approved by the FDA because it failed to show tumor reduction in Phase II clinical trials. As discussed further in Chapter 11, the drug's anti-infective activity was later demonstrated through *in vitro* and animal studies, and it was confirmed as a viable treatment for visceral leishmaniasis in subsequent Phase II clinical trials [24].

Prompted by the need to refurbish their pipelines at lower costs and to drive and sustain future profits, drug companies have turned to drug repositioning as a means of drug rediscovery. Currently, at least 24 existing drugs are being remarketed for new uses by the pharmaceutical industry, and at least 17 existing drugs are undergoing clinical and animal testing for new uses. However, the successful repositioning of drugs remains mostly serendipitous, with physicians and pharmaceutical companies mainly relying on chance observations and educated guesses [24]. In order to achieve its full potential, a more systematic approach to drug repositioning is required. A rational approach to drug repositioning may include a cross-disciplinary focus on the elucidation of the mechanisms of disease, allowing the matching of disease pathways with appropriately targeted therapeutic agents. Numerous publicly accessible databases are built for drug–target information containing structures, drug–target interactions, drug side effects, transcriptional responses, and drug–disease relationships, and hence provide a great resource for the development of computational approaches for drug repositioning (see also Chapters 5 and 6 in this book). These approaches can be categorized as structure-based, when the discovery of repositioning opportunities initiates from structural information about drugs and targets.

7.4. CHEMICAL AND PROTEIN STRUCTURE-BASED APPROACHES

There are several examples of drugs or co-factors that can bind to receptors that are sequentially and structurally unrelated, or where the same receptor can be inhibited by several drugs. For instance, G-protein coupled receptors (GPCRs) such as the 5-hydroxytryptamine subtypes 1, 2, and 4–7 (5-HT$_{1,2,4-7}$) are unrelated to the 5-HT$_{3A}$ receptor, an ion channel, by sequence and structure. However, both types of receptors are inhibited by serotonin and serotonergic drugs [27]. Another drug that is able to bind both GPCRs and ion channels is the opioid methadone, which interacts not only with the μ-opioid receptor but also with the N-methyl-D-aspartic acid (NMDA) receptor [28]. Three different enzymes, thymidylate synthase (TS), dihydrofolate reductase (DHFR), and glycinamide ribonucleotide formyltransferase (GART), are all inhibited by antifolate drugs [29]. In all of the above cases, the receptors have no substantial sequence identity and are structurally unrelated. The ability of chemically similar drugs to bind proteins without obvious sequence or structural similarity arises from the specific interactions between drugs and proteins. Such interactions include electrostatic interactions formed by polar/charged chemical groups, hydrophobic interactions between hydrophobic/aromatic groups, hydrogen bond interactions, a high degree of shape complementary, and other entropic effects. These specific interactions can be captured by ligand similarity comparison or binding site similarity comparison approaches.

7.4.1. Ligand Similarity-Based Approaches

The idea of ligand similarity analysis comes from the "similar property principle" (SPP) [30], which states that similar molecules should have similar biological activities. The computational basis of ligand similarity approaches is to extract a set of chemical features in order to generate similarity descriptors for each drug, and then calculate a similarity score for each pair of drugs. Subsequently, all drugs in the drug set are clustered based on the extracted features. Drugs in the same cluster are predicted to interact with the same group of proteins. Generally, methods are distinguished by using different descriptors and similarity criteria. These descriptors are generated based on different location-specific molecular details that include conformational, topological, or physicochemical properties. Based on the dimensionality of these properties, similarity descriptors can be classified as one-dimensional (1D), two-dimensional (2D), or three-dimensional (3D) descriptors.

1D descriptors are derived from global molecular properties such as molecular weight, molar refractivity, and logP. They are simple descriptors and cannot distinguish molecules effectively. The most widely used descriptors in ligand screening processes are 2D descriptors, which are generated based on the two-dimensional qualitative or quantitative properties of targeted molecules. There are many different types of 2D descriptors, including structural keys, molecular fingerprints, real value descriptors, and feature trees. Structural keys and molecular fingerprints are so-called binary descriptors. In binary descriptors, the properties of the targeted molecule are represented by a Boolean array set to "1" or "0," which indicates whether or not the molecule contains a particular functional group, a specific bond, or a certain number of functional groups or specific bonds [31–33].

7.4.1.1. Structural Keys
Structural keys are developed for substructure search systems. The values of the Boolean array for a structure represent the presence or absence of a specific 2D fragment from a fragment dictionary or a pattern dictionary [34]. This fragment dictionary is predefined and includes a list of fragments that are of interest. For molecules in the same database, structural keys are usually all the same size since each bit in the array must represent the same specific fragment/pattern in the dictionary. In order to achieve maximum screening efficiency, two principles should be obeyed when creating the fragment dictionary; independence of occurrence and equal distribution of frequency. A lack of either independence or equal frequency will introduce bias and redundancy. As a consequence, structural properties will not be properly identified, and unwanted results will be obtained during substructure screening. Therefore, dictionary building has generally been an intellectual, manual process that needs careful selection on the basis of the rules described above. Molecular ACCess System (MACCS) keys [35], which are the most commonly used structural keys, were developed by MDL (Molecular Design Limited) back in the late 1970s. MACCS keys come in 166 bit and 960 bit forms. When using MACCS, it is possible to take into account the frequency of occurrence of each fragment instead of a simple presence or absence call [31]. However, even MACCS keys cannot avoid the fundamental disadvantage of structural keys—the lack of generality due to the requirement for a predefined fragment dictionary. If only a few dictionary fragments are contained within a database, structures in the database will be poorly characterized and similar structures will not be identified in a substructure search.

7.4.1.2. Molecular Fingerprints
Compared with structural keys, molecular fingerprints [32, 33, 36] are more abstract and do not need such a predefined fragment/pattern dictionary. Patterns for the molecular fingerprint are generated from the molecule itself. The pattern could be a sequence of linked atoms

with a specific length N. Each atom and bond in this pattern has a numeric value, based on the element type, bond type, and other properties, which form a unique $2 \times N - 1$ valued term. Every pattern in this molecule up to a path length limit is generated. Since these patterns differ from molecule to molecule and the number of patterns is huge for any structure of non-trivial size, it is not possible to assign a particular bit to each pattern, as in the design of structural keys. Instead, a pseudorandom number generator is used to generate an integer for each pattern using the $2 \times N - 1$ valued term as a seed. A modulo operation [37] is performed on this integer divided by the number of bits in the fingerprint to calculate the location of the bit that represents this pattern. Subsequently, this bit will be set to 1. Notably, the bit location of a pattern is determined through a pseudorandom generator; thus a particular bit may not represent a single specific pattern in a fingerprint, but several patterns. Therefore, the fingerprint can indicate that a pattern is missing with 100% certainty when the bit is 0, but it can only indicate that a pattern is present with some probability due to the overlap of bit location. The shorter the length of the fingerprint, the greater the overlap. Such collisions will reduce the accuracy of the fingerprint compared with a structural key. However, since a fingerprint contains a much greater number of patterns than a structural key, the overall efficiency of characterization is increased [33].

Compared with structural keys, there are other advantages to fingerprints. The first is that one fingerprinting system serves all databases and all types of molecules without a predefined set of fragments. The second is the efficiency of the fingerprints. A typical molecule usually has very few fragments in the dictionary built for structural keys, causing structural keys to be very sparse. In contrast, the method of creating a fingerprint makes it more compact without losing specificity. The third advantage is that the patterns that code for a fingerprint are highly overlapping. More information can be generated from complex structures and therefore result in more accurate characterization. The most commonly used fingerprints are the Daylight fingerprint [38] and the UNITY fingerprint [39].

7.4.1.3. Real Value Descriptors   Both structural keys and fingerprints are binary descriptors and can be screened by a simple Boolean operation. The Tanimoto coefficient (Tc) is able to measure similarity between sample sets and is defined as the size of the intersection divided by the size of the union of the sample sets. Here, the Tc of similarity is calculated by counting the number of set bits that are common to each string.

The use of a simple Boolean operation makes them extremely fast for molecular similarity comparison. Real value descriptors such as VolSurf [40] and GRid-INdependent Descriptors (GRIND) [41] are derived from 3D structures, more specifically, from a 3D molecular interaction field (MIF) map. The MIF can be viewed as spatial grid points with attractive and repulsive forces between the molecule and an interacting partner. Real value descriptors extract the information into physicochemically relevant, quantitative numerical values. In VolSurf, the volumes and surfaces of grid points at different energy levels are calculated and summed to generate different types of descriptors. These descriptors include size and shape descriptors, descriptors of hydrophilic regions/hydrophobic regions, interaction energy moments, mixed descriptors referring to the balance between hydrophilic and hydrophobic, hydrogen bonding capacity, and molecular polarizability. In GRIND [41], virtual receptor sites (VRS), where groups of a potential receptor would interact favorably with the ligand, are defined according to the MIF. The VRS regions provide an ideal complementarity for small molecules and represent interactions between small molecules and proteins. Geometric relationships between the VRS regions are encoded by the interactions and distances between each pair of nodes in VRS regions to form GRIND.

Cruciani et al. carried out a comprehensive comparison between UNITY fingerprints, ISIS keys, VolSurf, GRIND, and logP on various databases to examine their clustering behavior from the viewpoint of both pharmacodynamics and pharmacokinetics [42]. VolSurf appears to be the best descriptor to optimize the pharmacokinetic profiles of pharmaceutically relevant compounds. The ranking of descriptor suitability for pharmacodynamics aspects was as follows; UNITY fingerprints > GRIND ≥ ISIS keys > VolSurf descriptors > logP.

7.4.1.4. Feature Keys While structural keys, fingerprints, and real value descriptors are all linear descriptors, that is, bit strings or integer strings, feature trees represent a chemical structure as a reduced topological graph [43–45]. Each node represents a functional group with its physicochemical properties. An edge appears between two nodes if atoms in one node connect with atoms in another node in the chemical structure. Such a representation focuses on structural features that are relevant to drug–receptor binding and the topology between them. The similarity between two reduced graph representations can be identified using clique detection methods [46], split-search and match-search algorithms [43], or dynamic programming [44]. The downside is that matching two graphs is slower than matching two strings. Gillet et al. developed a method to combine the reduced graphs and fingerprints by converting the reduced graphs into pseudo-SMILES (Simplified Molecular Input Line Entry Specification) representations [45]. Daylight fingerprints were then generated from the pseudo-SMILES strings. Gillet et al.'s method was investigated using data derived from the World Drug Index (http://www.daylight.com/products/wdi.html), and shown to be effective for similarity searching and to retrieve more diverse active compounds than those found using Daylight fingerprints.

7.4.1.5. 3D Descriptors The spatial arrangement of functional groups in chemical structures is important for drug–target binding. 3D descriptors are designed to capture such structural information. The most commonly used descriptors are distances and/or angles between atoms, ring centroids, and planes. For example, in the Tripos Unity 3D substructure system [31], ranges of distances are divided into a number of bins, and discrete sets of bits are defined to represent pairs of features (atom types) in different bins. There are two types of 3D features used in the Unity system; rigid features based on distances, and angles measured in a single conformation generated by CONCORD [47] (from 2D chemical structure and flexible features recording all possible distances that a pair of features can achieve). The Unity 3D descriptors are based on atom types and cannot distinguish the same atoms in different chemical groups and different environments. In order to distinguish the behavior of atoms, another type of 3D descriptor has been developed to encode structures in terms of distances and angles between potential pharmacophoric points, including hydrogen bond donors or acceptors, sites of potential positive or negative charge, and hydrophobic atoms. Such descriptors can be generated using a program known as 3D-FEATURE [31]. This program defines various 2D environments according to the rules encoded in the Daylight SMARTS language [48], and relates specific atoms in a given environment to a classification of one or more types of pharmacophoric point. DISCO [49] is another program to generate 3D descriptors. In DISCO, distances between pairs of pharmacophoric points are used to set a string, like in 2D fingerprints. The similarity measuring methods used with 2D fingerprints can also be used in 3D descriptor screening.

The results of compound screening are strongly influenced by changing similarity descriptors. It is surprising to find that 2D descriptors are more effective than 3D descriptors in similarity searching, even though 3D descriptors usually encode more structural information [31, 49]. The major problem associated with 3D descriptors is the conformational flexibility in chemical structures. Inappropriate handling of conformational flexibility can result in poor performance of 3D descriptors. However, the complementarity between 2D and 3D descriptors for chemical structure representation is being recognized by an increasing number of people [50–53]. As described by Shanmugasundaram et al. in their compound identification work for known targets, the candidate compounds selected by four different descriptors after hit-directed nearest-neighbor (HDNN) searching only have an approximately 15% overlap [54]. These four descriptors are 3D, 2D, 2D topological BCUTs (2-DT), and molecular fingerprints. Most identified hits are selected by only one of the alternative methods. The authors suggest that multiple searches based on a variety of molecular representations would provide an effective way to identify more hits during ligand similarity searches. It would therefore be beneficial to design novel algorithms and similarity methods that benefit from their complementary nature.

7.4.1.6. Case Studies with Ligand Similarity Comparison Chemical descriptors and similarity searching methods can be used to predict side effects and polypharmacology, and to reposition chemical agents based on the hypothesis that two similar molecules tend to have similar properties and bind to the same group of proteins. Keiser et al. recently proposed a Similarity Ensemble Approach (SEA) to identify the relationships between protein receptors, quantitatively based on the chemical similarity among their ligands [55]. They extracted ligands from compound databases that annotate molecules by their therapeutic or biological category, such as MDL Drug Data Report (MDDR) [56]. After filtering, 246 targets and a total of 65,241 unique ligands remained, with a median and mean of 124 and 289 ligands per target, respectively. All pairs of ligands between two targets were compared according to pairwise Tc scores [57], which were calculated based on standard 2D topological Daylight fingerprints [58] using default settings of 2048-bit array lengths and path lengths of 2–7 atoms. Keiser et al. found that for most ligand pairs, the Tc was low, that is, in the 0.2 to 0.3 range, even when comparing a set to itself. These pairs were considered to exhibit insubstantial similarity. Thus, in order to compare protein targets, only Tc's above a threshold between ligands across sets were summed, giving a raw score. Furthermore, the authors fitted the raw score to an extreme distribution model to quantify the statistical significance of the ligand similarity. They predicted that methadone, emetine, and loperamide (Imodium®) can antagonize the muscarinic M3, $\alpha 2$ adrenergic, and neurokinin NK2 receptors, respectively. These predictions were subsequently confirmed experimentally [55]. Keiser et al. also calculated the sequence similarity among these protein targets using PSI-BLAST and found that many ligand sets with enzyme targets have similar ligand binding profiles, but are dissimilar in terms of sequence. Noeske et al. developed a self-organizing map approach (SOM) [59] to provide a nonlinear 2D projection of multidimensional chemical space represented by CATS2D [60] descriptors. This approach aided the discovery of the cross-activities of metabotropic glutamate receptor antagonists. These antagonists were predicted to interact with human dopamine D2-like receptors, the histamine H1 receptor, and the muscarinic acetylcholine receptor. Their binding activities were confirmed in pharmacological assays, though only weak binding constants in the low to medium micromolar range were determined [59].

From ligand-based similarities, Hert et al. built chemoinformatics networks for more than 1,600 protein targets derived from the MDDR [56] and WOMBAT [61] databases, and compared them with bioinformatics networks based on the BLAST similarity between sequences [62]. Ligand-based similarities between different proteins were calculated through two different statistical techniques; the SEA [55] and a Bayesian Model [63]. Five 2D fingerprints (Daylight [38], Unity [39], MDL Keys [64], ECFP_4 [65], and FCFP_4 [65]) and two 3D fingerprints (CATS [60] or FEPOPS [66]) were used to describe the chemical structures in ligand sets. Unexpectedly, the chemoinformatics networks were stable to chemical representation. The networks based on five 2D fingerprints were similar and their correlation coefficients varied from 0.783 to 0.940. Thus, even though the overlap between different fingerprints to identify similar chemical compounds was fairly low (~15%) [54], they were able to capture the same information from different ligand sets, and likely afford similar relationships among protein targets when comparing the ligand sets as a whole. Correlations between these 2D fingerprints and 3D fingerprints were lower than those among 2D fingerprints, probably due to the different ways in which the fingerprints are designed. The chemoinformatics and bioinformatics networks differed substantially. Many targets highly related by sequence were unrelated by ligands, and vice versa. Such differences may be caused by the global representation of sequence similarity. Topological network analysis showed that chemoinformatics networks are small-world, which means that most nodes are not directly connected to one another, but they can be reached from each other by a small number of hubs. This property makes chemoinformatics networks more similar to social networks than bioinformatics networks.

7.4.1.7. *Limitations of Ligand-Based Methods*

It is well known that a small change in chemical structure can sometimes dramatically change molecular properties. In such cases, approaches based on chemical similarity no longer work. To explain the dissimilarity of activity among similar molecules, Gerald Maggiora introduced the concept of "activity landscapes" [67]. The landscape can appear as gently rolling hills or rugged canyons where "activity cliffs" occur. In the range of a gently rolling hill, small changes in chemical structure only have a slight effect on molecular activity. In such cases, the basic hypothesis of chemical similarity approaches still remains true. However, in cliff regions, the structure–activity relationship is discontinuous and therefore similarity analysis is meaningless [68].

Another issue in chemical similarity searching is that the activity landscape varies with changes in the chemical descriptors used to represent the chemical structure. Neighboring compounds in one chemical-space representation may not be neighbors in another. Such a lack of invariance has been observed in several studies [54] and will result in inaccurate ligand similarity predictions. Fortunately, Hert's work [62] shows that the chemoinformatics networks for protein targets remain stable to changes in chemical representation.

A further issue is the accuracy of input data for chemoinformatics studies. Recent work reported a significant error rate in the medicinal chemistry literature [61] and several popular public databases of bioactive molecules [69, 70], and also highlighted the importance of chemical data curation in quantitative structure–activity relationship (QSAR) modeling. In a recent study, Fourches et al. [69] proposed a general chemical dataset curation workflow and suggested several important rules when using chemical data. Descriptors calculated indirectly from curated 2D chemical structures from SMILES are preferred. Thoroughly curated chemical data on both chemical structure and associated target property values will provide a remarkable contribution to the field of chemoinformatics in the same way that the Protein Data Bank (PDB) does for the structural biology community.

7.4.2. Ligand Binding Site Similarity-Based Approaches

One hundred years ago, the Nobel Laureate organic chemist Emil Fischer introduced a "lock and key" model to explain enzyme specificity [71]. The geometric shape complementarity and physicochemical complementarity provide the basic principle for most drug–target screening methods based on binding site comparison: Similar binding sites usually mean similar ligand binding. Binding site similarity analysis provides information about whether binding sites are common among proteins and what parts of binding sites are important for binding. When 3D structures of the protein targets of interest are available, structural bioinformatics methods can be employed to compare protein–ligand binding sites, thereby providing valuable insight into likely promiscuity and selectivity both within and across gene families [3]. Binding sites are usually pockets or crevices on the protein surface. Therefore, the detection and characterization of protein–ligand binding sites is the first step in binding site comparison. Binding site detection and characterization methods are usually developed to describe geometric shape, physicochemical properties, energetic properties (solvation, hydrophobicity, and electrostatics), and sequence information. A recent review [72] gives a detailed summary of these methods. Here, we will focus on the second step; comparison of binding site similarity. Indeed, through the use of binding site comparison software, it is possible to identify all potential off-targets of a particular drug on a proteome-wide scale. It is likely that some of these off-targets will represent viable drug targets, therefore providing opportunities to repurpose that particular drug to target different pathways and to treat different diseases. Many groups have been actively employing this methodology with the ultimate intention of repurposing a number of different drugs, as we will describe in the following section.

As with chemical similarity comparison, MIF descriptors can be used in protein binding site comparison. Similarity indices were originally derived to compare the electrostatic fields/potentials of small molecules obtained from quantum mechanics calculations [73]. Alternative expressions of similarity indices were then developed to compare the MIFs computed by classical molecular mechanics of both small molecules and protein structures [74, 75]. Electrostatic potential-based similarity comparison was applied to a large-scale classification of the Pleckstrin homology (PH) domain family [74]. In this method, the similarity index for two binding pockets was calculated by an analytical expression of the scalar product of two electrostatic potentials over a spherical layer of superimposed binding pockets. The binding pockets were represented by an angular extent of the functional region (usually ranging from 10° to 90°), a thickness value of the spherical layer, and a vector pointing to the location of the functional sites. Similarity analysis showed that the electrostatic properties of the PH domains are generally conserved despite extreme sequence divergence within the family, indicating common phospholipid binding sites. Electrostatic properties of protein structures were calculated with a continuum solvation model by finite difference solution of the Poisson–Boltzmann equation [76], or analytically as a multipole expansion [75] that permits rapid comparison of very large datasets. A simplified analytical expression can reproduce electrostatic potential similarities calculated from the linear Poisson–Boltzmann equation [74]. In order to test the application of this method on high-throughput homology models, the similarity indices of the electrostatic potentials calculated from model structures were compared with those calculated from crystal structures [74]. Strong correlation between the two sets of similarity indices indicates the robustness of this method to homology models. Following the same idea, a web server, webPIPSA [77], was released to provide an automatic workflow to describe, compare, and analyze electrostatic potentials for protein structures or homology models of proteins from different species. Electrostatic potential comparison can identify electrostatic features that are important for binding and catalysis. Wade et al. [75] identified conserved potentials responsible for electrostatic substrate-steering fields and found that they act as the primary determinants of biomolecular association rates. Such applications indicate the important role of electrostatic potential in the binding process of both charged and nonpolar ligands.

The FLAP algorithm (Fingerprints for Ligands and Proteins) provides a different way of comparing two binding sites using a common reference framework of four-point pharmacophore fingerprints and a molecular-cavity shape [78]. This method starts from MIFs produced by running different GRID probes over the target binding sites and mapping their energetic interactions with the protein structure using a GRID force field [79, 80]. These probes should represent all possible functional groups for potential ligands in the binding sites. The GRID–MIFs are then condensed into a total of 100 or 200 pharmacophoric points by using a weighted energy-based and space-coverage function. These points are characterized by the type of energetic interaction, interaction energy value, and Cartesian coordinates for its position in the protein. All possible arrangements of tetrahedrons containing four pharmacophoric points are selected to represent the binding cavity. Each tetrahedron is represented by a vector containing 11 integers (six values of distances, the indices of four site points, and a value proportional to the sum of the energies of the four points). Vectors for all possible tetrahedrons in a binding site produce a large matrix, known as a 3D pharmacophore fingerprint of the binding site. The locations of vectors in the fingerprints are determined by the tetrahedron volume, type, and chirality. Similar fingerprints could also be generated for ligands based on the coordinates of each ligand atom. Thus, FLAP provides a common reference framework for both ligands and proteins to compare protein and ligand pharmacophore fingerprints, pairwise ligand fingerprints, and pairwise protein pharmacophore fingerprints. During similarity searching, conformational flexibility of the ligand in the binding site is considered by allowing fluctuations of pharmacophoric points. This approach was tested to cluster the active sites of specific protein kinases into distinct subfamilies [81]. The prediction of protein kinase clusters was consistent with the classification of protein kinase subfamilies. This method also produced favorable results for kinase specificity prediction and high-throughput protein virtual screening.

The PharmMapper server is a free web-based tool for identifying potential drug targets for any given small molecule via a "reverse" pharmacophore mapping approach [82]. This server collects 3D pharmacophore models describing the binding modes of known ligands at the binding sites of protein–ligand complexes selected from the DrugBank [83], BindingDB [84], PDBbind [85], and PDTD [86] databases. The pharmacophore models were extracted by LigandScout [87] and deposited in PharmTargetDB. A set of pharmacophoric features was created to reflect the specific ligand–receptor interaction at each binding site, including hydrophobic center, positively charged center, negatively charged center, hydrogen bond acceptor vector, hydrogen bond donor vector, aromatic plane, and one optional feature. The query molecule is aligned onto each pharmacophore model of each protein in the target list using a combination of geometric hashing and a genetic algorithm [88]. The top ranked proteins are then selected as potential targets of the query molecule. In a benchmark study, the PharmMapper method detected 29% of the experimentally confirmed protein targets of tamoxifen among the top 100 predicted candidates, and 71% among the top 300 predicted candidates, therefore indicating its reliability [82].

Pharmacophore models may be used to guide the design of compounds that can inhibit two or more specific proteins simultaneously, in cases where the simultaneous inhibition of these proteins is found to have the desired effect on phenotype. One such example is the design of a series of dual inhibitors of acetylcholinesterase (AChE) and the serotonin transporter (SERT) by Toda et al. in 2003 [2, 89]. Firstly, the authors derived a model of the AChE binding site from the X-ray crystal structure of AChE with the bound inhibitor donepezil. They then combined this model with the pharmacophores of rivastigmine (another AChE inhibitor) and fluoxetine (a SERT inhibitor), and used this combined pharmacophore model to guide compound design. Similarly, in 2004, Aronov and Murcko derived a pharmacophore of molecular features common to the binding of promiscuous kinase inhibitors from protein structural information [2, 90]. When queried against a test set, their pharmacophore was able to successfully identify promiscuous kinase inhibitors. High-throughput screening (HTS) of thousands of compounds against these selected targets can also detect a single compound that will inhibit them simultaneously. However, since HTS against multiple targets is extremely time-consuming and expensive, structure-based drug design would be a more sensible approach to take.

Relibase is an object-oriented database system designed to show detailed information about particular protein entries or ligands in the PDB [91]. The binding site environment within 7 Å around every ligand is pre-calculated and stored. Ligand binding site similarity is evaluated by superimposing homologous protein structures onto a reference binding site. Another object-oriented database, Cavbase [92], fully integrates with Relibase and assigns descriptors to binding sites with generic pseudocenters encoding cavity properties. Each pseudocenter represents one type of property that is important in protein–ligand binding, including hydrogen bond donor, hydrogen bond acceptor, mixed donor/acceptor, and hydrophobic aliphatic and aromatic π interactions. A clique detection algorithm is implemented to detect a common motif between two cavities. Multiple clique solutions are generated and scored according to the property-based surface patches shared by different clique solutions. The best scoring solution is produced among all generated comparisons. Such a study provides a new classification of protein structures in terms of cavity similarity. Following the pseudocenter definitions developed in Cavbase, a smooth molecular surface was constructed in the SiteEngine method [93], and only pseudocenters that represent at least one surface exposed atom were retained. For each query protein, the surface region within 4 Å of the binding partner is referred to as the binding site. The binding site is then superimposed on a similar surface region of another protein by the efficient hashing and matching of triangles defined by triplets of pseudocenters. All possible transformations are listed and scored according to the similarity of the physicochemical properties and shapes of triangles on aligned surface regions. The top ranked solutions are then selected for comparison between the query protein and the other protein. This method can be extended to compare protein–protein interfaces and to recognize complexes with similar binding organization and biological functions. Both methods can be useful in drug discovery and the prediction of side effects. A triangular transformation is also implemented in the SuMo (Surfing the Molecules) software, in which protein structures are represented by a set of stereochemical groups. Graphs of triangles of chemical groups are then used to detect similarities between binding sites [94].

In 2004, Brakoulias and Jackson developed a geometric matching method that proceeds by identifying equivalent heavy atom constellations between pairs of binding sites [95]. Matching atom–atom correspondences are those that occur in the same relative spatial orientation and have the same element type. Similarity is measured by an atom–atom score, that is, the number of atoms comprising the largest possible matching constellation. In 2005, Morris et al. developed a binding site comparison method that uses the coefficients of a real spherical harmonics expansion to describe the shape of a protein binding site [96]. In 2008, Yeturu and Chandra presented the algorithm PocketMatch, in which each binding site is represented by 90 lists of sorted distances that capture its shape and chemical nature [97]. In order to obtain a similarity score for a pair of binding sites, the sorted arrays are aligned using an incremental alignment method. After validating their method using the PDBbind database of experimentally determined protein–ligand complexes, they integrated it into a target identification pipeline for *M. tuberculosis* [98]. They used PocketMatch to compare the binding sites of their shortlisted *M. tuberculosis* targets with those of the human proteome, and removed those shortlisted targets that showed significant similarity to human proteins, since targeting them could result in adverse side effects. Another approach for pocket comparison was developed based on a shape matching and object recognition method using shape context descriptors [99]. Atoms in the binding pocket are grouped into certain atom types that define their physical chemical properties. In order to consider the flexibility of a side chain, side chain atoms are encoded by a representative atom in the side chain. The shape of the pocket with respect to a given atom lining the cavity is described by a shape context descriptor, the occurrence of different atom types within spheres of radius r centered on the given point. A similarity score is assigned to each pair of atoms from two pockets to measure the match of their shape contexts. The best alignment between two pockets is obtained by using the Procrustes algorithm [100], starting from equivalent atoms in two pockets with a similarity score lower than a given threshold, to minimize the overall similarity score. The two pockets are superimposed according to their best alignment. Finally, the root mean square deviation (RMSD) of Cartesian coordinates between superimposed pockets is added to the overall similarity score to take into account the 3D geometrical features between the compared pockets. The method was validated using a set of 17 inhibitors with K_d measured across 189 kinases, and it retrieved targets with $K_d < 10 \ \mu M$ at 10% receiver operating characteristic (ROC) enrichment [99].

Xie and Bourne recently developed the efficient and robust ligand binding site comparison software, structural matching algorithm for off-target prediction (SMAP) [101, 102], which is based on a sequence order independent profile-profile alignment (SOIPPA) algorithm [103]. Protein structures are represented by Cα atoms only, making it computationally efficient and applicable to low resolution structures and homology models on a proteome-wide scale. The structure is then Delaunay tessellated and partitioned into a set of tetrahedra. Each Cα atom is characterized by a geometric potential depending on the atom's distance to the environmental boundary and the distances and directions to neighboring Cα atoms. It has been shown that both the location and the boundary of the ligand binding site can be accurately predicted using the geometric potential [104]. Figure 7.2 shows the steps to determine the geometric potentials for Cα atoms in the ligand binding site. Besides the geometric potential, each Cα atom is assigned a probability distribution and a position-specific score matrix (PSSM) of 20 amino acids, which are taken directly from a PSI-BLAST database search, using the sequence of the structure as a query. In doing so, both the geometric and evolutionary properties of functional sites are included in the descriptors. The protein is then scanned and aligned to the functional site of the query protein using the SOIPPA, which is based on a fast, maximum weighted sub-graph (MWSG) algorithm [105]. The MWSG finds the most similar surface patch without *a priori* knowledge of the location and boundary of functional sites [106]. This feature makes SMAP appropriate to practical problems since typically the boundary of the ligand binding site is not clearly defined and depends on the bound ligand.

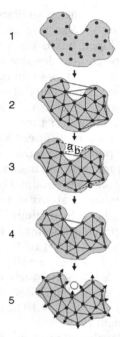

FIGURE 7.2. Overview of the Geometric Potential algorithm for ligand binding site characterization and prediction [104]. The solid body and circles indicate an all-atom and Cα atom representation, respectively. Open circles are virtual atoms determined by the algorithm. (1) The protein structure is represented as Cα atoms. (2) Cα atoms are Delaunay tessellated. The convex hull is determined at the same time. (3) The environmental boundary (solid lines) is determined from the Delaunay tessellation by peeling off the tetrahedra (triangles labeled a, b, and c) with edge lengths longer than 30 Å (black dashed lines) starting from the convex hull. (4) Portions of the protein boundary are overlapped with the environmental boundary and determined from the Delaunay tessellation by removing tetrahedra with a circumscribed sphere radius larger than 7.5 Å. (5) Shape descriptors such as residue surface direction and geometric potential for each Cα atom position are computed and ligand binding sites and virtual atoms (open circle) are predicted.

Finally, the aligned surface patches are ranked by a scoring function that combines evolutionary, geometric, and physical information. The statistical significance of the binding site similarity is then rapidly computed using a unified statistical model derived from an extreme value distribution [107]. SMAP was evaluated on a benchmark set and a control group that included 247 and 101 non-redundant protein chains of diverse folds with and without adenine binding pockets, respectively. The results showed that SMAP outperformed a number of existing algorithms in terms of ligand binding site alignment quality, and database search sensitivity and specificity [103].

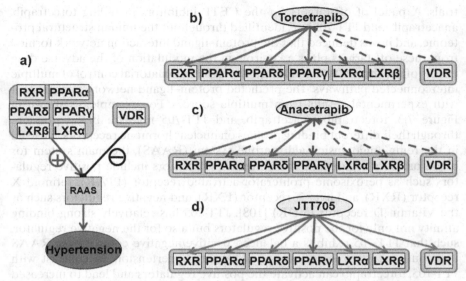

FIGURE 7.3. Effects of torcetrapib, anacetrapib, and JTT-705 on regulating the RAAS system through the combinational control of nuclear hormone receptors [102]. The dark gray solid, gray solid, and dashed lines between inhibitors and off-targets indicate strong, relatively strong, and weak binding affinities, respectively. The dark gray and black lines between off-targets and pathways or clinical indications represent positive and negative regulation, respectively. (a) Regulation control of nuclear hormone receptors on the RAAS system. (b) Binding profile of torcetrapib on nuclear hormone receptors. (c) Binding profile of anacetrapib on nuclear hormone receptors. (d) Binding profile of JTT-705 on nuclear hormone receptors.

The ability of SMAP to establish cross-fold ligand–drug relationships and its application to drug discovery has been proven by several recent studies. For example, by providing a list of potential off-targets using SMAP, Xie et al. elucidated a possible molecular mechanism for the observed side effects of selective estrogen receptor modulators (SERMs), which are widely used to treat and prevent breast cancer and other diseases [101]. They discovered that the side effects may be caused by the inhibition of the sarcoplasmic reticulum Ca^{2+} ion channel ATPase (SERCA) protein transmembrane domain. Their prediction provided molecular insight into reducing the adverse effects of SERMs and was supported by both clinical and *in vitro* observations [101]. In another study, SMAP was applied to explore the molecular mechanisms behind the known side effects of torcetrapib, a cholesteryl ester transfer protein (CETP) inhibitor, by mapping the predicted off-target network to interconnected signal transduction, gene regulatory, and metabolic networks [102]. Torcetrapib was in development as a preventive therapy for cardiovascular disease. However, clinical studies indicated that it had off-target effects that resulted in hypertension, and it was withdrawn from Phase III clinical trials. A panel of off-targets for the CETP inhibitors including torcetrapib, anacetrapib, and JTT-705 was identified throughout the human structural proteome, and it was deduced that the protein–ligand interaction network formed from these off-targets plays a key role in the modulation of the adverse drug effects of the three CETP inhibitors, through combinatorial control of multiple interconnected pathways. The predicted protein–ligand network is consistent with experimental results from multiple sources. For example, as shown in Figure 7.3, torcetrapib, anacetrapib, and JTT-705 regulate blood pressure through their different binding profiles on nuclear hormone receptors involved in the renin-angiotension-aldosterone system (RAAS), the main system for blood pressure regulation. These hormone receptors include positive regulators such as peroxisome proliferator-activated receptor (PPAR), retinoid X receptor (RXR), and liver X receptor (LXR), and negative regulators such as the Vitamin D receptor (VDR) [108]. JTT-705 has relatively strong binding affinity not only for the positive regulators but also for the negative regulator, such that JTT-705 exhibits a balanced positive/negative control over RAAS and consequently a lesser chance of causing hypertension. In contrast with JTT-705, torcetrapib can activate the positive regulators and lead to increased blood pressure through upregulation of RAAS. Anacetrapib can only bind to RXR and PPARδ in their active conformations and PPARα and VDR in their inactive conformations. Thus, anacetrapib has less effect on both the positive and negative control of blood pressure, and its negative effect on blood pressure regulation may be less than that of torcetrapib.

The value of SMAP in drug repositioning has been demonstrated through the discovery that the commercially available drugs entacapone and tolcapone, which are prescribed for the treatment of Parkinson's disease, have the potential to treat MDR and XDR tuberculosis [109]. SMAP detected that the substrate binding site of *M. tuberculosis* enoyl-acyl carrier protein reductase (InhA), a drug target for the treatment of tuberculosis, is similar to that of human catechol-*O*-methyltransferase (COMT), a drug target used in the treatment of Parkinson's disease [109]. Although InhA and COMT belong to different structural folds, their binding site similarity indicated that safe pharmaceuticals such as entacapone, an inhibitor of COMT, could potentially be repurposed to directly inhibit InhA. More convincingly, enzyme kinetic assays confirmed that entacapone inhibits *M. tuberculosis* InhA with an MIC99 of approximately 260 μM and an IC_{50} value of approximately 80 μM, well below the toxicity concentration (500 μM) determined by an *in vitro* cytotoxicity model using a human neuroblastoma cell line [110]. In another study, SMAP results showed that the protein kinase, ATP grasp, and phosphoribosylaminoimidazole-succinocarboxamide synthesase-like superfamilies share highly significant similarities in their ligand binding sites [103]. The cross-reactivity between the protein kinase and ATP grasp superfamilies was later experimentally confirmed by Miller et al. [111], who repurposed libraries of protein kinase inhibitors to target carboxyltransferases, members of the ATP grasp superfamily. Most recently, this method identified a panel of protein kinases whose ATP binding sites are significantly similar to the inhibitor binding site in the HIV protease dimer [18]. In addition, the predicted protein kinase off-targets have favorable hydrogen bonding and electrostatic interactions with nelfinavir, an HIV protease inhibitor. By mapping the protein–ligand interaction network to the human PI3K/AKT signal transduction pathway, Xie et al. were able to rationalize the clinically observed pleiotropic effects of nelfinavir in human cancer and diabetes [18]. These encouraging results indicate that SMAP is a powerful tool for analyzing protein promiscuity at the binding site level and thus to facilitate multitarget drug design.

7.4.3. Structure-Based Virtual Ligand Screening

If 3D protein structures of a target of interest are available, then computational docking can be used to prioritize sets of compounds against the target— a method known as virtual screening. Structure-based virtual screening provides an efficient way to discover relationships between chemical ligands and targets through the simulation and modeling of their physical interactions. Traditional virtual screening starts with the 3D structure of the target of interest obtained either by X-ray crystallography, nuclear magnetic resonance (NMR) experiments, or homology modeling, to identify promising compounds that may bind to that target. In inverse virtual screening, a high number of protein structures are screened against the structure of a compound of interest in order to detect additional targets and novel uses for that compound. The docking process, which binds protein and ligand structures together, has been gaining significant attention in both traditional and inverse virtual screening. A docking program usually consists of two parts [112]; a searching method to explore the conformational space and a scoring function to evaluate the binding affinity. Searching and scoring are often highly coupled in docking; the searching algorithm should generate an optimum number of conformations, including native-like modes for ligands, and the scoring function should rank these conformations accurately and select the native-like binding modes.

The most commonly used searching methods are stochastic algorithms such as Monte Carlo (MC) methods and genetic algorithms. MC methods [113] are among the most widely used stochastic optimization techniques. These methods generate conformations randomly and accept or reject these conformations based on a Boltzmann distribution. Modeling starts with a high, effective temperature, which means a larger chance of acceptance. The effective temperature of the modeled system decreases over time until a minimized docking position is obtained. Genetic algorithms are another type of stochastic searching algorithm, and are derived from the evolutionary ideas of natural selection and genetics. Conformations are generated through mutations and crossover transformations between previous conformations. Genetic algorithms are implemented in a range of docking programs [114]. Energy minimization and molecular simulation can also provide powerful tools for conformational searching. Among the most commonly used docking programs, AutoDock [115], uses both MC-simulated annealing and a genetic algorithm for ligand conformational sampling. GOLD [116] utilizes a genetic algorithm for conformational search. Darwin [117] combines a genetic algorithm with a gradient minimization search strategy. Another type of searching algorithm is based on fragment reconstruction of the ligand molecule [118]. Fragments are generated by breaking rotational bonds, and these fragments are docked separately into the binding site. All possible connections of fragments with favorable energies are retained in order to reconstruct the ligand conformation. FlexX [119] and Dock [120] use such fragment-based methods to generate a large number of conformations in a short time. A third type of searching algorithm firstly generates low-energy conformations in the gas phase and then places these conformations into the binding pocket to produce more binding modes by perturbing six rotational and translational degrees of freedom in rigid conformations. Searching algorithms in Slide [121] and Fred [122] utilize this type of searching method.

Scoring functions measure the interactions between proteins and ligands in order to select the best conformation of a single ligand in the protein binding pocket, and to estimate the binding affinities of different protein–ligand complexes. Different types of interactions contribute to scoring functions, such as van der Waal's interactions, electrostatic interactions, dispersion interactions, hydrogen bonding interactions, hydrophobic effects, and solvation effects. Scoring functions in docking programs always make some assumptions and simplifications to constitute a compromise between accuracy and computational effort. Based on their strategy of simplification, scoring functions can be categorized as force-field-based, empirical-based, knowledge-based, or consensus scoring functions [123]. Force-field-based scoring functions obey energy landscape theory to describe the potential energy surface by summing up different energies between ligand and protein atoms. In principle, such functions are more accurate in estimating binding free energies. Similar to force-field functions, empirical-based functions are composed of a set of parameterized function terms. The coefficients of various terms are fitted by regression analysis to reproduce experimental data. Thus, the accuracy of this type of function depends on the datasets used in the regression analysis and fitting. In knowledge-based scoring functions, atomic interactions are defined by statistically accounting for molecular environments, such as distances between different types of atoms and the hydrophobic and solvation environments of atoms, from a database of protein–ligand complexes. The simplicity of such scoring functions makes them computationally efficient. Like empirical-based functions, the disadvantage of knowledge-based functions is the limitation resulting from protein–ligand complex structural databases. Considering the limitations of the above three types of scoring functions, consensus scoring functions may provide a better estimation of binding infinities by combining information from different scoring functions to balance errors in single scoring functions [124].

Many conventional docking algorithms treat the protein as rigid; however, in reality, binding sites adjust in order to accommodate structurally distinct ligands. On the other hand, many ligand binding sites are characterized by a degree of structural plasticity, and even similar ligands can differ in binding conformation and/or orientation. A recent study found that ligands can also use distinct conformations to bind both active and inactive conformations of the estrogen receptor, and induce corresponding changes in transcriptional activity [125]. This work suggests that protein–ligand interactions should be studied by coupling protein conformational states with ligand binding poses. Accordingly, many newer docking algorithms take into account receptor flexibility. However, the task of identifying the most stable conformation of the protein–ligand complex becomes much more computationally intensive due to the large number of degrees of freedom possessed by the receptor. Numerous different methods have been devised to address this problem, including docking into multiple receptor structures individually, averaging the coordinates of multiple receptor structures to create a single site for docking, softening a single receptor conformation in order to approximate flexibility, re-optimizing the conformation of the binding site during the docking process itself, and generating a representative ensemble from a molecular dynamics trajectory [126]. The high false positive rate associated with conventional virtual screening is significantly reduced when considering the flexibility of ligand–receptor complexes. For example, this protocol was used to identify drug-like inhibitors of an essential RNA-editing ligase in *Trypanosoma brucei*. Subsequent experiments validated most of the top ranked predictions [127]. The identified off-targets have strong implications for developing new multi-target drugs to treat this neglected yet deadly disease, African sleeping sickness, with both efficacy and a desired safety profile. On the one hand, the lead compound can be optimized to inhibit both *T. brucei* RNA-editing ligase and UDP-galactose 4′ epimerase, both of which are validated drug targets known to be required for *T. brucei* survival. On the other hand, the identification of the human off-targets, mitochondrial 2-enoyl thioester reductase and DNA ligase III beta, will greatly increase the success rate of drug development, since any potential side effects can be evaluated and minimized at an early stage.

Ideally, the performance of docking methods would be evaluated by assessing their ability to prospectively predict ligand binding affinities [128]. However, since this is still unachievable, docking methods are commonly evaluated using one or more of the following criteria; (1) their ability to discriminate actives from among a database of decoys ("enrichment"), (2) their ability to reproduce the correct bound conformation of the ligand ("pose fidelity"), and (3) their ability to produce scores that correlate well with the measured binding affinities of known ligands. Although existing methods often provide significant enrichment and produce accurate binding poses, docking scores notoriously show poor correlation with experimentally determined binding affinities across a series of compounds. Such limitations can be attributed to the simplicity of scoring functions, which are primarily designed for high-throughput analyses. While docking methods focus on a single bound conformation of the ligand, free energy methods generate thermodynamic averages through the use of conformational sampling. Unlike docking, free energy methods are not sensitive to the details of a single representative ligand conformation, and as a result can provide a much more accurate calculation of protein–ligand binding affinity. However, free energy methods are much more time-consuming and computationally intensive than docking methods, and the conformational searches tend to be less exhaustive [126].

Despite its shortcomings, the use of docking in virtual screening still has clear advantages over high-throughput screening. Indeed, virtual screening can access far more chemistry, much faster, and at a much lower cost. The top scoring compounds from virtual screening can then be tested rapidly, and although only a few of them are likely to actually bind the target, even a couple of novel hits can be extremely useful [128]. While docking may be useful for the virtual screening of a set of compounds against a single target, docking on a large scale against multiple targets is hindered by its high computational complexity during conformational searching, and a lack of practical methodologies to accurately estimate binding affinities [129]. In order to identify all possible proteins that can bind a specified ligand, it is not feasible to dock the ligand into all proteins in the whole structural genome, especially in those cases when both the location and the boundary of the binding site are unknown. Geometric properties of the protein structure, such as pockets and cavities, and evolutionary linkages between proteins across fold and function space can provide rational constraints to address this problem [103, 104]. Indeed, the prior identification of similar ligand binding sites across gene families will significantly reduce the search space that docking needs to address.

7.5. MOLECULAR ACTIVITY SIMILARITY-BASED METHODS

A bioactivity-guided mapping of chemical space may improve the correlation between chemical structure and bioactivity [130–132]. Recently, chemogenomics has emerged as a new discipline to systematically establish target relationships based on the biological similarity of their ligands [133–143]. Polypharmacology can be assessed by integrating *in silico* methods with ligand profiling against protein assays and gene expression arrays. For instance, by extracting data from gene ontologies and metabolic databases such as KEGG [144], it is possible to relate proteins that bind the same or similar compounds. Alternatively, gene expression profiles or phenotypic data, such as clinical side effects, can be used to cluster ligands by functional effects. Such methods facilitate the discovery of previously unknown molecular mechanisms [3].

As discussed in detail in Chapter 5, by using gene expression profiles corresponding to drug treatments, Connectivity Map [145] provides a genetic solution to establish the relationship among diseases, physiological processes, and drugs. The perturbation of mRNA expression assayed on DNA microarrays acts as a genomic signature to describe cellular responses to drug therapeutics. This signature is a list of genes rank-ordered according to their differential expression relative to the control (gene expression in the same condition without drug treatments). Genomic signatures for a broad range of FDA-approved drugs and non-drug bioactive compounds in different concentrations, duration times, and cell lines are collected to build the reference gene expression profile database. A query signature corresponding to a treatment is compared with reference signatures to identify small molecules with similar effects using a nonparametric, rank-based pattern-matching strategy based on the Kolmogorov–Smirnov statistic [146, 147]. This approach was validated by a histone deacetylase 4 (HDAC4) inhibitor experiment to recover the same group of HDAC4 inhibitors in the reference database, successfully identifying estrogen receptor agonists and antagonists and facilitating the repositioning of phenothiazine antipyschotics [145]. Since no structural information about drugs and targets is required by Connectivity Map, this method can be used to elucidate the mechanism of action of uncharacterized small molecules without known structures. As an example, the mechanism of the natural product gedunin, a heat shock protein inhibitor to abrogate the androgen receptor activation in prostate cancer cells, was discovered through the high connectivity scores of gedunin to multiple instances of heat shock protein inhibitors [148]. More interestingly, Connectivity Map can be used to identify small molecules that could induce or suppress diseases if the query signatures from disease states are available. Candidate drugs have also been suggested for diet-induced obesity, Alzheimer's disease, dexamethasone resistance, and glucocorticoid resistance in acute lymphoblastic leukemia [149].

A limitation of Connectivity Map is how to choose the subset of genes composing the signature from multiple gene expression profiles in different cell lines and experimental conditions for the same drug. Even though the most differentially expressed genes can be identified by backtracking expression changes onto known biological pathways, success is limited due to the complexity of such attempts. In order to overcome this problem, Iorio et al. developed an approach [150] to calculate a "consensus" synthetic gene expression profile by combining all of the transcriptional effects of the same drug across multiple treatments on different cell lines and/or at different concentrations. The ranked list of genes for the "consensus" synthetic gene expression profile is called the Prototype Ranked List (PRL). Contributions of each transcriptional response across different cell lines and different conditions are equally weighted and merged into the PRL by a hierarchical majority-voting scheme [151]. The PRL provides a single, unique signature, captures the consensus transcriptional response for a drug, and consistently reduces irrelevant effects due to toxicity, dosage, and cell line. A drug network can be constructed by connecting drug pairs whose consensus responses are similar. Using this method, Iorio et al. [151] constructed a drug similarity network from a dataset containing genome-wide expression profiles following treatment with more than a thousand compounds. Based on the drug similarity network, a web server, Mode of Action by Network Analysis (MANTRA, http://mantra. tigem.it), was then developed to explore the drug network for the classification of previously uncharacterized compounds. From their network they were able to identify known similarities in drug mode of action, therefore suggesting that it could be used for the identification of the mode of action of new compounds. By analyzing corresponding drug networks, known and uncharacterized HSP90 inhibitors, topoisomerase inhibitors, and cyclin-dependent kinase (CDK) inhibitors were correctly classified [151]. In addition, a novel activity predicted for fasudil, a well-characterized drug for cerebral vasospasm, known to promote cellular autophagy, was experimentally verified, enabling it to be exploited for disorders caused by protein misfolding, such as neurodegenerative diseases [150].

The perturbation of gene expression is a genetic response to drug treatment. Conversely, drug side effects are phenomenological observations attributed to genetic or biochemical changes, and they reflect a number of molecular activities including drug–drug interference, metabolic activities, drug kinetic effects, downstream pathway perturbations, and most importantly, drug–target interactions. Similar side effects of unrelated drugs indicate similar protein binding profiles or commonly shared protein targets [152, 153]. Thus, drug side effects can also be used as signatures to detect connections between drugs that are not inferred by their chemical similarity or the sequence and structural similarity of their primary targets. Campillos et al. developed a method to determine whether two drugs share a common target by measuring the phenotypic side effect similarity between two drugs [154]. The side effect concepts were extracted from the Unified Medical Language System (UMLS) [155] metathesaurus to build a dictionary of side effects. Text-mining techniques were used to search for matches to the dictionary from the side effect and indication area sections in the package inserts of individual drugs available from the FDA, manufacturers, and public websites. Side effects were encoded in a binary fashion to define a side effect signature for each drug. Similarity between two drugs was determined by the number of shared side effect concepts. A benchmark test showed an inverse correlation between side effect frequency and the likelihood of two drugs sharing a common target. Thus, the similarity score is weighted by the negative logarithm of the side effect frequency. Another weighting score was used to correct the independence between different side effects by a method analogous to the down-weighting scheme within multiple sequence alignments [156]. This method was tested on a reference set of 502 drugs with known targets. In the reference set, 6.9% of drug pairs were known to have common targets. 2678 pairs were predicted to share targets based on their side effect similarity, of which 956 (35.7%) were known to have common targets. Enrichment of true positives in the predicted result showed a clear correlation between side effect similarity and the possibility of two drugs sharing the same target [154]. The authors then applied their methodology to 746 marketed drugs and derived a network of 1018 side effect-driven drug–drug relations, 261 of which involved drugs that were chemically dissimilar and used in the treatment of different diseases. A number of their predictions were subsequently confirmed experimentally, therefore suggesting new uses for existing drugs. More recently, the authors have integrated this information into a freely available side effect resource (SIDER) that connects 888 drugs to 1,450 side effect terms [157].

Side effect similarity and structural similarity between drugs are used to explore drug–target relations in PROMISCUOUS [158], a database for network-based drug-repositioning. By integrating relationships between drugs, targets, and side effects, PROMISCUOUS provides a public resource to predict off-target effects, and to establish and analyze networks responsible for polypharmacology. Drugs, proteins, and side effects are connected through drug–target, drug side effect, protein–protein, and drug–drug relationships to form a comprehensive network consisting of 12,000 proteins and 104,000 associated interactions, as well as 21,500 relationships connecting 5000 drugs with 6500 target proteins. The integrated network visualization tool implemented in PROMISCUOUS allows an interactive analysis of the network and provides useful information for drug repositioning.

Many past examples have informed us that if two diseases share a common subset of therapies, then alternative drugs for one disease could be potential therapeutics for treating the other, including rivastigmine for the treatment of Alzheimer's disease and Parkinson's disease [159], and bevacizumab for the treatment of colorectal cancer and non-squamous non-small-cell lung cancer [160]. Based on this idea, Chiang and Butte implemented a network-based, guilt-by-association method to perform a systematic pairwise comparison for the treatment profiles of 726 diseases and 2022 drugs derived from the Drug-Disease Knowledge Base (DrDKB) [26]. Novel drug uses were predicted based on the overlap of treatment profiles between disease pairs. From the 5549 disease pairs that shared at least one FDA-approved drug in common under the FDA-approved view, a final total of 57,542 unique novel drug uses were suggested. Even though the underlying idea is oversimplified and lacking theoretical support, the drug uses suggested by this method were 12 times more likely to be in a clinical trial than those drug uses not suggested. The performance of this method was further validated by the enrichments in clinical trials of the predicted novel uses for rituximab and atorvastatin. Of 107 diseases that were predicted to be treated with rituximab, 59 were subject to ongoing clinical trials in 2009 with rituximab, and 6 of them are already known and in practice (found in DrDKB). Among 75 novel drug uses suggested for atorvastatin, 37 were found to be in ongoing atorvastatin clinical trials, and 6 are already known and in practice [26]. In addition to discovering more human disease relationships, Suthram et al. developed a disease comparison method by integrating disease-related mRNA expression and human PPI networks [161]. In this method, the gene expression data were selected from the National Center for Biotechnology Information (NCBI) Gene Expression Omnibus

(GEO) [162], and assigned to human disease conditions by connecting their Medical Subject Headings (MeSH) [163] terms to disease concepts through the UMLS [155]. For each disease, the gene expression data were first normalized using the Z-score transformation in order to allow the direct comparison of gene expression profiles across different microarray samples and diseases. The gene response score for a given disease was measured through a t-test statistic of the Z-transformed scores between the disease and the control samples. PPI data from humans were extracted from the Human Protein Reference Database (HPRD) [164]. Conserved functional modules in the human PPI network were identified by the PathBLAST family of network alignment tools [165]. Each module contains several genes presented in the gene expression profile. The mean of the gene response scores of the component genes in a module was assigned as the module response score. A vector of module response scores formed a signature for a certain disease. The similarity score for two diseases was calculated by the partial Spearman correlation between their signatures, and used to define the distance between these two diseases. Using this method, Suthram et al. constructed a disease correlation network based on 138 significant disease correlations between 54 human diseases, and they discovered a set of common pathways and processes dysregulated in at least half of the diseases [161]. These studies highlighted not only the importance of such an integrated approach in revealing disease relationships, but also the value of the resulting common molecular pathological pathways for therapeutic applications.

7.6. OTHER APPROACHES THROUGH DATA AND TEXT MINING

By exploiting information from pharmaceutical company screening sets and the medicinal chemistry literature, proteins can be related through the observed polypharmacology of large compound sets [3]. For instance, Paolini et al. integrated a number of diverse sources of medicinal chemistry structure–activity relationship data to produce a ligand–target matrix, which they subsequently used to link targets by drugs that bound to more than one of them [166]. With the availability of large-scale, integrated chemogenomics databases, such as that described by Paolini et al., it is possible to search across large datasets of structure–activity relationship data for compounds that are known to bind multiple targets [3]. This logic has been extended by Wermuth into a design strategy, known as the "selective optimization of side activities (SOSA) approach", which can be used for multitarget drug discovery [167]. The SOSA approach involves screening a limited number of structurally diverse drug molecules, and then optimizing the hits so that they show a stronger affinity for the new target(s) and a weaker affinity for the original target(s). Such a methodology provides a wealth of opportunities for the identification of lead series of compounds that have been shown by structure–

activity relationship data to exhibit interesting pharmacological profiles [3]. By consolidating pharmacological activity data with protein sequence and chemical structure, it is expected that more progressive prediction power can be achieved for polypharmacology [168].

As discussed in Chapters 5 and 6, there are currently a number of public repositories available, including ChEMBL [169], ChemDB [170], and PubChem [171], from which compounds can be downloaded for integration into the *in silico* pipeline. Furthermore, there are several publicly available databases that specifically focus on drug–target interactions, such as Drug-Bank [172], SuperTarget [173], Matador [173], and the Therapeutic Target Database (TTD) [174]. DrugBank, for instance, contains nearly 4800 annotated drug entries, including more than 1350 FDA-approved small molecule drugs, 123 FDA-approved biotech (protein/peptide) drugs, 71 nutraceuticals, and more than 3243 experimental drugs. Detailed information is given about each drug, including chemical, pharmacological, and pharmaceutical data. Furthermore, these drugs are linked to more than 2500 nonredundant protein targets, for which there is sequence, structure, and pathway information. By integrating the FDA-approved small molecule drugs from DrugBank with the aforementioned computational approaches, it may be possible to identify mechanisms of drug resistance, identify previously unknown drug targets, make predictions about alternative uses for known drugs, or even make predictions about any potential side effects at an early stage in drug development for experimental drugs.

7.7. CONCLUSION

The potential of polypharmacology in biomedical research and drug discovery is enormous. It will help biologists and chemists not only to identify multiple drug targets, but also to assess their druggability, to optimize lead compounds across genomes, to predict potential side effects at an early stage, and to repurpose old drugs for new uses, thereby improving the productivity of drug discovery and development. Even though *in vitro* and *in vivo* screening is increasingly being applied to polypharmacology, efficient *in silico* approaches may provide invaluable information concerning the underlying molecular mechanisms of drug actions. In *in vitro* screening, a proteome-wide experiment is rarely employed, except for focusing on off-targets or pathways of interest. Therefore, drug-phenotype responses may not be directly assessed. Moreover, whether or not a protein binds to a specific ligand depends not only on the protein promiscuity across the proteome, but also on the chemical properties of the ligand. Thus, two different compounds, even those that have been designed to bind the same primary target, do not necessarily share the same off-targets, or result in the same drug response. *In vivo* screening treats the biological system as a whole. Although relevant drug efficacy and side effects can be observed, it may not be straightforward to identify the mode of action of a drug. The lack of knowledge about drug–target interactions may hinder late stage drug development. Computational techniques and data models that enable the proteome-wide study of protein–ligand interactions and the correlation of molecular interactions with clinical outcomes will provide us with valuable clues as to the molecular basis of cellular function, thereby facilitating a shift in the conventional one-drug-one-target drug discovery process to a new paradigm of polypharmacology. A number of studies have proven that such a methodology is particularly useful for both understanding the molecular mechanisms of drug side effects, and repurposing safe pharmaceuticals to target different pathways and/or treat different diseases. In spite of tremendous advances in chemoinformatics and bioinformatics, predicting protein–ligand interactions on a proteome-wide scale is a long way from realization. The computational techniques discussed in this chapter each have their own limitations in terms of both their predictive power and target coverage. In order to progressively predict polypharmacological effects, it is important to integrate ligand- and phenotype-based approaches with target-based methodologies.

REFERENCES

1. Hopkins, A.L. (2007). Network pharmacology. *Nature Biotechnology, 25*, 1110–1111.
2. Hopkins, A.L., Mason, J.S., Overington, J.P. (2006). Can we rationally design promiscuous drugs? *Current Opinion in Structural Biology, 16*, 127–136.
3. Hopkins, A.L. (2008). Network pharmacology: The next paradigm in drug discovery. *Nature Chemical Biology, 4*, 682–690.
4. Roth, B.L., Sheffler, D.J., Kroeze, W.K. (2004). Magic shotguns versus magic bullets: Selectively non-selective drugs for mood disorders and schizophrenia. *Nature Reviews. Drug Discovery, 3*, 353–359.
5. Ho, R.L., Lieu, C.A. (2008). Systems biology: An evolving approach in drug discovery and development. *Drugs in R&D, 9*, 203–216.
6. Zimmermann, G.R., Lehar, J., Keith, C.T. (2007). Multi-target therapeutics: When the whole is greater than the sum of the parts. *Drug Discovery Today, 12*, 34–42.
7. Keiser, M.J., Setola, V., Irwin, J.J., Laggner, C., Abbas, A.I., Hufeisen, S.J., Jensen, N.H., Kuijer, M.B., Matos, R.C., Tran, T.B., Whaley, R., Glennon, R.A., Hert, J., Thomas, K.L., Edwards, D.D., Shoichet, B.K., Roth, B.L. (2009). Predicting new molecular targets for known drugs. *Nature, 462*, 175–181.
8. Overington, J.P., Al-Lazikani, B., Hopkins, A.L. (2006). How many drug targets are there? *Nature Reviews. Drug Discovery, 5*, 993–996.
9. Forrest, L.R., Zhang, Y.W., Jacobs, M.T., Gesmonde, J., Xie, L., Honig, B.H., Rudnick, G. (2008). Mechanism for alternating access in neurotransmitter transporters. *Proceedings of the National Academy of Sciences of the United States of America, 105*, 10338–10343.

10. O'Connor, K.A., Roth, B.L. (2005). Finding new tricks for old drugs: An efficient route for public-sector drug discovery. *Nature Reviews. Drug Discovery*, *4*, 1005–1014.

11. Zhu, J., Xie, L., Honig, B. (2006). Structural refinement of protein segments containing secondary structure elements: Local sampling, knowledge-based potentials, and clustering. *Proteins*, *65*, 463–479.

12. Apsel, B., Blair, J.A., Gonzalez, B., Nazif, T.M., Feldman, M.E., Aizenstein, B., Hoffman, R., Williams, R.L., Shokat, K.M., Knight, Z.A. (2008). Targeted polypharmacology: Discovery of dual inhibitors of tyrosine and phosphoinositide kinases. *Nature Chemical Biology*, *4*, 691–699.

13. Kitano, H. (2007). A robustness-based approach to systems-oriented drug design. *Nature Reviews. Drug Discovery*, *6*, 202–210.

14. Kinnings, S.L., Xie, L., Fung, K.H., Jackson, R.M., Xie, L., Bourne, P.E. (2010). The *Mycobacterium tuberculosis* druggome and its pharmaceutical implications. *PLoS Computational Biology*, *6*(11), e1000976.

15. Raman, K., Chandra, N. (2008). *Mycobacterium tuberculosis* interactome analysis unravels potential pathways to drug resistance. *BMC Microbiology*, *8*, 234.

16. Kennedy, T. (1997). Managing the drug discovery/development interface. *Drug Discovery Today*, *2*, 436–444.

17. Nobeli, I., Favia, A.D., Thornton, J.M. (2009). Protein promiscuity and its implications for biotechnology. *Nature Biotechnology*, *27*, 157–167.

18. Xie, L., Evangelidis, T., Xie, L., Bourne, P.E. (2011). Drug discovery using chemical systems biology: Weak inhibition of multiple kinases may contribute to the anticancer effect of nelfinavir. *PLoS Computational Biology*, *7*, e1002037.

19. Ashburn, T.T., Thor, K.B. (2004). Drug repositioning: Identifying and developing new uses for existing drugs. *Nature Reviews. Drug Discovery*, *3*, 673–683.

20. Renaud, R.C., Xuereb, H. (2002). Erectile-dysfunction therapies. *Nature Reviews. Drug Discovery*, *1*, 663–664.

21. Lange, R.P., Locher, H.H., Wyss, P.C., Then, R.L. (2007). The targets of currently used antibacterial agents: Lessons for drug discovery. *Current Pharmaceutical Design*, *13*, 3140–3154.

22. Billingsley, M.L. (2008). Druggable targets and targeted drugs: Enhancing the development of new therapeutics. *Pharmacology*, *82*, 239–244.

23. Oureshi, Z.P., Szeinbach, S.L., Seoane-Vazquez, E., Rodriguez-Mongulo, R. (2009). Market discontinuation of pharmaceuticals in the United States: Analysis of drugs approved by the FDA from 1939 to 2008. *Value in Health*, *12*, A81–A82.

24. Chong, C.R., Sullivan, D.J. Jr (2007). New uses for old drugs. *Nature*, *448*, 645–646.

25. DiMasi, J.A., Hansen, R.W., Grabowski, H.G. (2003). The price of innovation: New estimates of drug development costs. *Journal of Health Economics*, *22*, 151–185.

26. Chiang, A.P., Butte, A.J. (2009). Systematic evaluation of drug-disease relationships to identify leads for novel drug uses. *Clinical Pharmacology and Therapeutics*, *86*, 507–510.

27. Kroeze, W.K., Kristiansen, K., Roth, B.L. (2002). Molecular biology of serotonin receptors structure and function at the molecular level. *Current Topics in Medicinal Chemistry*, *2*, 507–528.

28. Callahan, R.J., Au, J.D., Paul, M., Liu, C., Yost, C.S. (2004). Functional inhibition by methadone of N-methyl-D-aspartate receptors expressed in *Xenopus oocytes*: Stereospecific and subunit effects. *Anesthesia and Analgesia*, 98, 653–659.

29. Widemann, B.C., Balis, F.M., Godwin, K.S., McCully, C., Adamson, P.C. (1999). The plasma pharmacokinetics and cerebrospinal fluid penetration of the thymidylate synthase inhibitor raltitrexed (Tomudex) in a nonhuman primate model. *Cancer Chemotherapy & Pharmacology*, 44, 439–443.

30. Johnson, M., Maggiora, G.M., eds. (1990). *Concepts and Applications of Molecular Similarity*. New York: John Wiley & Sons.

31. Brown, R.D., Martin, Y.C. (1996). Use of structure-activity data to compare structure-based clustering methods and descriptors for use in compound selection. *Journal of Chemical Information and Computer Sciences*, 36, 572–584.

32. Hert, J., Willett, P., Wilton, D.J., Acklin, P., Azzaoui, K., Jacoby, E., Schuffenhauer, A. (2004). Comparison of fingerprint-based methods for virtual screening using multiple bioactive reference structures. *Journal of Chemical Information and Computer Sciences*, 44, 1177–1185.

33. Xue, L., Stahura, F.L., Godden, J.W., Bajorath, J. (2001). Fingerprint scaling increases the probability of identifying molecules with similar activity in virtual screening calculations. *Journal of Chemical Information and Computer Sciences*, 41, 746–753.

34. McGregor, M.J., Pallai, P.V. (1997). Clustering of large databases of compounds: Using the MDL "Keys" as structural descriptors. *Journal of Chemical Information and Computer Sciences*, 37, 443–448.

35. Barcza, S., Kelly, L.A., Wahrman, S.S., Kirschenbaum, R.E. (1985). Structured biological data in the molecular access system. *Journal of Chemical Information and Computer Sciences*, 25, 55–59.

36. Bender, A., Glen, R.C. (2005). A discussion of measures of enrichment in virtual screening: Comparing the information content of descriptors with increasing levels of sophistication. *Journal of Chemical Information and Modeling*, 45, 1369–1375.

37. Cormen, T.H., Leiserson, C.E., Rivest, R.L., Stein, C. (2001). *Section 31.3: Modular Arithmetic. Introduction to Algorithms*, 2nd ed., 862–868. New York: MIT Press and McGraw-Hill.

38. Holm, L., Sander, C. (1996). Mapping the protein universe. *Science*, 273, 595–602.

39. Pearl, F.M., Martin, N., Bray, J.E., Buchan, D.W., Harrison, A.P., Lee, D., Reeves, G.A., Shepherd, A.J., Sillitoe, I., Todd, A.E., Thornton, J.M., Orengo, C.A. (2001). A rapid classification protocol for the CATH domain database to support structural genomics. *Nucleic Acids Research*, 29, 223–227.

40. Cruciani, G., Pastor, M., Guba, W. (2000). VolSurf: A new tool for the pharmacokinetic optimization of lead compounds. *European Journal of Pharmaceutical Sciences*, 11(Suppl 2), S29–S39.

41. Pastor, M., Cruciani, G., McLay, I., Pickett, S., Clementi, S. (2000). GRid-INdependent descriptors (GRIND): A novel class of alignment-independent three-dimensional molecular descriptors. *Journal of Medicinal Chemistry*, 43, 3233–3243.

42. Cruciani, G., Pastor, M., Mannhold, R. (2002). Suitability of molecular descriptors for database mining. A comparative analysis. *Journal of Medicinal Chemistry*, 45, 2685–2694.

43. Rarey, M., Dixon, J.S. (1998). Feature trees: A new molecular similarity measure based on tree matching. *Journal of Computer-Aided Molecular Design*, *12*, 471–490.

44. Rarey, M., Stahl, M. (2001). Similarity searching in large combinatorial chemistry spaces. *Journal of Computer-Aided Molecular Design*, *15*, 497–520.

45. Gillet, V.J., Willett, P., Bradshaw, J. (2003). Similarity searching using reduced graphs. *Journal of Chemical Information and Computer Sciences*, *43*, 338–345.

46. Takahashi, Y., Sukekawa, M., Sasaki, S. (1992). Automatic identification of molecular similarity using reduced-graph representation of chemical structure. *Journal of Chemical Information and Computer Sciences*, *32*, 639–643.

47. Rusinko III, A., Sheridan R.P., Nilakantan, R., Haraki, K.S., Bauman, N., Venkataraghavan R. (1989). Using CONCORD to construct a large database of three-dimensional coordinates from connection tables. *Journal of Chemical Information and Computer Sciences*, *29*, 251–255.

48. James, C.A., Weininger, D. (1995). In Daylight Software Manual, version 4.41, Daylight Chemical Information Systems Inc. CA: Irvine.

49. Matter, H. (1997). Selecting optimally diverse compounds from structure databases: A validation study of two-dimensional and three-dimensional molecular descriptors. *Journal of Medicinal Chemistry*, *40*, 1219–1229.

50. Briem, H., Kuntz, I.D. (1996). Molecular similarity based on DOCK-generated fingerprints. *Journal of Medicinal Chemistry*, *39*, 3401–3408.

51. Schuffenhauer, A., Gillet, V.J., Willett, P. (2000). Similarity searching in files of three-dimensional chemical structures: Analysis of the BIOSTER database using two-dimensional fingerprints and molecular field descriptors. *Journal of Chemical Information and Computer Sciences*, *40*, 295–307.

52. Sheridan, R.P., Kearsley, S.K. (2002). Why do we need so many chemical similarity search methods? *Drug Discovery Today*, *7*, 903–911.

53. Kinnings, S.L., Jackson, R.M. (2011). ReverseScreen3D: A structure-based ligand matching method to identify protein targets. *Journal of Chemical Information and Modeling*, *51*, 624–634.

54. Shanmugasundaram, V., Maggiora, G.M., Lajiness, M.S. (2005). Hit-directed nearest-neighbor searching. *Journal of Medicinal Chemistry*, *48*, 240–248.

55. Keiser, M.J., Roth, B.L., Armbruster, B.N., Ernsberger, P., Irwin, J.J., Shoichet, B.K. (2007). Relating protein pharmacology by ligand chemistry. *Nature Biotechnology*, *25*, 197–206.

56. (2006). MDL Drug Data Report, 2006.1, MDL Information Systems Inc., San Leandro, CA.

57. Chen, X., Reynolds, C.H. (2002). Performance of similarity measures in 2D fragment-based similarity searching: Comparison of structural descriptors and similarity coefficients. *Journal of Chemical Information and Computer Sciences*, *42*, 1407–1414.

58. James, C., Weininger, D., Delany, J. (2011). Daylight Theory Manual—Daylight Chemical Information Systems Inc., Mission Viejo, CA, 1992–2005.

59. Noeske, T., Sasse, B.C., Stark, H., Parsons, C.G., Weil, T., Schneider, G. (2006). Predicting compound selectivity by self-organizing maps: Cross-activities of metabotropic glutamate receptor antagonists. *ChemMedChem*, *1*, 1066–1068.

60. Fechner, U., Franke, L., Renner, S., Schneider, P., Schneider, G. (2003). Comparison of correlation vector methods for ligand-based similarity searching. *Journal of Computer-Aided Molecular Design, 17,* 687–698.

61. Olah, M., Mracec, M., Ostopovici, L., Rad, R., Bora, A., Hadaruga, N., Olah, I.., Banda, M., Simon, Z., Mracec, M., Oprea, T.I., Oprea, T.I., eds. (2005). WOMBAT: World of Molecular Bioactivity. In *Chemoinformatics in Drug Discovery.* New York: Wiley-VCH.

62. Hert, J., Keiser, M.J., Irwin, J.J., Oprea, T.I., Shoichet, B.K. (2008). Quantifying the relationships among drug classes. *Journal of Chemical Information and Modeling, 48,* 755–765.

63. Xia, X., Maliski, E.G., Gallant, P., Rogers, D. (2004). Classification of kinase inhibitors using a Bayesian model. *Journal of Medicinal Chemistry, 47,* 4463–4470.

64. Durant, J.L., Leland, B.A., Henry, D.R., Nourse, J.G. (2002). Reoptimization of MDL keys for use in drug discovery. *Journal of Chemical Information and Computer Sciences, 42,* 1273–1280.

65. Henikoff, S., Henikoff, J.G. (1994). Position-based sequence weights. *Journal of Molecular Biology, 243,* 574–578.

66. Jenkins, J.L., Glick, M., Davies, J.W. (2004). A 3D similarity method for scaffold hopping from known drugs or natural ligands to new chemotypes. *Journal of Medicinal Chemistry, 47,* 6144–6159.

67. Maggiora, G.M. (2006). On outliers and activity cliffs—Why QSAR often disappoints. *Journal of Chemical Information and Modeling, 46,* 1535.

68. Eckert, H., Bajorath, J. (2007). Molecular similarity analysis in virtual screening: Foundations, limitations and novel approaches. *Drug Discovery Today, 12,* 225–233.

69. Fourches, D., Muratov, E., Tropsha, A. (2010). Trust, but verify: On the importance of chemical structure curation in cheminformatics and QSAR modeling research. *Journal of Chemical Information and Modeling, 50,* 1189–1204.

70. Young, D., Martin, T., Venkatapathy, R., Harten, P. (2008). Are the chemical structures in your QSAR correct. *QSAR & Combinatorial Science, 27,* 1337–1345.

71. Lemieux, R.U., Spohr, U. (1994). How Emil Fischer was led to the lock and key concept for enzyme specificity. *Advances in carbohydrate chemistry and biochemistry, 50,* 1–20.

72. Henrich, S., Salo-Ahen, O.M., Huang, B., Rippmann, F.F., Cruciani, G., Wade, R.C. (2009). Computational approaches to identifying and characterizing protein binding sites for ligand design. *Journal of Molecular Recognition, 23,* 209–219.

73. EE, H., WG, R. (1987). Molecular similarity based on electrostatic potential and electric field. *International Journal of Quantum Chemistry, 32,* 105–110.

74. Blomberg, N., Gabdoulline, R.R., Nilges, M., Wade, R.C. (1999). Classification of protein sequences by homology modeling and quantitative analysis of electrostatic similarity. *Proteins, 37,* 379–387.

75. Wade, R.C., Gabdoulline, R.R., Ludemann, S.K., Lounnas, V. (1998). Electrostatic steering and ionic tethering in enzyme-ligand binding: Insights from simulations. *Proceedings of the National Academy of Sciences of the United States of America, 95,* 5942–5949.

76. Fogolari, F., Brigo, A., Molinari, H. (2002). The Poisson-Boltzmann equation for biomolecular electrostatics: A tool for structural biology. *Journal of Molecular Recognition, 15*, 377–392.

77. Richter, S., Wenzel, A., Stein, M., Gabdoulline, R.R., Wade, R.C. (2008). web-PIPSA: A web server for the comparison of protein interaction properties. *Nucleic Acids Research, 36*, W276–W280.

78. Baroni, M., Cruciani, G., Sciabola, S., Perruccio, F., Mason, J.S. (2007). A common reference framework for analyzing/comparing proteins and ligands. Fingerprints for Ligands and Proteins (FLAP): Theory and application. *Journal of Chemical Information and Modeling, 47*, 279–294.

79. Goodford, P.J. (1985). A computational procedure for determining energetically favorable binding sites on biologically important macromolecules. *Journal of Medicinal Chemistry, 28*, 849–857.

80. Carosati, E., Sciabola, S., Cruciani, G. (2004). Hydrogen bonding interactions of covalently bonded fluorine atoms: From crystallographic data to a new angular function in the GRID force field. *Journal of Medicinal Chemistry, 47*, 5114–5125.

81. Sciabola, S., Stanton, R.V., Mills, J.E., Flocco, M.M., Baroni, M., Cruciani, G., Perruccio, F., Mason, J.S. (2010). High-throughput virtual screening of proteins using GRID molecular interaction fields. *Journal of Chemical Information and Modeling, 50*, 155–169.

82. Liu, X., Ouyang, S., Yu, B., Liu, Y., Huang, K., Gong, J., Zheng, S., Li, Z., Li, H., Jiang, H. (2010). PharmMapper server: A web server for potential drug target identification using pharmacophore mapping approach. *Nucleic Acids Research, 38*, W609–W614.

83. Wishart, D.S., Knox, C., Guo, A.C., Cheng, D., Shrivastava, S., Tzur, D., Gautam, B., Hassanali, M. (2008). DrugBank: A knowledgebase for drugs, drug actions and drug targets. *Nucleic Acids Research, 36*, D901–D906.

84. Liu, T., Lin, Y., Wen, X., Jorissen, R.N., Gilson, M.K. (2007). BindingDB: A web-accessible database of experimentally determined protein-ligand binding affinities. *Nucleic Acids Research, 35*, D198–D201.

85. Wang, R., Fang, X., Lu, Y., Wang, S. (2004). The PDBbind database: Collection of binding affinities for protein-ligand complexes with known three-dimensional structures. *Journal of Medicinal Chemistry, 47*, 2977–2980.

86. Gao, Z., Li, H., Zhang, H., Liu, X., Kang, L., Luo, X., Zhu, W., Chen, K., Wang, X., Jiang, H. (2008). PDTD: A web-accessible protein database for drug target identification. *BMC Bioinformatics, 9*, 104.

87. Wolber, G., Langer, T. (2005). LigandScout: 3-D pharmacophores derived from protein-bound ligands and their use as virtual screening filters. *Journal of Chemical Information and Modeling, 45*, 160–169.

88. Schneidman-Duhovny, D., Dror, O., Inbar, Y., Nussinov, R., Wolfson, H.J. (2008). Deterministic pharmacophore detection via multiple flexible alignment of drug-like molecules. *Journal of Computational Biology, 15*, 737–754.

89. Toda, N., Tago, K., Marumoto, S., Takami, K., Ori, M., Yamada, N., Koyama, K., Naruto, S., Abe, K., Yamazaki, R., Hara, T., Aoyagi, A., Abe, Y., Kaneko, T., Kogen, H. (2003). A conformational restriction approach to the development of dual inhibitors of acetylcholinesterase and serotonin transporter as potential agents for Alzheimer's disease. *Bioorganic & Medicinal Chemistry, 11*, 4389–4415.

90. Aronov, A.M., Murcko, M.A. (2004). Toward a pharmacophore for kinase frequent hitters. *Journal of Medicinal Chemistry*, 47, 5616–5619.

91. Hendlich, M., Bergner, A., Gunther, J., Klebe, G. (2003). Relibase: Design and development of a database for comprehensive analysis of protein-ligand interactions. *Journal of Molecular Biology*, 326, 607–620.

92. Schmitt, S., Kuhn, D., Klebe, G. (2002). A new method to detect related function among proteins independent of sequence and fold homology. *Journal of Molecular Biology*, 323, 387–406.

93. Shulman-Peleg, A., Nussinov, R., Wolfson, H.J. (2005). SiteEngines: Recognition and comparison of binding sites and protein-protein interfaces. *Nucleic Acids Research*, 33, W337–W341.

94. Jambon, M., Imberty, A., Deleage, G., Geourjon, C. (2003). A new bioinformatic approach to detect common 3D sites in protein structures. *Proteins*, 52, 137–145.

95. Brakoulias, A., Jackson, R.M. (2004). Towards a structural classification of phosphate binding sites in protein-nucleotide complexes: An automated all-against-all structural comparison using geometric matching. *Proteins*, 56, 250–260.

96. Morris, R.J., Najmanovich, R.J., Kahraman, A., Thornton, J.M. (2005). Real spherical harmonic expansion coefficients as 3D shape descriptors for protein binding pocket and ligand comparisons. *Bioinformatics (Oxford, England)*, 21, 2347–2355.

97. Yeturu, K., Chandra, N. (2008). PocketMatch: A new algorithm to compare binding sites in protein structures. *BMC Bioinformatics*, 9, 543.

98. Raman, K., Yeturu, K., Chandra, N. (2008). targetTB: A target identification pipeline for *Mycobacterium tuberculosis* through an interactome, reactome and genome-scale structural analysis. *BMC Systems Biology*, 2, 109.

99. Milletti, F., Vulpetti, A. (2010). Predicting polypharmacology by binding site similarity: From kinases to the protein universe. *Journal of Chemical Information and Modeling*, 50, 1418–1431.

100. Rohlf, F.J., Slice, D. (1990). Extensions of the procrustes method for the optimal superimposition of landmarks. *Systematic Zoology*, 39, 40–59.

101. Xie, L., Wang, J., Bourne, P.E. (2007). In silico elucidation of the molecular mechanism defining the adverse effect of selective estrogen receptor modulators. *PLoS Computational Biology*, 3, e217.

102. Xie, L., Li, J., Xie, L., Bourne, P.E. (2009). Drug discovery using chemical systems biology: Identification of the protein-ligand binding network to explain the side effects of CETP inhibitors. *PLoS Computational Biology*, 5, e1000387.

103. Xie, L., Bourne, P.E. (2008). Detecting evolutionary relationships across existing fold space, using sequence order-independent profile-profile alignments. *Proceedings of the National Academy of Sciences of the United States of America*, 105, 5441–5446.

104. Xie, L., Bourne, P.E. (2007). A robust and efficient algorithm for the shape description of protein structures and its application in predicting ligand binding sites. *BMC Bioinformatics*, 8(Suppl 4), S9.

105. Ostergard, P.R.J. (2001). A new algorithm for the maximum-weight clique problem. *Nordic Journal of Computing*, 8, 424–436.

106. Smith, T.F., Waterman, M.S. (1981). Identification of common molecular subsequences. *Journal of Molecular Biology*, 147, 195–197.

107. Xie, L., Bourne, P.E. (2009). A unified statistical model to support local sequence order independent similarity searching for ligand-binding sites and its application to genome-based drug discovery. *Bioinformatics (Oxford, England)*, 25, i305–i312.

108. Kuipers, I., van der Harst, P., Navis, G., van Genne, L., Morello, F., van Gilst, W.H., van Veldhuisen, D.J., de Boer, R.A. (2008). Nuclear hormone receptors as regulators of the renin-angiotensin-aldosterone system. *Hypertension*, 51, 1442–1448.

109. Kinnings, S.L., Liu, N., Buchmeier, N., Tonge, P.J., Xie, L., Bourne, P.E. (2009). Drug discovery using chemical systems biology: Repositioning the safe medicine comtan to treat multi-drug and extensively drug resistant tuberculosis. *PLoS Computational Biology*, 5, e1000423.

110. Korlipara, L.V., Cooper, J.M., Schapira, A.H. (2004). Differences in toxicity of the catechol-O-methyl transferase inhibitors, tolcapone and entacapone to cultured human neuroblastoma cells. *Neuropharmacology*, 46, 562–569.

111. Miller, J.R., Dunham, S., Mochalkin, I., Banotai, C., Bowman, M., Buist, S., Dunkle, B., Hanna, D., Harwood, H.J., Huband, M.D., Karnovsky, A., Kuhn, M., Limberakis, C., Liu, J.Y., Mehrens, S., Mueller, W.T., Narasimhan, L., Ogden, A., Ohren, J., Prasad, J.V., Shelly, J.A., Skerlos, L., Sulavik, M., Thomas, V.H., Vanderroest, S., Wang, L., Wang, Z., Whitton, A., Zhu, T., Stover, C.K. (2009). A class of selective antibacterials derived from a protein kinase inhibitor pharmacophore. *Proceedings of the National Academy of Sciences of the United States of America*, 106, 1737–1742.

112. Verdonk, M.L., Berdini, V., Hartshorn, M.J., Mooij, W.T., Murray, C.W., Taylor, R.D., Watson, P. (2004). Virtual screening using protein-ligand docking: Avoiding artificial enrichment. *Journal of Chemical Information and Computer Sciences*, 44, 793–806.

113. Metropolis, N., Rosenbluth, A.W., Rosenbluth, M.N., Teller, A.H., Teller, E. (1953). Equation of state calculations for fast computing machines. *The Journal of Chemical Physics*, 21, 1087–1092.

114. Ziemys, A., Rimkute, L., Kulys, J. (2004). Nonlinear Analysis: Modelling and Control.

115. Morris, G.M., Huey, R., Olson, A.J. (2008). Using AutoDock for ligand-receptor docking. *Current Protocols in Bioinformatics*, 24, 8.14.1–8.14.40.

116. Jones, G., Willett, P., Glen, R.C., Leach, A.R., Taylor, R. (1997). Development and validation of a genetic algorithm for flexible docking. *Journal of Molecular Biology*, 267, 727–748.

117. Taylor, J.S., Burnett, R.M. (2000). DARWIN: A program for docking flexible molecules. *Proteins*, 41, 173–191.

118. Huang, D., Caflisch, A. (2009). Library screening by fragment-based docking. *Journal of Molecular Recognition*, 23, 183–193.

119. Rarey, M., Kramer, B., Lengauer, T., Klebe, G. (1996). A fast flexible docking method using an incremental construction algorithm. *Journal of Molecular Biology*, 261, 470–489.

120. Knegtel, R.M., Kuntz, I.D., Oshiro, C.M. (1997). Molecular docking to ensembles of protein structures. *Journal of Molecular Biology*, 266, 424–440.

121. Zavodszky, M.I., Kuhn, L.A. (2005). Side-chain flexibility in protein-ligand binding: The minimal rotation hypothesis. *Protein Science*, 14, 1104–1114.

122. Miteva, M.A., Lee, W.H., Montes, M.O., Villoutreix, B.O. (2005). Fast structure-based virtual ligand screening combining FRED, DOCK, and Surflex. *Journal of Medicinal Chemistry*, *48*, 6012–6022.

123. Huang, S.Y., Grinter, S.Z., Zou, X. (2010). Scoring functions and their evaluation methods for protein-ligand docking: Recent advances and future directions. *Physical Chemistry Chemical Physics*, *12*, 12899–12908.

124. Clark, R.D., Strizhev, A., Leonard, J.M., Blake, J.F., Matthew, J.B. (2002). Consensus scoring for ligand/protein interactions. *Journal of Molecular Graphics and Modelling*, *20*, 281–295.

125. Bruning, J.B., Parent, A.A., Gil, G., Zhao, M., Nowak, J., Pace, M.C., Smith, C.L., Afonine, P.V., Adams, P.D., Katzenellenbogen, J.A., Nettles, K.W. (2010). Coupling of receptor conformation and ligand orientation determine graded activity. *Nature Chemical Biology*, *6*, 837–843.

126. Gilson, M.K., Zhou, H.X. (2007). Calculation of protein-ligand binding affinities. *Annual Review of Biophysics and Biomolecular Structure*, *36*, 21–42.

127. Amaro, R.E., Schnaufer, A., Interthal, H., Hol, W., Stuart, K.D., McCammon, J.A. (2008). Discovery of drug-like inhibitors of an essential RNA-editing ligase in *Trypanosoma brucei*. *Proceedings of the National Academy of Sciences of the United States of America*, *105*, 17278–17283.

128. Irwin, J.J. (2008). Community benchmarks for virtual screening. *Journal of Computer-Aided Molecular Design*, *22*, 193–199.

129. Warren, G.L., Andrews, C.W., Capelli, A.-M., Clarke, B., LaLonde, J., Lambert, M.H., Lindvall, M., Nevins, N., Semus, S.F., Senger, S., Tedesco, G., Wall, I.D., Woolven, J.M., Peishoff, C.E., Head, M.S. (2006). A critical assessment of docking programs and scoring functions. *Journal of Medicinal Chemistry*, *49*, 5912–5931.

130. Koch, M.A., Schuffenhauer, A., Scheck, M., Wetzel, S., Casaulta, M., Odermatt, A., Ertl, P., Waldmann, H. (2005). Charting biologically relevant chemical space: A structural classification of natural products (SCONP). *Proceedings of the National Academy of Sciences of the United States of America*, *102*, 17272–17277.

131. Renner, S., van Otterlo, W.A., Dominguez Seoane, M., Mocklinghoff, S., Hofmann, B., Wetzel, S., Schuffenhauer, A., Ertl, P., Oprea, T.I., Steinhilber, D., Brunsveld, L., Rauh, D., Waldmann, H. (2009). Bioactivity-guided mapping and navigation of chemical space. *Nature Chemical Biology*, *5*, 585–592.

132. Wetzel, S., Klein, K., Renner, S., Rauh, D., Oprea, T.I., Mutzel, P., Waldmann, H. (2009). Interactive exploration of chemical space with Scaffold Hunter. *Nature Chemical Biology*, *5*, 581–583.

133. Bender, A., Young, D.W., Jenkins, J.L., Serrano, M., Mikhailov, D., Clemons, P.A., Davies, J.W. (2007). Chemogenomic data analysis: Prediction of small-molecule targets and the advent of biological fingerprint. *Combinatorial Chemistry & High Throughput Screening*, *10*, 719–731.

134. Bleicher, K.H. (2002). Chemogenomics: Bridging a drug discovery gap. *Current Medicinal Chemistry*, *9*, 2077–2084.

135. Bredel, M., Jacoby, E. (2004). Chemogenomics: An emerging strategy for rapid target and drug discovery. *Nature Reviews. Genetics*, *5*, 262–275.

136. Harris, C.J., Stevens, A.P. (2006). Chemogenomics: Structuring the drug discovery process to gene families. *Drug Discovery Today*, *11*, 880–888.

137. Jacoby, E. (2006). Chemogenomics: Drug discovery's panacea? *Molecular Biosystems*, *2*, 218–220.

138. Jacoby, E., Schuffenhauer, A., Floersheim, P. (2003). Chemogenomics knowledge-based strategies in drug discovery. *Drug News & Perspectives*, *16*, 93–102.

139. Kubinyi, H. (2006). Chemogenomics in drug discovery. Ernst Schering Research Foundation workshop, 1–19.

140. Mestres, J. (2004). Computational chemogenomics approaches to systematic knowledge-based drug discovery. *Current Opinion in Drug Discovery & Development*, *7*, 304–313.

141. Rognan, D. (2007). Chemogenomic approaches to rational drug design. *British Journal of Pharmacology*, *152*, 38–52.

142. Savchuk, N.P., Balakin, K.V., Tkachenko, S.E. (2004). Exploring the chemogenomic knowledge space with annotated chemical libraries. *Current Opinion in Chemical Biology*, *8*, 414–417.

143. Wuster, A., Madan Babu, M. (2008). Chemogenomics and biotechnology. *Trends in Biotechnology*, *26*, 252–258.

144. Kanehisa, M., Goto, S. (2000). KEGG: Kyoto encyclopedia of genes and genomes. *Nucleic Acids Research*, *28*, 27–30.

145. Lamb, J., Crawford, E.D., Peck, D., Modell, J.W., Blat, I.C., Wrobel, M.J., Lerner, J., Brunet, J.P., Subramanian, A., Ross, K.N., Reich, M., Hieronymus, H., Wei, G., Armstrong, S.A., Haggarty, S.J., Clemons, P.A., Wei, R., Carr, S.A., Lander, E.S., Golub, T.R. (2006). The Connectivity Map: Using gene-expression signatures to connect small molecules, genes, and disease. *Science*, *313*, 1929–1935.

146. Lamb, J., Ramaswamy, S., Ford, H.L., Contreras, B., Martinez, R.V., Kittrell, F.S., Zahnow, C.A., Patterson, N., Golub, T.R., Ewen, M.E. (2003). A mechanism of cyclin D1 action encoded in the patterns of gene expression in human cancer. *Cell*, *114*, 323–334.

147. Mootha, V.K., Lindgren, C.M., Eriksson, K.F., Subramanian, A., Sihag, S., Lehar, J., Puigserver, P., Carlsson, E., Ridderstrale, M., Laurila, E., Houstis, N., Daly, M.J., Patterson, N., Mesirov, J.P., Golub, T.R., Tamayo, P., Spiegelman, B., Lander, E.S., Hirschhorn, J.N., Altshuler, D., Groop, L.C. (2003). PGC-1alpha-responsive genes involved in oxidative phosphorylation are coordinately down-regulated in human diabetes. *Nature Genetics*, *34*, 267–273.

148. Gorre, M.E., Ellwood-Yen, K., Chiosis, G., Rosen, N., Sawyers, C.L. (2002). BCR-ABL point mutants isolated from patients with imatinib mesylate-resistant chronic myeloid leukemia remain sensitive to inhibitors of the BCR-ABL chaperone heat shock protein 90. *Blood*, *100*, 3041–3044.

149. Wei, G., Twomey, D., Lamb, J., Schlis, K., Agarwal, J., Stam, R.W., Opferman, J.T., Sallan, S.E., den Boer, M.L., Pieters, R., Golub, T.R., Armstrong, S.A. (2006). Gene expression-based chemical genomics identifies rapamycin as a modulator of MCL1 and glucocorticoid resistance. *Cancer Cell*, *10*, 331–342.

150. Iorio, F., Bosotti, R., Scacheri, E., Belcastro, V., Mithbaokar, P., Ferriero, R., Murino, L., Tagliaferri, R., Brunetti-Pierri, N., Isacchi, A., Di Bernardo, D. (2010). Discovery of drug mode of action and drug repositioning from transcriptional responses. *Proceedings of the National Academy of Sciences of the United States of America*, *107*, 14621–14626.

151. Iorio, F., Tagliaferri, R., Di Bernardo, D. (2009). Identifying network of drug mode of action by gene expression profiling. *Journal of Computational Biology*, *16*, 241–251.

152. Fliri, A.F., Loging, W.T., Thadeio, P.F., Volkmann, R.A. (2005). Analysis of drug-induced effect patterns to link structure and side effects of medicines. *Nature Chemical Biology*, *1*, 389–397.

153. Fliri, A.F., Loging, W.T., Volkmann, R.A. (2007). Analysis of system structure-function relationships. *ChemMedChem*, *2*, 1774–1782.

154. Campillos, M., Kuhn, M., Gavin, A.C., Jensen, L.J., Bork, P. (2008). Drug target identification using side-effect similarity. *Science*, *321*, 263–266.

155. Bodenreider, O. (2004). The Unified Medical Language System (UMLS): Integrating biomedical terminology. *Nucleic Acids Research*, *32*, D267–D270.

156. Gerstein, M., Sonnhammer, E.L., Chothia, C. (1994). Volume changes in protein evolution. *Journal of Molecular Biology*, *236*, 1067–1078.

157. Kuhn, M., Campillos, M., Letunic, I., Jensen, L.J., Bork, P. (2010). A side effect resource to capture phenotypic effects of drugs. *Molecular Systems Biology*, *6*, 343.

158. von Eichborn, J., Murgueitio, M.S., Dunkel, M., Koerner, S., Bourne, P.E., Preissner, R. (2010). PROMISCUOUS: A database for network-based drug-repositioning. *Nucleic Acids Research*, *39*, D1060–D1066.

159. Cummings, J., Winblad, B. (2007). A rivastigmine patch for the treatment of Alzheimer's disease and Parkinson's disease dementia. *Expert Review of Neuro-therapeutics*, *7*, 1457–1463.

160. Sandler, A., Gray, R., Perry, M.C., Brahmer, J., Schiller, J.H., Dowlati, A., Lilenbaum, R., Johnson, D.H. (2006). Paclitaxel-carboplatin alone or with bevacizumab for non-small-cell lung cancer. *The New England Journal of Medicine*, *355*, 2542–2550.

161. Suthram, S., Dudley, J.T., Chiang, A.P., Chen, R., Hastie, T.J., Butte, A.J. (2010). Network-based elucidation of human disease similarities reveals common functional modules enriched for pluripotent drug targets. *PLoS Computational Biology*, *6*, e1000662.

162. Barrett, T., Troup, D.B., Wilhite, S.E., Ledoux, P., Rudnev, D., Evangelista, C., Kim, I.F., Soboleva, A., Tomashevsky, M., Edgar, R. (2007). NCBI GEO: Mining tens of millions of expression profiles—Database and tools update. *Nucleic Acids Research*, *35*, D760–D765.

163. Fowler, J., Kouramajian, V., Maram, S., Devadhar, V. (1995). Automated MeSH indexing of the World-Wide Web. *Proceedings of The Annual Symposium on Computer Applications in Medical Care*, pp. 893–897.

164. Keshava Prasad, T.S., Goel, R., Kandasamy, K., Keerthikumar, S., Kumar, S., Mathivanan, S., Telikicherla, D., Raju, R., Shafreen, B., Venugopal, A., Balakrishnan, L., Marimuthu, A., Banerjee, S., Somanathan, D.S., Sebastian, A., Rani, S., Ray, S., Harrys Kishore, C.J., Kanth, S., Ahmed, M., Kashyap, M.K., Mohmood, R., Ramachandra, Y.L., Krishna, V., Rahiman, B.A., Mohan, S., Ranganathan, P., Ramabadran, S., Chaerkady, R., Pandey, A. (2009). Human protein reference database—2009 update. *Nucleic Acids Research*, *37*, D767–D772.

165. Sharan, R., Suthram, S., Kelley, R.M., Kuhn, T., McCuine, S., Uetz, P., Sittler, T., Karp, R.M., Ideker, T. (2005). Conserved patterns of protein interaction in mul-

tiple species. *Proceedings of the National Academy of Sciences of the United States of America*, *102*, 1974–1979.

166. Paolini, G.V., Shapland, R.H., van Hoorn, W.P., Mason, J.S., Hopkins, A.L. (2006). Global mapping of pharmacological space. *Nature Biotechnology*, *24*, 805–815.

167. Wermuth, C.G. (2006). Selective optimization of side activities: The SOSA approach. *Drug Discovery Today*, *11*, 160–164.

168. Metz, J.T., Johnson, E.F., Soni, N.B., Merta, P.J., Kifle, L., Hajduk, P.J. (2011). Navigating the kinome. *Nature Chemical Biology*, *7*, 200–202.

169. Overington, J. (2009). ChEMBL. An interview with John Overington, team leader, chemogenomics at the European Bioinformatics Institute Outstation of the European Molecular Biology Laboratory (EMBL-EBI). Interview by Wendy A. Warr. *Journal of Computer-Aided Molecular Design*, *23*, 195–198.

170. Chen, J., Swamidass, S.J., Dou, Y., Bruand, J., Baldi, P. (2005). ChemDB: A public database of small molecules and related chemoinformatics resources. *Bioinformatics (Oxford, England)*, *21*, 4133–4139.

171. Wheeler, D.L., Barret, T., Benson, D.A., Bryant, S.H., Canese, K., Church, D.M., Dicuccio, M., Edgar, R., Federhen, S., , Helmberg, W., Kenton, D.L., Khovayko, O., Lipman, D.J., Madden, T.L., Maglott, D.R., Ostell, J., Pontius, J.U., Pruitt, K.D., Schuler, G.D., Schriml, L.M., Sequeira, E., Sherry, S.T., Sirotkin, K., Starchenko, G., Suzek, T.O., Tatusov, R., Tatusova, T.A., Wagner, L., Yaschenko, E. (2005). Database resources of the National Center for Biotechnology Information. *Nucleic Acids Research*, *33*, D39–D45.

172. Wishart, D.S., Knox, C., Guo, A.C., Shrivastava, S., Hassanali, M., Stothard, P., Chang, Z., Woolsey, J. (2006). DrugBank: A comprehensive resource for in silico drug discovery and exploration. *Nucleic Acids Research*, *34*, D668–D672.

173. Gunther, S., Kuhn, M., Dunkel, M., Campillos, M., Senger, C., Petsalaki, E., Ahmed, J., Urdiales, E.G., Gewiess, A., Jensen, L.J., Schneider, R., Skoblo, R., Russell, R.B., Bourne, P.E., Bork, P., Preissner, R. (2008). SuperTarget and Matador: Resources for exploring drug-target relationships. *Nucleic Acids Research*, *36*, D919–D922.

174. Chen, X., Ji, Z.L., Chen, Y.Z. (2002). TTD: Therapeutic target database. *Nucleic Acids Research*, *30*, 412–415.

CHAPTER 8

Systematic Phenotypic Screening for Novel Synergistic Combinations: A New Paradigm for Repositioning Existing Drugs

MARGARET S. LEE

8.1. INTRODUCTION

The complexity of human disease results in numerous opportunities for disease pathology to circumvent the effectiveness of a drug against a single molecular target. Clinicians in therapeutic areas like oncology and infectious disease have long known that intensive initial therapy with combinations of drugs can often mean the difference in a sustained and durable response with limited emergence of resistance. Indeed, with the transition from the era of genomics to the era of personalized medicine comes the realization that even the most highly targeted agents can perform unexpectedly in the context of complex disease pathology [1]. It is clear that in many cases combinations of multiple targeted agents will be required to adequately address disease pathology and prevent the action of redundant pathways or resistance mechanisms from circumventing drug effectiveness. But the complexity and probability of success of bringing a single new molecular entity to the market makes the contemplation of a dual new chemical entity (NCE) clinical development plan a challenging case. Furthermore, dwindling pipelines and conservative regulatory posture add to the challenges.

So how can the pharmaceutical industry leverage the power of drug combinations in this current environment? One approach is to access the untapped value in combinations of drugs whose use in humans has already been shown to be safe and effective. The world's pharmacopeia of approved

Drug Repositioning: Bringing New Life to Shelved Assets and Existing Drugs, First Edition.
Edited by Michael J. Barratt and Donald E. Frail.
© 2012 John Wiley & Sons, Inc. Published 2012 by John Wiley & Sons, Inc.

drugs represents in some cases decades of clinical experience in many thousands of patients. In addition, there are a large number of drug candidates that have been shown to be safe and well tolerated but have failed to demonstrate adequate efficacy for approval. Together, this group of molecules represents an elite set of active pharmaceutical agents targeting some of the most important pathways known in human disease. By combining these elite molecules, the industry can tap into a complexity of millions of independent pairwise combinations, each with the potential to act synergistically in human disease.

Creating combinations of active ingredients to facilitate convenience or compliance is nothing new and has been leveraged in the pharmaceutical industry, in some cases with a high level of commercial success. For example Avandamet®, the fixed dose combination of metformin and rosiglitazone to treat type 2 diabetes combines two classes of oral antidiabetic drugs and provides patients with an alternative to multi-pill regimens. Similarly, multiple fixed dose combinations are used in antihypertensive therapy, for example, combinations of angiotensin-converting enzyme (ACE) inhibitors with calcium channel blockers (CCBs), which have been shown to improve patient compliance and convenience and reduce out-of-pocket costs [2]. Although such combinations have been used by the pharmaceutical industry as a component of drug life cycle management and can provide real benefit to patients, they are fundamentally not about the discovery of new unexpected combination biology.

It is a different case entirely to discover and create drug combinations which access an unexpected synergistic interaction that reveals new combination biology. Unlike fixed dose combinations employing a rational pairing of drugs already used concurrently, unexpected synergistic drug combinations demonstrate effects substantially greater than would be expected from adding together each individual activity. Some examples in this category include the antibiotic Bactrim®, the combination of sulfamethoxazole and trimethoprim [3], and the anti-HIV drug Atripla® [4], where three nucleotide/nonnucleotide reverse transcriptase inhibitors are combined in a single tablet. Synergistic combinations such as those embodied by Bactrim® and Atripla® have changed treatment paradigms and demonstrate how synergistic drug interactions can impact patients' lives [5].

This chapter will focus on the potential of combinations of existing drugs to provide unexpected synergies when used in combination in a different disease model. Included will be a discussion of the rationale and technologies that can be used to discovery unexpected combination biology as well as a review of some of the unique opportunities and challenges associated with the development and commercialization of repositioned drugs used in combinations.

8.2. FUNDAMENTAL APPROACHES

Combination space is large and complex. Imagine for a moment all possible unique pairwise combinations of the world's approved drugs, approximately

3000 active agents. That is almost 4.5 million unique pairs. In order to survey this space over multiple assays—cancer cell lines for instance—or multiple drug concentrations, it is quickly apparent that the numbers quickly become enormous. There are a number of technological innovations that have made accessing this space ever more possible, and these are discussed further below. However, the most effective first step in designing a combination discovery effort is careful consideration of the objectives of the experiment and tailoring the fundamental approach to achieve those objectives. One approach is to undertake a systematic survey of an entire set of drugs to find all possible pairwise synergistic interactions. In this approach, the combination space can be imagined as a cube with each single agent represented once on both the x- and y-axes with each pairwise combination at the intersection of any given x,y point. The cube can stretch out into the z-axis by replicating each combination test in a unique cellular assay system (Figure 8.1). This approach maximizes the potential to discover new and unexpected combination biology and is well aligned with early discovery objectives. The main disadvantage of this approach is the large number of data points needed to systematically survey a cube shaped space.

An alternative is to take a more focused approach, what is sometimes referred to as an enhancer screen in the author's laboratory. Here combination space can be imagined as a more rectangular shape where one axis consists of a small number of drugs of particular value that are surveyed broadly against a second axis of many drugs—the enhancers. This approach is well suited to the evaluation of existing drugs as potential combination partners for a new agent and can suggest potential co-therapy options or indeed combination regimens to avoid during clinical development. This approach best balances the ability to discover new combination biology with a focused approach to reduce the number of data points collected.

In addition to the scope and scale of a combination effort, consideration must be given to the sophistication of the hypothesis driving the experiment. For example, one could design a study using highly specific and selective drugs representing a defined set of drug targets along a particular disease pathway to test specific hypotheses about target interactions on a disease pathway. In this case, concentrations could be carefully tailored to maintain "on-target" effects making for a clear interpretation of the results. There is much to be learned about specific target interactions using this approach, but since the selection of targets and drugs is based on current understanding from the literature or empirical experimentation, the ability to discover new targets and unexpected combination biology is limited. Conversely, an approach that is more agnostic toward the targets being tested and instead relies on a phenotypic endpoint predictive of disease biology greatly enhances the probability of discovering unexpected synergistic targets by allowing disease biology to select the best interactions. A key disadvantage of the agnostic approach is the potential need for reverse pharmacology and target validation work to understand unexpected synergies.

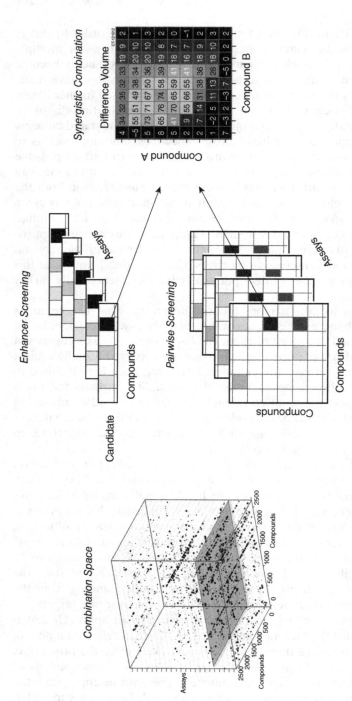

FIGURE 8.1. Exploring combination space. Combination space can be envisioned as a cube consisting of single agents represented on the x- and y-axes and unique screening assays on the z- axis. Sampling the entire plane of all possible pairs of agents in a given assay or set of assays can be referred to as pairwise screening. Sampling a rectangular space where a single or focused set of candidates is combined with a large set of agents in a given assay or set of assays can be referred to as enhancer screening. Synergies can be represented by spots on the cube or in a heat map format with size/color scaled to the magnitude of their deviation from the reference model. The difference volume represents the difference between the empirical data and the model surface for each square of the dose response matrix.

A final screen design consideration particularly relevant to repurposing existing drugs in combination stems from the pragmatic strategy of accelerating the timeline to clinical proof of concept in human studies. Approved drugs have been optimized to overcome a key set of development hurdles including safety, availability, metabolism, pharmacokinetics, stability, and many others. These properties endow approved drugs with elite status and can enable rapid entry into new clinical situations with limited additional nonclinical evaluation. One has only to look a bit farther back in the pipeline to find an additional set of elite compounds—those that have passed safety, availability, and manufacturing hurdles—yet failed late in development for reasons of efficacy or commercial considerations. While not approved drugs, this set represents a rich source of additional assets with human clinical experience and the potential for nascent activity in combination. In cases where approved drugs or late stage development candidates are inaccessible because of branded status, lack of commercial source, or difficulties in manufacturing, surrogates can often be selected from the plethora of potent, selective research-grade compounds that engage the same target. Once relevant combination biology has been discovered, confirmatory studies can be undertaken with the development candidate or approved drug.

8.3. KEYS TO SUCCESS

8.3.1. What's in a Model?

Interactions between two drugs can take many forms, and an extensive body of mathematical and theoretical literature has been presented on this topic. It should be noted that a robust debate over the best reference interaction models, their use and interpretation, and indeed uniform terminology on drug interactions has been ongoing for many decades and continues today. Readers who are interested in exploring the theoretical discussion of drug interactions and models to predict them are encouraged to refer to several excellent discourses on the topic [6–10]. For the purposes of this review, the discussion will focus on discovery and exploitation of the desirable aspects of drug interactions (i.e., antidisease effects) as opposed to the less desirable aspects (i.e., metabolic interactions, traditional "drug–drug interactions"). Although the theoretical models discussed here can in many cases be applied to the latter, such interactions are often easily identified and removed during the traditional and well-established pharmaceutical lead optimization process.

From the perspective of providing medical benefit, there are two useful ways in which one compound can influence the antidisease activity of another, which will hereafter be referred to as potency shifting and effect boosting (Figure 8.2A and [11]). In the case of potency shifting, the magnitude of a combination effect is typically evaluated on the basis of whether the addition of a second agent results in substantially less of the first agent needed to achieve the desired effect level. The evaluation of synergy in this context is particularly useful in the justification of clinically used combinations where one can define the point at which the combination provides clinical benefit that cannot be otherwise achieved by just increasing the dose of either single agent. The most commonly used model of dose additivity is that initially described by Loewe, where the model provides a null reference that is predicted by the expected response if the two compounds combined are in fact the same drug [10]. As an example consider two drugs, trimethoprim and sulfamethoxazole, the components of Bactrim®, which each achieves a single agent effect level of 50% at 1.3 µM and 31 µM, respectively, in an antibacterial assay (Figure 8.2B). The Loewe additivity model would then predict that if the combination of these two drugs was strictly additive, combining 0.63 µM of trimethoprim and 15.5 µM of sulfamethoxazole would also give an effect level of 50%. This would be analogous to combining 0.63 µM of trimethoprim with to 0.63 µM of trimethoprim, giving a total of 1.3 µM of trimethoprim and achieving a 50% effect level. By quantifying the deviation from the Loewe additivity model, one can then quantify the effect of the combination interaction. One common way in which such deviations are quantified is by using the combination index (CI) [12]. The CI is the ratio of the total effective drug dose of the combination compared with that of the single agents required to achieve

---

FIGURE 8.2. Recognizing combination effects. (A) Compound interactions can be described as potency shifting where the concentration required to achieve a specific effect is reduced, and effect boosting where the maximal effect achieved is increased. (B) Single agent responses of trimethoprim and sulfamethoxazole, the components of Bactrim®, in a bacterial growth inhibition assay. Trimethoprim has an EC50 of 0.63 µM, and sulfamethoxazole has an EC50 of 31 µM. (C) The empirical data of a combination of trimethoprim and sulfamethoxazole in an 8 × 8 dose response matrix where all possible doses and ratios of the combination are sampled. The single agent responses are depicted in the first column and bottom row of the response matrix. Each square represents a unique dose/ratio pair with the number in the square indicating the effect level achieved by that pair in a bacterial growth inhibition assay. Squares are also shaded in a heat map according to the magnitude of the effect level. The model surface indicates the derived reference model data for the situation where the two single agents are additive in combination. In this case the Loewe additivity model is calculated based on the two single agent responses. The difference volume represents the difference between the empirical data and the model surface for each square of the dose response matrix. The sum of the difference volume across all doses and ratios of the combination is equal to 1920% in this example. The isobologram at the 50% effect is depicted where the axes are normalized for the drug concentration of each single agent that achieves the 50% effect level. The diagonal line between the 100%/0% pairing of the two single agents represents the hypothetical additivity model at 50% inhibition. Arrows depict the direction of deviation from the additivity line indicating synergy or antagonism. The calculated dose ratios of both agents achieving the 50% effect level are connected by the isobol line indicating a high level of synergy.

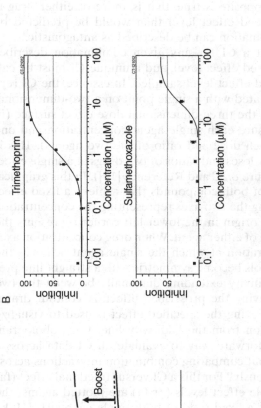

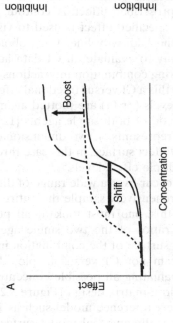

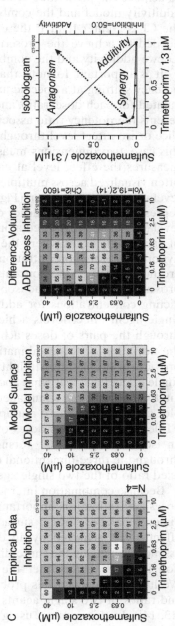

a given effect level. When the CI is less than 1, less of either drug is needed to achieve the proscribed effect level than would be predicted by the Loewe additivity model and the combination can be described as synergistic. When the CI is greater than 1, the opposite is true, that is, more of either drug is needed to achieve the proscribed effect level than would be predicted by Loewe additivity and the combination can be described as antagonistic.

It is important to note that a CI for any given combination describes potency shifting at a specific fixed effect level, and a unique CI must be calculated for each dose, ratio, and effect level sampled. In essence, the CI represents the potency ratio associated with a single point on a two-dimensional slice or iso-effect level through the three-dimensional dose effect surface (in this case, two dimensions measure each single agent concentration and one measures the effect level at each dose and ratio of the two agents). This is often visualized across multiple doses and ratios of two drugs at a single effect level using an isobologram (Figure 8.2C and Reference [10]). In this graphical representation, pairs of doses of both compounds that achieve a fixed effect level (isoboles) are plotted along the two axes representing the concentration of each single agent where the origin in the lower left corner represents the hypothetical zero concentration of either agent. When drug concentration axes are normalized to the concentration at which the single agent achieves the proscribed effect level, the isobols become symmetric with a straight line predicting concentrations for additivity extending diagonally between the two single agent effect levels achieving the proscribed effect. A contour drawn through the pairs of doses achieving the specified effect is used to visualize the deviation of the combination from the additivity line. The isobologram provides a simple and straightforward way to evaluate all CI data across a single effect level, but what about comparing combination interactions across multiple effect levels simultaneously? For this a CI versus fractional effect (fa) plot can be used, where multiple effect levels (or fa) are plotted against the CI derived for various doses of a fixed ratio of both single agents [12]. Like an isobologram, the CI versus fa plot represents a two-dimensional slice through the three-dimentional dose/ratio/effect surface, in this case through a fixed ratio of the two single agents at multiple effect levels.

Because combination interactions can occur over a wide range of different doses and ratios, it is important to comprehensively sample the entire three-dimensional dose effect surface. To do this, one must look at all possible effect levels achieved by all doses and ratios of the two single agents, in essence visualizing the three-dimentional surface of the combination interaction in ways that neither the isobologram nor CI versus fa plot depicts. We have approached this problem by evaluating all possible concentrations and ratios of two single agents in a full dose-matrix design (Figure 8.2C and [13, 14]). In this context, using a null-effect reference model such as Loewe additivity allows the calculation of a three-dimensional model surface predicted by the single agent response curves. This surface can then be compared with the three-dimensional dose effect surface empirically derived from tests of all doses and ratios of each of the single agents in combination. Simply subtracting the model surface predicted from the null-effect model from the observed, empirically derived surface allows the calculation of a difference volume representing deviation from the model. This difference volume can also be further scaled by the meaningful effect level associated with the particular assay, enabling the prioritization of synergistic interactions identified in a screen. In this context, it is often very helpful to collect a series of "self-crosses" or pairwise combinations of the same agents, to develop a statistical benchmark for the noise of the difference volume in the assay system. The method of utilizing difference volume from the model surface has the advantage of emphasizing the combination interaction across a broad range of concentrations and ratios, minimizing the effects of individual outliers, and facilitating the identification of combinations with robust combination effects. Furthermore, by using a set of shape models to characterize the morphology of the full response surfaces, one can infer a relationship between the dose matrix response shape of a combination and the connectivity of the targets engaged by the combination [13].

The discussion so far has focused on the Loewe additivity null-effect model, which is one of the best recognized and robust models for evaluating drug interactions. The approach of calculating the entire difference volume across full matrix dose response data has the advantage of flexibility in that it can be applied using a variety of null-effect reference models, and multiple models can be calculated and evaluated against a single set of empirically derived matrix data. Indeed given the ongoing debate regarding the best interaction models, it is very desirable to be able to evaluate multiple models to determine the best one for any given situation. For example, Bliss independence is another commonly used null-effect reference model that predicts an interaction of two agents where neither one interferes with the other and each contributes independently to the resulting effect [6]. Bliss independence is particularly useful in quantifying boosts in maximal effect level over that achievable by either single agent alone, although this model suffers from the theoretical consideration that pure mechanistic independence in complex and highly integrated biologic systems is likely a rare occurrence. A third useful reference model is that of Gaddum's noninteraction, also described as the "highest single agent" (HSA) model, which uses the highest effect level achieved by the most active single agent as the null reference [7]. Finally, the coalism model is used to describe interaction cases where there is a strong increase in effect level that occurs above a concentration threshold for either single agent and is independent of all single agent activity [10, 15]. Coalism describes the chemical genetics equivalent to a genetic synthetic lethal interaction; where neither drug has a substantial effect on its own but when combined there is a dramatic increase in maximal effect level.

An important consideration that goes hand in hand with selection of the most appropriate reference model is the level of experimental sampling required to ensure robustness. Factors to consider in this decision include the expected effect level and reproducibility of the single agent dose response, the complexity of the three-dimensional dose effect surface expected and whether the experiment is operating in an exploratory (screening) or confirmatory mode (Figure 8.3A,B). For screening approaches where the objective is to cover as much combination space as possible with acceptable false positive and false negative rates, lower density sampling approaches can be used and reference models that more robustly handle limited data can be employed. For example, the most sparsely sampled method would be to collect 4 points, a single concentration for each single agent, a combination of these two concentrations, and a negative control (untreated) reference (1×1 format). Reference models such as HSA can be useful in interpreting such sparse data, in particular when the concentrations of either single agent are selected as to produce no or low effect levels. Conversely, in situations where the objective is to carefully characterize a combination interaction for the purposes of decision making for further preclinical development, a higher density approach where the entire dose effect surface is characterized would be more appropriate. In this case, full sampling of both single agents across the dose response spectrum including the no effect concentration, EC50 and EC90 would provide the best null model prediction. Similarly, dose matrix sampling across multiple concentrations and ratios of the combination will best characterize the interaction surface. The Loewe additivity model has proven particularly robust in detecting combination interactions under these conditions.

8.3.2. Complex Biology

There are three key technological features required for successful combination screening effort. First is the ability to access complex disease biology through the use of phenotypic cell-based assays. Second is a robust screening operations platform with some important distinguishing capabilities enabling the construction and tracking of combination tests. Finally, a robust data collection, storage, and analysis platform that optimally incorporates existing knowledge about approved drugs and late stage development candidates is needed. In the following section each of these key factors will be discussed, with an emphasis on large-scale efforts to evaluate large numbers of combinations.

Efficient and high-throughput cell free assays have been the mainstay for target-based drug screening throughout the pharmaceutical industry and have been used successfully to discover potent and selective drugs against a variety of enzymatic targets. These assays, however, are generally not suitable for a combination high-throughput screen because they do not properly model the complexity of multi-target biology which a combination screening effort seeks to perturb. Therefore, a successful combination screening effort will employ cell-based phenotypic assays that preserve the biological complexity and relevant molecular pathway interactions of disease pathology [16]. Typically, phenotypic assays are evaluated for an endpoint that represents the culmination of a number of biological pathway interactions and optimally represents

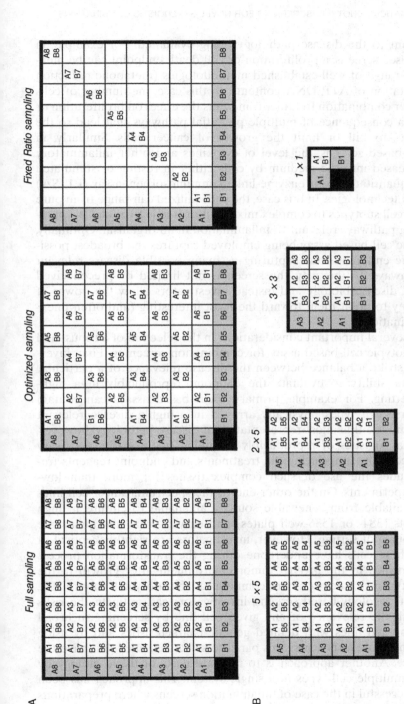

FIGURE 8.3. Experimental sampling in dose matrix formats. (A) The level of sampling in a dose matrix format can utilize full sampling of every possible dose and ratio, optimized sampling of a subset of doses and ratios, fixed ratio sampling on the "diagonal" of a dose matrix, as well as combinations of the latter two methods. (B) The number of doses and ratios and the shape of the dose matrix can be modified to fit the objectives of the screen and the response of the agents used. Combinations of two active agents require sampling at multiple doses, while silent agents can be sampled at a single relevant concentration. Lower resolution formats can be used for initial screening and higher resolution formats for confirmation and follow-up.

a state relevant to the disease pathology being evaluated. For example, in oncology-focused screens, a proliferation or cell death endpoint can be measured using a range of well-established methodologies (metabolic reduction assays, quantitation of ATP, DNA content). In this case, the number of cells remaining after combination treatment, and thus the effect on proliferation or cell death, is a consequence of multiple potential pathways that lead to the desired result—to kill or limit the growth of cancer cells. Similarly, in inflammation-based screens, the level of cytokines and other inflammatory mediators released into the medium by cells either in resting or stimulated states can be quantitated using enzyme-linked immunosorbent assay (ELISA) or bead-based technologies. In this case, the cells utilized can range from pure inflammatory cell subtypes to complex mixed cultures able to model the paracrine signaling pathways relevant to inflammation in an organism. Optimally, the phenotypic cell-based assay being employed captures the broadest possible phenotypic endpoint, thus capturing as many possible disease-relevant signaling pathways. In this way, the screen is not limited by preconceived notions about disease biology and instead investigators allow the power of systems biology to point them toward the most interesting (and often unexpected) combinations.

There are several important considerations in the selection of a robust and relevant phenotypic cell-based assay for combination screening. First, investigators must strike a balance between the disease relevance of a particular assay with the ability to evaluate the endpoint reproducibly in a high-throughput setting. For example, primary tissue-based assays can contain multiple diverse cell types physically arrayed in a highly disease relevant architecture and are thus most representative of disease pathology; however, the operational logistics of reproducibly obtaining tissue at the necessary scale and successfully introducing the treatments and endpoint reagents frequently precludes the use of such complex tissues for more than low-throughput experiments. On the other end of the spectrum, cancer cell lines are widely available from renewable sources, amenable to culture in high density formats (384- or 1536-well plates) and easy to treat and quantitate in a high-throughput setting. However, investigators are rightly skeptical of the changes these cells have undergone during the transformation process and their relevance to the *in vivo* tumor environment after growth in the serum- and oxygen-rich environment common to laboratory cell culture [17]. In the case of oncology-based screens, investigators can mitigate the risks associated with the relevance of any given cell line by screening in broad panels of many cell lines with defined genetic characteristics and by using the power of multiple tests across this panel to select activities that have the most relevance. Another approach is to recreate parts of tissue biology by co-culture of multiple cell types in a single system. This approach has been particularly successful in the case of inflammation screens where preparations of mixed white blood cells partially purified from whole blood or plasmapheresus by-products can be used to model the complex immunological interactions between cell populations *in vivo* [15, 18]. Similarly, multicellular culture systems can re-create the cell–cell interactions and drug penetration challenges relevant to the complex interplay of normal and tumor cells that comprise the tumor microenvironment [19, 20].

Despite their limitations, phenotypic cell-based assays have demonstrated their utility in the repositioning of single drugs in alternate indications. In one example, the topical antifungal agent ciclopirox olamine has been identified in a cell-based screen for decreased cell growth and viability in malignant leukemia, myeloma, and solid tumor cell lines [21]. This drug has since been reformulated into an oral preparation and is being evaluated in patients with relapsed and refractory hematological malignancies [22]. In another example, minocycline, a second-generation tetracycline analog with broad-spectrum antibacterial action, has demonstrated neuroprotective activity in several cell-based assays of neurological diseases and experimental models of neuronal injury including cerebral ischemia, amyotrophic lateral sclerosis, Parkinson's disease, Huntington's disease, and multiple sclerosis. These observations have led to the evaluation of minocycline in a growing number of human studies of neurodegenerative diseases [23]. By extension, these examples support the utility of cell-based phenotypic screening to the repurposing of approved drugs in combination.

So how does the investigator choose the right phenotypic cell-based assay for a combination high-throughput screen? Initially, the objectives of the screen and what biological features are most important to achieving those objectives should be considered. Is the target disease pathology based on a single genetic mutation or is the disease polygenic? Are interactions between multiple cell types responsible or is the disease driven by a single cell type? Are there phenotypic endpoints that are known to be directly linked to disease pathology? Are there endpoints that encompass the broadest possible spectrum of mechanisms that potentially impact disease biology? It is important to consider the questions of relevant biology early in the planning of any combination screen utilizing cell-based phenotypic assays, and there is no substitute for understanding how this biology will ultimately impact the discovery objectives of the screen. Optimally, cell-based assays and endpoints should capture the broadest possible sampling of molecular pathways to limit potential bias imposed by preconceived ideas regarding what pathways are most relevant. This is especially important in the context of combination drug screening since probing multiple pathways in concert can often reveal completely unexpected pathway connections.

Once investigators have developed an understanding of the most relevant biology for the screening objectives, consideration should be given to what assay endpoints related to this biology can be reasonably and reproducibly measured in a high-throughput setting. At this point it is important to understand the level of effect that must necessarily be achieved and how this compares with the expected noise of the screening assay. For example, in an oncology setting, success might depend on complete killing of cells, expressed as logarithmic changes in cell number that might be easily measured in the context of moderate noise levels (for example, 10–15%). Conversely, in an inflammation setting, even 50% reduction of particular inflammatory mediators might be all that is necessary for therapeutic benefit and thus detecting such effects necessitates an assay endpoint where noise levels are minimized. It is important to note that all screening efforts require a compromise between disease relevance and the logistical limitations on precision and accuracy that automated screening imposes. The key to selecting and optimizing (or rejecting) a phenotypic cell-based assay for combination screening is understanding what the successful output will look like and the probability of observing this effect clearly above the noise of the screening system. Other important strategic considerations in this respect include the level of false positive and false negative results that are tolerable and the amount of time and resources that are available to achieve the goal.

8.3.3. Screening Operations

High-throughput drug screening is a well-established and widely used technology for target-based and phenotypic assay-based drug discovery and evaluation and several excellent reviews cover this topic [24–30]. However, there are several key features distinguishing combination screen operations from that of single agents. The first is the laboratory information management system (LIMS) needed to generate and track combinations. In early screening efforts, available automation software was limited to the delivery of a single agent from one well on a compound source plate to its analogous well on a corresponding assay plate. The only way to generate combinations containing more than one agent in one assay well was to generate two sets of compound source plates with the appropriate single agents to be delivered sequentially to a single assay well. Although tractable (and heavily utilized in early screening efforts), this approach suffers from the limitation that all compound source plates for a combination screen must be specified and created in advance, limiting the ability to make changes to compounds and concentrations during the course of a screen and increasing the amount of compound waste. With the advent of acoustic liquid delivery and new compound management algorithms it has become possible to "cherry-pick" single agents from a standard set of compound source plates for introduction into a single assay well on an automated system [31, 32]. It is important to note that while there are "off-the-shelf" automation hardware platforms that are amenable to this approach, they are limited in number and lack sophisticated LIMS architecture to drive, monitor, and track complex combination screens.

The level of sampling of a combination interaction has important impacts on experimental design as well as the methodology used for interaction interpretation (see Figure 8.3A,B and section above). For most combination interaction models, "active" single agents will require sampling across multiple doses while "silent" agents can be sampled at a single relevant concentration. The most robust way to effectively sample active combination interaction is through the use of a dose matrix format where all possible doses and ratios of the two single agents are tested (Figure 8.3A). This dose matrix or "check-erboard" format requires substantial assay plate real estate and creates large datasets. Several methods have been employed to reduce the amount of combination sampling while retaining the ability to robustly evaluate any potential combination effect. In the author's laboratory, symmetrical matrices ranging from 10×10 to 1×1 have been utilized to evaluate combinations of active single agents (Figure 8.3A,B). In many cases, lower resolution matrices (e.g., 1×1 or 3×3) can be used for initial comprehensive screening and "hits" can be followed up in higher resolution formats (e.g., 8×8). In other cases, combination matrices can be sampled in an "optimized" format where only a subset of combination doses are collected across the most important points in the matrix for combination interpretation. This can range from approximately every other well to a fixed ratio of serial dilutions across the "diagonal" of the matrix (Figure 8.3A). It is important that concentration sampling of single agents and combinations allows both the determination of a robust curve fit for reference model calculation as well as dynamic range available to observe combination effects. For example, if one or both of the single agents tested achieves a minimum 95% effect level in an assay system with a top effect level of 100%, little dynamic range is left to observe a synergistic interaction. In this case single agents should be titrated across a range of concentrations so as to define the EC50 in the assay and leave room above this level for synergy to be observed. Conversely, when one of the single agents is silent and demonstrates little to no effect in the assay system, a single high dose of this agent can be combined with the dose-titrated active agent. This approach has the effect of dramatically diminishing the number of assay wells needed to sample "active–silent" combination space. When screening pairs of silent agents, a single high dose of each agent can be screened and any effect observed can be attributed to the combination. Furthermore, in the case of "silent–silent" screening, pooling strategies may also be employed to increase throughput and minimize necessary time and supplies.

Combination screening is not limited to the evaluation of pairwise combinations and indeed the use of higher order combination screening has been used to probe the robustness of biological systems [33]. In the author's laboratory, approaches including three-, four-, five-way, and higher order combinations have been routinely utilized. There are several important considerations when planning the generation of higher order combinations, the first of which being the density of sampling across the combination. When using a dose matrix format such as those described above, a three-way combination could be sampled in all possible doses and ratios of all three single agents resulting in a three-dimensional cube of data. The reader can quickly see that although this is the most systematic way of evaluating three-way synergy, the number of data points and complexity of data analysis become quite challenging. An alternative approach is the use of fixed ratio combinations serially diluted in two-dimensional dose matrices. In this approach, appropriate fixed ratios for each combination are selected that effectively sample across the synergy surface, then fixed doses are combined in a second dose matrix, enabling an accurate prediction of the mathematical synergy associated with a four-way combination with data from a two-dimensional format. By generating a set of pairwise, three-way and four-way combination data using fixed dose ratios, one can effectively evaluate combination interactions associated with a drug of interest and complex cocktails of treatment therapies currently in use. Furthermore, higher order combination evaluation may also assist in deconvoluting network interconnectivity and in understanding pathway addiction under particular genotypic conditions [33]. For an example of this approach, see Figure 8.4.

A final consideration in the operational design of any combination screen is whether to add compounds simultaneously or sequentially to the assay system. There are documented cases of combinations of compounds where sequential application elicits maximal balance of therapeutic benefit and side effect profile. Take for example the clinical regimen of gemcitabine and platinum drugs utilized in metastatic breast cancer [34], non-small cell lung cancer [35] and in esophageal cancer [36]. Preclinical evidence suggests that the sequential administration of gemcitabine and cisplatin confers schedule-dependent synergy *in vitro* [37]. Investigation of different schedules of administration of gemcitabine and cisplatin in the clinical setting reveals that administration of cisplatin 24 hours prior to gemcitabine led to the highest levels of gemcitabine triphosphate accumulation and total platinum levels in plasma [38] while administration of gemcitabine 24 hours prior to cisplatin led to the least toxicity [39]. These results have become the basis of the further evaluation of schedule-dependent administration of gemcitabine with platinum drugs on efficacy in metastatic breast cancer with and without trastuzumab [40, 41], and eosophageal cancer [36]. Given these findings, the use of temporal sequencing in combination screening has the potential to add an additional level of complexity for detecting relevant combination interactions. It stands to reason that in certain cases signaling pathways, cellular state (quiescent vs. activated), or epigenetic context must be perturbed in advance in order for a second agent to generate a synergistic disease-modifying effect. Thus, temporal sequencing in combination screening may have the capacity to identify combination interactions that would otherwise be missed when using only simultaneous addition. However, this added benefit comes at the cost of additional time and resource allocation for a temporal sequencing effort, which can easily triple the number of assay wells needed to evaluate any single pair of agents. Furthermore, the translation of any *in vitro* schedule dependence to a clinical treatment regimen would need to be explored preclinically and empirically confirmed in a patient setting. Despite these caveats and the relatively limited understanding of the rate and translatablility of sequence-dependent combination interactions, it is the author's expectation that there remain undiscovered synergistic interactions in this poorly explored portion of combination space.

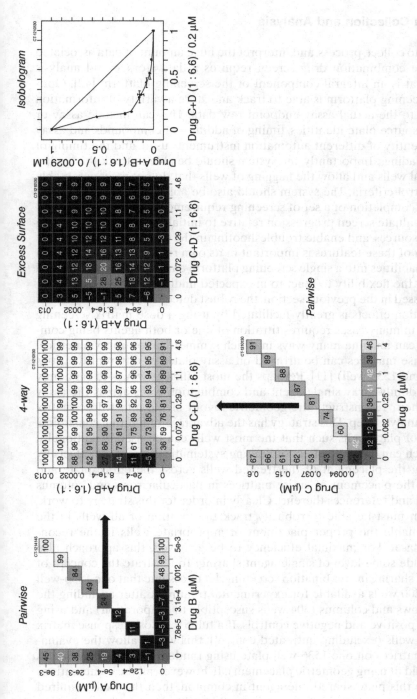

FIGURE 8.4. Higher order combinations. An example of a synergistic four-way combination using fixed ratio pairwise combinations is depicted. Synergistic pairwise combinations of drugs A and B and drugs C and D are sampled at a fixed ratio represented by the "diagonal" of each matrix. These fixed ratios of A + B and C + D are then serially diluted in a second matrix to create a response curve for reference model calculation. Responses for all possible doses and ratios of the two fixed dose combinations are collected in the dose matrix. The excess surface indicates deviation from the reference model surface in the four-way combination of drugs A + B + C + D. The isobologram depicts deviation from additivity at the 80% effect level.

8.3.4. Data Collection and Analysis

The ability to collect, process, and interpret the huge amount of data associated with a large combination drug screen requires a data storage and analysis platform that is an integral component of the screening platform [42]. Optimally, a screening platform is able to track and store a variety of information in addition to the actual assay endpoint raw data. This can include assay or compound source plate identities, timing of addition of compounds and assay reagents, identity of different automation instruments used, and the timing of endpoint readings. Importantly, the system should be able to track the quality of individual wells and allow the flagging of wells that do not meet acceptable quality control criteria. The system should also be able to catalog and report the level of completion of a set of screening requirements, allowing the investigator to evaluate screen progression relative to initial assumptions regarding time and resources, and enable troubleshooting in the case of systemic quality issues. Each of these features is important in its own right, but the integration of these capabilities into a single screening platform enables efficient and rapid results with the flexibility to react to unexpected findings.

As discussed in the previous section, the robust detection and interpretation of combination effects is greatly facilitated by using a dose matrix screening format and in many cases requires titration of one or both agents being combined. One can imagine many ways in which symmetrical or nonsymmetrical dose response matrices can be arrayed on assay plates of different densities (96-, 384-, and 1536-well) [11]. Perhaps the most efficient way is to randomly or semi-randomly array single agent and combination wells across the assay plate and then "reconstruct" the geometric layout of the intact dose matrix during the analysis step. This strategy has the advantage of limiting constraints on the use of plate wells such that the most wells can be used. Additionally, this approach can have the effect of limiting systematic plate-based effects by randomizing the placement of the treated wells across the entire plate and minimizing the placement of entire matrices in particular rows and columns (see [43, 44] and references therein). Clearly in order for this strategy to work, the platform must be able to robustly track the location of all wells in the matrix to enable the proper placement of appropriate wells in the reconstructed dataset. For maximal efficiency to be achieved, this approach also should include some level of single agent sharing. To illustrate the concept of single agent sharing in combination screening, let us assume that one 1536-well plate has 1200 wells available for experimental treatment after excluding the outer two rows and columns (304 wells susceptible to evaporation) and using 32 wells for positive and negative controls. If a full 5×5 dose response matrix requires 35 wells (excluding untreated control), this would allow the evaluation of 34 matrices on one 1536-well plate using random placement (whereas only 28 would fit using geometric placement). If, however, all the combinations included on this plate shared one agent in common, then the wells required for each subsequent combination matrix would be 30, allowing the evaluation of 40 full matrices on the same plate. This number can be further increased when replicate wells of the same combination are collected on the same plate. Using these parameters in a screen of 25,000 unique combinations (approximately 200 × 200 pairwise screen), in a single assay, 100s of plates can be saved with single agent sharing. One can quickly see how single agent sharing can greatly increase the efficiency at which assay plate wells are used and thus decrease the amount of expensive lab supplies and reagents needed to complete a screening program.

Efficiency in screening time is another important factor to consider in this process. The number of automation steps required to construct the combination matrices on any given plate will dictate how long it takes to complete each assay plate. For example, if a different compound source master plate must be loaded into the compound delivery system for each single agent utilized, this can add many minutes to the time necessary to complete the dosing of each plate. In the author's laboratory, dynamic real-time decision making and workflow optimization have been integrated into the LIMS architecture. In this approach, when an assay plate barcode is read by the platform, the LIMS dynamically determines an optimized unit of work for that plate. This work unit is not predetermined; rather the LIMS iterates an algorithm that optimizes both the single agents and combinations to be dosed on the assay plate based on outstanding work required to complete the screen. The algorithm surveys the screen attributes (e.g., combination dose-ratio points, number of replicate wells, intra- versus inter-plate replicates) and remaining work to optimize the number of combination matrices assigned to the assay plate based on single agent sharing, compound availability, and the minimal number of compound source plates required to dose the assay plate. This dynamic decision making facilitates the most efficient use of available assay plate wells, minimizes the time required to array combination matrices across the assay plate, and reduces compound consumption. By fine-tuning each of these parameters throughout screen production, screening throughput is increased while screening timeline and associated assay costs are reduced.

All of these improvements in time and cost savings can be negated by later bottlenecks in the time and resources required for evaluation of the screening data both for quality and assay controls and for combination effects. Thus, a seamless data transfer protocol into quality control and analytical methodology is required. Optimally quality control procedures should allow the ability to visually inspect plates at the whole plate and individual well level, evaluate positive and negative controls, examine systematic inter- and intra-plate effects, quantify variability, and apply pass–fail criteria to entire plates, individual wells, specific compounds, and combination matrices. Sophisticated algorithms can be employed that utilize automated quality scores to highlight data that must be further examined for quality by human investigators [45]. Quantitative methods of calculating combination interactions based on the reference models described above can then be applied to high quality data. One important feature of the use of repurposed drugs in combination screening is the ability to incorporate the vast body of existing clinical and research experience with these molecules into the evaluation of a combination effect. The ability to draw on this knowledgebase of information including, for example, potency at target, exposure levels, pharmacokinetics, tissue specificity, side effect profile, and metabolism profile, enables investigators to rapidly prioritize combinations with the most potential for rapid preclinical and clinical translation and the least potential for toxic side effects. In the author's laboratory we have incorporated a drug pharmacopeia library into our analysis platform software, enabling this type of triage to rapidly identify and prioritize the most interesting combinations warranting further follow-up.

8.4. OPPORTUNITIES AND CHALLENGES IN COMBINATION DRUG DEVELOPMENT

There are many aspects of combination drug development and ultimately commercialization that are shared with that of single molecules. One must still identify the correct therapeutic dose and demonstrate the safety and efficacy of any clinical candidate. There are, however, some key features of development and commercialization that are particularly important to combination drugs and are further distinguished when undertaking these activities with repurposed drugs in combinations. The following section will outline and discuss some the key differences and highlight where these differences produce opportunities for value generation as well as challenges to success.

8.4.1. Intellectual Property

The advent of screening repurposed agents in therapeutic assays outside the scope of their original indications has gained wide appeal in recent years with several newsworthy examples of success. Typically, such discoveries with repurposed single drugs result in patent claims for a new method of manufacture, delivery, or use [46]. The highly desired claims around composition of matter can be difficult to obtain with repurposed single drugs although strategies do exist to enhance patent protection and limit substitution to levels similar to a new unique molecular entity [46, 47]. In contrast, by combining two repurposed drugs to create a novel combination effect, one can generate and prosecute allowable composition of matter claims for the combination in a relatively straightforward manner. In this case, the demonstration of true mathematical synergy is a key component to overcoming examiner objections for obviousness. The patent estate of a combination of repurposed agents is often strengthened by claims for novel formulations, specific dissolution, release, or pharmacokinetic profiles, all of which have the potential to enhance the efficacy or convenience to the patient and serve to further reinforce the case against physician or patient substitution with individual components.

8.4.2. Reverse Pharmacology

The approach of phenotypic endpoint screening of drugs in combination results in both advantages and challenges in a drug discovery and development strategy [27]. Importantly, complex phenotypic assays for drug discovery represent a purely empirical approach, one where the biology of the system drives the discovery of novel pathway interactions. As has been demonstrated quite elegantly in genetic model systems such as yeast, fly, and worm, the selective power in phenotypic assay systems can lead to breakthrough discoveries otherwise not obtainable with strict hypothesis-driven approaches [48–50]. The power of this discovery approach does come with the addition of some important challenges to drug development. When using phenotypic endpoint screening, investigators do not know *a priori* what specific pathway is being perturbed to result in the phenotypic response. This is a necessary consequence of the cell-based assay approach—the complexity is needed to successfully probe complex networked systems, but substantial follow-up is often required to better understand the pathways and targets that are driving the effect. This outcome can be mitigated to some extent by screening highly selective targeted agents at concentrations within the range of the potency at their known
• target. However, restricting a screening effort in this way can reduce the potential for discovery of "off-target" effects, which can be an important component in expanding the utility of repurposed agents. While the discovery of such off-target effects undoubtedly poses challenges, investigators can often generate a reasonable hypothesis about relevant targets and pathways based on existing information that is associated with repurposed agents. This can form a basis for further evaluation through the use of additional assay systems, chemical genetic approaches, additional combination pairings, and overexpression or knockdown of relevant targets/pathways. In cases where no reasonable hypothesis can be formulated, targets and pathways can often be elucidated by employing system-wide approaches such as genomic or proteomic profiling or target interaction purification [51–53].

8.4.3. Preclinical Translation

When determining how to go about evaluating synergistic combinations in complex translational models of disease, it is important to consider upfront the key objectives of the combination study. Investigators should determine whether demonstration of mathematical synergy is the key objective versus the evaluation of the efficacy of a potential therapeutic. For the former, investigators will need to plan for enough dose levels of each single drug to calculate an appropriate reference model for the determination of a combination interaction. In this case, investigators may be inclined to reduce the dose of either or both drugs to sub-efficacy levels in order to demonstrate translation of the synergy mechanism. Although this is the best way to demonstrate true mathematical synergy, study designs such as this may be criticized for limiting the efficacy of either agent in a way that is not representative of clinical use. Furthermore, since translational models often require labor-intensive procedures or *in vivo* investigations, the dose-intensive nature of combination effect reference models can be at odds with the practicality of performing the experiment. In cases where the objective is improved outcome and strict demonstration of synergy is less important, study designs may start with a high and low dose of either agent, or even a single high dose when the maximal effect of an agent falls short of the desired level of efficacy. In cases where one or both agents is very active, alternative study designs focused on improving the treatment regimen (e.g., dose frequency and schedule) or reducing toxicity may be employed to demonstrate an improved outcome [54, 55]. When a combination demonstrates broad synergy in initial models across multiple doses and ratios, the selection of doses to evaluate in translational models offers many options. Conversely, in the case of synergy at only restricted doses or ratios, follow-up study doses must be carefully chosen and may utilize other factors such as relative level and timing of exposure to either agent after dose administration *in vivo*.

Investigators contemplating a combination screening program may ask what is the rate of translation of synergistic interactions from *in vitro* to *in vivo* models. This is very difficult to quantify. Many factors must be considered in the probability of translation of any combination interaction from primary discovery to disease models. For example, both agents must reach the appropriate tissue at the right concentration and with the right timing to elicit a combination effect. The impact of metabolism of both agents in the model system must also be considered. Thus, the administration of the individual agents at the appropriate times and by relevant routes is an integral part of any translational experimental design. In this respect, the incorporation of pharmacokinetic and/or pharmacodynamic evaluations can be very useful in interpreting the results of translational experiments. Investigators must also consider the magnitude of the synergy observed *in vitro* and what impact the translational model system may have on the ability to observe that effect. The dynamic range of effect measurable in the translational model, and the relative variability in measurement of the endpoint are factors that can impact the ability to observe the translation of synergy.

8.4.4. Embodiment of the Drug Product

A multi-targeted synergistic interaction can be a very powerful insight into disease biology, but how is this concept developed into a tangible drug product? Strategically one can imagine multiple ways in which a combination of two active agents can be created as a single commercial entity. One of the most straightforward ways is to develop the two active ingredients into a single fixed dose formulation, an approach that has been widely used in the case of "rational" pairings of approved drugs [15]. This strategy can be particularly useful when specific dose levels and ratios of the two active agents will be used in a particular indication and there is little need for dose titration or customization of the ratio for individual patients. In addition, this approach can provide a level of convenience and adherence to the patient, minimizing the number of pills that must be taken and ensuring the correct timing of administration of each drug, the latter being of particular significance in cases where the combination effect is dependent on the temporal action of either agent. In some indications, physicians require a greater level of flexibility in tailoring the dose or ratio of a combination product to each individual patient and thus might find that single fixed ratio co-formulated drug forms pose a limitation to the clinical benefit of their patients. The field of oncology is a good example of this case, where oncologists routinely combine multiple agents into a single regimen and frequently utilize dose modifications to maintain the level of clinical benefit while minimizing serious side effects (for example see References [56–58]). In cases such as this, a synergistic interaction may be more effectively developed as a single agent adjunctive indicated for use with a second drug or therapeutic regimen. When considering these two approaches specifically for repurposed drugs, an evaluation of factors necessary for commercial success should be integrated into the decision. A single fixed ratio formulation of two repurposed generic agents can be at risk for substitution with the single agent components unless the co-formulation facilitates clinical benefit such as aligned pharmacokinetics or improved schedule [46]. When repurposing a drug combination using a single agent adjunctive strategy, key product enhancements such as a substantial change in the kinetics of drug exposure (e.g., sustained release) or a switch in route of administration (e.g., from oral to intravenous or transdermal) may be required to provide an additional clinical benefit and thus protect from the threat of substitution.

The third and perhaps most challenging approach to embodying a combination insight is the creation of a single new multi-targeted chemical entity that harnesses the effect initially discovered with two separate agents. In this case, it is critical that the two (or more) targets/pathways engaged in the synergy are known such that traditional medicinal chemistry approaches can be combined with synergy analysis to identify and optimize chemical scaffolds and pharmacophores. Here one would likely utilize a combined approach of both cell-free targeted assays as well as cell-based phenotypic assays to develop a clear structure–activity relationship describing the activity and synergy of a multi-targeted agent. While clearly representing the more time-consuming path to embodiment, this approach represents the strongest protection against the threat of substitution. When repurposed drugs are used in the initial screening effort, investigators can build on what is known about the drugs and targets to design a successful multi-targeted agent development program. Furthermore, one could also consider this approach as a second-generation embodiment of a combination initially developed as either a fixed dose combination or single agent adjunctive. This approach had seen some early success at the preclinical stage [59, 60].

It is important to note that in the case of repurposed agents in combination, the matter of pharmacokinetics and tissue exposure can represent an important development challenge as well as an opportunity for innovation. Most drugs have been heavily optimized for the route of administration and indication for which they have been approved, ensuring the best efficacy and safety profile for that indication. When an alternative effect is discovered in a new potential indication, it is frequently the case that this new use requires different dosing, tissue exposure, or route of administration to achieve the appropriate efficacy and safety profile. Similarly, a change in route of administration can result in substantially different pharmacology for a known drug [46]. This issue can be amplified in the case of repurposed agents in combination. Here, the combination presentation must deliver both active ingredients to the right tissue at the right concentration/ratio and over the right timing in order to achieve the most efficacious combination effect with the least safety liability. Differences in pharmacokinetic profile, tissue accumulation, metabolism, and elimination can often be challenging to align, particularly when individual drugs have been optimized for a different indication. Here, clever changes to route of administration and pharmacokinetic profile of a synergistic combination can provide substantial medical benefit to patients while also generating new intellectual property and serving as a strong barrier to substitution. Such changes can be embodied through novel formulations and delivery vehicles (see Reference [61] and below).

8.4.5. Clinical Development

There are many scenarios for the clinical evaluation of two drugs in combination, requiring each program to be evaluated on its specifics on a case by case basis and several recent reviews discuss specific cases in pain, immunotherapy, oncology, infectious disease, diabetes, hypertension, migraine, and chronic obstructive pulmonary disease (COPD) [62–69]. This section will focus on highlighting some of the key considerations specific to combination clinical development with a particular focus on repurposed agents. There are a number of regulatory guidelines and regulations in the United States and worldwide that can be interpreted to apply to combination clinical development. Indeed, recently the FDA has developed guidance for industry focused on combination drug development in specific focus areas including HIV/AIDs treatments [70] and is evaluating draft guidance on the co-development of combinations of two or more investigational drugs [71]. In the United States, new combination drugs may be approved through either the 505(b)(1) or 505(b)(2) regulatory pathway of the Federal Food, Drug, and Cosmetics Act (Chapter V: Drugs and Devices, section 505). Further U.S. regulations specifically applicable to combinations of drugs include the Code of Federal Regulations, Title 21, (CFR 21) Volume 5, sections 300.50 and 314.54. For combinations of repurposed drugs, the decision between the 505(b)(1) and 505(b)(2) pathway must take into account several factors including the patent ownership and status of the components, ownership or right of reference to approval data for the components, and the extent to which the reference drug(s) are modified. Advantages of the 505(b)(2) route include the need for substantially less clinical development cost and time through reliance on safety and efficacy data utilized in the initial approval of one or both components of the combination. Depending on the amount of new data generated and the nature of the difference from the reference drug(s), 505(b)(2) approvals can enjoy 3 or 5 years of market exclusivity post approval and are even eligible for additional exclusivities associated with orphan drug status and pediatric drug approval [72]. For further information on the 505(b)(2) approach and market exclusivity, see Chapter 4.

It should be noted that obtaining regulatory approval for repurposed drugs and combinations is not without potential risks. For example, when utilizing the 505(b)(2) pathway, sponsors must include patent certifications and applications may be delayed due to patent or exclusivity protection of the reference drug. In addition, sponsors filing a 505(b)(2) application must provide notice of certain patent certifications to the holders of the patent and new drug application (NDA) of the reference drug(s). With respect to safety, it is important that sponsors do not assume that safety signals acceptable for a drug's original indication will also be acceptable in a new treatment setting, especially if the new use proposes different doses, exposures, or treatment durations. In a recent case, Horizant™, a transported prodrug of the approved drug gabapentin, faced several unexpected safety hurdles during its NDA review for approval in restless leg syndrome. These included the need to submit a risk evaluation and mitigation strategy (REMS) driven by a requirement based on the original indication (epilepsy) as well as the need to address concerns regarding the observation of a rare tumor type in some preclinical models [31].

One of the more challenging aspects of combination drug development can be the design of a clinical development plan that effectively demonstrates the value of combining two or more drugs into a single dosage form. The 505(b)(2) application route is intended to eliminate unnecessary duplication of preclinical and some clinical studies for drugs that have been demonstrated to be safe and effective by FDA approval. A key component of this route especially relevant for combination drugs is the "determination of which studies are necessary to support the change or modification from the listed drug(s)." CFR 21 300.54 states that "Two or more drugs may be combined in a single dosage form when each component makes a contribution to the claimed effects and the dosage of each component (amount, frequency, duration) is such that the combination is safe and effective for a significant patient population requiring such concurrent therapy as defined in the labeling for the drug." In this case, fixed dose combinations of two agents already approved in the same indication and concurrently used as part of a therapeutic regimen are common examples of the use of the 505(b)(2) pathway. Some notable examples of combination drugs recently approved via the 505(b)(2) pathway include Jalyn™ (dutasteride/tamsulosin), Tribenzor™ (olmesartan/amlodipine/hydrochlorothiazide), Tekamlo™ (aliskiren/amlodipine),

Nuedexta® (dextromethorphan/quinidine), Exforge® (amlodipine/valsartan/hydrochlorothiazide), Amturnide™ (aliskiren/amlodipine/hydrochlorothiazide), and Twynsta® (telmisartan/amlodipine) (source: Drugs@FDA monthly drug approval reports). The demonstration of bioequivalence between the individually administered agents and the components administered in combination is often sufficient basis for approval. There are numerous cases of such "rational" combination drugs approved on this basis that are part of a line extension or life cycle management approach for pharmaceutical companies. Most of the combination products in the FDA Orange book [73] fall into this category of rational combination drugs (approved via either the 505(b)(1) or 5050(b)(2) pathway) and typically do not add substantial therapeutic benefit over the two agents administered separately with the possible exception of an increased level of compliance afforded by the convenience of one pill versus two or more. Special cases of the CFR 21 300.54 general rule are "where a component is added: (1) To enhance the safety or effectiveness of the principal active component; and (2) To minimize the potential for abuse of the principal active component." There are few examples of approved combination products of this kind that generally provide a level of meaningful clinical benefit that exceeds the simple addition of their individual parts. Some examples of such combinations are seen in infectious disease, most notably the widely used antibacterial combination Bactrim® (trimethoprim/sulfamethoxazole) which elicits a strongly synergistic activity by targeting two nodes of the folate synthetic pathway in bacteria (Figure 8.2C) [3]. A number of HIV drugs combining nucleoside -reverse transcriptase inhibitors, non-nucleoside reverse transcriptase inhibitors and viral protease inhibitors have also recently been approved including Atripla® which may elicit better efficacy than the individual components through enhanced compliance and ease of use [74]. Another variation of this is combinations meant to minimize side effects or abuse, examples of which include Tredaptive® (niacin/larapiprant) [75] and Embeda™ (morphine/naltrexone) [76] respectively.

Clinical trials to demonstrate that a combination of two or more drugs provides meaningful clinical benefit over the administration of the single agents can be very challenging to design, execute and evaluate. In fact, the demonstration of true combination effects in excess of reference models in the clinic is rare. In most cases, the evaluation of strict mathematical synergy in a randomized clinical trial is impractical given the large patient numbers and comparator arms required to power statistical significance. Most studies rely on comparisons to one of the single agents or to historical efficacy data to evaluate drug combination effects. This can be an effective approach, especially in cases where one agent is expected to have little to no effect on its own and is thus dispensable for a practical comparison or cannot be tested alone for ethical reasons. The combination of gemcitabine and platinum based chemotherapy is a good example where the clinical benefit of the combination exceeds that of the single agents. There is a strong body of preclinical evidence supporting the synergistic effect of combination gemcitabine with platinum drugs [37]. Furthermore, the sequential addition of the platinum drug prior to gemcitabine is demonstrated to induce maximal cytotoxicity possibly through the schedule dependent inhibition of platinum induced DNA adduct formation by gemcitabine [37, 39, 77]. These results have been effectively translated into the clinical setting in metastatic breast cancer, ovarian cancer and nonsmall cell lung carcinoma with numerous studies demonstrating that the concurrent or sequence dependent treatment with gemcitabine and cisplatin or carboplatin give higher response rates when compared to historical use of either single agent [34, 35, 41, 78]. Another example of clinical synergy is that of perindopril addition to CCB therapy in the prevention of cardiac events and mortality in patients with coronary artery disease [79]. It is well described in the literature that ACE inhibitors and CCBs synergize in hypertension, reducing blood pressure with the potential to reduce secondary cardiac events. In the EUROPA trial and subsequent post hoc analysis, investigators evaluated >2000 patients on long-term CCB therapy comparing the addition of perindopril or placebo and found statistically significant improvements in outcomes with the addition of the second drug. Interestingly, in the post hoc analysis, investigators were able to compare four subpopulations who received placebo, perindopril, CCB, or the combination. Although the powering of the study was not sufficient to demonstrate statistical synergy, in this subset analysis a comparison of hazard ratios suggesting a clinical synergy greater than the effect the single agents was observed [79]. Given the investment of time, money, and patient resources needed for the evaluation of clinically meaningful combination interactions, it is beneficial to utilize *in vitro* and *in vivo* preclinical synergy evaluations to prioritize high potential combinations for further clinical investigation. Using *in vitro* high-throughput screening approaches, optimal pairs of agents and potential indications can be rapidly prioritized for hypothesis-directed clinical evaluation.

8.5. CASE STUDIES

In order to explore some of the complex and nuanced aspects of the discovery and development of combinations of repurposed drugs, we will now examine some specific examples of synergistic combinations discovered using systematic combination screening.

8.5.1. Synavive™—The Fixed Dose Combination of Prednisolone and Dipyridamole

The robust anti-inflammatory effects of glucocorticoids are well known and have been applied broadly in many settings to treat a diverse set of diseases. Despite these strong positive effects, the long-term utility of glucocorticoids is limited by their undesirable side effects that include increased serum glucose, induction of osteoporosis and glaucoma, suppression of the hypothalamus–pituitary–adrenal (HPA) axis, and behavioral and sleep alterations. Chronic treatment of patients with relatively low doses of steroids can lead to these adverse effects and efforts to dissociate the anti-inflammatory activity of glucocorticoids from their adverse effects have been a focus of medicinal chemistry and modified release development efforts with mixed success [80]. Synavive™ is a novel combination product candidate being developed by Zalicus, Inc., with a multi-target mechanism of action designed to enhance the anti-inflammatory benefits of glucocorticoids without amplifying the associated dose-dependent side effects. It is comprised of a unique formulation of the glucocorticoid prednisolone and the antithrombotic drug dipyridamole that blocks platelet activation and aggregation [81], in a fixed dose combination product for the treatment of anti-inflammatory conditions including rheumatoid arthritis (RA). This example will be used to highlight the development of a complex co-formulation of two approved generic agents designed to align pharmacokinetics and pharmacodynamics for optimum synergy. Importantly, this case demonstrates the ability to obtain a strong intellectual patent estate for a combination of repurposed drugs. The discovery and development of Synavive™ has resulted in issued patents and applications providing coverage until 2028. These include issued patents for method of use (U.S. Patent and Trademark Office [USPTO] #7,253,155) and composition of matter patent (USPTO #7,915,265), as well as a number of applications covering additional methods, pharmaceutical compositions, and therapeutic regimens in the United States and elsewhere in the world. In addition, this case demonstrates some approaches to reverse pharmacology to elucidate molecular mechanism of action.

The unexpected synergistic interaction between prednisolone and dipyridamole was discovered in a high-throughput screen designed to identify anti-inflammatory drug combinations having multi-target pathway mechanisms [16]. The primary screening assay was designed to examine both intercellular and intracellular signaling networks by monitoring the production of the pro-inflammatory cytokine tumor necrosis factor (TNF)-alpha in co-cultures of primary human peripheral blood mononuclear cells (PBMCs) following stimulation with either lipopolysaccharide (LPS) or phorbol ester plus ionomycin (PMA/I). This approach enabled a broad survey of multiple aspects of inflammatory signaling in a single assay while utilizing a pathologically relevant endpoint. Importantly, the phenotypic cell based assay used in this screening effort allowed access to a high level of biological complexity, enhancing the probability of uncovering multi-target molecular mechanisms. Using a systematic high throughput combination screening approach, 20,000 unique pairwise combinations composed of 600 approved drugs were tested in the primary screen. In this screen a number of combinations demonstrated synergy in excess of the Loewe additivity model and the combination of prednisolone and dipyridamole was observed to synergistically suppress the production of

TNF-alpha from both PMA/I and LPS-stimulated PBMCs. Isobolographic analysis of this combination demonstrated a CI of 0.31 and a synergistic effect resulting in a 10-fold and 5-fold reduction of the concentration of prednisolone and dipyridamole respectively needed to achieve a 70% inhibition of TNF-alpha secretion [18]. When evaluated in an acute LPS challenge inflammation model *in vivo*, the combination of prednisolone and dipyridamole suppressed the level of TNF-alpha in rat serum. Moreover, in an acute model of chemical hypersensitivity induced ear swelling, the combination of low-dose prednisolone with dipyridamole demonstrated equivalent efficacy to a 10-fold greater dose of prednisolone alone, indicating a 10-fold amplification of the low-dose prednisolone anti-inflammatory effect by dipyridamole in this model. Disease activity was also suppressed by the combination in both collagen and adjuvant induced arthritis models with low-dose prednisolone plus dipyridamole treatment demonstrating reduction in erythema, joint swelling, joint space narrowing, erosions, ankylosis, pannus formation and bone and cartilage damage (Figure 8.5 and Reference [18]). The ability of dipyridamole to amplify the anti-inflammatory effects of low-dose predinisolone did not extend to classical glucocorticoid adverse effects as measured using *in vivo* safety assays including elevated liver tyrosine aminotransferase, suppression of the HPA axis, suppression of thymus and adrenal gland weights, and altered expression of osteoporosis markers (Figure 8.5 and [18]). Thus, the combination appears to selectively amplify prednisolone anti-inflammatory activity without enhancing adverse effects typically associated with higher doses of glucocorticoids.

Discovery of the synergistic multi-target interaction between prednisolone and dipyridamole was achieved though phenotypic cell-based screening, as opposed to a traditional cell-free target-based screening approach. Further exploration of this multi-target interaction was therefore required to determine the molecular mechanism of action. Glucocorticoid molecular pharmacology has been well studied and these compounds are known to elicit diverse effects via the nuclear hormone receptor NR3C1. Free receptor resides in the cytoplasm until activation by glucocorticoid followed by translocation into the nucleus and direct binding to glucocorticoid-responsive elements that both activate and repress transcription depending on a variety of factors including promoter structure and presence of transcriptional co-activators and co-repressors. The activated glucocortioid receptor can also modulate transcription through mechanisms that are independent of DNA binding or transcription (for detailed review of glucocorticoid action, see References [82, 83] and references therein). Dipyridamole is an antithrombotic agent that inhibits phosphodiesterases and equilabrative nucleoside transporters to increase intracellular levels of cyclic adenosine and guanosine monophosphate that block platelet activation and aggregation. Dipyridamole is used therapeutically in combination with low-dose aspirin for the prevention of secondary stroke [81]. A survey of the literature reveals that dipyridamole attenuates pro-inflammatory gene expression in cell-based models of platelet-monocyte inflammation *in vitro* [84]. This insight, together with the known action of

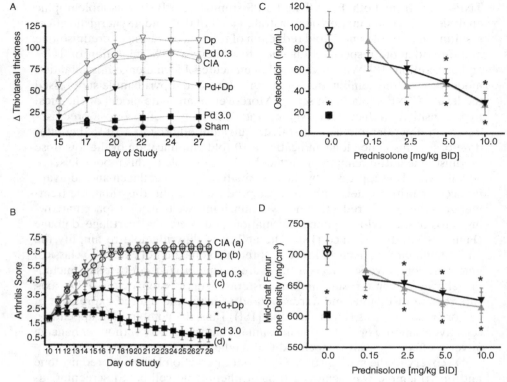

FIGURE 8.5. Dipyridamole enhances the effect of low-dose prednisolone without altering its safety profile. (A) Collagen-induced arthritis (CIA) was developed in Lewis rats for 10 days before oral daily dosing with compounds as indicated (mg/kg) for the next 17 days. Change in hind limb tibiotarsal joint diameter relative to the day 3 measurement is reported over the course of the study and (B) CIA was induced in Louvain rats for 10 days and test agents were administered orally once daily from days 10 to 28, as indicated (mg/kg). Arthritis severity was scored daily based on erythema and swelling. *$P < 0.001$ versus the CIA control; a$P = 0.0003$, b$P = 0.001$, c$P = 0.15$, d$P = 0.12$ versus the combination at day 28. (C and D) BL/6 mice were dosed twice daily with test agents for a total of 8 weeks to measure effects on markers of bone homeostasis. (C) Serum was collected at the end of the study and osteocalcin was measured by ELISA. (D) End-of-study mid-shaft femur bone density was measured by flurochrome labeling, sectioning, and peripheral quantitative computed tomography. Prednisolone alone (gray curve); prednisolone in combination with dipyridamole twice daily (black curve); dipyridamole alone and vehicle control are indicated with open triangle and open circle, respectively; subcutaneous dexamethasone (5 mg/kg once daily) positive control is indicated with a black square. *$P < 0.05$ versus the vehicle control. Dipyridamole was dosed at 37.5 mg/kg twice daily (allometrically scaled from a rat total daily dose of 150 mg/kg). Error bars are ±standard deviation, and statistical comparison is by analysis of variance with Tukey. Dp, dipyridamole; Pd, prednisolone. Reprinted with permission from figures 2–5 in Reference [18].

glucocorticoids, allowed investigators to begin a series of hypothesis generation and testing aimed at elucidation of the molecular mechanism of Synavive™. The combination of prednisolone and dipyridamole was evaluated for regulation of inflammatory mediators in stimulated chondrocytes and macrophages. These experiments revealed that in addition to suppression of TNF-alpha, the combination of prednisolone and dipyridamole also synergistically suppresses the secretion of a unique set of cytokines, chemokines, and proteases by mouse bone-derived macrophages. These include RANTES, IL-6, MIP-1alpha, MDC, and matrix metalloproteinase-9, exceeding the effect of either single agent alone [85]. Interestingly, RANTES and MMP-9 are both up-regulated in the synovioum of RA patients [86–89]. Further molecular mechanistic experiments have led to the discovery that the combination of prednisolone and dipyridamole, but not the individual components alone, can up-regulate expression of glucocorticoid-induced leucine zipper (GILZ) and dual-specificity phosphatase-1 (DUSP/MKP1) mRNA in LPS-stimulated mouse macrophages, supporting a hypothesis where suppression of MAP kinase pathway signaling may play a role in the anti-inflammatory activity of this combination [18].

Synavive™ is currently in Phase II clinical development and has demonstrated treatment benefit over placebo in Phase II studies in RA, hand osteoarthritis (HOA), and knee osteoarthritis (KOA). This combination has been generally well tolerated in clinical studies to date, with no serious adverse events reported from subjects taking Synavive™ [90–92]. Based on these initial clinical results and the mechanism of a low-dose glucocorticoid with amplified immune-inflammatory benefits, Synavive™ has the potential to be used in immune-inflammatory diseases including RA, osteoarthritis (OA), lupus, polymyalgia rheumatica ulcerative colitis, and Crohn's disease.

Synavive™ was tested in RA in a 6-week, randomized, blinded placebo-controlled study of 59 patients with a Disease Activity Score of 28 Joints (DAS28) score of >4.5 and a C-reactive protein (CRP) level of >2.2 mg/L [90]. Patients were randomized 1:1 to receive Synavive™ (3 mg of prednisolone plus 200 mg dipyridamole for the first week of treatment and 3 mg prednisolone plus 400 mg of dipyridamole for the following 5 weeks of treatment) or placebo, disease activity was measured by DAS28 scores and American College of Rheumatology 20 Response (ACR20) responses, and CRP levels were assessed. At day 42, 63% of Synavive™-treated patients achieved an ACR20 response as compared with 30% of placebo-treated patients ($P = 0.025$) with a mean decrease in DAS28 scores of −1.6 and −0.7 for Synavive™ and placebo, respectively ($P = 0.02$). Synavive™-treated patients achieved a rapid reduction in CRP levels with a median decrease from baseline of 50% and 19% for Synavive™- and placebo-treated patients, respectively ($P = 0.024$), and demonstrated a significant improvement in fatigue compared with placebo with scores of −27.2 and −14.3 for Synavive™ and placebo, respectively ($P = 0.03$), as measured using a visual analog scale (VAS). Synavive™ was generally well tolerated with most commonly reported adverse events including headache, gastrointestinal symptoms, and dizziness.

In a previous blinded, randomized, placebo-controlled trial of Synavive™, the combination was studied in patients suffering from HOA who had the presence of more than one swollen joint and more than one tender joint, a Kellgren–Lawrence score of two or more on radiographs and a self-reported hand pain of at least 30 mm on the AUSCAN VAS [91]. In this 6-week, proof-of-concept study, 83 patients were randomized 1:1 to the combination or placebo. Study drug was administered in a divided dose regimen with 2 mg of prednisolone and 100 mg of dipyridamole administered at 8 a.m. and 1 mg of prednisolone and 100 mg of dipyridamole at 1 p.m. on days 1–7, and 2 mg of prednisolone and 200 mg of dipyridamole administered at 8 a.m. and 1 mg of prednisolone and 200 mg of dipyridamole at 1 p.m. on days 8–42. The combination demonstrated a statistically significant superiority versus placebo in the AUSCAN pain score (primary endpoint) and both the VAS joint pain and VAS patient global scales in the intent-to-treat population. The combination was also consistently superior to placebo in the per-protocol population. The most frequently reported adverse event in this study was headache and this event was most frequently observed in the first days of treatment. Headache during the first days of treatment has been previously associated with the administration of dipyridamole and also with other cardiovascular pharmaceuticals acting through vasodilatation and was expected based on the repurposing of dipyridamole in this combination treatment.

Synavive™ was also studied in a double blind placebo-controlled trial of patients with KOA who had knee pain of 30–80 mm on Western Ontario and McMaster Universities Arthritis Index (WOMAC) VAS knee pain with at least 10 mm of flare following the discontinuation of nonsteroidal anti-inflammatory drug (NSAID)/coxib treatment (COMET-1, [92]). Three doses of Synavive™ were studied in the main trial, 2.7 mg prednisolone with 90, 180, or 360 mg of dipyridamole, and compared with prednisolone alone at 2.7 mg for a total of 14 weeks (98 days) including an initial 2-week dipyridamole titration phase. In a safety extension phase of the trial, all subjects received 1 of the 2 higher doses of Synavive™ and were monitored for long-term glucocorticoid tolerability and duration of response. This study enrolled 279 patients in the main trial and 74% of the eligible completers (141 patients) continued in the safety extension. The high-dose Synavive™ group demonstrated significant reductions in median WOMAC pain, function, and stiffness scores versus placebo with day 98 reductions greater than placebo and prednisolone alone groups by 17.2–19.5 and 5.5–8.6 mm, respectively. WOMAC 70% response rates were significantly greater for the highest dose of Synavive™ versus placebo on all three subscales at day 98 with similar trends in hand pain reduction in the subset of OA subjects with hand pain scores of 30 mm or greater. As in the hand OA trial, the most commonly reported adverse event was headache with a 4–5% dropout rate in each treatment arm.

At the time of this writing, the SYNERGY trial, a 12-week, five-arm global, double blind placebo-controlled study of Synavive™ in RA is planned for initiation in 2011 (ClinicalTrials.gov NTC01369745). This planned Phase IIb trial will evaluate the safety and efficacy of Synavive™ in subjects with moderate to severe RA and will include both a core study of approximately 250 subjects and a 12-month extension study to evaluate long-term safety and durability of response.

Initial studies of Synavive™ employed fixed ratio formulations of immediate-release prednisolone and dipyridamole. Based on the known pharmacokinetic profiles of prednisolone and dipyridamole, these early proof-of-concept studies employed split dosing of the immediate-release components to pharmacologically align the exposure of both drugs and enable the synergistic action of the combination. Furthermore, based on the known side effect profile of dipyridamole, namely headache during the initial phase of dosing, various titration schemes were employed to gradually increase exposure to this drug and limit the side effect profile. These approaches demonstrate how existing information for approved drugs can be effectively utilized to design appropriate dosing regimens for the initial clinical proof-of-concept studies of repurposed combination drugs. A modified-release, once-daily capsule formulation of Synavive™ for arthritis is currently being developed (Figure 8.6). This uniquely engineered formulation seeks to align the release profile of both prednisolone and dipyridamole to provide co-exposure of the two drugs and also maximize the dipyridamole exposure while minimizing the vasodilatory side effects including headache. This aligned release formulation will include prednisolone in both immediate-release and delayed-release forms as well as dipyridamole in a modified-release form. This formulation may provide greater synergy through co-exposure and an improved tolerability profile while also allowing for convenient once-daily dosing.

8.5.2. Adenosine A2A Receptor Agonist Synergies

Another example of a completely unexpected synergistic drug combination discovered using Zalicus combination high-throughput screening comes from a screen to discover novel glucocorticoid enhancers in hematological malignancies. In this case both approved drugs and targeted molecular probes representing the mechanisms of approved drugs or clinical stage compounds were used to enhance the effect of dexamethasone in multiple myeloma cell lines. Glucocorticoids have historically been a major component of combination therapy regimens in B-cell malignancies including multiple myeloma and continue to be used together with new targeted multiple myeloma drugs including immunomodulatory agents thalidomide and lenalidomide and the proteasome inhibitor bortezomib. Although significant advances have been made in the treatment of this complex disease, the disease remains incurable, accounting for 20% of the deaths related to cancers of the blood and bone marrow [93, 94]. The following example highlights how the evaluation of surrogates for

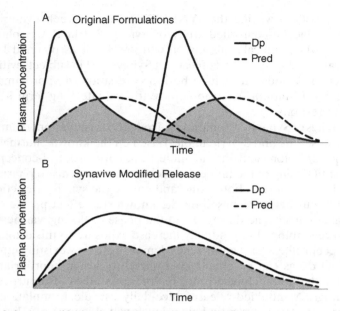

FIGURE 8.6. A modified-release, once-daily formulation of Synavive™. (A) Original formulations of immediate release prednisolone and dipyridamole administered twice daily enable some alignment of the exposure of both drugs. (B) A modified-release formulation of Synavive™ is being developed that will include prednisolone in both immediate-release and delayed-release forms as well as dipyridamole in a modified-release form. The formulation is designed to align the release profile of both dipyridamole and prednisolone to provide co-exposure while minimizing the vasodilatory side effects of dipyridamole, including headache, and allow for a convenient once-daily dosing.

drugs in development can uncover completely unexpected synergistic combination biology that can then be applied to a development program. Furthermore, this program demonstrates how synergistic combination biology can confer selectivity to a specific subset of disease pathology. Lastly, this example shows how three-way and higher order combination experiments can be explored to understand how a synergistic combination might be further deployed in a clinical setting with multiple therapeutic options. These results highlight how a single targeted mechanism can be envisioned as a single agent adjunctive to established therapeutic practice.

Combination high-throughput screening was used to identify compounds that synergize with dexamethasone to inhibit the proliferation of multiple myeloma cell lines *in vitro* [95]. In this screen, a total of 2841 unique combinations were evaluated in four multiple myeloma cell lines. Multiple compounds were identified that synergize with dexamethasone including known anticancer drugs and combinations of targets not previously studied in multiple myeloma. One compound of particular interest, Chloro-IB-MECA, an adenosine receptor agonist selective for adenosine A3 receptors but with some cross reactivity with A1, A2A, and A2B receptor subtypes at higher concentrations [96], potentiated the antiproliferative effect of dexamethasone at various concentrations and ratios in myeloma cells. This led to the further evaluation of adenosine receptor agonists in combination with dexamethasone and other multiple myeloma drugs using quantitative synergy analysis in a panel of 10 myeloma cell lines [97]. Potent, highly synergistic, inhibition of proliferation, was demonstrated with combinations of A2A agonists, including CGS-21680 and HE-NECA [96], when paired with multiple drugs including dexamethasone, lenalidomide, bortezomib, melphalan, doxorubicin, histone deacytylase (HDAC) inhibitors, and heat shock protein (HSP) 90 inhibitors at clinically relevant concentrations. These combinations exceeded Loewe additivity and demonstrated both substantial increases in efficacy over maximal single agent levels and significant potency shifting with many CIs in the range of 0.1 to 0.3. Synergistic antiproliferative effects were observed broadly across several multiple myeloma cell lines and when using cell lines unresponsive to standard MM drugs. The molecular pharmacology of the adenosine receptor agonists tested, which have varying selectivity and cross reactivity to different adenosine receptor subtypes, limited the ability of these experiments to conclusively identify the specific receptor subtype responsible for this unexpected synergy. Therefore, an elegant set of chemical biology and genetic experiments including antagonist studies and siRNA knockdown was utilized to demonstrate that the adenosine receptor (AdR) subtype responsible for synergy was the A2A subtype. A selective A2A antagonist but not A1, A2B, and A3 selective antagonists blocked the synergy and antiproliferative activity of 2-hexynyl-5′-N-ethylcarboxamido adenosine (HE-NECA), demonstrating that the effect is mediated via the A2A receptor. Transfection with siRNA directed against the adenosine A2A receptor isoform caused a concomitant reduction in the antiproliferative effects of HE-NECA, while siRNAs directed against the A1, A2B, and A3 adenosine receptor isoforms showed no diminished response [95, 97]. These combinations exert their antiprolifertive effect through rapid synergistic induction of apoptosis as evidenced by Annexin V staining that is not observed with either single agent alone. The synergistic antiproliferative effects of A2A combinations are highly selective for MM cells and are not observed in normal cell types including human PBMCs, aortic smooth muscle cells (AoSMCs), human umbilical vein endothelial cells (HUVECs), or human coronary artery endothelial cells (HCAECs) at concentrations 2–3 orders of magnitude greater than the IC_{50} on myeloma cell lines [98]. Evaluation of A2A agonists in combination with dexamethasone or melphalan in a panel of 83 tumor cell lines revealed that combination activity for these combinations is highly selective for B-cell malignancies. The synergistic antiproliferative effects of A2A agonist combinations translate into xenograft models of MM with no significant body weight loss. Mice bearing subcutaneous MM.1S tumors show a statistically significant reduction in tumor volume after treatment with the combination of dexamethasone and an A2A agonist as compared with either single agent alone [99]. Similar results are observed in an H929 xenograft model [100].

This body of work demonstrates a number of important features of combination screening discovery. First, an enhancer screening mode, one where a panel of agents is used to selectively increase the potency or activity of a selected mechanism (in this case glucocorticoid activity in hematological malignancies), can be an efficient way to discover unexpected synergies relevant to a specific indication/therapeutic strategy. Furthermore, this approach demonstrates how quantitative combination analysis in both a mechanistically agnostic and a hypothesis-driven approach can be used to "boot-strap" from an initial screening insight to a robust understanding of combination biology. In this case, the initial discovery was that adenosine receptor agonists enhance glucocorticoid activity in myeloma cell lines. Further evaluation of this synergy using panels of different chemical perturbigens and cell types revealed the breadth of this synergy with additional multiple myeloma drugs. Furthermore, hypothesis-driven quantitative combination analysis including either selective adenosine receptor antagonists or siRNA knockdown was used to clearly define the molecular targets responsible for the synergistic interaction. Finally, the robust synergy of these combinations and their striking selectivity for B-cell malignancies uncovered an important insight into combination biology in the context of specific disease pathology.

This work has uncovered a set of important biological insights into the molecular mechanism of a synergy relevant to a selected aspect of disease biology. Combination evaluation can also be effectively used to transform this information from an interesting phenomological insight into a robust drug development program. In the initial work, selective targeted molecular probes for specific mechanisms such as adenosine A2A receptor were used for convenient and potent screening *in vitro*. Research stage probe molecules for the adenosine receptor such as Chloro-IB-MECA, HE-NECA, and CGS-21680 were easily accessible tools for the early analysis where subtype selective A2A agonists were identified as a key component of the synergy. A review of the literature reveals several adenosine A2A receptor agonists approved or in development for different indications [96]. These include the recently approved drug regadenoson, a pharmacologic stress agent indicated for radionuclide myocardial perfusion imaging (MPI) in patients unable to undergo adequate exercise stress. In addition, apadenoson and binodenoson are both selective adenosine A2A receptor agonists in Phase III development for MPI, and ATL313 is an A2A agonist in early development for topical treatment of certain ophthalmic diseases including glaucoma [96, 101].

In an effort to translate the initial observation of synergy with adenosine A2A receptor agonists and myeloma drugs into a potential development program, the preclinical evaluation of ATL313 in combination with myeloma drugs was undertaken [102]. ATL313 is a very potent A2A receptor agonist with binding affinity for the human receptor in the low single digit nM range and at least 80-fold selectivity for A2A over other adenosine receptor subtypes [102–104]. ATL313 potently synergizes with glucocorticoids, bortezomib, lenalidomide, melphalan, and doxorubicin as well as emerging drug classes including HDAC inhibitors and HSP90 inhibitors to inhibit the proliferation of myeloma cell *in vitro*. Furthermore, ATL313, in combination with dexamethasone, demonstrates synergistic antitumor effects compared with either single agent in MM.1S xenografts with no significant body weight loss. In xenograft studies, treatment with ATL313 in combination with dexamethasone results in a statistically significant survival advantage as compared with either agent alone [102]. Microarray analysis of drug-induced gene expression changes suggests that combination-specific changes in gene expression may impact cell survival in multiple myeloma cells (R. Rickles, personal communication). These studies showed a number of genes down-regulated specifically by combination drug treatment including IRF4 and MYC and several downstream targets of these transcription factors. These genes play key roles in cell metabolism and growth including glycolysis, lipid synthesis, and cell cycle regulation [105]. The transcription factors MAF and PIM-2, genes known to play a role in multiple myeloma cell proliferation and viability [106, 107], are also down-regulated. Combination drug treatment up-regulates the leucine zipper protein GILZ, a gene known to play a role in glucocorticoid-induced cell death [108]. These studies provide early insights into how A2A agonist combinations potently kill multiple myeloma cells and will serve as the basis for future explorations of the molecular mechanism of this synergy.

These results demonstrate how an initial screening program based on research probes can be leveraged to define a potential new therapeutic area for a class of agents already approved or in late stage development for a completely unrelated indication. This case also serves as an example of how a synergistic combination biological insight can be embodied as a single agent adjunctive to an existing therapeutic regimen. Adenosine A2A receptor agonists show potent synergy with not only dexamethasone but also a number of drugs approved for use alone and in combination to treat multiple myeloma. Furthermore, work in the author's laboratory has demonstrated that three-way and four-way combinations of adenosine A2A receptor agonists, dexamethasone, lenalidomide, and bortezomib demonstrate additional mathematical synergy and increased cell killing in combination at clinically relevant concentrations (R. Rickles, personal communication). Thus, one could envision an adenosine A2A receptor agonist as a single agent indicated for use in combination with existing therapeutic regimens in myeloma. The approach would mitigate the need for development of multiple fixed dose combination products while also striving to give oncologists the dosing flexibility they require to treat multiple myeloma patients most effectively.

8.6. CONCLUDING REMARKS

In an industry that has been heavily focused on highly selective targeted agents, what level of interest is there for the development of repurposed drug combinations? Like the old adage goes "Beauty is in the eye of the beholder" and one investigator's "dirty drug" can be another investigator's "multi-targeted agent." The value of any combination of repurposed drugs will be based on the underlying mechanism, the level of meaningful medical benefit it provides to the patient, and the balance of acceptable risk associated with the side effect profile. This coupled with a vision to apply this benefit to the appropriate patient population and an innovative approach to the clinical development and approval path can result in valuable assets for an organization. There is no doubt that combinations of approved drugs have generated return on investment for pharmaceutical companies. In 2010, combination drugs accounted for nearly 15% of the top 200 approved prescription drugs by retail sales with $4.7 billion in revenue from the number 4 ranked Advair Diskus® [109]. As discussed above, currently approved combination drugs are primarily fixed dose combinations of agents already used concomitantly in the same indication. There is a tremendous amount of potential in the pharmaceutical industry's pharmacopeia of stalled or deprioritized programs whose failure occurred after significant investment in understanding the target, exposure, and safety profile of these agents. When considering the new level of mechanistic coverage that can be achieved by combining these agents, the potential for latent value is great indeed. It is important that pharmaceutical companies evaluate their shelved assets with an objective eye, one that is not tainted by reminders of the difficult decision to end a program. Given the complexity of disease biology and the relative conservation of critical pathways across multiple cellular types, it stands to reason that drugs whose efficacy was not sufficient as a single agent might be enhanced by engaging a second disease target. The resurrection of such shelved assets through combination repurposing has the potential to add great value with limited initial investment.

Given the complexity of disease biology and the recognition that in many cases the disruption of a single target or pathway will not be sufficient to treat disease [110], the case for combinations of drugs has never been stronger. The appropriate pairing of drugs and the generation of fixed dose combination forms can not only improve patient convenience and compliance but has also demonstrated real medical benefit. Despite this, only a fraction of possible combination space has been systematically explored and the scope of investments made to utilize combinations in the repurposing of existing drugs is far outweighed by the latent potential in this space. High-throughput combination screening enables both the systematic evaluation of large portions of combination space and the focused evaluation of key combination insights relevant to disease pathology and drug development. This technology makes it possible for the pharmaceutical industry to probe biological complexity and discover combination approaches that have the potential to bring real medical benefit to patients. Furthermore, combination screening can be utilized to rapidly and systematically discover latent value in existing drug assets and further expand the use of safe, biologically active molecules into unexpected indications. While the path for development of combination drugs is not without challenges, it also offers many opportunities for successful innovation, particularly in the case of repurposed drugs. In this era of personalized and evidence-based medicine, further investment in identifying synergistic combinations of existing drugs for new indications is likely to bring medical benefit to patients and value to the pharmaceutical industry.

ACKNOWLEDGMENTS

The author would like to thank Drs. Richard Rickles, Glenn Short, and Grant Zimmermann, and Mr. Jebediah Ledell for critical reading of the manuscript and helpful discussions on the content.

REFERENCES

1. Gonzalez-Angulo, A.M., Hennessy, B.T., Mills, G.B. (2010). Future of personalized medicine in oncology: A systems biology approach. *J. Clin. Oncol.*, *28*, 2777–2783.

2. Lewanczuk, R., Tobe, S.W. (2007). More medications, fewer pills: Combination medications for the treatment of hypertension. *Can. J. Cardiol.*, *23*, 573–576.

3. Schiffman, D.O. (1975). Evaluation of an anti-infective combination. Trimethoprim-sulfamethoxazole (Bactrim, Septra). *JAMA*, *231*, 635–637.

4. Feng, J.Y., Ly, J.K., Myrick, F., Goodman, D., White, K.L., Svarovskaia, E.S., Borroto-Esoda, K., Miller, M.D. (2009). The triple combination of tenofovir, emtricitabine and efavirenz shows synergistic anti-HIV-1 activity in vitro: A mechanism of action study. *Retrovirology*, *6*, 44.

5. Hughes, B. (2009). Tapping into combination pills for HIV. *Nat. Rev. Drug Discov.*, *8*, 439–440.

6. Bliss, C. (1939). The toxicity of poisons applied jointly. *Ann. Appl. Biol.*, *26*, 585–615.

7. Berenbaum, M.C. (1989). What is synergy? *Pharmacol. Rev.*, *41*, 93–141.

8. Chou, T.C. (2006). Theoretical basis, experimental design, and computerized simulation of synergism and antagonism in drug combination studies. *Pharmacol. Rev.*, *58*, 621–681.

9. Greco, W.R., Bravo, G., Parsons, J.C. (1995). The search for synergy: A critical review from a response surface perspective. *Pharmacol. Rev.*, *47*, 331–385.

10. Loewe, S., Muischnek, H. (1926). Effect of combinations: Mathematical basis of the problem. *Arch. Exp. Pathol. Pharmakol.*, *114*, 313–326.

11. Lehar, J., Stockwell, B.R., Giaever, G., Nislow, C. (2008). Combination chemical genetics. *Nat. Chem. Biol.*, *4*, 674–681.

12. Chou, T.C., Talalay, P. (1984). Quantitative analysis of dose-effect relationships: The combined effects of multiple drugs or enzyme inhibitors. *Adv. Enzyme Regul.*, *22*, 27–55.

13. Lehar, J., Zimmermann, G.R., Krueger, A.S., Molnar, R.A., Ledell, J.T., Heilbut, A.M., Short, G.F., 3rd, Giusti, L.C., Nolan, G.P., Magid, O.A., Lee, M.S., Borisy, A.A., Stockwell, B.R., Keith, C.T. (2007). Chemical combination effects predict connectivity in biological systems. *Mol. Syst. Biol.*, *3*, 80.

14. Lehar, J., Krueger, A.S., Avery, W., Heilbut, A.M., Johansen, L.M., Price, E.R., Rickles, R.J., Short, G.F., 3rd, Staunton, J.E., Jin, X., Lee, M.S., Zimmermann, G.R., Borisy, A.A. (2009). Synergistic drug combinations tend to improve therapeutically relevant selectivity. *Nat. Biotechnol.*, *27*, 659–666.

15. Zimmermann, G.R., Lehar, J., Keith, C.T. (2007). Multi-target therapeutics: When the whole is greater than the sum of the parts. *Drug Discov. Today*, *12*, 34–42.

16. Borisy, A.A., Elliott, P.J., Hurst, N.W., Lee, M.S., Lehar, J., Price, E.R., Serbedzija, G., Zimmermann, G.R., Foley, M.A., Stockwell, B.R., Keith, C.T. (2003). Systematic discovery of multicomponent therapeutics. *Proc. Natl Acad. Sci. U.S.A.*, *100*, 7977–7982.

17. Sharma, S.V., Haber, D.A., Settleman, J. (2010). Cell line-based platforms to evaluate the therapeutic efficacy of candidate anticancer agents. *Nat. Rev. Cancer*, *10*, 241–253.

18. Zimmermann, G.R., Avery, W., Finelli, A.L., Farwell, M., Fraser, C.C., Borisy, A.A. (2009). Selective amplification of glucocorticoid anti-inflammatory activity through synergistic multi-target action of a combination drug. *Arthritis Res. Ther.*, *11*, R12.

19. Hanahan, D., Weinberg, R.A. (2011). Hallmarks of cancer: The next generation. *Cell*, *144*, 646–674.

20. Kim, S.H., Kuh, H.J., Dass, C.R. (2011). The reciprocal interaction: Chemotherapy and tumor microenvironment. *Curr. Drug Discov. Technol.*, *8*, 102–106.

21. Eberhard, Y., McDermott, S.P., Wang, X., Gronda, M., Venugopal, A., Wood, T.E., Hurren, R., Datti, A., Batey, R.A., Wrana, J., Antholine, W.E., Dick, J.E., Schimmer, A.D. (2009). Chelation of intracellular iron with the antifungal agent ciclopirox olamine induces cell death in leukemia and myeloma cells. *Blood*, *114*, 3064–3073.

22. Sukhai, M.A., Spagnuolo, P.A., Weir, S., Kasper, J., Patton, L., Schimmer, A.D. (2011). New sources of drugs for hematologic malignancies. *Blood*, *117*, 6747–6755.

23. Plane, J.M., Shen, Y., Pleasure, D.E., Deng, W. (2010). Prospects for minocycline neuroprotection. *Arch. Neurol.*, *67*, 1442–1448.

24. Black, C.B., Duensing, T.D., Trinkle, L.S., Dunlay, R.T. (2011). Cell-based screening using high-throughput flow cytometry. *Assay Drug Dev. Technol.*, *9*, 13–20.

25. Macarron, R., Banks, M.N., Bojanic, D., Burns, D.J., Cirovic, D.A., Garyantes, T., Green, D.V., Hertzberg, R.P., Janzen, W.P., Paslay, J.W., Schopfer, U., Sittampalam, G.S. (2011). Impact of high-throughput screening in biomedical research. *Nat. Rev. Drug Discov.*, *10*, 188–195.

26. Macarron, R., Hertzberg, R.P. (2011). Design and implementation of high throughput screening assays. *Mol. Biotechnol.*, *47*, 270–285.

27. Michelini, E., Cevenini, L., Mezzanotte, L., Coppa, A., Roda, A. (2010). Cell-based assays: Fuelling drug discovery. *Anal. Bioanal. Chem.*, *398*, 227–238.

28. Bickle, M. (2010). The beautiful cell: High-content screening in drug discovery. *Anal. Bioanal. Chem.*, *398*, 219–226.

29. Elliott, N.T., Yuan, F. (2010). A review of three-dimensional in vitro tissue models for drug discovery and transport studies. *J. Pharm. Sci.*, *100*, 59–74.

30. Ling, X.B. (2008). High throughput screening informatics. *Comb. Chem. High Throughput Screen.*, *11*, 249–257.

31. Schaeffer, S. (2011). *For want of a nail*, in *BioCentury*. A1–A5.

32. Schmitt, R., Traphagen, L., Hajduk, P. (2010). High throughput cherry-picking of solvated samples. *Comb. Chem. High Throughput Screen.*, *13*, 482–489.

33. Lehar, J., Krueger, A., Zimmermann, G., Borisy, A. (2008). High-order combination effects and biological robustness. *Mol. Syst. Biol.*, *4*, 215.

34. Heinemann, V. (2002). Gemcitabine plus cisplatin for the treatment of metastatic breast cancer. *Clin. Breast Cancer*, *3*(Suppl 1), 24–29.

35. Hanna, N.H., Einhorn, L.H. (2002). The value of platinum compounds in non-small-cell lung cancer. *Clin. Lung Cancer*, *3*, 249–253.

36. Kroep, J.R., Pinedo, H.M., Giaccone, G., Van Bochove, A., Peters, G.J., Van Groeningen, C.J. (2004). Phase II study of cisplatin preceding gemcitabine in patients with advanced oesophageal cancer. *Ann. Oncol.*, *15*, 230–235.

37. Bergman, A.M., Ruiz Van Haperen, V.W., Veerman, G., Kuiper, C.M., Peters, G.J. (1996). Synergistic interaction between cisplatin and gemcitabine in vitro. *Clin. Cancer Res.*, *2*, 521–530.

38. van Moorsel, C.J., Kroep, J.R., Pinedo, H.M., Veerman, G., Voorn, D.A., Postmus, P.E., Vermorken, J.B., van Groeningen, C.J., van der Vijgh, W.J., Peters, G.J. (1999). Pharmacokinetic schedule finding study of the combination of gemcitabine and cisplatin in patients with solid tumors. *Ann. Oncol.*, *10*, 441–448.

39. Kroep, J.R., Peters, G.J., van Moorsel, C.J., Catik, A., Vermorken, J.B., Pinedo, H.M., van Groeningen, C.J. (1999). Gemcitabine-cisplatin: A schedule finding study. *Ann. Oncol.*, *10*, 1503–1510.

40. Loesch, D., Asmar, L., McIntyre, K., Doane, L., Monticelli, M., Paul, D., Vukelja, S., Orlando, M., Vaughn, L.G., Zhan, F., Boehm, K.A., O'Shaughnessy, J.A. (2008). Phase II trial of gemcitabine/carboplatin (plus trastuzumab in HER2-positive disease) in patients with metastatic breast cancer. *Clin. Breast Cancer*, *8*, 178–186.

41. Chew, H.K., Doroshow, J.H., Frankel, P., Margolin, K.A., Somlo, G., Lenz, H.J., Gordon, M., Zhang, W., Yang, D., Russell, C., Spicer, D., Synold, T., Bayer, R., Hantel, A., Stiff, P.J., Tetef, M.L., Gandara, D.R., Albain, K.S. (2009). Phase II studies of gemcitabine and cisplatin in heavily and minimally pretreated metastatic breast cancer. *J. Clin. Oncol.*, *27*, 2163–2169.

42. Shaffer, C. (2005). Automating compound management systems. *Drug Discov. Devel.*, *8*, 36–41.

43. Dragiev, P., Nadon, R., Makarenkov, V. (2011). Systematic error detection in experimental high-throughput screening. *BMC Bioinformatics*, *12*, 25.

44. Makarenkov, V., Zentilli, P., Kevorkov, D., Gagarin, A., Malo, N., Nadon, R. (2007). An efficient method for the detection and elimination of systematic error in high-throughput screening. *Bioinformatics*, *23*, 1648–1657.

45. Shun, T.Y., Lazo, J.S., Sharlow, E.R., Johnston, P.A. (2011). Identifying actives from HTS data sets: Practical approaches for the selection of an appropriate HTS data-processing method and quality control review. *J. Biomol. Screen.*, *16*, 1–14.

46. Cavalla, D. (2009). APT drug R&D: The right active ingredient in the right presentation for the right therapeutic use. *Nat. Rev. Drug Discov.*, *8*, 849–853.

47. Cavalla, D. (2005). Therapeutic switching: A new strategic approach to enhance R&D productivity. *IDrugs*, *8*, 914–918.

48. Putcha, G.V., Johnson, E.M., Jr (2004). Men are but worms: Neuronal cell death in C elegans and vertebrates. *Cell Death Differ.*, *11*, 38–48.

49. St Johnston, D. (2002). The art and design of genetic screens: *Drosophila melanogaster. Nat. Rev. Genet.*, *3*, 176–188.

50. Pulverer, B. (2001). Trio united by division as cell cycle clinches centenary Nobel. *Nature*, *413*, 553.

51. Speers, A.E., Adam, G.C., Cravatt, B.F. (2003). Activity-based protein profiling in vivo using a copper(i)-catalyzed azide-alkyne [3 + 2] cycloaddition. *J. Am. Chem. Soc.*, *125*, 4686–4687.

52. Speers, A.E., Cravatt, B.F. (2004). Profiling enzyme activities in vivo using click chemistry methods. *Chem. Biol.*, *11*, 535–546.

53. Speers, A.E., Cravatt, B.F. (2004). Chemical strategies for activity-based proteomics. *Chembiochem*, *5*, 41–47.

54. Cardoso, I., Martins, D., Ribeiro, T., Merlini, G., Saraiva, M.J. (2010). Synergy of combined doxycycline/TUDCA treatment in lowering Transthyretin deposition and associated biomarkers: Studies in FAP mouse models. *J. Transl. Med.*, *8*, 74.

55. Cao, S., Durrani, F.A., Rustum, Y.M. (2005). Synergistic antitumor activity of capecitabine in combination with irinotecan. *Clin. Colorectal Cancer*, *4*, 336–343.

56. Raftery, L., Goldberg, R.M. (2010). Optimal delivery of cytotoxic chemotherapy for colon cancer. *Cancer J.*, *16*, 214–219.

57. Renouf, D., Moore, M. (2010). Evolution of systemic therapy for advanced pancreatic cancer. *Expert Rev. Anticancer Ther.*, *10*, 529–540.

58. Hudis, C.A., Schmitz, N. (2004). Dose-dense chemotherapy in breast cancer and lymphoma. *Semin. Oncol.*, *31*, 19–26.

59. Lai, C.J., Bao, R., Tao, X., Wang, J., Atoyan, R., Qu, H., Wang, D.G., Yin, L., Samson, M., Forrester, J., Zifcak, B., Xu, G.X., DellaRocca, S., Zhai, H.X., Cai, X., Munger, W.E., Keegan, M., Pepicelli, C.V., Qian, C. (2010). CUDC-101, a multitargeted inhibitor of histone deacetylase, epidermal growth factor receptor, and human epidermal growth factor receptor 2, exerts potent anticancer activity. *Cancer Res.*, *70*, 3647–3656.

60. Cai, X., Zhai, H.X., Wang, J., Forrester, J., Qu, H., Yin, L., Lai, C.J., Bao, R., Qian, C. (2010). Discovery of 7-(4-(3-ethynylphenylamino)-7-methoxyquinazolin-6-yloxy)-N-hydroxyheptanam ide (CUDc-101) as a potent multi-acting HDAC, EGFR, and HER2 inhibitor for the treatment of cancer. *J. Med. Chem.*, *53*, 2000–2009.

61. Mayer, L.D., Janoff, A.S. (2007). Optimizing combination chemotherapy by controlling drug ratios. *Mol. Interv.*, *7*, 216–223.

62. Mao, J., Gold, M.S., Backonja, M.M. (2011). Combination drug therapy for chronic pain: A call for more clinical studies. *J. Pain*, *12*, 157–166.

63. Perez-Gracia, J.L., Berraondo, P., Martinez-Forero, I., Alfaro, C., Suarez, N., Gurpide, A., Sangro, B., Hervas-Stubbs, S., Ochoa, C., Melero, J.A., Melero, I. (2009). Clinical development of combination strategies in immunotherapy: Are we ready for more than one investigational product in an early clinical trial? *Immunotherapy*, *1*, 845–853.

64. Srinivas, N.R. (2009). Is there a place for drug combination strategies using clinical pharmacology attributes?—Review of current trends in research. *Curr. Clin. Pharmacol.*, *4*, 220–228.

65. Barnett, A.H. (2009). Translating science into clinical practice: Focus on vildagliptin in combination with metformin. *Diabetes Obes. Metab.*, *11*(Suppl 2), 18–26.

66. Ferrari, R. (2008). Optimizing the treatment of hypertension and stable coronary artery disease: Clinical evidence for fixed-combination perindopril/amlodipine. *Curr. Med. Res. Opin.*, *24*, 3543–3557.

67. Taylor, F., Smith, T. (2006). Use of combination therapy in migraine: A review of the clinical evidence. *Postgrad. Med.*, *Spec No*, 27–31.

68. Donohue, J.F. (2005). Combination therapy for chronic obstructive pulmonary disease: Clinical aspects. *Proc. Am. Thorac. Soc.*, *2*, 272–281; discussion 290–271.

69. Baddley, J.W., Pappas, P.G. (2005). Antifungal combination therapy: Clinical potential. *Drugs*, *65*, 1461–1480.

70. Division of Antiviral Drug Products in the Center for Drug Evaluation and Research (CDER) (2006). *Fixed dose combinations, co-packaged drug products, and single-entity versions of previously approved antiretrovirals for the treatment of HIV*, Food and Drug Administration.

71. Office of Medical Policy in the Center for Drug Evaluation and Research (CDER) (2010). *Codevelopment of two or more unmarketed investigational drugs for use in combination*, Food and Drug Administration.

72. Drug Information Branch, Division of Communications Management in the Center for Drug Evaluation and Research (CDER) (1999). *Applications covered by section 505(b)(2)*. Food and Drug Administration.

73. U.S. Dept. of Heath and Human Services, Food and Drug Administration (31st, 2011). *Approved Drug Produces with Therapeutic Equivalence Evaluations*.

74. Deeks, E.D., Perry, C.M. (2010). Efavirenz/emtricitabine/tenofovir disoproxil fumarate single-tablet regimen (Atripla(R)): A review of its use in the management of HIV infection. *Drugs*, *70*, 2315–2338.

75. Sanyal, S., Kuvin, J.T., Karas, R.H. (2010). Niacin and laropiprant. *Drugs Today (Barc.)*, *46*, 371–378.

76. Raffa, R.B., Pergolizzi, J.V., Jr (2010). Opioid formulations designed to resist/deter abuse. *Drugs*, *70*, 1657–1675.

77. Ledermann, J.A., Gabra, H., Jayson, G.C., Spanswick, V.J., Rustin, G.J., Jitlal, M., James, L.E., Hartley, J.A. (2010). Inhibition of carboplatin-induced DNA interstrand cross-link repair by gemcitabine in patients receiving these drugs for platinum-resistant ovarian cancer. *Clin. Cancer Res.*, *16*, 4899–4905.

78. Crino, L., Scagliotti, G., Marangolo, M., Figoli, F., Clerici, M., De Marinis, F., Salvati, F., Cruciani, G., Dogliotti, L., Pucci, F., Paccagnella, A., Adamo, V., Altavilla, G., Incoronato, P., Trippetti, M., Mosconi, A.M., Santucci, A., Sorbolini, S., Oliva, C.,

Tonato, M. (1997). Cisplatin-gemcitabine combination in advanced non-small-cell lung cancer: A phase II study. *J. Clin. Oncol.*, *15*, 297–303.

79. Bertrand, M.E., Ferrari, R., Remme, W.J., Simoons, M.L., Deckers, J.W., Fox, K.M. (2010). Clinical synergy of perindopril and calcium-channel blocker in the prevention of cardiac events and mortality in patients with coronary artery disease. Post hoc analysis of the EUROPA study. *Am. Heart J.*, *159*, 795–802.

80. Jacobs, J.W., Bijlsma, J.W. (2009). Innovative combination strategy to enhance effect and diminish adverse effects of glucocorticoids: Another promise? *Arthritis Res. Ther.*, *11*, 105.

81. Kim, H.H., Liao, J.K. (2008). Translational therapeutics of dipyridamole. *Arterioscler. Thromb. Vasc. Biol.*, *28*, s39–s42.

82. Lowenberg, M., Stahn, C., Hommes, D.W., Buttgereit, F. (2008). Novel insights into mechanisms of glucocorticoid action and the development of new glucocorticoid receptor ligands. *Steroids*, *73*, 1025–1029.

83. Cole, T.J. (2006). Glucocorticoid action and the development of selective glucocorticoid receptor ligands. *Biotechnol. Annu. Rev.*, *12*, 269–300.

84. Weyrich, A.S., Denis, M.M., Kuhlmann-Eyre, J.R., Spencer, E.D., Dixon, D.A., Marathe, G.K., McIntyre, T.M., Zimmerman, G.A., Prescott, S.M. (2005). Dipyridamole selectively inhibits inflammatory gene expression in platelet-monocyte aggregates. *Circulation*, *111*, 633–642.

85. Fraser, C., Wang, Y., Finelli, A., Keith, C.T., Zimmermann, G. (2007). Inhibition of macrophage and chondrocyte inflammatory mediators by CRx-102, a novel synergistic combination drug candidate. *EULAR Meet. Abstr.*, *66*, 141.

86. Makowski, G.S., Ramsby, M.L. (2005). Autoactivation profiles of calcium-dependent matrix metalloproteinase-2 and -9 in inflammatory synovial fluid: Effect of pyrophosphate and bisphosphonates. *Clin. Chim. Acta*, *358*, 182–191.

87. Yao, T.C., Kuo, M.L., See, L.C., Ou, L.S., Lee, W.I., Chan, C.K., Huang, J.L. (2006). RANTES and monocyte chemoattractant protein 1 as sensitive markers of disease activity in patients with juvenile rheumatoid arthritis: A six-year longitudinal study. *Arthritis Rheum.*, *54*, 2585–2593.

88. Stanczyk, J., Kowalski, M.L., Grzegorczyk, J., Szkudlinska, B., Jarzebska, M., Marciniak, M., Synder, M. (2005). RANTES and chemotactic activity in synovial fluids from patients with rheumatoid arthritis and osteoarthritis. *Mediators Inflamm.*, *2005*, 343–348.

89. Peake, N.J., Foster, H.E., Khawaja, K., Cawston, T.E., Rowan, A.D. (2006). Assessment of the clinical significance of gelatinase activity in patients with juvenile idiopathic arthritis using quantitative protein substrate zymography. *Ann. Rheum. Dis.*, *65*, 501–507.

90. Kirwan, J., George, E., Otsa, K., Clarke, S., Reid, D.M., Li, J., Lessem, J., Podrebarac, T.A. (2007). A phase 2a trial to evaluate CRx-102 for the treatment of active rheumatoid arthritis. *EULAR Meet. Abstr.*, *66*, 444.

91. Kvien, T.K., Fjeld, E., Slatkowsky-Christensen, B., Nichols, M., Zhang, Y., Proven, A., Mikkelsen, K., Palm, O., Borisy, A.A., Lessem, J. (2008). Efficacy and safety of a novel synergistic drug candidate, CRx-102, in hand osteoarthritis. *Ann. Rheum. Dis.*, *67*, 942–948.

92. Huttner, K., Shergy, W.J., Romney, C., Randle, J.C.R. (2009). CRx-102 (prednisolone/dipyridamole combination) enhances glucocorticoid (GC) efficacy and reduces

adverse effects in OA therapy: 3–12 month results. *Arthritis Rheum.*, *60*(Suppl 10), 1943.

93. Richardson, P.G., Mitsiades, C., Schlossman, R., Munshi, N., Anderson, K. (2007). New drugs for myeloma. *Oncologist*, *12*, 664–689.

94. Laubach, J., Richardson, P., Anderson, K. (2011). Multiple myeloma. *Annu. Rev. Med.*, *62*, 249–264.

95. Rickles, R.J., Pierce, L.T., Giordano, T.P., 3rd, Tam, W.F., McMillin, D.W., Delmore, J., Laubach, J.P., Borisy, A.A., Richardson, P.G., Lee, M.S. (2010). Adenosine A2A receptor agonists and PDE inhibitors: A synergistic multitarget mechanism discovered through systematic combination screening in B-cell malignancies. *Blood*, *116*, 593–602.

96. Jacobson, K.A., Gao, Z.G. (2006). Adenosine receptors as therapeutic targets. *Nat. Rev. Drug Discov.*, *5*, 247–264.

97. Rickles, R.J., Pierce, L.T., Giordano, T.P., 3rd, Tam, W.F., Avery, W., Farwell, M., Crowe, D., Chen, M., Brown, A., Kansra, V., Nawrocki, S.T., Carew, J.S., Giles, F.J., Lee, M.S. (2008). Adenosine A2A and beta-2 adrenergic receptor agonism: Novel selective and synergistic multiple myeloma targets discovered through systematic combination screening. *Blood*, *112*, Abstract 384.

98. Rickles, R.J., Tam, W.F., Necheva, A., Giordano, T.P., 3rd, Borisy, A., Lee, M.S. (2009). Adenosine A2A and beta-2 adrenergic receptor agonist synergy in B-cell malignancies: Selectivity, breadth of activity and effects of chronic exposure. *Blood*, *114*, Abstract 3762.

99. McMillin, D.W., Rickles, R.J., Negri, J., Delmore, J., Ooi, M.G., Farwell, M., Crowe, D., Chen, M., Avery, W., Kansra, V., Anderson, K.C., Lee, M.S., Mitsiades, C. (2008). Synergistic activity of adenosine A2A and beta-2 adrenergic receptor agonists in myeloma cells in the context of tumor-stromal interactions. *Blood*, *112*, Abstract 2663.

100. Rickles, R.J., Pierce, L.T., Giordano, T.P., 3rd, Avery, W., Farwell, M., Crowe, D., Tam, W.F., Chen, M., Kansra, V., McMillin, D.W., Anderson, K.C., Mitsiades, C., Lee, M.S. (2008). Preclinical evaluation of CRx-501, a potent selective A2A agonist as a novel drug candidate for the treatment of multiple myeloma. *Blood*, *112*, Abstract 252.

101. Ballantyne, C.E. (2011). Clinical Data, I. *Quarterly report for the period ending December 31, 2010.*

102. Rickles, R.J., Padval, M., Giordano, T.P., 3rd, Rieger, J.M., Lee, M.S. (2010). ATL313, a potent and selective A2A agonist as a novel drug candidate for the treatment of multiple myeloma. *Blood*, *116*, Abstract 2990.

103. Alam, M.S., Kurtz, C.C., Wilson, J.M., Burnette, B.R., Wiznerowicz, E.B., Ross, W.G., Rieger, J.M., Figler, R.A., Linden, J., Crowe, S.E., Ernst, P.B. (2009). A2A adenosine receptor (AR) activation inhibits pro-inflammatory cytokine production by human CD4+ helper T cells and regulates Helicobacter-induced gastritis and bacterial persistence. *Mucosal Immunol.*, *2*, 232–242.

104. Lappas, C.M., Rieger, J.M., Linden, J. (2005). A2A adenosine receptor induction inhibits IFN-gamma production in murine CD4+ T cells. *J. Immunol.*, *174*, 1073–1080.

105. Shaffer, A.L., Emre, N.C., Lamy, L., Ngo, V.N., Wright, G., Xiao, W., Powell, J., Dave, S., Yu, X., Zhao, H., Zeng, Y., Chen, B., Epstein, J., Staudt, L.M. (2008). IRF4 addiction in multiple myeloma. *Nature*, *454*, 226–231.

106. Hurt, E.M., Wiestner, A., Rosenwald, A., Shaffer, A.L., Campo, E., Grogan, T., Bergsagel, P.L., Kuehl, W.M., Staudt, L.M. (2004). Overexpression of c-maf is a frequent oncogenic event in multiple myeloma that promotes proliferation and pathological interactions with bone marrow stroma. *Cancer Cell*, *5*, 191–199.

107. Asano, J., Nakano, A., Oda, A., Amou, H., Hiasa, M., Takeuchi, K., Miki, H., Nakamura, S., Harada, T., Fujii, S., Kagawa, K., Endo, I., Yata, K., Sakai, A., Ozaki, S., Matsumoto, T., Abe, M. (2011). The serine/threonine kinase Pim-2 is a novel anti-apoptotic mediator in myeloma cells. *Leukemia*, *25*, 1182–1188.

108. Ayroldi, E., Riccardi, C. (2009). Glucocorticoid-induced leucine zipper (GILZ): A new important mediator of glucocorticoid action. *FASEB J.*, *23*, 3649–3658.

109. Bartholow, M. (2011). *Top 200 Drugs of 2010*, in *Pharmacy Times*.

110. Kummar, S., Chen, H.X., Wright, J., Holbeck, S., Millin, M.D., Tomaszewski, J., Zweibel, J., Collins, J., Doroshow, J.H. (2010). Utilizing targeted cancer therapeutic agents in combination: Novel approaches and urgent requirements. *Nat. Rev. Drug Discov.*, *9*, 843–856.

████████ CHAPTER 9

Phenotypic *In Vivo* Screening to Identify New, Unpredicted Indications for Existing Drugs and Drug Candidates

MICHAEL S. SAPORITO, CHRISTOPHER A. LIPINSKI, and
ANDREW G. REAUME

9.1. INTRODUCTION

Drug repositioning of clinical stage drug candidates and approved drugs has emerged as a viable but underutilized strategy for extracting more utility from compounds and filling the pharmaceutical industry innovation gap [1, 2]. As discussed in detail elsewhere in this book, multiple experimental platforms including *in silico*, *in vitro*, and cell-based biological approaches have been described for drug repositioning [3–5]. However, many of the new indications discovered for drugs occur through serendipitous observations in *in vivo* biological settings and not through the use of systematic *in vitro*-based screening approaches [1, 2, 6, 7]. The *in vivo* settings that provide the most fruitful platforms for drug repositioning include both pre- and post-marketing human clinical trials and preclinical experimental animal models of disease [1, 2, 7]. Phenotypic animal models of disease can be relevant to disease pathology, responsive to a broad range of approved drugs, and clinically translatable. Evaluating preclinical and clinical stage drug candidates through a multi-therapeutic platform of phenotypic disease models may provide the best systemized approach for repositioning these types of drugs and candidates. This chapter will provide examples of drug repositioning discoveries, the processes, and observations that drove those discoveries, and describe an optimized preclinical *in vivo* efficacy platform for drug repositioning.

Drug Repositioning: Bringing New Life to Shelved Assets and Existing Drugs, First Edition.
Edited by Michael J. Barratt and Donald E. Frail.
© 2012 John Wiley & Sons, Inc. Published 2012 by John Wiley & Sons, Inc.

9.2. SETTINGS FOR *IN VIVO* DRUG REPOSITIONING

A study of specific examples of drug repositioning and the stage of drug development where the discovery of the new utility occurred can be instructive in understanding the potential of drug repositioning as a strategy for filling depleted drug pipelines and defining the best biological systems for detecting new indications from drugs or drug candidates. Repositioning in *in vivo* settings generally occurs in one of three areas: (1) observations made in post-approval clinical studies, (2) observations in pre-marketing clinical studies, or (3) observations in preclinical animal models of disease.

9.2.1. Post-Approval Clinical Studies

Examination of off-label use of drugs provides a powerful metric for the potential of drug repositioning. It is estimated that at least 20% of drugs are prescribed for indications other than the ones for which they were approved. When considering cardiac, anticonvulsant, and psychotherapeutic drugs, the off-label prescribing rate increases to nearly 80% [8]. These off-label applications are supported by clinical observations made in small post-approval, post-marketing trials or based on anecdotal reports from physicians. Some well-known examples include the antidepressant bupropion, which is frequently prescribed for the treatment of obesity and attention deficit hyperactivity disorder (ADHD) [9–11], the anticonvulsant topiramate, used for bipolar disorder and eating disorders [12, 13], and the analgesic opioid buprenorphine for the treatment of refractory depression [14].

One interesting story of a recent mechanism-independent drug discovery is the one that describes the discovery of gabapentin (Neurontin®) and follow-on compounds for the treatment of neuropathic pain and other central nervous system (CNS) disorders. Gabapentin, a structural analog of the neurotransmitter gamma-aminobutyric acid (GABA), was originally developed as an anticonvulsant based on the concept that the compound would mimic GABA responses in the CNS [15]. Following its market approval, gabapentin was fortuitously found to attenuate pain responses and produce anxiolytic activity in rodent models. It was subsequently approved for use in post-herpetic neuralgia [16]. A more potent analog of gabapentin (pregabalin; Lyrica®) was subsequently approved for use in the treatment of neuropathic pain and fibromylagia [17]. Although both compounds were designed to activate the GABA receptor, recent studies have shown that they both drive their pharmacological responses independent of GABA receptor activation. In fact, in post-approval studies, both compounds were found to bind to the $\alpha2$-δ subunit of voltage-gated calcium channels, and it is now believed that this target mediates the anticonvulsant, analgesic, and other effects of this class of compounds [18], which has led to new drug discovery efforts around this molecular target [19].

These examples show that post-approval, off-label data are informative in characterizing the incidence of multi-therapeutic area utility of drugs and drug targets and the potential for drug repositioning, and show that *in vivo* data alone are sufficient to drive efforts for the discovery and development of next-generation compounds. However, relying on anecdotal reports of efficacy in clinical settings is not an efficient or systematic process for drug repositioning and driving chemistry efforts. Moreover, off-label uses do not address the repositioning potential of preclinical and development stage drugs including those that were abandoned due to lack of efficacy during development.

9.2.2. Preapproval Clinical Studies

Some of the more classic examples of drug repositioning include those drugs that were repositioned in clinical settings prior to approval. Two of the better-known examples include the phosphodiesterase 5 (PDE5) inhibitor sildenafil (Viagra®), a compound developed as an antihypertensive that produced improved erectile function in clinical trial patients, and finasteride (Propecia®), a 5-alpha-reductase inhibitor repositioned from a benign prostatic hyperplasia treatment to one for male pattern baldness [20]. In the preapproval setting, observations for new therapeutic potential are relatively rare, given (1) the recruitment criteria involved in clinical trial design, (2) the relatively limited sample size, (3) the often limited treatment duration, and (4) the often restricted range of endpoints that are measured. The vast majority of therapeutic potential is missed in clinical studies because drug activity can only be detected in disease conditions that are either excluded by trial design or are rare among the patient population as to make therapeutic effect difficult to detect. For example, compounds with undiscovered analgesic activity may only be revealed in patients that are experiencing pain, and compounds that normalized blood glucose levels would only be detected in diabetic patients. Such opportunities are limited based on measured parameters included in clinical trial designs.

9.2.3. Predevelopment *In Vivo* Studies

The most efficient way to describe the full therapeutic potential of a compound is to comprehensively evaluate its pharmacology in *in vivo* models of disease. Although it is difficult to determine the exact number of compounds repositioned based on preclinical *in vivo* findings, there are numerous well-described and informative examples of compounds that were repositioned, or that were originally discovered, based on functional findings in *in vivo* models. Two compounds that were discovered recently based on *in vivo* functional activity are ezetimibe (Zetia®) and modafinil (Provigil®). Ezetimibe was identified through its ability to block cholesterol absorption in hamsters and is now approved as a cholesterol-lowering agent [21], while modafinil, a compound that increased wakefulness in rats, is now approved for the treatment of narcolepsy and excessive sleepiness due to sleep apnea and shift-work sleep disorder, as well as an adjunct to antipsychotic medications [22]. In both of

TABLE 9.1. Examples of Drugs Discovered or Repositioned Based on *In Vivo* Phenotype

Drug	Phase of Discovery or Repositioning	Original Indication	Phenotype	Mechanism	Reference
Modafinil	Preclinical	NA	Increased locomotion and wakefulness in rats	Unknown	[22]
Ezetimibe	Preclinical	NA	Decreased cholesterol absorption	NPC1L1; (discovered post-approval)	[21, 105]
Sildenafil	Phase II/III	Anti-hypertensive	Increased erectile function	PDE5	[100]
Bupropion	Post-approval	Depression	Smoking cessation	Dopamine–norepinephrine uptake blocker	[9, 106]
Topirimate	Post-approval; off-label	Anti-convulsant	Multiple CNS	Multiple targets	[13, 107–110]
Buprenorphine	Post-approval	Analgesic; opioid addiction	Depression	Opioid receptor agonist; partial agonist	[14]
Finasteride	Phase II/III	Prostate hypertrophy	Hair growth	5-alpha reductase inhibitor	[20]
Minoxidil	Phase II/III	Anti-hypertensive	Hair growth	Potassium channel activator	[101, 111]
Gabapentin	Preclinical/ post-approval	Anti-convulsant	Neuropathic pain; anxiety	GABA receptor agonist; Voltage dependent calcium channels	[16]

these instances, the pharmacological activity was discovered in animal models independent of a known mechanism of action or molecular target.

Table 9.1 shows a list of approved drugs that were discovered based on functional activity in *in vivo* models independent of a known mechanism of action.

9.3. *IN VIVO* MODELS

The examples described above show that some drugs can have a broad, unpredicted therapeutic potential and that an *a priori* understanding of drug mechanisms is not essential to the repositioning of these compounds to new indications. Although the typical drug discovery paradigm prior to the early 1980s included an early *in vivo* phenotypic evaluation step with general behavioral observation as a key component of the drug discovery process, the current pharmaceutical industry drug discovery paradigm is oriented toward molecular targets and molecular mechanisms and not designed to benefit from *in vivo* observations that might reveal an otherwise unpredicted potential therapeutic benefit [23]. Current target-based drug discovery efforts in the pharmaceutical industry are heavily oriented toward drug interactions with molecular targets in *in vitro* and cell-based systems [24, 25]. Certainly this approach has been fruitful in some areas. For example, targeting 3-hydroxy-3-methylglutaryl-coenzyme (HMG-CoA) reductase led to the valuable addition of the statin class of cholesterol-lowering agents. Selective serotonin reuptake inhibitors (SSRIs) have revolutionized the treatment of depression. Also, the discovery of the bcr-abl inhibitor imatinib (Gleevec ®) has led to the effective treatment of chronic myelogenous leukemia [26]. These successes, however, may have led to an overconfidence and overemphasis on molecular target-focused drug discovery strategy. Contrary to the expectations for improved discovery productivity with the current target-based discovery paradigm, the rate of new drug approvals has been consistently flat or in decline for the last 15 years [27]. Some have suggested that the great success stories of the target-based paradigm (such as statins and SSRIs) may represent exceptions rather than the rule for the effectiveness of pure mechanism-based drug discovery [24, 25]. In fact, when examining drug approvals between 1999 and 2008 of first-in-class, small molecules, 28 out of 50 (56%) were discovered using phenotypic screening approaches and 17 (34%) were discovered using target-based approaches [28]. These observations have been driving the consensus that many drug responses are the result of drug interaction with multiple targets, modulation of biological networks, or simply driven through undefined mechanisms [29].

One of the deficiencies of single molecular target-driven approaches utilizing *in vitro* and cell-based approaches is that they tend to be hyperfocused on a single therapeutic area with *in vivo* efficacy testing occurring at a much later stage of the drug discovery paradigm. There are many indications and many drugs that do not fit into the single molecular target-based drug discovery paradigm. Antipsychotic medications are a classic example of this phenomenon [30]. It has been suggested that most of the drugs approved for CNS disorders evoke their therapeutic response through interaction with multiple targets [31]. Moreover, there are many notable drugs known to possess potent biological activity but with unknown or incompletely understood molecular mechanisms of action. Indeed, many of the most widely used drugs would remain undiscovered if molecular target-based drug discovery paradigms were relied on at the time of their discovery. For example, the antidiabetic agent metformin, which is a current first line of defense therapy after diet and exercise and is the most widely prescribed agent for diabetes was identified in the absence of any known mechanism. Although there is currently some understanding of cellular signaling events that drive metformin's antidiabetic activity, the molecular target for metformin is not known [32].

Recently, there has been a growing realization that complementary or even alternative approaches to molecular target-based drug discovery are required to reinvigorate pharmaceutical industry drug pipelines. These approaches may in fact utilize strategies and models established prior to the current molecular target-driven approaches and that rely on "systematic serendipity" to identify pharmacological activity [33]. Unlike *in silico*, *in vitro*, or cell-based approaches, these *in vivo* approaches are not biased or restricted by any known molecular target activity of the compound. Such approaches can detect pharmacological activity of compounds that are either selective for a specific molecular target, interact with multiple targets, or modulate complex biological networks. These *in vivo* approaches can be considered to be "non-hypothesis"-driven methodologies but can be systematized and designed to incorporate robust empirical observational science.

A powerful and complete way to more fully understand the pharmacological potential of a therapeutic agent is to complete an evaluation of the compound in a battery of disease-relevant, clinically translatable *in vivo* models. Such models can fall into two broad categories; those designed to determine molecular target interaction *in vivo* (target-based models) and those designed to reflect the disease state (pathology-based or functional models). Table 9.2 provides examples of mechanism- and pathology-based *in vivo* models and their predictive limitations.

9.3.1. Target-Based *In Vivo* Models

Target-based models are designed to determine the effects of a compound in an *in vivo* paradigm in which a molecular target/mechanism of interest plays a prominent role in the biological response. These models are an off-shoot of the molecular target drug discovery paradigm and rely on either pharmacological or genetic disruption of the molecular target and then determining if the compound repairs the disruption. Most molecular target-based models are designed in order to test drug–target interactions *in vivo* and in most cases may not reflect the pathology of human disease. These models are good proxies

TABLE 9.2. Examples of *In Vivo* Models Used in Drug Discovery

Model	Type	Disease	Clinically Approved Mechanism/Reference Compound	Preclinical/Clinical Read-Out	Predictive Limitations	Ref.
Cholinergic antagonism	Mechanism-based validity	Alzheimer's disease	Cholinesterase inhibitors/Tacrine	Cognition improvement/cognition improvement	Selective for cholinergic mimetics	[37, 112]
db/db mouse	Pathological (phenotypic) validity	Type 2 diabetes	Multiple mechanisms/Metformin, rosiglitazone, GLP-1	Glucose regulation/glucose regulation	None	[39, 54]
Forced swim test	Predictive validity	Depression	Serotonin-norepinephrine reuptake/Imipramine; fluphenazine	Increased struggle/improved mood	Most anti-depressants are active	[47]
Unilateral 6-hydroxydopamine (6-OHDA lesion model)	Mechanism-based validity	Parkinson's disease	Dopamine receptor agonism/l-dopa, pramipexole	Increased unilateral rotations/improved locomotor function	Selective for dopaminergic agonists	[113]
2,4,6-trinitro benzenesulfonic acid TNBS-induced colitis	Pathological (phenotypic) validity	Inflammatory bowel disease; ulcerative colitis	TNF-alpha inhibition/infliximab	Colitis score/colitis symptoms	Multiple active preclinical compounds	[114, 115]

for pharmacokinetics (PK) and *in vivo* target interaction, but by design are unlikely to detect phenotypic changes driven outside the molecular target's primary pathway of action.

As an example, cholinergic antagonists such as scopolamine are used to evoke cognitive dysfunction in rodents and produce a pharmacological model of memory impairment and Alzheimer's disease (AD) [34]. Although these models were originally developed because of the hypothesis that cholinergic deficiencies were a primary cause of cognitive dysfunction in AD, they have evolved into ones that are used to assess the *in vivo* target effects of cholinomimetics [34]. Disruption of cholinergic transmission by administration of muscarinic antagonists such as scopolamine elicits a well-described cognitive disturbance that in the past was believed to reflect a cognitive deficit associated with AD [35]. Administration of compounds that increase cholinergic transmission by blocking acetylcholinesterase, such as donepezil (ARICEPT®), or by directly activating muscarinic cholinergic receptors, overcomes these cholinergic disturbances and improves cognitive function [35, 36]. These cholinergic antagonist models rely on an underlying assumption that cholinergic pathways are a key cause of cognitive decline in AD. However, these models do not replicate the pathology of AD. In fact, the role of the cholinergic system dysfunction in cognitive deficits in AD has been questioned, and drugs that affect muscarinic cholinergic receptors have exhibited limited efficacy in the clinic [37].

9.3.2. Pathology-Based *In Vivo* Models

In contrast to target/mechanism-based models, pathology-based models are designed to more faithfully replicate at least some aspects of the pathophysiology of a specified disease and are responsive to a broader range of therapeutic agents for that disease, independent of their mechanism of action. These models, also referred to as functional or phenotypic models, rely on disease pathophysiology and/or their pharmacological responsiveness rather than addressing specific drug–target interactions. These can be traditional pharmacological models that use an external insult to generate a phenotype, or a genetic model that replicates a pathology utilizing genetic modifications. The read-outs from these models are typically disease-related pathologies and tend to better reflect those observed in clinical trials in humans. Although it is certainly true that not all human diseases can be modeled well in animal systems, where such models exist, they are said to have good face validity. Because of their design—the emphasis on mimicking human diseases, their broad responsiveness to approved drugs, and the relationship of read-outs in both the animals and humans—phenotypic models tend to be more clinically translatable than target-based models.

There are good examples of animal models that reflect the pathology of a given disease and produce pharmacological findings that are translatable to the clinic. One such set of models represents type 2 diabetes. Type 2 diabetes is a heterogeneous disease of disrupted glucose homeostasis that is characterized by elevated blood glucose. It typically presents as insulin receptor insensitivity that is followed by degeneration of insulin secreting pancreatic β-cells. Selective inbreeding of animals that spontaneously develop a type 2 diabetes-like phenotype has generated a number of strains that are currently used for type 2 diabetes research [38]. For example, one genetic model, the db/db mouse, exhibits many features of clinical stage type 2 diabetes [39]. These features include a progressive decrease in insulin receptor sensitivity, steadily increasing blood glucose levels, compensatory elevations in serum insulin followed by a degeneration of insulin secreting pancreatic β-cells, a precipitous drop in serum insulin levels and increased HbA1c levels over time [39]. These type 2 diabetic mice are responsive to a broad range of clinically approved pharmacological agents and the activities that these agents evoke in db/db mice correspond with their human clinical effects. For example, metformin, an inhibitor of gluconeogenesis, rosiglitazone an activator of peroxisome proliferator activated receptor γ (PPARγ), and exendin-4, a glucagon-like peptide-1 (GLP-1) receptor agonist, elicit dramatic improvements in metabolic function including sustained reductions in blood glucose in this model [40–42]. These drugs are of distinct structure, impact glucoregulatory mechanisms via different pathways, and are all effective in managing glucose levels in type 2 diabetic patients. As a result, these type 2 diabetes models, as well as other *in vivo* models of this disease, are considered clinically translatable phenotypic models.

There are also a number of examples of pharmacological models that do not have direct or face validity, but that have predictive validity for a disease. Examples of this type are particularly prevalent among models of psychiatric disease. For instance, rodents in a conditioned avoidance response or with induced deficits in prepulse inhibition respond to both typical (haloperidol) and atypical (clozapine) antipsychotics, and are predictive of positive antipsychotic pharmacological activity in the clinic [43–45]. In addition, forced helplessness models such as the forced swim test and tail suspension test respond to multiple antidepressants including tricyclics and the SSRI classes, and are also highly predictive of clinical antidepressant activity [46, 47].

Most *in vivo* models of course do not fall neatly into one of these categories. Frequently, *in vivo* models capture only some aspect of the disease pathology, but are responsive to a broad range of clinically approved drugs. It is the broad pharmacological responsiveness to a range of clinically approved drugs that is the most important feature for a valid phenotypic animal model.

9.4. ADVANTAGES OF COMPOUND SCREENING IN PHENOTYPIC *IN VIVO* MODELS

9.4.1. Broad Target Screening

Most diseases can be affected by through pharmacological modulation of different physiological and cellular pathways. Moreover, within each pathway there may be multiple nodes or molecular targets that can regulate the pharmacological response. For instance, blood glucose levels in type 2 diabetic patients can be affected by increasing pancreatic insulin secretion (sulfonylureas), increasing insulin receptor sensitivity (glitazones), affecting gluconeogenesis (metformin) or reducing glucose absorption (acarbose) [48–52]. Each of these independent processes can be regulated by multiple targets that lie within the pathway. For example, insulin secretion can be increased by administration of insulin secretagogues such as sulfonylureas and incretins [49]. Incretins, such as GLP-1, can be administered exogenously, or endogenous GLP-1 levels can be increased by administration of drugs such as sitagliptin that inhibit dipeptidyl peptidase-4 (DPP4), the enzyme primarily responsible for degradation of GLP-1 [53]. Each of these major antidiabetic pathways contains multiple potential druggable targets (Figure 9.1). Indeed, there are numerous putative molecular targets for the treatment of type 2 diabetes that have yet to be validated in clinical studies [54]. At the time of writing, a

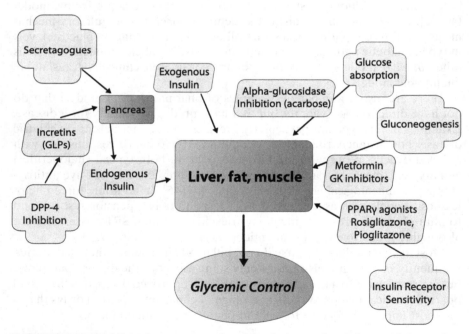

FIGURE 9.1. Antidiabetic agents regulate blood glucose levels by multiple mechanisms. Type 2 diabetes is a disease that is treated through the use of drugs that work by affecting different pathways. Drugs approved for the use in the treatment affect blood glucose levels by (1) increasing insulin secretion either directly (sulfonylureas) or indirectly (GLP-1; DPP4 inhibitors), (2) inhibiting glucose absorption (α-glucosidase inhibitors), (3) gluconeogenesis, (4) increasing insulin receptor sensitivity. Within each of these pathways are multiple drug targets that regulate or potentially could regulate them.

Prous Integrity search for treatments under the investigation for type 2 diabetes found 97 molecular targets that are currently being studied for this disease [55].

By screening a biologically active compound through an array of diabetes disease models one is essentially probing for interactions of the compound with one or more of these glucoregulatory pathways. More specifically, by screening a biologically active compound through an array of pathology-based diabetes models as a means of interrogating for potential new therapeutic activity, one is in effect probing for activity against at least 97 potential targets [54, 55]. By extension, when screening across a broad range of animal models of disease where disease function can be modulated by multiple pathways and targets, the number of pathways multiplies, as does the opportunity for detecting a beneficial functional activity. This type of functional screening is useful for identifying activities of drug-like compounds with poorly defined mechanisms, and compounds that may interact with multiple targets or pathways whose activities would not be identified in *in vitro* or cell-based systems. Moreover, when screening a compound that is highly selective toward a specific target, one is effectively interrogating that target for potential roles outside of its currently understood disease association.

In addition to diabetes, other disease areas are similarly associated with multiple pathways and by extension, multiple molecular targets. Inflammatory diseases represent one such broad condition. Broadly speaking, inflammation is highly complex and is driven by a multitude of physiological factors including vascular changes, cellular infiltration, immune system activation and expression of cytokines, and other mediators [56]. Many disease states are associated with inflammatory responses including inflammatory bowel disease, rheumatoid arthritis, and multiple sclerosis [57–59]. In fact, inflammation is increasingly considered a primary etiological component of a number of other disease states including metabolic disease, neurodegenerative diseases, and even psychiatric diseases [57, 60, 61].

Inflammation is the end product of activation of multiple cellular and extracellular processes [62]. These pathways can be modulated by diverse pharmacological agents that differ in chemical structure and mechanism of action. Examples of classes of compounds that affect inflammation include newer generation nonsteroidal anti-inflammatory drugs (NSAIDs) such as celecoxib, which selectively inhibits COX-2, older generation NSAIDs (e.g., indomethacin) that inhibit both COX-1 and -2, and the even less selective immunosuppressant corticosteroids (e.g., prednisone) [63–65]. Newer generation tumor necrosis factor (TNF)-alpha neutralizing agents etanercept (a monoclonal antibody) and infliximab (a soluble TNF-alpha receptor) are now used widely for treatment of several inflammatory conditions including psoriasis, Crohn's disease, and arthritic conditions [66, 67]. These examples serve to illustrate the complexity and diversity of the inflammatory processes. Because of this complexity, it should be expected that therapeutics for inflammatory conditions may especially lend themselves to identification by phenotypic screening approaches. As an example, PPARγ agonists such as pioglitazone (Actos), a drug first approved as diabetes therapeutic, affects inflammatory pathways that are also thought to be involved in conditions such as inflammatory bowel disease [68]. Another example involves the potential utility of statins in the treatment of the multiple sclerosis, a demyelinating autoimmune disease with an inflammatory component. It is now believed that the molecular target of statins, HMG-CoA reductase, may indeed modulate inflammatory processes, and the anti-inflammatory properties of these compounds may in part provide cardiovascular benefits associated with their use [69]. Other marketed drugs or drugs in development for indications outside of inflammation may have mechanisms that directly or indirectly impact inflammatory pathways and may be useful in one or several inflammatory diseases.

9.4.2. CNS Diseases

CNS diseases may also be especially amenable to phenotypic screening approaches. The list of CNS drugs originally identified by empirical observation, as opposed to modern day molecular target-driven approaches, is extensive and includes most of the CNS drugs already described in this chapter. In addition, in many instances the molecular targets through which these drugs are mediating their therapeutic effect were unknown at the time of their approval. Thus, as previously described, gabapentin was approved as an anticonvulsant and was designed to mimic the actions of the neurotransmitter GABA. The pharmacological effects of gabapentin are now known to be driven through inhibition of α2-δ subunit of voltage-gated calcium channels [15]. Modafinil, an approved drug for narcolepsy, elicits a wake-promoting effect through a mechanism that is still undefined [70]. It is now understood that many CNS drugs act through multiple pathways to evoke their responses [30]. The atypical antipsychotics such as clozapine and duloxetine elicit their psychotropic activity through interaction with more than one molecular target. The antipsychotic activities of clozapine are evoked through inhibition of dopaminergic and serotonergic receptors [71, 72], and the antidepressant and other activities of duloxetine are driven by inhibition of both serotonergic and dopaminergic transporters [72]. Clearly the CNS is a highly complex, highly networked organ with multiple built-in redundancies that make it difficult to adequately correct pharmacological imbalances through drugs identified using single molecular target-driven drug discovery approaches. The highly complex nature of CNS diseases and the history of empirical observations that drive CNS drug discovery are characteristics that make diseases such as schizophrenia, depression, anxiety, and alertness particularly amenable to *in vivo* phenotypic screening [16]. Indeed, there are many CNS screens that are not so much models of disease as broad indicators of potential positive or negative pharmacological effects. The Irwin test, for example, can be used to detect positive effects such as alertness or improved motor coordination, or negative effects such as hyperactivity, motor dyscoordination, or sympathetic activation [73].

Electroencephalography, while from a screening perspective only moderate in throughput, is a powerful model capable of detecting general changes in wakefulness and circadian rhythmicity, specific changes in cortical activity (e.g., frequency shifts) indicative of psychoactive effects including cognitive benefit, and both pro- and anticonvulsant activity [74]. These types of changes are independent of target and are particularly powerful in identifying the function of compounds that modulate CNS activity by interaction with multiple CNS pathways. The complex behavioral outcomes of these models to many known pharmacological agents would rarely be predicted, much less complex behavioral outcomes would not be detected, using *in vitro*, cell-based, or *in silico* systems.

By screening a compound through an array of *in vivo* models of a variety of disease states, a multitude of pathways and targets within that those pathway are screened simultaneously. Moreover, in contrast to *in vitro* and cell-based systems, by screening drugs through an intact *in vivo* system it is possible to uncover drug activities and pharmacological responses that are the result of a simultaneous modulation of multiple targets and pathways, and activities that are driven by modulation of complex biological networks.

9.4.3. Network Modulation and Polypharmacology

An alternative drug discovery and development paradigm now emerging is based on the concept of complex biological networks and pathway-based drug discovery. These concepts have been reviewed earlier in the book (see Chapters 5 and 7) and elsewhere [29, 75, 76], so will not be discussed in detail here. Briefly, the concept is that biological systems are highly networked and robust, and that in most cases, affecting a single molecular target that lies within this network will have poorly predictable biological outcomes. Moreover, this hypothesis postulates that compounds that produce one effect will also produce many effects and that this unpredictable activity can be exploited for new therapeutic utility. In fact, broad activities of "selective" compounds have been observed in preclinical and clinical settings. Some of these target-selective drugs with multiple activities are listed in Table 9.4 and are described in other sections in this chapter. Two examples include the lipid-lowering statins, which are selective HMG-CoA that elicit beneficial effects in autoimmune diseases including rheumatoid arthritis and multiple sclerosis, and the selective COX-2 inhibitors such as the anti-inflammatory agent celecoxib, which is also used for the treatment of familial adenomatus polyps and the prevention of colorectal cancer [77, 78].

In vivo phenotypic approaches including the *thera*TRACE® platform that is described in the next section are particularly amenable for detecting compounds that affect biological networks. Unlike *in vitro* systems, *in vivo* phenotypic model outcomes are affected by the full complement of network complexity including PK, phamacodynamic (PD), and network modulatory functions.

9.5. DESIGN OF AN OPTIMAL DRUG REPOSITIONING PLATFORM

9.5.1. Evolution of High-Throughput Focused Phenotypic Strategies

The implementation of hypothesis-driven target-based drug discovery has coincided with a steady decline in the number of clinically approved new molecular entities [25]. Prior to the 1980s, observations of therapeutic benefit of test compounds in *in vivo* biological systems were an important driver of drug discovery. Currently, the systematic screening of drug-like compounds through *in vivo* systems in order to detect beneficial therapeutic activity is an underutilized approach for identifying and characterizing drug activity. There are, however, several drug repositioning examples that have used *in vivo* models to uncover new indications. These screening strategies have used different formats to uncover novel drug activities. A currently prominent format consists of screening a library of drugs in a single disease model with the aim of identifying a meaningful therapeutic activity. This approach was used effectively in identifying a potential antimalarial compound from a library of compounds [79]. In this example, approximately 2700 approved drugs or development stage drug candidates were screened for inhibition of *Plasmodium falciparum* growth. This screening led to identification of the nonsedating antihistamine astemizole and its primary human metabolite, desmethylastemizole, as submicromolar inhibitors of three different *P. falciparum* strains with potent oral activity in two mouse parasite suppression tests (for a more detailed discussion of this case study, see Chapter 11). This important finding demonstrates that a drug can produce unpredicted activity in completely unrelated therapeutic areas. This example of a high-throughput, screening-based repositioning strategy serves as a *bona fide* drug discovery approach, although this particular platform is obviously limited to a single therapeutic area.

9.5.2. Low-Throughput, Broad Spectrum Strategies

Using the above example of screening through a single model, it follows that evaluating a large number of approved or development stage drugs through multiple predictive models should yield a far larger number of repositioning opportunities. One study has attempted to identify the potential of such an approach [75]. In this study, a small number of approved drugs were evaluated in several *in vivo* and cell-based models for their effects on a number of diverse cell pathways. The drugs tested in that study included statins, glitazones, salicylates, retinoids, and calcium channel blockers. The set of *in vivo* and cell-based models included insulin-mediated glucose utilization, hippocampal neurogenesis, liver collagen synthesis, lymphocyte proliferation, and microglial proliferation. In this limited evaluation, it was found that nearly every tested drug showed an effect in at least one of the models that had not been predictable based on the original indication or known molecular target interactions [75]. These findings confirm that drugs even with only one primary biological activity can elicit many biological responses at a systems/whole organism level.

Importantly, this study highlights the possibilities of examining drugs for completely unrelated indications.

This approach of testing a series of compounds in an array of diverse, therapeutically distinct models with the goal of identifying novel activities achieves the broad therapeutic strategy needed for effective drug repositioning; however, it is low throughput, costly, and inefficient for evaluating broad therapeutic potential of a relatively large number of compounds.

9.5.3. *thera*TRACE®: A High-Throughput, Broad Therapeutic Area Approach

The repositioning strategies described above have limitations relating to either the breadth of therapeutic areas that were examined, or the number of compounds that can be reasonably and efficiently evaluated in practical time frames. In order to maximize the probability of identifying clinically relevant drug effects, a platform that enables screening large numbers of compounds through a broad therapeutic range of clinically translatable phenotypic animal models is required. Ideally, such a platform should capture the high-throughput capability that is described above in the screening for potential antimalarial compounds and the quality and hit-rate frequency that was reported in the aforementioned limited *in vivo* screening study [75]. A platform designed to meet these criteria was created by Melior Discovery and coined "*thera*TRACE®." This platform utilizes a multiplexed strategy capable of evaluating the broad therapeutic potential of drugs and drug candidates in a relatively short period of time. In this multiplexing approach, a drug candidate is tested in groups of animals that are subjected to multiple sequential and parallel pharmacological tests. For example, a group of animals might be treated with a test agent for 6 weeks, simultaneously fed a high fat diet over that period of time while monitoring multiple metabolic parameters. Such parameters would include measurement of blood glucose levels in a glucose tolerance test, fat pad development, and metabolism-related hormones including adiponectin, insulin, and leptin. In addition, this same group of animals may be tested for other pharmacologically unrelated responses, such as pain responsiveness in a formalin chemical analgesia test, gastrointestinal motility, and/or psychotherapeutic alterations. Such a multiplexed format must be designed and validated so that the multiplexed animal models perform as they would in an independent, nonmultiplexed, format. Therefore, the challenge and key to success with this platform is the understanding of the models that can be combined and in which sequence those models are run in order not to compromise the clinical translatability of each model. For instance, in the assay combination described above, two reference compounds, metformin and rosiglitazone, have been shown to regulate blood glucose and affect fat pad deposition in the high fat diet-fed mice in the same way they do when evaluated in a standalone format. Further, these mice exhibit normal baseline nociceptive and forced swim test results, responding normally to the positive control compounds indomethacin and imipramine, respectively.

The *thera*TRACE® platform utilizes measurements that would be typically used in clinical settings to indicate efficacy including observation, biochemical, physiological, and behavioral changes. In nearly all cases, multiple types of measurements are made from the same group of animals. For example, in a model of Parkinson's disease induced by 1-methyl-4-phenyl-1,2,3,6-tetrahydropyridine (MPTP) administration, striatal dopamine content, substantia nigra cell markers, and locomotor behavior are all measured in the same animals. In this example, the pattern of responses in these overlapping and functionally related measurements allows for the identification and separation of potential symptomatic agents from potential neuroprotective agents. As an example, a symptomatic agent such as l-dopa would positively affect locomotor response without affecting dopaminergic markers, whereas a neuroprotective compound would affect locomotor parameters and preserve dopaminergic markers. In another example, dexamethasone and tacrolimus were compared in a 2,4-dinitrofluorobenzene (DNFB) model of contact hypersensitivity. Both compounds reduced visual inflammatory readouts. However, dexamethasone did not affect scratching behavior and the compounds produced differential inhibition expression of interferon γ (IFN γ), and interleukins 4 (IL-4) and 5 (IL-5) [80]. These studies emphasize that multiple read-outs from the same model can produce a much more thorough understanding of the pharmacology and potential therapeutic benefit of drugs.

The predictive power of the *thera*TRACE® platform is driven by multiple factors. First, as mentioned above, there are multiple clinically translatable outputs for most *in vivo* assays. Second, each assay is powered such that a statistically meaningful endpoint can be measured for each biological output. Finally, there are multiple redundant assays for each therapeutic area. Assay redundancy is a particularly powerful mechanism for detecting potential therapeutic activity. For instance, there are multiple inflammatory models within the platform including a collagen-induced arthritis model, an inflammatory bowel disease model, and an ovalbumin pulmonary inflammation model. In addition, there are multiple inflammatory ancillary assays including a lipopolysaccharide (LPS)-cytokine stimulation model, and a thioglycollate monocyte infiltration model. Potential anti-inflammatory compounds would be expected to produce not only changes in multiple outputs in one model, but would be expected to affect more than one of the inflammation models. In the above example, the pattern of responses across inflammation models is important both for increasing confidence in and interpreting potential mechanisms of the compound as well as in identifying the relevant inflammatory therapeutic applications.

To date 300 compounds have passed through the *thera*TRACE® platform. Nearly all of these are small molecules with a well-described biological activity, and the majority of these compounds had been previously developed through to at least Phase II clinical trials. It has been our experience (unpublished) that approximately 30% of the compounds that enter the platform exhibit a new activity that was not previously known based on reported biological activity including known molecular target and original therapeutic area. This "hit rate" is consistent with hit rates that were described for approved drugs in a limited *in vivo* model system and is also consistent with off-label prescription rates [8, 75]. Further, this discovery rate underscores the significant potential for undiscovered disease relevant activity in candidate drugs and already developed therapeutics.

The *thera*TRACE® multiplexed *in vivo* platform described here is "agnostic" to known or postulated mechanisms associated with the drug candidate. For drugs or drug candidates that have been tested in the platform, most of the new biological activities detected were not predictable based on known activities of the compound. Moreover, in each instance where an appropriate model resided in the platform, the *thera*TRACE® platform confirmed the known therapeutic activities of the compound. In the majority of these instances, modulation of the primary target can be ascribed as at least partially causative in driving the new response. As described in Section 9.6, it is our belief that up to 90% of the otherwise unpredicted biological activities that are uncovered by the array of models in *thera*TRACE® are the result of at least a partial on-target activity.

9.5.4. Design of the *thera*TRACE® Platform

The *thera*TRACE® platform is a biological assay system that has been established in mice. Mice are small, specifically bred for pharmacological research, easily obtainable, well characterized, and adaptable to the high-throughput multiplexed screening methodologies described below. Mice are also the preferred species for other practical reasons including the amount of compound that is required for testing. The *thera*TRACE® process integrates three essential steps in the discovery process: (1) a PK evaluation to optimize the dosing paradigm including determining the optimal route of administration, optimal dose interval, and optimal dosing frequency; (2) a dose-level finding step to ensure that the test compound is evaluated at dose levels within the safety limits of the compound; and (3) an efficacy step in which the test compound is evaluated, at a minimum of three dose levels, in a broad spectrum of clinically translatable animal models of disease. The output from this entire process is a characterization of the broad therapeutic potential and alternative therapeutic indications for the tested compound. This process is illustrated in Figure 9.2.

9.5.4.1. PK Optimization
Therapeutic activity is dependent on a combination of PK and pharmacodynamic (PD) function of a drug, absent of any confounding adverse activities. Full understanding of the PK and the tolerability of the compound are essential parameters required to optimize a thorough, high-quality and broad spectrum efficacy evaluation. In the *thera*TRACE® evaluation, a pre-efficacy PK study and a dose-finding study are utilized to determine the optimal route of administration, frequency of dosing, interval

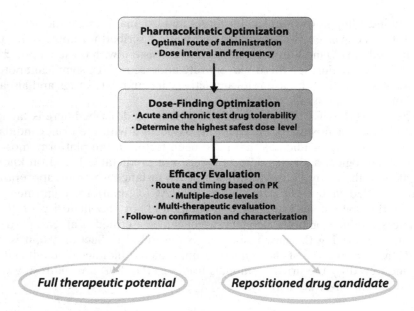

FIGURE 9.2. *thera*TRACE®. This multiplexed, multi-therapeutic phenotypic *in vivo* platform is used to identify the therapeutic potential of preclinical drug candidates and to reposition development stage and approved drugs. *thera*TRACE® occurs in three steps: (1) a pharmacokinetic optimization step, (2) dose-finding step, and (3) an efficacy evaluation step. The efficacy models included in the platform are phenotypic and are responsive to a broad range of pharmacological agents. A follow-on step is typically added to confirm findings found in the platform screen, to compare with an approved drug to that particular therapeutic indication and to fully understand the pharmacology of the compound. The *thera*TRACE® platform is unbiased with regard to the original indication or molecular target of the compound. *Reprinted with permission from Elsevier: Drug Discovery Today, Volume 8: pages 89–95 (Saporito and Reaume), 2011.* Note: All experiments are conducted in accordance with the National Institutes of Health regulations of animal care covered in "Principles of Laboratory Animal Care," National Institutes of Health publication 85–23 and approved by the Institutional Animal Care and Use Committee.

between administration and response measurements and dose levels for efficacy evaluations. The PK and dose-finding studies occur in the same species and often the same strains as the efficacy evaluations. In the PK optimization studies, a compound is evaluated via multiple routes of administration including oral, intraperitoneal (IP) subcutaneous, and intravenous. Blood levels of drug are measured over time. The dose route that produces the best overall exposure parameters including peak drug levels (C_{max}) and half-life ($t_{1/2}$) is selected for use in subsequent analysis.

An example of a compound repositioned using the *thera*TRACE® platform is provided by MLR-1023, a compound that was originally developed to increase mucosity as a treatment for gastric ulcer [81]. In the *thera*TRACE®

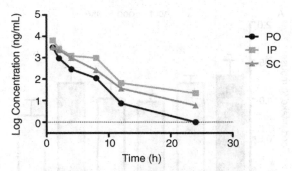

FIGURE 9.3. MLR-1023 pharmacokinetics. MLR-1023 is a repositioned drug candidate. In this mouse pharmacokinetic optimization study, IP administration produced optimal exposure. Although the compound was orally bioavailable, for dose-finding and efficacy studies, the compound was dosed IP to maximize exposure levels and duration.

platform, MLR-1023 was found to reduce glucose levels in acute rodent models of hyperglycemia, and in chronic studies it elicited effects on multiple diabetic parameters [82]. MLR-1023 is now in clinical development for the treatment of type 2 diabetes. Prior to testing in the *thera*TRACE® platform, the PK profile of MLR-1023 was determined and these data are shown in Figure 9.3. These PK data were critical in designing an optimized dosing regimen for dose-finding evaluation and efficacy studies. Specifically, these PK data show (1) that although MLR-1023 was orally bioavailable, IP administration produced a slightly better overall exposure duration and higher C_{max} level, (2) that the compound had a $t_{1/2}$ of approximately 2 hours, and (3) that the T_{max} was 1 hour. These data were applied in the design of the dose-finding and efficacy studies. For subsequent dose-finding and efficacy studies, MLR-1023 was administered via IP administration, with acute measurements occurring within a time frame that encompassed the T_{max} time point (1 hour). Since the compound was minimally detectable in blood 12 hours after administration, a twice per day dosing regimen was established for chronic studies.

9.5.4.2. Dose-Finding Optimization

With MLR-1023 and other compounds, dose-finding studies are conducted prior to the evaluation in the *thera*TRACE® platform. These dose-finding studies are conducted in order to determine the safe dose levels of the test compound for subsequent efficacy analysis. Since a drug is administered repeatedly in long-duration studies, the dose-finding stage is designed to determine both acute and repeat dose tolerability of a test compound. In these studies, the compound is administered to mice at 5 or more dose levels for at least 5 days using the dosing conditions established in the PK study. Parameters such as food intake, weight gain, and gross behavioral changes are monitored at the T_{max} after each administration and at Tmin time points. These measurements are rapid, readily conducted, and extremely sensitive to adverse drug reactions. An example of a feeding

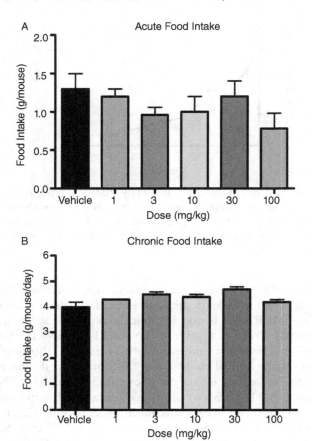

FIGURE 9.4. MLR-1023 dose-finding studies. In dose-finding studies, general behavioral parameters, food intake, and weight gain are measured as indices of compound tolerability. In this study, MLR-1023 was administered acute (A) and daily for 5 consecutive days (B). Food intake is an exquisitely sensitive marker for animal well-being and drug tolerability. In this study, MLR-1023 was well tolerated to a dose level of 100 mg/kg.

activity in a dose-finding study is shown in Figure 9.4. In this example, MLR-1023 was tested at dose levels up to 100 mg/kg via IP administration and using dosing parameters established in the PK optimization study. MLR-1023 did not affect acute or long-term feeding behavior. MLR-1023 also did not produce any changes in overt behavior or appearance, did not alter weight gain, and therefore was well tolerated. These data indicated that MLR-1023 could be administered safely up to a dose level of 100 mg/kg.

It is important to note that these PK and dose-finding efficacy optimization studies are not intended to replace preclinical development stage PK and maximum tolerated dose studies. In this context, the results are used to optimize design of subsequent evaluations in the multiplexed *thera*TRACE® platform. In some instances, compounds have existing PK and tolerability data that allow for the bypass of these first two steps of the *thera*TRACE® process. These types of data are particularly useful when effective dose levels in the original *in vivo* models are equivalent to those that drive an *in vivo* response. This equivalence in effective dose-levels may be evidence of an "on-target" activity.

9.5.4.3. Multiplexed Efficacy Model Strategy

The compilation of efficacy models in the *thera*TRACE® platform is ideally suited for detecting pharmacological activities that might not otherwise be predicted or not readily apparent based on the known biology of the target and thus elude detectability by standard, hypothesis-based, screening practices. Since this is an *in vivo* platform, the models used in the *thera*TRACE® platform take into account PK complexity, molecular target kinetics, pathway modulations, and activities that are independent of the original target and unique to the molecules tested. The models are pathology-based with responses that can be driven by drug interactions with single or multiple targets, or modulate complex biological networks. In most instances these are the same models that are used throughout the pharmaceutical industry on a standalone basis to determine if a compound warrants entry into clinical development. Strict criteria have been used to select models included in the platform. The selected models have demonstrated clinical relevance and translatability, are relatively facile to conduct and responsive to approved drugs for their respective modeled disease, or provide data that support findings in other disease models. Table 9.3 lists the therapeutic areas that are included in the *thera*TRACE® platform with representative models, their respective disease indications, and therapeutically relevant measurements.

9.5.4.4. Interpretation of theraTRACE® Results

A "hit" in the *thera*TRACE® platform is defined as an effect in an assay that shows statistically significant dose dependence, ideally across a number of related disease relevant models. As discussed previously in this chapter, a key feature of the *thera*TRACE® platform is the built-in redundancy of animal models. For example, there are multiple metabolic disease models and metabolic measures that are tightly linked. Thus, a compound that shows antidiabetic activity may be expected to affect metabolic parameters in more than one animal model of disrupted metabolism. For example, MLR-1023 was evaluated in the full *thera*TRACE® platform and displayed activity in the metabolic disease area, specifically in lowering blood glucose levels in an oral glucose tolerance test. In addition, with long-term daily administration MLR-1023 elicited a dose-dependent reduction in other metabolic disease tests including a reduction in weight gain, fat pad development, and serum leptin levels in a diet-induced obesity model. The significant dose-related effect of the drug in the oral

TABLE 9.3. Therapeutic Areas and Assays Included in the *thera*TRACE® Platform

Therapeutic Area	Assays	Specific Disease State
Psychotherapeutic	• Tail suspension test • Forced swim test • Chronic mild stress • Irwin test • Automated open-field analysis • Rotarod • Startle prepulse inhibition • Fear conditioning • Novel object recognition	• Depression • General CNS activity • Locomotor function and coordination • Schizophrenia • Cognition
Neurology	• Pentylenetetrazole-induced seizure • Maximal electroshock • Sleep/Wake cycle	• Epilepsy • Circadian rhythm/wake and sleep-promoting activities
Neurodegeneration	• MPTP • 6-hydroxydopamine • Experimental autoimmune encephalomyelitis (EAE)	• Parkinson's disease • Multiple sclerosis
Pain	• Hot plate • Tail-flick • Hargreaves • Formalin • Von Frey/Carrageenan • Chronic constrictive injury	• Thermal nociception • Chemical nociception • Inflammatory pain • Neuropathic pain
Diabetes	• Oral glucose tolerance test • db/db mouse model • ob/ob mouse • Streptozotocin-mediated type 1 diabetes	• Type 2 diabetes • Type 1 diabetes
Metabolic disease	• Diet-induced obesity • ob/ob mouse • Home cage activity (telemetry)	• Obesity • Energy utilization
Gastrointestinal disorders	• Colonic propulsion • Stress-induced fecal production • Morphine-induced constipation • Acetylcholine writhing • Gastrointestinal transit • Dextran sulfate sodium (DSS)-induced colitis	• Irritable bowel syndrome • Inflammatory bowel disease
Urogenital	• Diuretic-mediated micturition • Urinary output	• Urinary incontinence

TABLE 9.3. (*Continued*)

Therapeutic Area	Assays	Specific Disease State
Inflammation	• Collagen-induced arthritis • Experimental autoimmune encephalomyelitis • Lipopolysaccharide-systematic inflammation • Pulmonary inflammation • Lipopolysaccharide pulmonary inflammation • DSS-induced colitis	• Rheumatoid arthritis • Multiple sclerosis • General inflammatory responses (cytokine measurements) • Allergic reaction • Asthma • Inflammatory bowel disease
Immunology/ Allergic response	• Thioglycollate-mediated monocyte infiltration • Delayed type hypersensitivity	• Allergic reaction/ immunological function
Dermatology	• Oxazolone contact hypersensitivity • DNFB contact hypersensitivity • Chronic DNFB	• Atopic dermatitis • Psoriasis
Cardiovascular	• Cardiovascular telemetry • Tail cuff • Blood clotting	• Hypertension; cardiovascular function • Coagulation
Other	• Hormonal, cytokine, clinical chemistry, cell counts • Electrophysiology	• Multiple general pharmacological responses • Sleep wake, seizure potential, general CNS physiology

glucose tolerance test, along with the activities in related therapeutic animal models, provided confidence that the observed activity was a true potential beneficial therapeutic response.

Test compounds that demonstrate activity in the *thera*TRACE® platform ("hits") are retested independently in the same and other therapeutically related models, not included in the platform, in order to confirm and characterize the response, as well as to strengthen a preclinical pharmacology package to support entry into the drug development process. MLR-1023 was retested in an oral glucose tolerance test outside of the *thera*TRACE® platform and compared with metformin, a reference compound that is known to be effective in this model and is approved and widely prescribed for the treatment of type 2 diabetes (Figure 9.5). In this follow-on study, MLR-1023 produced identical glucose lowering to that shown in the *thera*TRACE® platform. Additional studies with MLR-1023 in other models of type 2 diabetes with chronic dosing paradigms and in other species confirmed and extended those original findings [83]. Indeed, in these follow-on studies MLR-1023 elicited a faster onset and

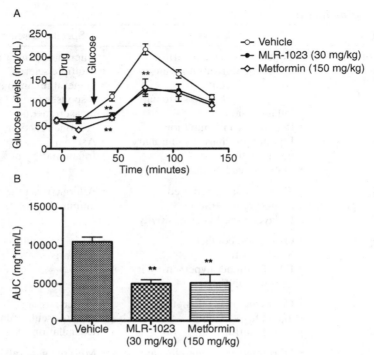

FIGURE 9.5. MLR-1023 lowered blood glucose levels in an oral glucose tolerance test. In the *thera*TRACE® platform, MLR-1023 elicited a significant blood glucose-lowering response in an oral glucose tolerance test, a phenotypic model of type 2 diabetes and glucose regulation. The data in this figure shows the effects of MLR-1023 in a follow-on oral glucose tolerance test and with a comparison to metformin, an approved drug for type II diabetes. In this follow-on study, MLR-1023 elicited a significant blunting of the glucose departure in this OGTT with greater potency and equivalent efficacy to that of metformin.

more robust blood glucose lowering than the clinically approved type 2 agents, metformin and rosiglitazone. MLR-1023 is now in clinical development for the treatment of type 2 diabetes.

9.6. RESULTS FROM PHENOTYPIC SCREENING STUDIES

As discussed above, the drug discovery paradigm as it exists in the pharmaceutical industry is heavily oriented toward designing drugs that interact with a single molecular target with high potency and selectivity. These target-driven approaches place less emphasis (at least initially) on high quality chemical structure, PK, and safety considerations as early medicinal chemistry efforts are focused on optimizing potency and selectivity. Target-driven approaches are limited by known pharmacological activity of that target. However, as has been discussed above, the breadth of biologic activity regulated by a molecular target often extends well beyond the known pathology associated with it. Thus, drug interaction with a specific target, interaction with multiple target subtypes, and widespread tissue distribution of targets coupled with PK and distribution phenomenon virtually guarantee unpredicted effects of molecular target directed drugs. Indeed, these unpredicted activities are what drive the majority of drug repositioning events.

9.6.1. On-Target Activities

For drugs that are highly selective to a drug target and for which the pharmacological activity of that drug can be directly attributed to a given drug-target interaction, the drug repositioning event can also be described as a molecular target repositioning event. There are many examples of this type of "target" repositioning wherein the target has also been associated with a new therapeutic area. Examples of on-target drug repositioning are described in Table 9.4. As described above, sildenafil was repositioned to erectile dysfunction treatment after serendipitous findings in early anti-hypertensive preclinical studies [84]. This finding was not only a drug-repositioning finding, but motivated a broader repositioning of the molecular target, PDE5, as a target for erectile dysfunction. After this discovery, other PDE5 inhibitors were in turn repositioned to this indication. Tadalafil, another PDE5 inhibitor that was being developed for inflammation and cardiovascular disease, relied upon the sildenafil clinical findings for repositioning as a treatment for erectile dysfunction [85]. Based on these clinical findings, this target is now clearly associated with smooth muscle relaxation and vascular dilation [85]. PDE5 has since been found to be the predominant phosphodiesterase in the corpus cavernosum [86]. More recently sildenafil and other PDE5 inhibitors may have beneficial effects in other therapeutic areas including pulmonary hypertension, coronary vasospasm and benign prostatic hyperplasia and are being assessed in small clinical trials for these conditions [87]. This PDE5 example shows how the functional pharmacology of a compound can drive molecular target repositioning. The selective HMG-CoA reductase inhibitor atorvastatin provides another example and its potential utility as a treatment for multiple sclerosis. In an experimental autoimmune model of multiple sclerosis (MS), atorvastatin attenuated EAE-mediated paralysis in mice [88]. This effect was driven by inhibition of HMG-CoA mediated immune responses. These preclinical findings led to a clinical study of atorvastatin in MS patients. In that study, atorvastatin slowed the clinical progression of MS and reduced the number brain lesions [89]. HMG-CoA reductase is now considered to be a potential target for the treatment of MS.

These two examples are representative of "on-target" repositioning. Indeed, most repositioning of drugs with well-defined molecular targets can be attributed to on-target effects. In addition to the examples described above, other

TABLE 9.4. Mechanisms Associated with Drug Repositioning: On-Target versus Off-Target Repositioning

Compound Name	Original Target or Mechanism of Action	Original Indication	Alternative Indication	Mechanism of Alternative Indication	Reference
Celecoxib	COX-2 antagonist	Osteoarthritis and rheumatoid arthritis	Adenomatous polyposis; multiple cancers	On-target	[116]
Dapoxetine	Serotonin reuptake inhibitor (SSRI)	Depression (discontinued)	Premature ejaculation	On-target	[1]
Finasteride	Testosterone 5alpha-reductase inhibitor	Benign prostatic hypertrophy	Hair loss; marketed as Propecia®	On-target	[20]
Fluoxetine	SSRI	Depression	Premenstrual dysphoria;	On-target	[117]
Gabapentin	α2delta of L-type Ca2+ ion channels	Epilepsy	Pain, anxiety	Unknown	[16]
Lidocaine	Na channel blocker	Local anesthetic	Corticosteroid-dependent asthma	Unknown	[118]
Mifepristone	Progesterone antagonist;	Pregnancy termination	Cushing's syndrome	Off-target; glucocorticoid antagonist	[94]
Minoxidil	Potassium channel activator	Severe hypertension	Hair loss	Unknown	[101, 119]
Paclitaxel	Beta tubulin inhibitor	Cancer	Restenosis	On-target	[120]
Raloxifene	Selective estrogen receptor modulator	Osteoporosis	Breast and prostate cancer	On-target	[121]
Ropinirole	Dopamine receptor (D2, D3) agonist	Antihypertensive (discontinued)	Parkinson's disease/restless leg syndrome	On-target	[1]
Sildenafil	PDE5 inhibitor	Angina (discontinued)	Erectile dysfunction, pulmonary atrial hypertension	On-target	[100]
Simvastatin	HMG-CoA reductase	Cholesterol lowering	Multiple Sclerosis (immunomodulatory)	On-target	[88]
Topiramate	Multiple CNS targets	Epilepsy	Obesity, alcohol dependence, bipolar disorder,	Unknown;	[13]
Telmisartan	Angiotensin II type I antagonist	Antihypertensive	Diabetes	Off-target, PPAR agonist	[91]

278

on-target drug repositioning examples include raloxifene a selective estrogen receptor antagonist originally developed for osteoporosis and now also used for treatment of breast cancer [90]; and ropinirole, a D2 receptor agonist developed as an anti-hypertensive and now used as a treatment for Parkinson's disease [1]. On-target drug repositioning is an important concept to consider for drug repositioning by phenotypic screening. Drugs that have been developed through some phase of clinical development and that act via interaction with a single target have been chemically optimized to interact with that target. Thus, if new therapeutic activity is uncovered and the mechanism is confirmed to be mediated as an on-target activity then no further optimization of that compound may be required prior to initiation of clinical studies in the new indication.

9.6.2. Off-Target Activities

Examples of drug repositioning events that can be attributed to off-target mediated responses for "highly selective" drugs are rare and indicate activity at a previously unidentified target, presumably one missed by the extensive battery of selectivity panels employed during early candidate development in the pharmaceutical industry. An example of this type of off-target mediated response is illustrated by the antihypertensive drug telmisartan (see Table 9.4). Telmisartan was originally developed as an inhibitor of angiotensin type 2 receptors and was found to also activate PPARγ receptors and improve insulin sensitivity in experimental animals [91]. This unique dual target activity has been extended to clinical trials in which telmisartan functions as an antihypertensive with the ability to regulate insulin sensitivity in type 2 diabetics [92]. Another example is illustrated by mifepristone. Originally developed as a progesterone receptor antagonist and an abortifacient [93], it was repositioned as a treatment for Cushing's syndrome on the basis of its interaction with glucocorticoid receptors [94].

9.7. COMPOUND SELECTION FOR DRUG REPOSITIONING

In selecting ideal candidates for repositioning, it is instructive to consider drug repositioning examples with particular attention focused on chemical structure, drug-like characteristics, original indication, and stage of development that the compound reached.

Examination of off-label applications of drugs shows that those drugs that evoke CNS activity as their primary indication produce the broadest potential use. These drugs have high volumes of distribution, which translates into good tissue penetrance (including brain penetrance) and good drug-like qualities including "rule of 5" compliance [95]. CNS-active compounds may exhibit a high rate of repositioning because of their preponderance of target promiscuity and the interrelatedness of many of these CNS indications [30].

Nonetheless, many CNS drugs have been repositioned to non-CNS indications. For instance, thalidomide, a drug originally developed as a sedative and a treatment for morning sickness, and with well-described disastrous consequences [96], was repositioned for the treatment of erythema nodosum laprosum, an inflammatory condition of leprosy, and, more recently, as a treatment for multiple myeloma [97]. Moreover, a number of SSRI compounds including duloxetine are used in the treatment of fibromyalagia [98].

For *in vivo* phenotypic screening, there are certain guiding principles that emerge for choosing the most suitable candidates. Compounds with high volumes of distribution and thereby good tissue penetrance exhibit higher hit rates than compounds with low volumes of distribution. Accordingly, such filtering tends to exclude biologics. A recent meta-analysis of studies that screened libraries of U.S. Food and Drug Administration (FDA)-approved drugs for use in orphan and rare diseases described chemical characteristics of small molecule drugs that produce alternative activities. In this evaluation, it was found that promiscuous drugs were statistically more hydrophobic, with higher molecular weight and AlogP than those drugs that were selective for that particular disease [99].

Anti-infectives (antibacterials, antivirals, and antifungals) tend to be poor substrates for broad therapeutic area repositioning outside of the realm of infectious diseases. These compounds are typically designed to interact with targets specific for infective agents and therefore are less likely to likely to interact predictably with mammalian targets, or alter mammalian networks.

Finally, most oncology therapeutics are less likely to elicit beneficial effects in therapeutic areas outside of neoplastic disease. These compounds are for the most part cytotoxic or cytostatic agents and, moreover, frequently have well-described adverse effects that are often not compatible with non-oncologic indications.

Moving beyond these biology considerations, one can also consider aspects of commercial potential when choosing the ideal repositioning candidates. For example, from an intellectual property and exclusivity strategy perspective, actively marketed drugs including generics have very limited exclusivity potential, and thereby market potential, as the existing marketed drug may be prescribed off-label by physicians for the new indication regardless of "method-of-use" patents that may be obtained. In this scenario, the holder of a "method-of-use" patent for the new indication is dependent on the fact that the supplier of the drug for its original indication cannot promote the new use. This limitation of "method-of-use" patents does not exist for compounds that have never received market approval.

Most small molecule drug candidates, which clear the above-listed filtering criteria, are otherwise biologically active and well tolerated in humans, are good repositioning candidates, and have proven to have a surprisingly high rate of exhibiting novel therapeutic potential in phenotypic screens. As mentioned earlier, of the roughly 300 compounds that Melior Discovery has tested in the *thera*TRACE® platform, approximately 30% show potential new therapeutic utility. This high frequency of new indications discovery is consistent with hit rates found in phenotypic screening protocols and off-label prescription rates [8, 75, 99].

Melior Discovery has focused on compounds that have been discontinued in the clinical trial process for reasons of efficacy for their original indication. Clinical efficacy failures may suggest that the compound elicited insufficient modulation of its molecular target. However, suboptimal target modulation does not appear to be the key driver for clinical efficacy failures. For example, sildenafil, minoxidil, and ropinirole were abandoned for their original indications in clinical efficacy studies but repositioned to new indications that were driven by on-target effects [1, 100, 101]. In these instances, the molecular target was not optimal for the original indication but was better suited to the newly found indication. This again illustrates the concept of molecular target repositioning using highly selective target-directed compounds.

In instances where the original clinical trial data are available, a repeat of a Phase I clinical trial may be avoided with such compounds, assuming appropriate present-day requirements are met by the original package. Avoidance of Phase I studies can lead into rapid entry into a Phase II efficacy trial for the new indication. As discussed in detail in Chapter 1 of this book, drug repositioning of these discontinued clinical candidates can dramatically shorten the time of the drug discovery process and greatly reduce the risk of early clinical failures [1].

As mentioned in the preceding section, MLR-1023 was a discontinued Phase II clinical stage compound originally developed for the treatment of gastric ulcers [81]. Using the *thera*TRACE® platform, MLR-1023 was repositioned as a type 2 diabetes treatment. Follow-on studies in multiple type 2 diabetes models confirmed and extended the results, and a full pharmacological profile of MLR-1023 in diabetes models has been established. Based on those new findings, a new investigational new drug (IND) was granted by the FDA [102]. The design of Phase II studies in type 2 diabetes have tremendously aided by the PK and safety data that were generated in the original gastric ulcer clinical studies [103].

9.8. EXCLUSIVITY STRATEGIES FOR REPOSITIONED DRUGS IDENTIFIED BY PHENOTYPIC SCREENING

A full discussion of marketing exclusivity strategies for newly repositioned drugs is beyond the scope of this chapter. Nonetheless, there are aspects of exclusivity strategy that overlap with drug repositioning methods and specifically phenotypic screening methodology. In many instances where a new therapeutic use is indentified for a compound, "method-of-use" patents are a primary means for a company to seek market exclusivity for the product in the new indication. This type of a patent is ideal for compounds that have not otherwise had market approval and there are no other compounds of the same mechanism that are marketed. In these instances, method-of-use provides extensive and long-lasting marketing exclusivity for the new drug. This type of patent strategy was successfully utilized for MLR-1023. In this instance, MLR-1023 was never marketed for the original indication (gastric ulcer) and the composition-of-matter for this compound had expired. The findings of a glycemic control response were sufficiently novel and unexpected to acquire a method-of-use patent for MLR-1023 for the treatment of certain metabolic disease indications. In fact, since the compound has never been marketed, it is viewed by the FDA as a "new chemical entity" and the exclusivity provided by the method-of-use is as powerful as that provided by composition of matter patents.

Recently, a growing challenge for seeking patents on any new inventions, whether in the pharmaceutical industry or otherwise, is to meet the U.S. patent and trade offices rising bar of non-obvious inventions [104]. Phenotypic screening approaches of compounds that are systematically interrogated across a broad array of *in vivo* models independent of a mechanism-based hypothesis have frequently uncovered new potential therapeutic utilities that were not predicted based on *a priori* understanding of the mechanism. This process of identifying unexpected therapeutic uses through phenotypic screening thus confers a significant advantage in passing the more stringent tests of "non-obviousness" and therefore potentially provides better substrate for method-of-use patents.

9.9. SUMMARY

Drug action is a highly complex function mediated by a composite of PK properties, including absorption, distribution, metabolism, and elimination, and PD complexity including target kinetics, interaction with related and unrelated molecular targets, and modulation of complex biological networks. These features make it difficult to predict whether a drug might have alternative therapeutic benefits based solely on chemical structure and known drug actions or activities and particularly as our understanding of systems pharmacology for complex diseases is often incomplete. Thus, in nearly all cases, the full therapeutic potential of a molecular target is incompletely understood. The concept that many drug actions are driven through polypharmacology and modulation of complex biological networks is gaining acceptance (see Chapters 5 and 7). Thus, accurately predicting potential alternative therapeutic activity of existing drugs using *in silico*, *in vitro* or cell-based systems has significant limitations. Evaluating drugs through an *in vivo* phenotyping platform occurs in a target-independent fashion and does not require an *a priori* understanding of the drug's mechanism. Evaluation of unique chemical entities in *in vivo* model systems has proven valuable in identifying drug leads and development stage drug candidates.

In this chapter we have described strategies for developing a multi-therapeutic *in vivo* phenotypic platform that is capable of identifying the broad therapeutic potential of drugs and drug candidates, and one such platform coined *thera*TRACE®. The *thera*TRACE® platform is being utilized successfully in repositioning drugs that have reached various stages of preclinical and clinical development. This platform has been developed to maximize likelihood of detecting activity in major marketable disease fields. The method speeds up the process of serendipity. While the platform has wide therapeutic area representation, it has revealed that certain therapeutic areas including metabolic disease, psychotherapeutics, and inflammation, are "hot spots" for identifying new therapies by this strategy, possibly as a result of the complex, incompletely understood pathways underlying these areas of physiology.

The ideal compounds to evaluate for drug repositioning are those that have demonstrated high quality PK properties with a good human safety profile preferably up to at least the Phase II clinical development, but that have not been marketed. With such compounds, rapid entry into proof of concept clinical trials is possible with significant shortening of the development process. In addition, method-of-use patents can be used as a rigorous exclusivity strategy of these compounds, especially when they are first in mechanistic class. This approach can be used to complement existing drug discovery approaches, identifying novel clinical targets for drugs in development or identifying novel therapeutics for a diverse set of diseases, thus replenishing depleted drug pipelines.

REFERENCES

1. Ashburn, T.T., Thor, K.B. (2004). Drug repositioning: Identifying and developing new uses for existing drugs. *Nature Reviews Drug Discovery, 3*, 673–683.

2. Dimond, P.F. (2010). Drug repositioning gains in popularity. *Genetic Engineering and Biotechnology News, 30*, 3–5.

3. Li, H., Liu, A., Zhao, Z., Xu, Y., Lin, J., Jou, D., Li, C. (2011). Fragment-based drug design and drug repositioning using multiple ligand simultaneous docking (mlsd): Identifying celecoxib and template compounds as novel inhibitors of signal transducer and activator of transcription 3 (STAT3). *Journal of Medicinal Chemistry, 54*, 5592–5596.

4. Swamidass, S.J. (2011). Mining small-molecule screens to repurpose drugs. *Briefings in Bioinformatics, 12*, 327–335.

5. Ekins, S., Williams, A.J., Krasowski, M.D., Freundlich, J.S. (2011). In silico repositioning of approved drugs for rare and neglected diseases. *Drug Discovery Today, 16*, 298–310.

6. Tobinick, E.L. (2009). The value of drug repositioning in the current pharmaceutical market. *Drug News & Perspectives, 22*, 119–125.

7. Tartaglia, L.A. (2006). Complementary new approaches enable repositioning of failed drug candidates. *Expert Opinion on Investigational Drugs, 15*, 1295–1298.

8. Radley, D.C., Finkelstein, S.N., Stafford, R.S. (2006). Off-label prescribing among office-based physicians. *Archives of Internal Medicine, 166,* 1021–1026.

9. Tonnesen, P., Tonstad, S., Hjalmarson, A., Lebargy, F., Van Spiegel, P.I., Hider, A., Sweet, R., Townsend, J. (2003). A multicentre, randomized, double-blind, placebo-controlled, 1-year study of bupropion SR for smoking cessation. *Journal of Internal Medicine, 254,* 184–192.

10. Wilens, T.E., Haight, B.R., Horrigan, J.P., Hudziak, J.J., Rosenthal, N.E., Connor, D.F., Hampton, K.D., Richard, N.E., Modell, J.G. (2005). Bupropion XL in adults with attention-deficit/hyperactivity disorder: A randomized, placebo-controlled study. *Biological Psychiatry, 57,* 793–801.

11. Anderson, J.W., Greenway, F.L., Fujioka, K., Gadde, K.M., McKenney, J., O'Neil, P.M. (2002). Bupropion SR enhances weight loss: A 48-week double-blind, placebo- controlled trial. *Obesity Research, 10,* 633–641.

12. Rozen, T.D. (2001). Antiepileptic drugs in the management of cluster headache and trigeminal neuralgia. *Headache, 41*(Suppl 1), S25–S32.

13. Teter, C.J., Early, J.J., Gibbs, C.M. (2000). Treatment of affective disorder and obesity with topiramate. *Annals of Pharmacotherapy, 34,* 1262–1265.

14. Bodkin, J.A., Zornberg, G.L., Lukas, S.E., Cole, J.O. (1995). Buprenorphine treatment of refractory depression. *Journal of Clinical Psychopharmacology, 15,* 49–57.

15. Bryans, J.S., Wustrow, D.J. (1999). 3-substituted GABA analogs with central nervous system activity: A review. *Medical Research Reviews, 19,* 149–177.

16. Singh, L., Field, M.J., Ferris, P., Hunter, J.C., Oles, R.J., Williams, R.G., Woodruff, G.N. (1996). The antiepileptic agent gabapentin (Neurontin) possesses anxiolytic-like and antinociceptive actions that are reversed by D-serine. *Psychopharmacology, 127,* 1–9.

17. Dworkin, R.H., Kirkpatrick, P. (2005). Pregabalin. *Nature Reviews Drug Discovery, 4,* 455–456.

18. Belliotti, T.R., Capiris, T., Ekhato, I.V., Kinsora, J.J., Field, M.J., Heffner, T.G., Meltzer, L.T., Schwarz, J.B., Taylor, C.P., Thorpe, A.J., Vartanian, M.G., Wise, L.D., Zhi-Su, T., Weber, M.L., Wustrow, D.J. (2005). Structure-activity relationships of pregabalin and analogues that target the alpha(2)-delta protein. *Journal of Medicinal Chemistry, 48,* 2294–2307.

19. Taylor, C.P., Angelotti, T., Fauman, E. (2007). Pharmacology and mechanism of action of pregabalin: The calcium channel alpha2-delta (alpha2-delta) subunit as a target for antiepileptic drug discovery. *Epilepsy Research, 73,* 137–150.

20. Chen, C., Puy, L.A., Simard, J., Li, X., Singh, S.M., Labrie, F. (1995). Local and systemic reduction by topical finasteride or flutamide of hamster flank organ size and enzyme activity. *Journal of Investigative Dermatology, 105,* 678–682.

21. Clader, J.W. (2004). The discovery of ezetimibe: A view from outside the receptor. *Journal of Medicinal Chemistry, 47,* 1–9.

22. Duteil, J., Rambert, F.A., Pessonnier, J., Hermant, J.F., Gombert, R., Assous, E. (1990). Central alpha 1-adrenergic stimulation in relation to the behaviour stimulating effect of modafinil; studies with experimental animals. *European Journal of Pharmacology, 180,* 49–58.

23. Drews, J. (2000). Drug discovery: A historical perspective. *Science, 287,* 1960–1964.

24. Brown, D. (2007). Unfinished business: Target-based drug discovery. *Drug Discovery Today*, *12*, 1007–1012.

25. Sams-Dodd, F. (2005). Target-based drug discovery: Is something wrong? *Drug Discovery Today*, *10*, 139–147.

26. Deininger, M.W., Druker, B.J. (2003). Specific targeted therapy of chronic myelogenous leukemia with imatinib. *Pharmacological Reviews*, *55*, 401–423.

27. Munos, B. (2009). Lessons from 60 years of pharmaceutical innovation. *Nature Reviews Drug Discovery*, *8*, 959–968.

28. Swinney, D.C., Anthony, J. (2011). How were new medicines discovered? *Nature Reviews Drug Discovery*, *10*, 507–519.

29. Hopkins, A.L. (2008). Network pharmacology: The next paradigm in drug discovery. *Nature Chemical Biology*, *4*, 682–690.

30. Enna, S.J., Williams, M. (2009). Challenges in the search for drugs to treat central nervous system disorders. *Journal of Pharmacology and Experimental Therapeutics*, *329*, 404–411.

31. Spedding, M., Jay, T., Costa E Silva, J., Perret, L. (2005). A pathophysiological paradigm for the therapy of psychiatric disease. *Nature Reviews Drug Discovery*, *4*, 467–476.

32. Miller, R.A., Birnbaum, M.J. (2010). An energetic tale of AMPK-independent effects of metformin. *Journal of Clinical Investigation*, *120*, 2267–2270.

33. Schlueter, P.J., Peterson, R.T. (2009). Systematizing serendipity for cardiovascular drug discovery. *Circulation*, *120*, 255–263.

34. Terry, A.V., Jr (2006). Muscarinic receptor antagonists in rats. In *Animal Models of Cognitive Impairment*, eds. Levin, E.D., Buccafusco, J.J., Boca Raton, FL: CRC Press.

35. Buccafusco, J.J., Terry, A.V., Jr, Webster, S.J., Martin, D., Hohnadel, E.J., Bouchard, K.A., Warner, S.E. (2008). The scopolamine-reversal paradigm in rats and monkeys: The importance of computer-assisted operant-conditioning memory tasks for screening drug candidates. *Psychopharmacology*, *199*, 481–494.

36. Bartolomeo, A.C., Morris, H., Buccafusco, J.J., Kille, N., Rosenzweig-Lipson, S., Husbands, M.G., Sabb, A.L., Abou-Gharbia, M., Moyer, J.A., Boast, C.A. (2000). The preclinical pharmacological profile of WAY-132983, a potent M1 preferring agonist. *Journal of Pharmacology and Experimental Therapeutics*, *292*, 584–596.

37. Martorana, A., Esposito, Z., Koch, G. (2010). Beyond the cholinergic hypothesis: Do current drugs work in Alzheimer's disease? *CNS Neuroscience & Therapeutics*, *16*, 235–245.

38. Chagnon, Y.C., Bouchard, C. (1996). Genetics of obesity: Advances from rodent studies. *Trends in Genetics*, *12*, 441–444.

39. Baribault, H. (2010). Mouse models of type II diabetes mellitus in drug discovery. *Methods in Molecular Biology*, *602*, 135–155.

40. Connor, S.C., Hughes, M.G., Moore, G., Lister, C.A., Smith, S.A. (1997). Antidiabetic efficacy of BRL 49653, a potent orally active insulin sensitizing agent, assessed in the C57BL/KsJ db/db diabetic mouse by non-invasive 1H NMR studies of urine. *The Journal of Pharmacy and Pharmacology*, *49*, 336–344.

41. Fujita, H., Fujishima, H., Koshimura, J., Hosoba, M., Yoshioka, N., Shimotomai, T., Morii, T., Narita, T., Kakei, M., Ito, S. (2005). Effects of antidiabetic treatment with

metformin and insulin on serum and adipose tissue adiponectin levels in db/db mice. *Endocrine Journal, 52,* 427–433.

42. Young, A.A., Gedulin, B.R., Bhavsar, S., Bodkin, N., Jodka, C., Hansen, B., Denaro, M. (1999). Glucose-lowering and insulin-sensitizing actions of exendin-4: Studies in obese diabetic (ob/ob, db/db) mice, diabetic fatty Zucker rats, and diabetic rhesus monkeys (Macaca mulatta). *Diabetes, 48,* 1026–1034.

43. Elmer, G.I., Kafkafi, N. (2009). Drug discovery in psychiatric illness: Mining for gold. *Schizophrenia Bulletin, 35,* 287–292.

44. Swerdlow, N.R., Geyer, M.A. (1998). Using an animal model of deficient senso-rimotor gating to study the pathophysiology and new treatments of schizophrenia. *Schizophrenia Bulletin, 24,* 285–301.

45. Wadenberg, M.L. (2010). Conditioned avoidance response in the development of new antipsychotics. *Current Pharmaceutical Design, 16,* 358–370.

46. Cryan, J.F., Mombereau, C., Vassout, A. (2005). The tail suspension test as a model for assessing antidepressant activity: Review of pharmacological and genetic studies in mice. *Neuroscience and Biobehavioral Reviews, 29,* 571–625.

47. Petit-Demouliere, B., Chenu, F., Bourin, M. (2005). Forced swimming test in mice: A review of antidepressant activity. *Psychopharmacology, 177,* 245–255.

48. Bischoff, H. (1995). The mechanism of alpha-glucosidase inhibition in the manage-ment of diabetes. *Clinical and Investigative Medicine, 18,* 303–311.

49. Davies, M.J. (2002). Insulin secretagogues. *Current Medical Research and Opinion, 18*(Suppl 1), s22–s30.

50. Hundal, R.S., Krssak, M., Dufour, S., Laurent, D., Lebon, V., Chandramouli, V., Inzucchi, S.E., Schumann, W.C., Petersen, K.F., Landau, B.R., Shulman, G.I. (2000). Mechanism by which metformin reduces glucose production in type 2 diabetes. *Diabetes, 49,* 2063–2069.

51. Rosen, E.D., Spiegelman, B.M. (2001). PPARgamma: A nuclear regulator of metabolism, differentiation, and cell growth. *Journal of Biological Chemistry, 276,* 37731–37734.

52. Thornberry, N.A., Weber, A.E. (2007). Discovery of JANUVIA (Sitagliptin), a selective dipeptidyl peptidase IV inhibitor for the treatment of type 2 diabetes. *Current Topics in Medicinal Chemistry, 7,* 557–568.

53. Drucker, D.J. (2007). Dipeptidyl peptidase-4 inhibition and the treatment of type 2 diabetes: Preclinical biology and mechanisms of action. *Diabetes Care, 30,* 1335–1343.

54. Rendell, M. (2004). Advances in diabetes for the millennium: Drug therapy of type 2 diabetes. *Medscape General Medicine, 6,* 9–14.

55. Lipinski, C.A. (2011). Prous Integrity Search of Targets for Type II Diabetes.

56. Serhan, C.N. (2009). Systems approach to inflammation resolution: Identification of novel anti-inflammatory and pro-resolving mediators. *Journal of Thrombosis and Haemostasis, 7*(Suppl 1), 44–48.

57. Amor, S., Puentes, F., Baker, D., van der Valk, P. (2010). Inflammation in neurode-generative diseases. *Immunology, 129,* 154–169.

58. Harris, E.D. (1997). *Rheumatoid Arthritis.* Philadelphia: W.B. Saunders.

59. Fiocchi, C. (2004). Inflammatory bowel disease: New insights into mechanisms of inflammation and increasingly customized approaches to diagnosis and therapy. *Current Opinion in Gastroenterology, 20,* 309–310.

60. Nishimura, S., Manabe, I., Nagai, R. (2009). Adipose tissue inflammation in obesity and metabolic syndrome. *Discovery Medicine*, *8*, 55–60.

61. Leonard, B.E. (2010). The concept of depression as a dysfunction of the immune system. *Current Immunology Reviews*, *6*, 205–212.

62. Serhan, C.N., Ward, P.A. (1999). *Molecular and Cellular Basis of Inflammation*. Current Inflammation Research, Totowa, NJ: Humana Press.

63. Chen, Y.F., Jobanputra, P., Barton, P., Bryan, S., Fry-Smith, A., Harris, G., Taylor, R.S. (2008). Cyclooxygenase-2 selective non-steroidal anti-inflammatory drugs (etodolac, meloxicam, celecoxib, rofecoxib, etoricoxib, valdecoxib and lumiracoxib) for osteoarthritis and rheumatoid arthritis: A systematic review and economic evaluation. *Health Technology Assessment*, *12*, 1–278, iii.

64. Bovill, J.G. (2003). Pharmacology and clinical action of COX-2 selective NSAIDs. *Advances in Experimental Medicine and Biology*, *523*, 201–214.

65. Vane, J.R., Botting, R.M. (1998). Anti-inflammatory drugs and their mechanism of action. *Inflammation Research*, *47*(Suppl 2), S78–S87.

66. Siddiqui, M.A., Scott, L.J. (2005). Infliximab: A review of its use in Crohn's disease and rheumatoid arthritis. *Drugs*, *65*, 2179–2208.

67. Woolacott, N.F., Khadjesari, Z.C., Bruce, I.N., Riemsma, R.P. (2006). Etanercept and infliximab for the treatment of psoriatic arthritis: A systematic review. *Clinical and Experimental Rheumatology*, *24*, 587–593.

68. Wang, D., DuBois, R.N. (2010). Therapeutic potential of peroxisome proliferator-activated receptors in chronic inflammation and colorectal cancer. *Gastroenterology Clinics of North America*, *39*, 697–707.

69. Sorrentino, S., Landmesser, U. (2005). Nonlipid-lowering effects of statins. *Current Treatment Options in Cardiovascular Medicine*, *7*, 459–466.

70. Gerrard, P., Malcolm, R. (2007). Mechanisms of modafinil: A review of current research. *Neuropsychiatric Disease and Treatment*, *3*, 349–364.

71. Meltzer, H.Y., Huang, M. (2008). In vivo actions of atypical antipsychotic drug on serotonergic and dopaminergic systems. *Progress in Brain Research*, *172*, 177–197.

72. Bymaster, F.P., Dreshfield-Ahmad, L.J., Threlkeld, P.G., Shaw, J.L., Thompson, L., Nelson, D.L., Hemrick-Luecke, S.K., Wong, D.T. (2001). Comparative affinity of duloxetine and venlafaxine for serotonin and norepinephrine transporters in vitro and in vivo, human serotonin receptor subtypes, and other neuronal receptors. *Neuropsychopharmacology*, *25*, 871–880.

73. Irwin, S. (1968). Comprehensive observational assessment: Ia. A systematic, quantitative procedure for assessing the behavioral and physiologic state of the mouse. *Psychopharmacologia*, *13*, 222–257.

74. Gruner, J.A., Mathiasen, J.R., Flood, D.G., Gasior, M. (2011). Characterization of pharmacological and wake-promoting properties of the dopaminergic stimulant sydnocarb in rats. *Journal of Pharmacology and Experimental Therapeutics*, *337*, 380–390.

75. Hellerstein, M.K. (2008). Exploiting complexity and the robustness of network architecture for drug discovery. *Journal of Pharmacology and Experimental Therapeutics*, *325*, 1–9.

76. Hellerstein, M.K. (2008). A critique of the molecular target-based drug discovery paradigm based on principles of metabolic control: Advantages of pathway-based discovery. *Metabolic Engineering*, *10*, 1–9.

77. Chalubinski, M., Broncel, M. (2010). Influence of statins on effector and regulatory immune mechanisms and their potential clinical relevance in treating autoimmune disorders. *Medical Science Monitor*, *16*, RA245–RA251.

78. Sinicrope, F.A. (2006). Targeting cyclooxygenase-2 for prevention and therapy of colorectal cancer. *Molecular Carcinogenesis*, *45*, 447–454.

79. Chong, C.R., Chen, X., Shi, L., Liu, J.O., Sullivan, D.J., Jr (2006). A clinical drug library screen identifies astemizole as an antimalarial agent. *Nature Chemical Biology*, *2*, 415–416.

80. Inagaki, N., Shiraishi, N., Igeta, K., Itoh, T., Chikumoto, T., Nagao, M., Kim, J.F., Nagai, H. (2006). Inhibition of scratching behavior associated with allergic dermatitis in mice by tacrolimus, but not by dexamethasone. *European Journal of Pharmacology*, *546*, 189–196.

81. Lipinski, C.A., Stam, J.G., Pereira, J.N., Ackerman, N.R., Hess, H.J. (1980). Bronchodilator and antiulcer phenoxypyrimidinones. *Journal of Medicinal Chemistry*, *23*, 1026–1031.

82. Reaume, A., Saporito, M.S. (2010). Methods and formulation for modulating lyn kinase activity and treating related disorders, *USPTO*, Melior Discovery, Inc.: USA.

83. Ochman, A., Lipinski, C.A., Reaume, A., Handler, J.A., Saporito, M.S. (2011). MLR-1023 is a repositioned drug candidate for type II diabetes that elicits a rapid-onset and durable improvement in glucose homeostasis and preserves pancreatic β-cells in mice. *In preparation*.

84. Boolell, M., Gepi-Attee, S., Gingell, J.C., Allen, M.J. (1996). Sildenafil, a novel effective oral therapy for male erectile dysfunction. *British Journal of Urology*, *78*, 257–261.

85. Corbin, J.D., Francis, S.H. (2002). Pharmacology of phosphodiesterase-5 inhibitors. *International Journal of Clinical Practice*, *56*, 453–459.

86. Wallis, R.M., Corbin, J.D., Francis, S.H., Ellis, P. (1999). Tissue distribution of phosphodiesterase families and the effects of sildenafil on tissue cyclic nucleotides, platelet function, and the contractile responses of trabeculae carneae and aortic rings in vitro. *American Journal of Cardiology*, *83*, 3C–12C.

87. Giovannoni, M.P., Vergelli, C., Graziano, A., Dal Piaz, V. (2010). PDE5 inhibitors and their applications. *Current Medicinal Chemistry*, *17*, 2564–2587.

88. Youssef, S., Stuve, O., Patarroyo, J.C., Ruiz, P.J., Radosevich, J.L., Hur, E.M., Bravo, M., Mitchell, D.J., Sobel, R.A., Steinman, L., Zamvil, S.S. (2002). The HMG-CoA reductase inhibitor, atorvastatin, promotes a Th2 bias and reverses paralysis in central nervous system autoimmune disease. *Nature*, *420*, 78–84.

89. Weber, M.S., Zamvil, S.S. (2008). Statins and demyelination. *Current Topics in Microbiology and Immunology*, *318*, 313–324.

90. Moen, M.D., Keating, G.M. (2008). Raloxifene: A review of its use in the prevention of invasive breast cancer. *Drugs*, *68*, 2059–2083.

91. Benson, S.C., Pershadsingh, H.A., Ho, C.I., Chittiboyina, A., Desai, P., Pravenec, M., Qi, N., Wang, J., Avery, M.A., Kurtz, T.W. (2004). Identification of telmisartan as a unique angiotensin II receptor antagonist with selective PPARgamma-modulating activity. *Hypertension*, *43*, 993–1002.

92. Yamana, A., Arita, M., Furuta, M., Shimajiri, Y., Sanke, T. (2008). The angiotensin II receptor blocker telmisartan improves insulin resistance and has beneficial

effects in hypertensive patients with type 2 diabetes and poor glycemic control. *Diabetes Research and Clinical Practice, 82*, 127–131.

93. Chabbert-Buffet, N., Meduri, G., Bouchard, P., Spitz, I.M. (2005). Selective progesterone receptor modulators and progesterone antagonists: Mechanisms of action and clinical applications. *Human Reproduction Update, 11*, 293–307.

94. Castinetti, F., Conte-Devolx, B., Brue, T. (2010). Medical treatment of Cushing's syndrome: Glucocorticoid receptor antagonists and mifepristone. *Neuroendocrinology, 92*(Suppl 1), 125–130.

95. Lipinski, C.A., Lombardo, F., Dominy, B.W., Feeney, P.J. (2001). Experimental and computational approaches to estimate solubility and permeability in drug discovery and development settings. *Advanced Drug Delivery Reviews, 46*, 3–26.

96. Wu, K.L., Sonneveld, P. (2002). Thalidomide: New uses for an old drug. *Nederlands Tijdschrift Voor Geneeskunde, 146*, 1438–1441.

97. Melchert, M., List, A. (2007). The thalidomide saga. *International Journal of Biochemistry and Cell Biology, 39*, 1489–1499.

98. Arnold, L.M. (2007). Duloxetine and other antidepressants in the treatment of patients with fibromyalgia. *Pain Medicine, 8*(Suppl 2), S63–S74.

99. Ekins, S., Williams, A.J. (2011). Finding promiscuous old drugs for new uses. *Pharmaceutical Research, 28*, 1785–1791.

100. Langtry, H.D., Markham, A. (1999). Sildenafil: A review of its use in erectile dysfunction. *Drugs, 57*, 967–989.

101. Fenton, D.A., Wilkinson, J.D. (1983). Topical minoxidil in the treatment of alopecia areata. *British Medical Journal, 287*, 1015–1017.

102. Reaume, A.G. (2008). Melior Signs Option Agreement with Pfizer. Press release. http://www.meliordiscovery.com

103. Reaume, A.G. (2009). Melior Discovery Announces IND Approval for Novel Diabetes Drug MLR1023. Press release. http://www.meliordiscovery.com

104. Furrow, M.E. (2008). Pharmaceutical patent life-cycle management after KSR v. Teleflex. *Food and Drug Law Journal, 63*, 275–320.

105. Garcia-Calvo, M., Lisnock, J., Bull, H.G., Hawes, B.E., Burnett, D.A., Braun, M.P., Crona, J.H., Davis, H.R., Jr, Dean, D.C., Detmers, P.A., Graziano, M.P., Hughes, M., Macintyre, D.E., Ogawa, A., O'Neill, K.A., Iyer, S.P., Shevell, D.E., Smith, M.M., Tang, Y.S., Makarewicz, A.M., Ujjainwalla, F., Altmann, S.W., Chapman, K.T., Thornberry, N.A. (2005). The target of ezetimibe is Niemann-Pick C1-Like 1 (NPC1L1). *Proceedings of the National Academy of Sciences, 102*, 8132–8137.

106. McIntyre, R.S., Mancini, D.A., McCann, S., Srinivasan, J., Sagman, D., Kennedy, S.H. (2002). Topiramate versus bupropion SR when added to mood stabilizer therapy for the depressive phase of bipolar disorder: A preliminary single-blind study. *Bipolar Disorders, 4*, 207–213.

107. Johnson, B.A., Ait-Daoud, N., Bowden, C.L., DiClemente, C.C., Roache, J.D., Lawson, K., Javors, M.A., Ma, J.Z. (2003). Oral topiramate for treatment of alcohol dependence: A randomised controlled trial. *Lancet, 361*, 1677–1685.

108. Mikaeloff, Y., de Saint-Martin, A., Mancini, J., Peudenier, S., Pedespan, J.M., Vallee, L., Motte, J., Bourgeois, M., Arzimanoglou, A., Dulac, O., Chiron, C. (2003).

Topiramate: Efficacy and tolerability in children according to epilepsy syndromes. *Epilepsy Research, 53*, 225–232.

109. Van Ameringen, M., Mancini, C., Patterson, B., Bennett, M. (2006). Topiramate augmentation in treatment-resistant obsessive-compulsive disorder: A retrospective, open-label case series. *Depression and Anxiety, 23*, 1–5.

110. Van Ameringen, M., Mancini, C., Pipe, B., Oakman, J., Bennett, M. (2004). An open trial of topiramate in the treatment of generalized social phobia. *Journal of Clinical Psychiatry, 65*, 1674–1678.

111. Kosman, M.E. (1980). Evaluation of a new antihypertensive agent. Minoxidil. *JAMA: The Journal of the American Medical Association, 244*, 73–75.

112. Stone, W.S., Croul, C.E., Gold, P.E. (1988). Attenuation of scopolamine-induced amnesia in mice. *Psychopharmacology, 96*, 417–420.

113. Metz, G.A., Tse, A., Ballermann, M., Smith, L.K., Fouad, K. (2005). The unilateral 6-OHDA rat model of Parkinson's disease revisited: An electromyographic and behavioural analysis. *European Journal of Neuroscience, 22*, 735–744.

114. Maharshak, N., Hart, G., Ron, E., Zelman, E., Sagiv, A., Arber, N., Brazowski, E., Margalit, R., Elinav, E., Shachar, I. (2010). CCL2 (pM levels) as a therapeutic agent in inflammatory bowel disease models in mice. *Inflammatory Bowel Diseases, 16*, 1496–1504.

115. Triantafillidis, J.K., Papalois, A.E., Parasi, A., Anagnostakis, E., Burnazos, S., Gikas, A., Merikas, E.G., Douzinas, E., Karagianni, M., Sotiriou, H. (2005). Favorable response to subcutaneous administration of infliximab in rats with experimental colitis. *World Journal of Gastroenterology, 11*, 6843–6847.

116. Koehne, C.H., Dubois, R.N. (2004). COX-2 inhibition and colorectal cancer. *Seminars in Oncology, 31*, 12–21.

117. Pearlstein, T., Yonkers, K.A. (2002). Review of fluoxetine and its clinical applications in premenstrual dysphoric disorder. *Expert Opinion on Pharmacotherapy, 3*, 979–991.

118. Hunt, L.W., Frigas, E., Butterfield, J.H., Kita, H., Blomgren, J., Dunnette, S.L., Offord, K.P., Gleich, G.J. (2004). Treatment of asthma with nebulized lidocaine: A randomized, placebo-controlled study. *Journal of Allergy and Clinical Immunology, 113*, 853–859.

119. Messenger, A.G., Rundegren, J. (2004). Minoxidil: Mechanisms of action on hair growth. *British Journal of Dermatology, 150*, 186–194.

120. Schwertz, D.W., Vaitkus, P. (2003). Drug-eluting stents to prevent reblockage of coronary arteries. *Journal of Cardiovascular Nursing, 18*, 11–16.

121. Vogel, V.G., Costantino, J.P., Wickerham, D.L., Cronin, W.M., Cecchini, R.S., Atkins, J.N., Bevers, T.B., Fehrenbacher, L., Pajon, E.R., Jr, Wade, J.L., 3rd, Robidoux, A., Margolese, R.G., James, J., Lippman, S.M., Runowicz, C.D., Ganz, P.A., Reis, S.E., McCaskill-Stevens, W., Ford, L.G., Jordan, V.C., Wolmark, N. (2006). Effects of tamoxifen vs raloxifene on the risk of developing invasive breast cancer and other disease outcomes: The NSABP Study of Tamoxifen and Raloxifene (STAR) P-2 trial. *JAMA: The Journal of the American Medical Association, 295*, 2727–2741.

CHAPTER 10

Old Drugs Yield New Discoveries: Examples from the Prodrug, Chiral Switch, and Site-Selective Deuteration Strategies

ADAM J. MORGAN, BHAUMIK A. PANDYA, CRAIG E. MASSE, and SCOTT L. HARBESON

10.1. INTRODUCTION

Drug repositioning approaches are flexible, diverse, and dynamic. They can be customized to accommodate the goals and needs of the organizations implementing them. For example, repositioning can provide an approach [1] to capitalize on low risk opportunities by leveraging existing expertise on an in-house or in-licensed entity. In contrast, some biotechnology companies have developed repositioning approaches in the form of new technology platforms applied to generic, in-licensed, or *de novo* entities. Despite the varied applications of drug repositioning as well as the numerous technologies to implement them, a commonality among them is the goal to rapidly extract value from existing agents while improving the odds of successful development.

When applied to previously approved drugs and advanced clinical agents, repositioning approaches typically require less investment, shorter development time, and less risk for late stage clinical failure than typical pharmaceutical research and development (R&D) [2]. Through the examination of individual case studies, three repositioning strategies will be evaluated herein: (1) prodrugs: chemically modified analogs of approved agents which, upon administration, are metabolized *in vivo* into the parent drug molecule; (2) chiral switch: single enantiomer variants of previously approved chiral drug

Drug Repositioning: Bringing New Life to Shelved Assets and Existing Drugs, First Edition.
Edited by Michael J. Barratt and Donald E. Frail.
© 2012 John Wiley & Sons, Inc. Published 2012 by John Wiley & Sons, Inc.

mixtures; and (3) site-selective deuteration: deuterium-labeled analogs of previously approved drugs.

10.2. PRODRUG APPROACH

10.2.1. Introduction

One of the most common methods employed for drug repositioning has been through the development of chemically modified analogs of approved agents which, upon administration, are metabolized *in vivo* into the parent drug molecule [3]. This prodrug strategy has been successfully applied to an array of previously approved agents across a wide range of therapeutic indications and chemical scaffolds. Prodrugs have demonstrated numerous clinically relevant enhanced properties including, but not limited to, increased bioavailability, improved PK profiles, more convenient dosing regimens, dramatic changes in tissue distribution, and decreased adverse events.

In addition to improving the pharmaceutical profile of the existing agent, the prodrug approach also provides additional intellectual property advantages. The prodrug variants are considered new chemical entities (NCEs) by the U.S. Patent Office and thus are granted appropriate protection. Furthermore, as described by the Hatch–Waxman amendments, the U.S. Food and Drug Administration (FDA) indicates that drugs for which no active ingredient (including any ester or salt of the active ingredient) has been previously approved are granted 5-year market exclusivity. Therefore, prodrugs of previously approved agents are viewed by the FDA as new molecular entities (NMEs) imparting the same extent of exclusivity as traditionally developed new therapeutic agents [4]. The atypical antipsychotic paliperidone palmitate (Figure 10.1e), however, represents an interesting exception to this rule. The FDA states that simple carboxylate ester derivates of previously approved drugs do not earn the designation of NME. As such, the palmitate ester of paliperidone was classified as a new formulation and granted a shorter period of exclusivity [4c]. Furthermore, the FDA requires suitable evidence for safety and tolerability for the approval of all new drug applications (NDAs). This can be presented as new data received from Phase I clinical trials or by way of previously documented safety data. Companies developing prodrugs of their own parent agents may leverage internal safety data of the active metabolite for a traditional 505b(1) path to market. Alternatively, as described in detail in Chapter 4, other companies can proceed via a 505b(2) path, referring to the safety and tolerability data produced by the parent drug developer or other institution [5]. Either course can present a significantly accelerated path to market by circumventing the need for completely independent safety and tolerability studies.

A classic example of a prodrug with enhanced properties over its active metabolite is the naturally occurring amino acid levodopa (L-Dopa) [6].

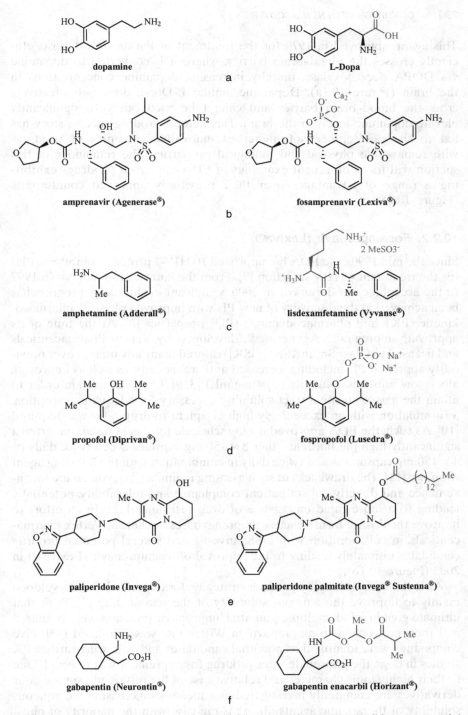

FIGURE 10.1. Prodrug case studies: (a) dopamine/L-Dopa, (b) amprenavir/fosamprenavir, (c) amphetamine/lisdexamfetamine, (d) propofol/fospropofol, (e) paliperidone/paliperidone palmitate, (f) gabapentin/gabapentin enacarbil.

This agent, approved in 1970 for the treatment of Parkinson's disease, efficiently crosses the blood–brain barrier, where it is converted to dopamine via DOPA decarboxylase, thereby increasing dopamine concentrations in the brain (Figure 10.1a). Dopamine, unlike L-Dopa, does not effectively cross the blood–brain barrier and cannot be used orally to significantly elevate dopamine levels in the brain. This natural prodrug success story has led to the development of numerous innovative examples of prodrugs with remarkable physical and biological properties. The remainder of this section will focus on recent examples of FDA-approved prodrugs exhibiting a range of advantages over their previously approved counterparts (Figure 10.1).

10.2.2. Fosamprenavir (Lexiva®)

Since the mid 1990s, the FDA has approved 10 HIV-1 protease inhibitors (PIs) for the treatment of HIV infection [7]. From the launch of saquinavir in 1997 to the acceptance of darunavir in 2006, significant evolutionary progress has been achieved in the discovery of new PIs with improved physical, pharmacokinetic (PK), and pharmacodynamic (PD) properties [8]. At the time of its approval, amprenavir (Agenerase®, developed by Vertex Pharmaceuticals and licensed to GlaxoSmithKline [GSK]) offered many advantages over previously approved PIs including increased antiviral activity, as well as improved, albeit low, aqueous solubility (0.04 mg/mL) [3, 9]. Unfortunately, in order to attain the gastrointestinal tract solubility necessary for adequate absorption, a formulation with an exceedingly high excipient-to-drug ratio was required [10]. As such, the FDA approved dosing schedule for Agenerase® imparted a significantly high pill burden: either 8×150 mg capsules dosed twice daily or 4×150 mg capsules dosed twice daily in combination with the boosting agent ritonavir [11]. The drawbacks of such a dosing regimen go beyond mere inconvenience and directly impact patient compliance and tolerability, potentially leading to a more rapid emergence of drug resistance [12]. In an effort to improve the dosage form of active amprenavir, researchers at Vertex Pharmaceuticals, in collaboration with GSK, investigated several potential prodrug candidates ultimately leading to the approval of fosamprenavir (Lexiva®) in 2003 (Figure 10.1b).

As is the case with many prodrug strategies, fosamprenavir was developed mainly to improve the aqueous solubility of the parent drug [3]. With that ultimate goal in mind, multiple potential amprenavir prodrugs were prepared and their conversion to amprenavir in Wistar rats was evaluated [13]. Five compounds were identified as potential candidates and, following further PK studies in dogs, the phosphate ester prodrug fosamprenavir was selected. Due to their highly ionic character and relative ease of hydrolysis, phosphate ester derivatives are commonly investigated as a means of increasing the aqueous solubility of therapeutic agents [3]. As is the case with the majority of phosphate ester prodrugs, endogenous alkaline phosphatases located within the intestinal epithelium efficiently hydrolyze fosamprenavir, releasing the active drug and leaving minimal intact prodrug in the systemic circulation. In fact, within 15 minutes of oral administration, detectable plasma levels of amprenavir are attained with peak concentrations (C_{max}) achieved at 1.5–2.5 hours [14]. In a Phase II trial of antiretroviral therapy in naïve HIV-1 patients, equimolar doses of fosamprenavir and amprenavir were shown to exhibit equivalent plasma amprenavir exposure. Interestingly, however, the cohort dosed with fosamprenavir presented significantly reduced C_{max} levels, as well as elevated trough levels. Furthermore, a dramatically improved aqueous solubility of 54 mg/mL at pH 3.3 [10] provided a marked enhancement in GI tract solubility [14]. These factors ultimately led to the development of a solid tablet formulation of fosamprenavir containing 700 mg of active ingredient resulting in a much more convenient dosing regimen: either two tablets dosed twice daily or two tablets dosed once daily in combination with the boosting agent ritonavir [15].

Shortly after its approval in 2003, Lexiva® began to replace Agenerase® as GSK shifted resources toward this superior therapeutic agent [16]. The benefits to both patient and drug proprietor are clearly evident in the repositioning strategy described in this example (Table 10.1). The launch of Lexiva® provided patients with a much more convenient dosing form, improving both adherence and tolerability likely leading to a slower onset of drug resistance. Likewise, by discontinuing Agenerase®, GSK was able to extend their patent life by 3 years with Lexiva® [17]. In 2008, Lexiva® reached peak global sales of $296 million declining in recent years due to the approval of new HIV-1 PIs such as darunavir (Prezista®), which offer enhanced activity and improved resistance profiles [18].

TABLE 10.1. Comparison of Agenerase® and Its Prodrug Successor Lexiva®

	Agenerase®	Lexiva®
Prodrug functionality	–	Phosphate ester
API	Amprenavir	Fosamprenavir
FDA approval[a]	1999	2003
Originator	Vertex	Vertex/GSK
Expected patent expiration[b]	Discontinued	2017
Peak global sales (year)[c]	$79 million (2000)	$296 million (2008)
Therapeutic class	HIV-1 protease inhibitors	
Key advantages		
• Aqueous solubility	0.04 mg/mL	54 mg/mL
• Approved unboosted dosing	8 capsules bid	2 tablets bid
• Approved boosted dosing[d]	4 capsules bid	2 tablets qd

[a] Drugs@FDA.
[b] Based on FDA Orange Book data for longest possible coverage.
[c] Sales figures obtained from Thomson Reuters Integrity[SM] database.
[d] Ritonavir (Norvir®, 100 mg) dosed concomitantly.

10.2.3. Lisdexamfetamine (Vyvanse®)

According to the National Resource Center on ADHD, "Attention-deficit/ hyperactivity disorder (ADHD) is a condition affecting children and adults that is characterized by problems with attention, impulsivity, and overactivity." It affects between 5% and 8% of school age children, and between 2% and 4% of adults. ADHD is the current diagnostic label for a condition that has been recognized and studied for over a century [19]. Although there is no known cure for ADHD, symptoms of the disorder can, in many cases, be effectively controlled with a combination of medication, psychotherapy, and education. The two most widely recognized medications for the treatment of ADHD include the psychostimulants methylphenidate (MPH) (Ritalin®) and amphetamine (Adderall®, Figure 10.1c). Administration of these agents results in increased levels of dopamine and norepinephrine, addressing the hypothesis that the root cause of this disorder involves dysregulation of these two neurotransmitters [20]. A significant drawback of both Ritalin® and Adderall® is their potential for misuse and abuse. Reports of their misuse have been attributed to the grinding of various formulations and either oral or intranasal administration resulting in a sensation of euphoria [21]. Furthermore, both, MPH and amphetamine are classified as schedule II controlled substances by the U.S. Drug Enforcement Administration (DEA). Therefore, midday doses must be administered by a school nurse, potentially causing additional social stigma for these already atypical children [21].

To address the issues associated with amphetamine treatment, New River Pharmaceuticals set out to develop an inactive prodrug analog that would result in prolonged exposure to dextroamphetamine (*d*-amphetamine). A series of amino acid-linked analogs of *d*-amphetamine were prepared and evaluated, ultimately leading to the identification of the L-lysine conjugate lisdexamfetamine (Vyvanse®) shown in Figure 10.1c [22]. Results from non-clinical *in vitro* and *in vivo* studies indicate that lisdexamfetamine is readily absorbed through the small intestine and subsequently converted to active *d*-amphetamine in the blood [23]. Interestingly, while both rat and human whole blood samples were shown to effectively convert lisdexamfetamine to *d*-amphetamine, white blood cells and plasma were deemed ineffective. Enzymes located on red blood cells are therefore most likely responsible for the hydrolysis of lisdexamfetamine ultimately leading to an observed delayed exposure of *d*-amphetamine [23]. In fact, in a study of 12 healthy adult stimulant abusers, prodrug administration resulted in a significantly lower exposure to *d*-amphetamine over the first 4 hours (AUC_{0-4h}) compared with dosing *d*-amphetamine sulfate directly (165.3–231.1 ng/mL vs. 245.5–316.8 ng/mL) [21]. Similarly, lisdexamfetamine administration exhibited a dramatically increased T_{max} over *d*-amphetamine sulfate (3.78–4.25 hours vs. 1.88–2.74 hours) [21]. Furthermore, in an effort to assess the relative abuse potential for lisdexamfetamine versus *d*-amphetamine, intranasal administration of the two agents was compared in rats. Results from this study indicate that a 95% reduction in AUC_{last}, a 96% reduction in C_{max}, and a 12-fold increase in T_{max} are attained upon intranasal dosing of the prodrug [24]. From this study it was determined that misuse of lisdexamfetamine via intranasal administration would result in minimal exposure to d-amphetamine, providing a dramatically reduced abuse potential.

In 2005, New River Pharmaceuticals entered into a collaborative agreement with Shire for the commercialization of Vyvanse®, which was subsequently launched in 2007 for the treatment of ADHD in adults and children ages 6–17 [25]. Shire was originally expected to attain patent protection for amphetamine through 2018 via the development of an extended-release formulation (Adderall XR®). This approach proved less successful than anticipated as generic forms ultimately became available in the United States as early as 2009 [26]. The release of the prodrug derivative of amphetamine (Vyvanse®), however, provided Shire with an improved amphetamine alternative with a patent life extending out to 2023 [27]. Although still classified as a schedule II controlled substance by the DEA, this prolonged release analog of amphetamine not only showed dramatic evidence for reduced abuse potential, but it also negated the requirement for midday dosing [21]. For these reasons, global sales of Vyvanse® have continued to grow since its release, amassing over $500 million in sales in 2009 alone [28] (Table 10.2).

10.2.4. Fospropofol (Lusedra®)

Many conventional surgical procedures require the use of general anesthesia as a means of attaining unconsciousness, as well as relaxation of both the skeletal muscles and reflex actions of the body. While highly effective and typically safe, the use of general anesthesia is avoided if possible due to the

TABLE 10.2. Comparison of Adderall® and Its Prodrug Successor Vyvanse®

	Adderall®	Vyvanse®
Prodrug functionality	–	Lysine amide
API	Dexamphetamine (mixture)	Lisdexamfetamine
FDA approval[a]	1996	2007
Originator	Shire	Shire
Expected patent expiration[b]	Generic	2023
Peak global sales (year)[c]	$1.1 billion (2008)	>$500 million (2009)
Therapeutic class	Dopamine and norepinephrine regulators	
Key advantages		
• Abuse potential[d]	1032 ng·mL/h	56 ng·mL/h
• Approved dosing	qd-bid	qd

[a] Drugs@FDA.
[b] Based on FDA Orange Book data for longest possible coverage.
[c] Sales figures obtained from Thomson Reuters Integrity^{SM} database.
[d] As inferred by reduced intranasal exposure in rats [24].

potential for significant adverse events and prolonged recovery time. Fortunately, with the advent of new and improved medical techniques and devices, more and more conventional surgical procedures are being replaced with minimally invasive methods, escalating the use of mild procedural sedation methods [29]. The administration of therapeutic agents for the attainment of procedural sedation is common practice among a variety of diagnostic routines as well as outpatient surgical procedures. These sedative drugs typically result in less overall discomfort, faster recovery time, and fewer side effects as compared with those used for general anesthesia [29]. In order to be considered an ideal agent for procedural sedation (moderate sedation), a drug must meet certain accepted criteria including: (1) a predictable PK/PD profile; (2) the ability to attain amnesia, analgesia, and anxiolysis; (3) rapid onset of action and ultimately a prompt recovery of both physical and cognitive function [30]. Although classical agents for sedation used in endoscopic procedures include both benzodiazepines and opioids, these drugs are not ideal agents due to their delayed onset, unpredictable PK/PD due to interpatient metabolic variability, as well as hangover effects [30a].

In 1986, an injectable emulsified formulation of the sedative–hypnotic agent propofol (Diprivan®, Figure 10.1d) was first launched by Imperial Chemical Industries (now Astra Zeneca) in the United Kingdom [29]. This agent offered several advantages over benzodiazepine and opioid-induced sedation including rapid onset of action (<1 minute), predictable PK/PD profile, and an improved dose titration as well as a fast sedation recovery period. The mechanism of action of this drug is believed to be attributed to a wide range of pharmacological effects: propofol exhibits allosteric modulation of γ-aminobutyric acid (GABA) receptors in the brain [31], is involved in the endocannabinoid system [32], and serves as a sodium channel blocking agent [33]. In practice, moderate levels of sedation can be achieved with propofol either through a single bolus dose or via controlled infusion.

A significant drawback of propofol, however, relates to the sensitive dose–response relationship of this agent [34]. As such, small increases in the dose of propofol can result in dramatic changes in pharmacological effect, ultimately resulting in a higher potential for misjudged levels of sedation. With deeper levels of sedation come heightened cardiopulmonary risks and the possible need for distinctive methods of sedation recovery [29]. For these reasons, certain states have placed limitations on the personnel allowed to administer propofol [35]. Furthermore, approximately 30% of patients receiving a bolus administration of propofol report significant injection-site pain, likely due to the acidic properties of this compound [36]. The original lipid emulsion formulation of propofol did not include any preservative ingredients, leading to clusters of reported deaths associated with microbial contamination [37]. By pulling their initial formulation and relaunching a new formulation including the preservative agent ethylenediaminetetraacetic acid (EDTA), AstraZeneca maintained their propofol market while causing the FDA to require all future formulations of propofol to include preservative agents. On one hand, this benefited AstraZeneca by hindering the production of generic versions of the original formulation. On the other hand, AstraZeneca was fairly specific in their claims for the use of EDTA as the preservative agent, opening the door for direct generic competition from formulations including other preservatives such as benzyl alcohol or sodum metabisulfite [37].

These disadvantages of propofol administration led researchers at Pro-Quest Pharmaceutical to investigate the development of prodrug analogs with the aim of improving solubility, prolonging single-dosed sedation, and alleviating injection-site pain. The methylene-bridged phosphate ester prodrug fospropofol disodium (Lusedra®) was ultimately identified and subsequently launched by Eisai in 2009 (Figure 10.1d) [29]. Upon intravenous administration, fospropofol is immediately exposed to the alkaline phosphatases responsible for the generation of the active metabolite [29]. This conversion, however, is not as rapid as one would expect from the metabolism rates of other phosphate ester prodrugs. In fact, the prodrug analog of propofol exhibits a slower onset of action (T_{max} = 3–7.2 minutes for the prodrug vs. immediate T_{max} for propofol), a reduction in maximum concentration (C_{max}), and a slower elimination of active drug. This ultimately contributes to a prolonged sedation profile compared with that of the parent agent [38]. Further benefits of fospropofol over its parent counterpart include reduction in injection-site pain likely due to capping of the phenolic hydroxyl group, as well as resistance of the sterile aqueous formulation to microbial contamination [29].

One issue this prodrug strategy was unable to address, however, was the sensitive dose–response relationship attributed to potential oversedation. In fact, the interpatient variability regarding the bioavailability and conversion of this prodrug to active metabolite instills an elevated level of caution associated with its administration [29]. This disadvantage aside, fospropofol (Lusedra®) provides significant improvements over the parent agent including an enhanced PK/PD profile, prolonged duration of sedation, and the ability for sterile aqueous formulation (Table 10.3). These attributes have led to the widespread use of Lusedra® for monitored anesthesia care sedation in an array of diagnostic and outpatient surgical procedures [29]. In recent years, the halting of production of Diprivan® by AstraZeneca combined with recalls of generic propofol due to contamination has led to shortages of this widely used agent [39]. Through the development of the prodrug fospropofol, Eisai was able to gain entry into the propofol market with an exclusive agent expected to remain under patent protection until 2018 [40].

10.2.5. Paliperidone Palmitate (Invega® Sustenna®)

In 2006, the FDA approved the use of paliperidone (Invega®, Figure 10.1e) for both short-term and long-term maintenance treatment of schizophrenia [41]. As a member of the class of drugs known as atypical antipsychotics, paliperidone is believed to achieve its therapeutic effects via antagonism of dopamine (D2) receptors, serotonin (5-HT2$_A$) receptors, α_1, and α_2 adrenergic

TABLE 10.3. Comparison of Diprivan® and Its Prodrug Successor Lusedra®

	Diprivan®	Lusedra®
Prodrug functionality	–	Phosphate ester
API	Propofol	Fospropofol
FDA approval[a]	1989	2008
Originator	AstraZeneca	ProQuest
Expected patent expiration[b]	Generic	2018
Peak global sales (year)[c]	$507 million (2000)	N/A
Therapeutic class	Allosteric modulaters of GABA$_A$ receptors	
Advantages		
• Injection-site pain	Reported	Not reported
• Formulation	Lipid emulsion	Aqueous solution

[a] Drugs@FDA.
[b] Based on FDA Orange Book data for longest possible coverage.
[c] Sales figures obtained from Thomson Reuters Integrity^{SM} database.

receptors as well as histamine receptors [41]. Although this extended-release oral formulation of paliperidone is dosed only once a day ($t_{1/2}$ = ~24 hours) [42], a large degree of patient noncompliance is still reported. In fact, after two years of treatment only approximately 25% of patients can be classified as fully compliant due to several factors, including complex drug regimens, cognitive dysfunctions, and adverse effects [43]. To address this issue of noncompliance, Johnson and Johnson launched a palmitate ester prodrug of paliperidone in the United States in 2009 (Figure 10.1e).

Due to the poor water solubility associated with the prodrug, paliperidone palmitate (Invega® Sustenna®) was ultimately formulated as an aqueous suspension using proprietary NanoCrystal® technology developed by Elan Pharma International, Ltd [41]. Upon intramuscular (i.m.) injection of the suspension, the prodrug slowly dissolves and is subsequently hydrolyzed to the active metabolite ultimately entering the systemic circulation. Systemic exposure can be measured after 1 day and continues for up to 126 days [41]. The demonstrated 30-day half-life ($t_{1/2}$) for plasma paliperidone upon 50 mg eq. dosing of the prodrug supported the use of this agent as a long-term therapy option for patients suffering from schizophrenia. Furthermore, results from clinical studies comparing monthly administration of paliperidone palmitate with biweekly dosing of resperidone long acting injection (RLAI) demonstrated noninferiority of paliperidone palmitate [44]. As such, the current recommended prescribing procedure for Invega® Sustenna® involves an initial dose of 150 mg eq. followed by a second 100 mg eq. dose one week later. Maintenance therapy can then be achieved with monthly injections of 75 mg equivalents, modifying the dose from 25 to 150 mg eq. as needed [45]. The ability to achieve similar therapeutic benefits with monthly injections of the prodrug as opposed to daily oral administration of paliperidone will

TABLE 10.4. Comparison of Invega® and Its Prodrug Successor Invega® Sustenna®

	Invega®	Invega® Sustenna®
Prodrug functionality	–	Palmitate ester
API	Paliperidone	Paliperidone palmitate
FDA approval[a]	2006	2009
Originator	Ortho McNeil (Janssen/Johnson & Johnson)	Janssen(Johnson & Johnson)
Expected patent expiration[b]	2014	2017
Peak global sales (year)[c]	$424M (2010)	N/A
Therapeutic class	Multiple receptor antagonists (D2, 5HT2$_A$, α1 + α2 adrenergic, and histamine)	
Key advantages		
• $t_{1/2}$ (paliperidone)	~24 hours	~30 days
• Approved dosing	QD Tablet	Monthly injection

[a] Drugs@FDA.
[b] Based on FDA Orange Book data for longest possible coverage.
[c] Sales figures obtained from Thomson Reuters Integrity^{SM} database.

undoubtedly lead to improvements in patient compliance as well as overall market share for Johnson and Johnson (Table 10.4).

10.2.6. Gabapentin Enacarbil (Horizant®)

Gabapentin (Figure 10.1f), approved by the FDA in 1993 under the brand name Neurontin®, was originally developed for the treatment of epilepsy and has since been applied to a number of alternative indications, including neuropathic pain and hot flashes [46]. Structurally, gabapentin is an analog of the neurotransmitter GABA. However, the efficacy associated with gabapentin is believed to result from a different mechanism of action: arresting the formation of new synapses as well as imparting calcium trafficking effects via binding to voltage-dependent calcium channel subunits α2δ1 and α2δ2 [47]. A significant drawback of gabapentin relates to its PK profile. The zwitterionic nature of gabapentin at physiologic pH limits its diffusion into cellular membranes. As such, gabapentin exhibits a non-dose-proportional relationship due to saturation in the human intestine resulting in high interpatient variability, dose-limited PK, as well as sub-therapeutic exposures in some patients [48]. Furthermore, in order to maintain therapeutic levels, the recommended administration of gabapentin is 3–4 times daily due to its relatively short half-life ($t_{1/2}$ = 5–7 hours) [48]. Such dosing regimens are commonly associated with higher rates of noncompliance. To address the issues of non-dose-proportionality, as well as dosing inconvenience, researchers at XenoPort, Inc. developed a prodrug analog of gabapentin designed specifically to take advantage of nutrient transporters located within the human intestine [48].

On April 6, 2011, XenoPort received approval for the use of gabapentin enacarbil (Horizant®) for the treatment of moderate to severe restless legs syndrome (RLS) (Figure 10.1f), a neurological disorder classified as an urge to move the legs in association with leg discomfort and unpleasant sensations [46]. Symptoms typically worsen during periods of rest and are partially or fully relieved by movement. Horizant® represents a nondopaminergic approved treatment option for these patients with potentially reduced dopamine-related adverse events. This monoanionic (at physiological pH) prodrug analog of gabapentin was specifically designed to be absorbed in the GI tract by serving as a substrate for the high capacity nutrient transporters MCT-1 (monocarboxylate transporter 1) and SMVT (sodium-dependent multivitamin transporter) [48]. Once absorbed, the prodrug is readily converted to gabapentin via nonspecific esterases, providing therapeutic exposure to the active metabolite. Due to these characteristics of gabapentin enacarbil, no evidence for intestinal saturation was observed providing a dose-proportional relationship lacking with the parent agent [46]. Furthermore, the improved bioavailability of the prodrug has permitted the formulation of gabapentin enacarbil as an extended release 600 mg tablet (Horizant®) exhibiting a significant increase in time to maximum exposure (T_{max} = 8.4 hours vs. 2.7 hours for gabapentin) [49]. As such, the FDA-approved dosing of Horizant® for the treatment of RLS is one tablet daily at 5 p.m. [50].

The repositioning strategy outlined in this case study provided XenoPort with a therapeutic agent approved by the FDA in an indication unique to the prodrug form of gabapentin (Table 10.5). This granted access to a new market with a significantly reduced risk of competition from generic gabapentin. With a patent life extending out to 2022, gabapentin enacarbil can be expected to gain approval in a number of indications associated with current gabapentin therapy.

TABLE 10.5. Comparison of Neurontin® and Its Prodrug Successor Horizant®

	Neurontin®	Horizant®
Prodrug functionality	–	Carbamate
API	Gabapentin	Gabapentin enacarbil
FDA approval[a]	1993	2011
Originator	Pfizer	Xenoport
Expected patent expiration[b]	Generic	2022
Peak global sales (year)[c]	$2.7 billion (2004)	N/A
Therapeutic class	Arrestors of new synapse formation and modulators of calcium trafficking	
Key advantages		
• T_{max} (gabapentin)	2.7 hours	8.4 hours
• Dose response	Nonproportional	Proportional

[a] Drugs@FDA.
[b] Based on FDA Orange Book data for longest possible coverage.
[c] Sales figures obtained from Thomson Reuters Integrity^{SM} database.

10.2.7. Conclusions

As depicted in the above examples, the prodrug strategy to drug repositioning offers a unique approach to drug discovery with its own set of advantages and challenges. Often viewed as NMEs by the FDA, prodrug analogs have been developed by many companies as an effective way of resurrecting life into a parent agent with a looming patent expiration. Alternatively, this approach can be employed by rival pharmaceutical companies in an effort to improve upon the parent agent and directly compete or overtake market share. In some cases, prodrug analogs may exhibit significantly dissimilar physical properties, resulting in improvements in aqueous solubility, formulation, bio-availability, PK profiles, and even pill burden. Whether it be the discovery of a monthly injection treatment option to overcome patient noncompliance or the development of an agent engineered to take advantage of specific absorption mechanisms, prodrugs can provide unique opportunities to address a range of issues, resulting in substantial benefits to both the patient and the drug developer.

10.3. CHIRAL SWITCH APPROACH

10.3.1. Introduction

Interrogating biological space to elicit a therapeutic response is the central goal of drug discovery. Living systems are comprised of chiral environments developed from the systematic assembly of naturally containing chiral molecules. Amino acids, sugars, nucleosides, and nucleotides are all examples of these biomolecules utilized for processes that are stereospecific, preferring one stereoisomer over another. Early drug discovery efforts utilized either achiral small molecules or racemic mixtures of chiral molecules to produce a therapeutic response. Although successful as first-generation therapies, further understanding of the complexities of biological processes required more sophisticated approaches. Advances in chemical synthesis has allowed for a more thorough analysis of the influence of stereochemistry on biological processes. Single enantiomer small molecule drugs have since been shown to be a more powerful approach for tackling a variety of indications and needs.

Single enantiomer drugs may have a number of potential advantages over their racemic counterparts [51]. Lower doses of the single isomer may provide the same efficacy as the racemic mixture [52]. This requires that one enantiomer is the active eutomer and the other is the inactive or less active distomer. Alternatively each enantiomer may have activity but for different pharmacologies. The use of single enantiomer drugs in the latter scenario may also lead to a reduction in off-target effects. The metabolism and PK profile of each enantiomer may also differ. Thus dosing the desired eutomer may reduce the formation of reactive metabolites that may be toxic or limit efficacy of the drug. Utilizing only the eutomer may allow for an increase in tolerability over larger doses and thus improve the therapeutic impact. Ultimately all of these advantages associated with single enantiomer drug development may reduce the amount of side effects and adverse events while improving efficacy and safety as compared to the racemate.

Regulatory agencies have also recognized the impact of stereochemistry in the safety and efficacy of new therapeutics [53]. For example, the current approval process for racemic mixtures involves evaluating each enantiomer separately for safety and efficacy along with the combination [54]. This requires the preparation of each isomer in quantities sufficient for animal toxicology studies. The advances in enantioselective chemical synthesis have rendered it plausible for the manufacturing cost of a single enantiomer drug to compete with that of preparing a racemic mixture.

Since 1990, the annual FDA approval of single enantiomers has surpassed that of racemates and achiral new molecular entities (NMEs). Further indication of the pharmaceutical industry's paradigm shift is the application of the chiral switch strategy on the existing pharmacopeia of racemic drug substances. The chiral switch approach involves developing single enantiomer components of marketed racemic drugs [55]. The FDA does not consider chiral switch compounds as NMEs (CHE1), which are defined as containing active ingredients never approved in the United States. Instead chiral switch drugs are categorized as derivatives of existing drugs (CHE2) or new formulations (CHE3) and benefit from 3 rather than 5 years of market exclusivity [55]. Unfortunately there are no set guidelines that would predict which category (CHE2 or CHE3) a new agent would be placed in and thus each is evaluated independently.

The patentability of the chiral switch strategy continues to be debated and evaluated by the USPTO and the European Patent Office (EPO) on a case-by-case basis. Many chiral switch filings are made under the selection invention designation. This type of invention is defined as one that selects a group of new members from a previously known class on the basis of superior properties [55]. Alternatively separate fillings on the superior properties of each enantiomer are also being pursued. Although this area of patent law continues to evolve, both of these types of filings have been granted in the United States and ultimately have led to the successful launch of chiral switch drugs.

Several pharmaceutical companies have even used the chiral switch approach to direct their corporate strategy. They have benefited from the favorable regulatory and intellectual property environments surrounding this strategy as well as the demonstrable advantage of the single enantiomer over the racemate. Sepracor Pharmaceuticals (now Sunovion) has been a leader in advancing the chiral switch strategies. Their efforts have resulted in the successful approval and launch of desloratadine (Clarinex®), fexofenadine (Allegra-R®), levalbuterol (Xopenx®), and eszopiclone (Lunesta®). The following case studies (Figure 10.2) are provided as other successful examples of this approach to drug discovery.

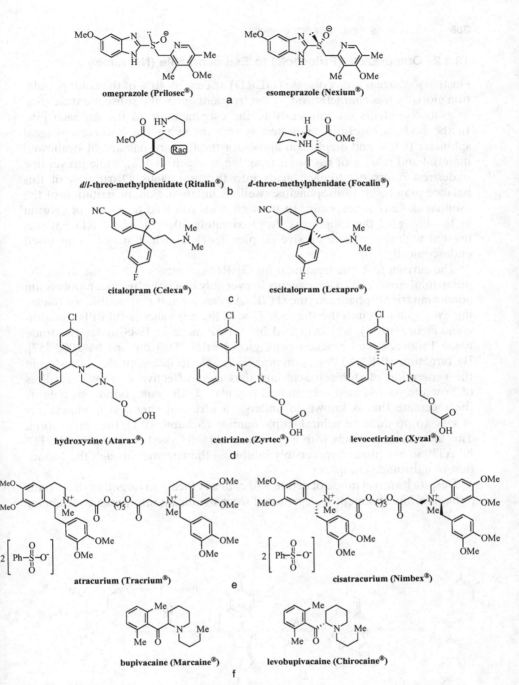

FIGURE 10.2. Chiral switch case studies: (a) benzimidazole proton pump inhibitors omeprazole and esomeprazole, (b) DAT reuptake inhibitors d,l-threo-methylphenidate and d-threo-methylphenidate, (c) selective serotonin reuptake inhibitors (SSRI) citalopram and escitalopram, (d) UCB's franchise of histamine H1 receptor antagonists, (e) rationally designed tetrahydroisoquinolinium NMBs, (f) topical analgesics.

10.3.2. Omeprazole (Prilosec®) to Esomeprazole (Nexium®)

Gastroesophageal reflux disease (GERD) affects 20–40% of the adult population globally. It is characterized by the frequent entry and subsequent clearing of gastric contents intermittently to the esophagus from the stomach [56]. In the body, a carefully calibrated system involving the lower esophageal sphincter (LES) and diaphragm allows for the forward passage of swallowed material and release of gas or air from the stomach (belch), while preventing undesired reflux of stomach acids into the esophagus. Disruption of this balance may result in esophagitis, swelling, inflammation, or irritation of the esophagus. Chronic exposure to stomach acids can lead to breaks or erosion in the lining of the esophagus. Approximately 40–60% of GERD patients present with this type of erosive esophagitis (EE), which may be diagnosed endoscopically [56].

The current first-line treatment for GERD symptoms is daily use of proton pump inhibitors (PPI). These agents irreversibly block the hydrogen/potassium adenosine triphosphate enzyme (H^+/K^+ ATPase) that is responsible for releasing hydrogen ions into the stomach. One of the most successful PPIs, omeprazole (Figure 10.2a), was launched by AstraZeneca in 1988 under the trade name Prilosec® and reached peak global sales (\$6.3 billion) by 2000 [57]. By targeting H^+/K^+ ATPase, omeprazole is able to intercept the final step in the generation of stomach acid and thus is an effective therapy regardless of how the gastric acid secretion is stimulated. The compound was sold as the racemate that is known to undergo a series of chemical modifications *in vivo* to produce an achiral sulphenamide (Scheme 10.1), the active form. This intermediate reacts with a cysteine residue (Cys 813) present in the H^+/K^+ ATPase machinery, irreversibly inhibiting the enzyme through the formation of a disulfide complex.

Despite its novel mode of action and clinical efficacy in targeting the proton pump machinery, omeprazole suffered from significant interpatient variability

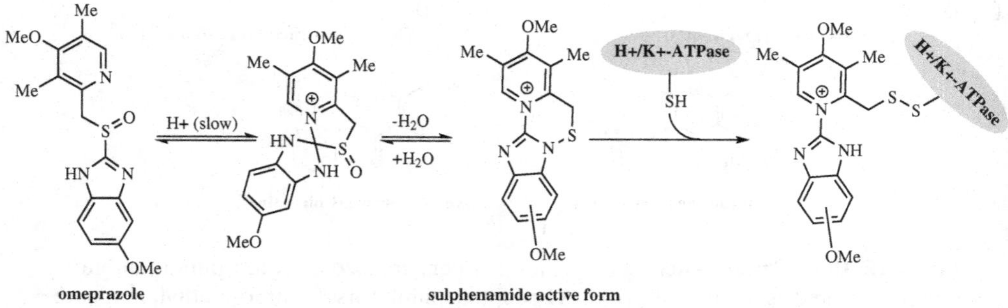

Scheme 10.1. Omeprazole molecular mechanism of action.

[57] requiring larger or repeated doses. Human liver microsome studies (HLM) demonstrated that the CYP3A4 and CYP2C19 isozymes of the cytochrome P450 super family are responsible for omeprazole's metabolism [58]. The CYP2C19 enzyme is not equally distributed in all human populations as evident by its absence in 3% of Caucasian and 15–20% of Asian populations. Ultimately this genetic variation results in striations of therapeutic benefit of omeprazole within the population as mean plasma concentration (AUC) has been directly linked to its therapeutic benefit [59].

Investigations into the metabolism of omeprazole by CYP2C19 in extensive and poor metabolism patients (EM vs. PM) revealed a 7.5-fold increase in mean plasma concentration (AUC) of (R)-omeprazole in PM compared with EM [60]. This is in contrast to the AUC of (S)-omeprazole (esomeprazole), which had only a threefold increase for PM over EM. Similar disparities were seen in terms of the clearance. The (R)-omeprazole demonstrated a 10-fold difference in clearance between PM and EM groups while the (S)-omeprazole did not demonstrate any difference in clearance rates [60]. AstraZeneca recognized that capitalizing on this CYP450-derived stereochemical metabolism preference may lead to an improved PPI with respect to bioavailability. Esomeprazole reduced interpatient variability and helped standardize dose.

In an open-label, crossover study, 130 patients received either omeprazole or esomeprazole daily for 5 days [61]. Esomeprazole (40 mg) more effectively maintained intragastric pH > 4 in patients with symptoms of GERD over those taking once daily omeprazole (40 mg). Intragastric pH (24 hours) was monitored on days 1 and 5. In the esomeprazole treatment group, the patient's intragastric pH remained above 4 for 2 hours longer on day 1 than those in the omeprazole group and 1.5 hours longer on day 5. Significantly less interindividual variation, with respect to the percentage of time with intragastric pH > 4, was observed in the esomeprazole group. These studies led AstraZeneca scientists to suggest that equal doses of racemate versus single isomer drug are not equivalent. The company subsequently set its standard dose for esomeprazole to 40 mg.

When evaluated in four different large multicenter double-blind randomized trials (6708 treatment patients total) esomeprazole (40 or 20 mg) was shown to have greater consistency of healing rates across all grades of baseline disease versus omeprazole (20 mg) [62]. Esomeprazole was also shown to reduce the incidence of GERD relapse as well as the time to recurrence (34 vs. 78 days) versus placebo in patients with healed esophagitis. The positive efficacy and safety clinical data led to the FDA approval of esomeprazole (Nexiuim®) in 2000 as a new PPI for GERD and EE. Since 2005, Nexium has consistently reported annual global sales over $4.5 billion [63].

More recently esomeprazole and omeprazole were compared in a multicenter, double-blind, parallel-group trial for the healing of EE in 1148 patients with endoscopically confirmed EE [64]. Patients were given either esomeprazole (40 mg) or omeprazole (20 mg). Primary outcomes were healing at 8 weeks and secondary outcomes included diary and investigator assessments of heartburn symptoms. Healing rates with the enantiopure drug were significantly higher than those with the racemate at both 4 weeks (61% vs. 48%) and 8 weeks (88% vs. 77%) in patients with moderate to severe EE at baseline.

Adverse events associated with nonsteroidal anti-inflammatory drugs (NSAIDs) and *Helicobacter pylori* infection are the two leading causes of peptic ulceration [65, 66]. Esomeprazole (40 mg, qd or bid) has been shown to be superior to omeprazole (20 mg, bid) when given in conjunction with amoxicillin (1000 mg, bid) and clarithromycin (500 mg, bid) as 7-day triple therapy for the eradication of *H. pylori* infection [67]. Patients positive for *H. pylori* infection with active duodenal ulcers also benefited from this single enantiomer treatment. In this population, an esomeprazole containing 7-day triple therapy followed by 3 weeks of placebo was shown to be as effective as omeprazole containing triple therapy followed by 3 weeks of daily omeprazole treatment [68]. The healing rates and infection eradication rates were comparable among the two treatment groups.

The omeprazole to esomeprazole chiral switch has been one of the most successful in the pharmaceutical industry (Table 10.6). Upon approval of esomeprazole (Nexium®, 40 mg), AstraZeneca priced the single enantiomer dose lower than omeprazole (Prilosec®, 20 mg), thus re-capturing the PPI market from its own product. This type of evergreening has led to consecutive years of multibillion dollar sales for each product for AstraZeneca. Although

TABLE 10.6. Comparison of Prilosec® and Its Chiral Switch Successor Nexium®

	Prilosec®	Nexium®
Stereochemistry	(*R/S*)	(*S*)
API	Omeprazole	Esomeprazole
FDA approval[a]	1989	2001
Originator	Astra Zeneca	AstraZeneca
Expected patent expiration[b]	Generic/OTC	2018
Peak global sales (year)[c]	$6.3 billion (2000)	$5.5 billion (2008)
Therapeutic class	Proton pump inhibitors (PPIs) for GERD	
Key advantages		
• PK data	Polymorph. metab. (CYP2C19)	$>t_{1/2}$ and AUC than racemate.
• Clinical data	• Comparison study demonstrated (*S*)-enantiomer superior for maintaining gastric pH > 4 longer. • Triple therapy study for *H. pylori* treatment with (*S*)-enantiomer shortened treatment time over racemate	

[a] Drugs@FDA.
[b] Based on FDA Orange Book data for longest possible coverage.
[c] Sales figures obtained from Thomson Reuters Integrity^{SM} database.

Nexium® demonstrated a measurable and significant improvement versus its racemic counterpart, the industry was vilified for taking advantage of the consumer [69].

10.3.3. *d,l*-threo-Methylphenidate HCl (Ritalin®) to *d*-threo-Methylphenidate HCl (Focalin®)

ADHD is the most commonly diagnosed and studied psychiatric disorder in children, affecting an estimated 3–5% of all children in America [70]. It is a neurobehavioral disorder that disrupts a person's ability to stay on a task and to exercise age-appropriate inhibition. Current research suggests that ADHD symptoms are caused by imbalances in neurotransmitter levels in the brain. As discussed earlier in this chapter, disruptions in dopamine signaling have been shown to be associated with ADHD symptoms [71]. The recommended treatment protocol involves a combination of behavioral modification at home and in the classroom along with oral medications such as methylphenidate (MPH) or dextroamphetamine.

MPH was first synthesized in 1944 [72] and the diastereomerically enriched racemate was evaluated as a stimulant [73] (Figure 10.2b). Two decades later it began to be evaluated for the treatment of ADHD in children. As understanding and acceptance of the disorder grew in the medical community, the prescription rates of MPH rose through the 1990s. Abuse and addiction have also been linked with the illicit use of MPH; therefore, it has been categorized as a Class II substance along with cocaine and amphetamines [74]. Similar to these drugs, MPH's primary target is the dopamine transporter (DAT) [75]. It is thought to increase brain levels of dopamine by blocking reuptake of the neurotransmitter and thus increasing its concentration at the presynaptic neuron. The net increase in dopamine levels is thought to alleviate the symptoms of ADHD although the exact therapeutic mechanism is still under investigation.

Recent advances in chemical synthesis [76] have allowed for the independent evaluation of each enantiomer of *threo*-methylphenidate [77]. Rodent and primate models with radiolabeled MPH have demonstrated that binding of *d-threo*-methylphenidate (*d*-MPH, Focalin®) to DATs was selective, saturable, and reversible, while binding of *l-threo*-methylphenidate (*l*-MPH) was unselective. The influence of each enantiomer on behavior has also been evaluated. Several studies suggest that efficacy resides solely with *d*-MPH. Seminal work by Ding and coworkers, through the use of positron emission tomography (PET) and microdialysis with radiolabeled agents, demonstrated a greater uptake in human and baboon basal ganglia of [^{11}C]-*d-threo*-methylphenidate when compared with [^{11}C]-*l-threo*-methylphenidate [78]. Localization in the basal ganglia is indicative of more selective binding to DATs. One hypothesis proposed to explain the difference in efficacy between enantiomers was that the absorption of *l*-MPH is poor due to presystemic metabolism. Ding and coworkers have demonstrated that radiolabeled *l*-MPH

TABLE 10.7. Comparison of Ritalin® and Its Chiral Switch Successor Focalin®

	Ritalin®	Focalin®
Stereochemistry	$(R,R/S,S)$	(R,R)
API	d/l-methylphenidate (MPH)	d-methylphenidate
FDA approval[a]	1955	2001
Originator	Ciba	Novartis
Expected patent expiration[b]	Generic	2019
Peak global sales (year)[c]	N/A	$440 million (2009)
Therapeutic class	Attention deficit hyperactivity disorder (ADHD) agents	
Key advantages		
• Pharmacology	• Radiolabel studies in monkey and human brains demonstrate that d-MPH localizes in the areas of the brain associated with dopamine transport while l-MPH disperses randomly throughout the brain. • Metabolism and brain penetration is equal for each enantiomer	
• Clinical data	• Single enantiomer therapy was more effective in improving the overall clinician's rating than racemate in comparison studies with ADHD children.	

[a] Drugs@FDA.
[b] Based on FDA Orange Book data for longest possible coverage.
[c] Sales figures obtained from Thomson Reuters Integrity[SM] database.

or its metabolites are absorbed and enter the brain after oral dosing in rats [79]. Clinical trials in children with ADHD have demonstrated that d-MPH and d,l-MPH have comparable efficacy, safety, and tolerability [80]. Furthermore, a comparison study between the racemate and d-MPH demonstrated that the single enantiomer was superior in clinical ratings of overall improvement [81] (Table 10.7).

10.3.4. Citalopram (Celexa®) to Escitalopram (Lexapro®)

Clinical depression is the leading cause of disability as measured by the World Health Organization's Years Living with Disability metric (YLD) and the fourth leading contributor to the global burden of disease [82]. Depression affects approximately 121 million people globally but fewer than 25% of those affected have access to treatments [82]. Symptoms of depression include chronic depressed mood, loss of interest or pleasure, feelings of guilt or low self-worth, disturbed sleep or appetite, low energy, and poor concentration. Long-range studies have demonstrated that depression is a chronic disease with significant levels of remission [83].

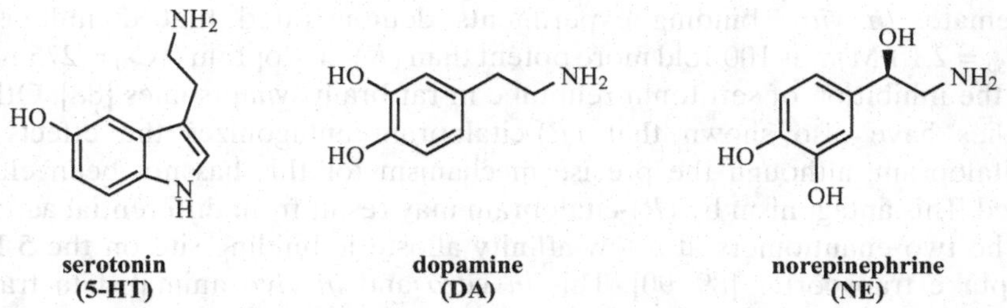

serotonin
(5-HT)

dopamine
(DA)

norepinephrine
(NE)

FIGURE 10.3. Endogenous neurotransmitters: serotonin, dopamine, norepinephrine.

The central amine theory of depression suggests that deficiencies in neurotransmitters such as dopamine, serotonin and norepinephrine (Figure 10.3) are responsible for the observed symptoms [84]. A tremendous amount of work has revealed that many biochemical and genetic pathways are involved in connecting neurotransmitter levels with disease pathology [85]. Chronic antidepressant use is thought to up-regulate the cAMP signaling cascade and eventually the expression of the CREB transcription factor [86]. Prolonged execution of these events may ultimately lead to a change in the evolution of neuronal pathways.

Antidepressant therapies have evolved from broad-spectrum agents such as tricyclic antidepressants (TCA) and monoamine oxidase inhibitors (MAOI) to targeted therapies such as selective serotonin reuptake inhibitors (SSRI) and most recently dual action serotonin–norepinephrine reuptake inhibitors (SNRI) [87]. The latter two categories of therapies are considered first-line due to their improved efficacy and safety profiles. In general SSRI and SNRI therapies are accompanied by fewer side effects and are more tolerable. The goal of all of these therapies is to increase the population of neurotransmitters at the synapse. Many of these approaches rely on binding the neurotransmitter's transporter, which leads to a conformational change that prevents the neurotransmitter from passing through the synapse and thus preventing reuptake so prolonging their biological effects.

Citalopram (Figure 10.2c) is a selective and potent SSRI launched by Lundbeck in 1989 under the brand name Cipramil® in Denmark [88]. Following successful launches throughout Europe and Canada, it was introduced by Forrest Labs to the United States in 1998 under the brand name Celexa®. Subsequently, an orally disintegrating tablet developed by Valeant has also been approved in the United States. Along with major depressive disorder (MDD) it has also been approved for anxiety in Europe and is being evaluated in clinical trials (Phase II/III) for bipolar disorder, Huntington's disease, and alcoholism in the United States. Its mode of action is in line with other SSRI therapies displaying nanomolar potency for human serotonin receptors and transporters [88].

Evaluation of each enantiomer of citalopram revealed that escitalopram (Lexapro®, [S]-enantiomer) had improved potency and specificity over the racemate. *In vitro* binding experiments demonstrated that escitalopram (IC_{50} = 2.1 nM) was 100-fold more potent than (*R*)-citalopram (IC_{50} = 275 nM) for the inhibition of serotonin reuptake in rat brain synaptsomes [88]. Other studies have also shown that (*R*)-citalopram antagonizes the effects of escitalopram, although the precise mechanism for this has not been elucidated. This antagonism by (*R*)-citalopram may result from differential actions of the two enantiomers at a low-affinity allosteric binding site on the 5-HT reuptake transporter [89, 90]. This *in vitro* and *in vivo* animal data translated to a measureable clinical difference between citalopram and escitalopram [91].

Escitalopram was as effective as other SSRIs in treating MDD patients and more effective in comparison with those treated with SNRIs such as duloxetine and venlafaxine XR [87]. The racemate and single enantiomer have also been evaluated in comparison studies. In a 6-week multicenter prospective randomized double-blind study of 322 patients (mean age, 35 years) escitalopram (10 mg) proved to be superior over citalopram (10 mg or 20 mg) [92]. Clinical metrics of depression (MADRS, CGI-S, CGI-I) were used to demonstrate the statistically significant improvement of the escitalopram (10 mg) arm over the two citalopram arms (10 mg or 20 mg). Severely depressed patients saw the greatest improvement. In 2001, Lundbeck launched escitalopram as Cipralex® in Denmark and eventually in Europe. Forest Labs obtained FDA approval in 2002 to market it as Lexapro® in the United States (Table 10.8).

10.3.5. Cetirizine (Zyrtec®) to Levocetrizine (Xyzal®)

Seasonal hay fever or allergic rhinitis, an allergic inflammation of the nasal airways and symptoms include itching, sneezing, and nasal congestion, affects as many as 30–60 million people in the United States alone [93]. Rhinitis sufferers may also experience swelling of the eyes as well as middle ear effusions. Rhinitis is thought to be triggered by the body's response to the presence of allergens such as pollen or dust that catalyzes a series of pro-inflammatory events culminating in the release of inflammatory mediators such as histamine and tryptase [93]. These in turn stimulate the production of other mediators as well as trigger processes that lead to the observed symptoms of congestion [93].

A general goal of rhinitis therapies is to reduce or prevent the inflammatory events that lead to symptoms. In lieu of removing all potential allergens, antagonist approaches have provided a method of managing symptoms in the presence of suboptimal conditions. These approaches attempt to intercept the actions of the endogenous signaling molecules participating in the inflammatory cascade [94]. Histamine is responsible for increasing vascular permeability, which allows fluid release from capillaries to tissues and ultimately congestion, runny nose and water eyes. First-generation antihistamine drugs were plagued with sedative side effects [94]. This was later revealed to be the

TABLE 10.8. Comparison of Celexa® and Its Chiral Switch Successor Lexapro®

	Celexa®	Lexapro®
Stereochemistry	(R/S)	(S)
API	Citalopram	Escitalopram
FDA approval[a]	1998	2002
Originator	Lundbeck/Forest	Lundbeck/Forest
Expected patent expiration[b]	Generic	2023
Peak global sales (year)[c]	$1.5 billion (2003)	$1 billion (2010)/$2.2 billion (2010)
Therapeutic class	Antidepressants (SSRI)	
Key advantages		
• Pharmacology	• Escitalopram is 100-fold more potent than (R)-citalopram.	
	• (R)-citalopram antagonizes the activity of escitalopram. Differential actions of the two enantiomers at a low affinity allosteric binding site on the 5-HT reuptake transporter is thought to be responsible.	
• Clinical data	• Comparison studies demonstrated that escitalopraom was more effective in improving all clinical metrics than citalopram in adult MDD patients.	
	• Adverse event incident rate was lower with escitalopram.	

[a] Drugs@FDA.
[b] Based on FDA Orange Book data for longest possible coverage.
[c] Sales figures obtained from Thomson Reuters Integrity^{SM} database.

result of the penetration of these agents through the blood–brain barrier and subsequent interference with brain chemistry.

Cetirizine (Zyrtec®) (Figure 10.2d) is now an over-the-counter (OTC) remedy for seasonal and persistent allergic rhinitis available in the United States. It was first launched as a prescription medication for this indication by UCB Pharmaceuticals in 1987. Cetirizine is derived from another UCB product, hydroxyzine, one of the original first-generation antihistamines [95]. Hydroxyzine was launched in 1956 by UCB in Europe and marketed in the United States by Pfizer. Whereas hydroxyzine itself results in significant sedative effects due to its central nervous system (CNS) penetration, its major human methylphenidate (metabolite, cetirizine, transits the blood-brain barrier poorly. As such, when cetirizine is dosed directly, the side effects related to sedation are not observed [95].

Further expanding the antihistamine franchise, UCB investigated the activity of each enantiomer of cetirizine separately and determined that (R)-cetirizine, levocetirizine, was the eutomer (active enantiomer) [95]. Studies using human H_1 receptors transfected into hamster ovary cells demonstrated that levocetirizine had a 30-fold higher receptor affinity than dextrocetirizine (the less potent *[S]*-enantiomer, or "distomer", of cetirizine) [95]. Levocetirizine distribution is confined to the plasma as indicated by a low volume of distribution (V_d = 0.3–0.41 L/kg) [95]. Volume of distribution (V_d) relates drug concentration in blood or plasma to overall drug in the body. Levocetirizine's low V_d contrasts with other approved antihistamines such as loratadine and ebastine [95]. Low values for this metric suggest that organs and systems not involved in the desired therapeutic effect are not exposed to the drug, which may improve the tolerability of the agent.

The observed preclinical potency, selectivity, and toxicity yielded measurable clinical benefits as evidenced by the comparison studies of levocetirizine, cetirizine, and dextrocetirizine [96]. Both cetirizine and levocetirizine were superior to dextrocetirizine; however, only levocetirizine demonstrated a faster onset and a greater postdose effect [97]. A large (28K patients) randomized double-blind crossover comparison study evaluated the impact of cetirizine, levocetirizine, and dextrocetirizine on the histamine-induced skin allergy in healthy adults [97]. Inhibition of histamine-induced wheal and flare, inflammation within the skin, was used as a primary read-out. Levocetirizine (2.5 mg) had comparable antihistamine activity as cetirizine (5.0 mg) and was superior to dextrocetirizine, which had no activity. Plasma concentrations of levocetirizine (AUC) were greater than cetirizine (Table 10.9). Encouraged by these results, UCB filed for and was granted FDA approval in 2007 for levocetirizine, marketed as Xyzal®.

TABLE 10.9. Comparison of Zyrtec® and Its Chiral Switch Successor Xyzal®

	Zyrtec®	Xyzal®
Stereochemistry	(*R/S*)	(*R*)
API	Cetirizine	Levocetirizine
FDA approval[a]	1986	2007
Originator	UCB	UCB
Expected patent expiration[b]	Generic/OTC	2013
Peak global sales (year)[c]	$117 million (2009)	N/A
Therapeutic class	Antihistamines	
Key advantages		
• Pharmacology	• Levocetirizine is a competitive agonist of histamine H_1 receptor.	
	• Binding studies have demonstrated a twofold greater affinity of levocetirizine compared to cetirizine.	
• Clinical data	• Levocetirizine has a faster onset and a more sustained efficacy as evident by clinical studies.	

[a] Drugs@FDA.
[b] Based on FDA Orange Book data for longest possible coverage.
[c] Sales figures obtained from Thomson Reuters Integrity^{SM} database.

10.3.6. Atracurium (Tracrium®) to Cisatracurium (Nimbex®)

The introduction of neuromuscular blocking agents (NMB) represented a significant advance in anesthetic sciences and has had an immediate impact on the success of surgical practices. NMBs relax skeletal muscle, allowing for intubation and access to body cavities [98]. Recently these agents have also found applications in outpatient and pediatric applications. NMBs are divided by their mode of action: depolarizing or nondepolarizing. Nondepolarizing agents are competitive antagonists of nicotinic acetylcholine receptors (nAChR) at the neuromuscular junction. Inhibition of these receptors prevents polarization of the cell membrane, resulting in relaxation of muscle. Examples of this class include mivacurium, pancuronium, and cisatracurium. The majority of the clinical NMBs are members of this class. Depolarizing NMBs are agonists of nAChR that cause contractions known as fasciculation and have longer receptor residency causing persistent depolarization and desensitization [99]. Due to a greater side effect profile, few agents with this mode of action have been developed. Succinylcholine is the only depolarizing NMB agent used clinically.

Atracurium besylate (Figure 10.2e) was the first rationally designed nonsteroidal NMB. It undergoes chemodegradation to inactive forms *in vivo* [100]. It was first prepared in the academic labs of the Strathcylde University [101] and later licensed to The Wellcome Foundation, which developed and launched the drug as a mixture of 10 stereoisomers (Tracrium) in the United Kingdom [102]. The design of atracurium was based on the importance of *bis*-quaternary structure for neuromuscular blocking efficacy. Degradation of atracurium occurs via nonenzymatic Hoffman elimination under mildly alkaline conditions at physiological pH and temperature (Scheme 10.2). The degradation products are not antagonists for nAChR and thus the programmed decomposition leads to a measurable and reliable off-rate of the NMB agent. The half-life of the agent is thus expectedly short, 17–20 minutes, which allows the anesthesiologist to plan dosing around the expected surgery time.

Atracurium was quickly superseded by cisatracurium when the active isomer of the mixture was discovered as the $(1R, 2R, 1'R, 2'R)$-*cis-cis* configuration (Table 10.10) [103]. This isomer makes up only 15% of the original mixture and thus dosing it as a single stereoisomer was expected to improve both efficacy and safety. Common side effects associated with the tetrahydroisoquinolinium class of NMBs include hypotension, reflex tachycardia, and cutaneous flushing resulting from a rapid release of histamine after administration of the NMB agent. Supratherapeutic dosing of cisatrucurium ($8\times$ ED95), on the other hand, does not result in increased histamine production, resulting in a significantly improved adverse event profile [104]. Both the single isomer and the mixture have also been evaluated in neurosurgical mechanically ventilated patients. Cisatracurium was superior over the mixture as measured by reduced intracranial pressure, cerebral perfusion, and lower overall blood pressure [105]. Furthermore, lower dosing of cisatracurium

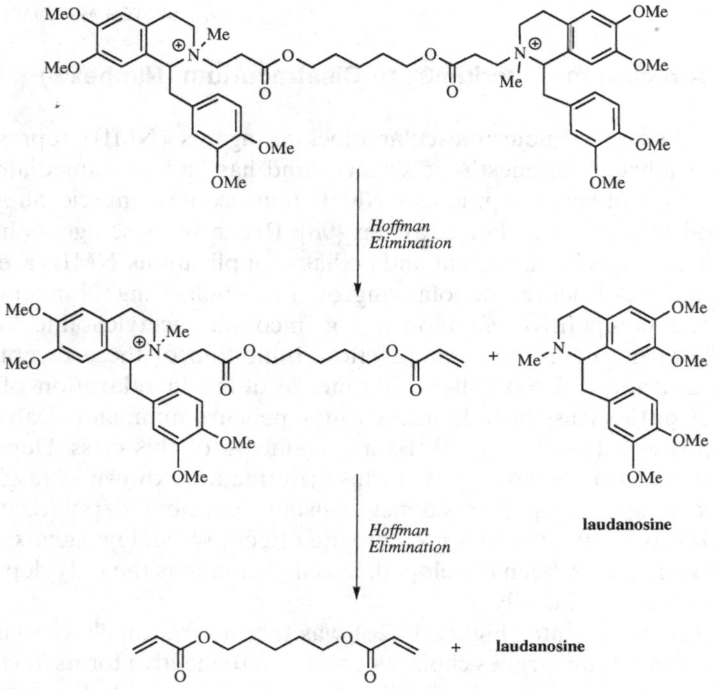

Scheme 10.2. Rationally designed *in vivo* chemodegradation of atracurium.

TABLE 10.10. Comparison of Tracrium® and Its Chiral Switch Successor Nimbex®

	Tracrium®	Nimbex®
Stereochemistry	Multiple	(R-cis, R-cis)
API	Atracurium	Cisatracurium
FDA approval[a]	1983	1995
Originator	The Wellcome Foundation	GSK
Expected patent expiration[b]	Generic	2012
Peak global sales (year)[c]	N/A	N/A
Therapeutic class	Depolarizing neuromuscular blocking agents (NMB)	
Key advantages		
• Pharmacology	• Nicotinic acetylcholine receptor antagonist (nAChR)	
	• Rationally designed bis-quaternary warhead decomposes at a measurable and reproducible rate to allow for precise dosing.	
• Clinical data	• Single stereoisomer is threefold more potent than mixture with slower onset and reduced histamine releasing profile.	
	• Lower dosing allows for less exposure to reactive metabolite.	

[a] Drugs@FDA.
[b] Based on FDA Orange Book data for longest possible coverage.
[c] Sales figures obtained from Thomson Reuters Integrity^SM database.

results in the reduction of the amount of laudanosine, a major metabolite related to increased seizure events in animals [104].

10.3.7. Bupivacaine (Marcaine®/Sensorcaine®) to Levobupivacaine (Chirocaine®)

Reducing the abuse potential of analgesics has been a standing goal in this therapeutic class. This has spurred the evolution of agents from the original cocaine (1884) to tetracaine (1941) to bupivacaine (1967) and most recently ropivacaine (1996). All of these compounds share the same pharmacophore and thus capitalize on similar modes of action.

Bupivacaine (Marcaine) (Figure 10.2f) has been used as a topical anesthetic for many years [106]. When administered intravenously, however, the agent causes cardiac toxicity. Bupivacaine is approved as a racemic mixture and studies on the individual enantiomers have demonstrated that the therapeutic activity and improved safety resides with the (S)-enantiomer, levobupivacaine (Chirocaine®) [106]. In an effort to study the enantiospecific cardiotoxicity, effects on the action potential of each enantiomer on guinea-pig papillary muscle were evaluated. Less of the (R)-bupivacaine was needed to elicit a reduced maximal rate in the action potential amplitude of the membrane. The time for the membrane potential to recover was also extended [107]. Further, *in vivo* rat studies examined the influence of agent stereochemistry on the cell firing rate (CFR) and subsequent cardiovascular system. Although similar in many cardiac metrics (i.e., blood pressure, heart rate), the (R)-bupivacaine-treated rats exhibited higher rates of severe bradycardia, hypotension, and eventual death compared with the levobupivacaine rats [108].

Along with the pharmacological differences, the two enantiomers also have unique PK profiles specifically with regard to metabolism, exposure, distribution, and elimination. In animal studies, (R)-bupivacaine was found to have a higher clearance than levobuvacaine [106]. This observation was correlated in healthy humans exhibiting higher mean total plasma clearance for the (R)-enantiomer. In a study of patients undergoing minor surgery, levobupivacaine had higher peak plasma concentrations than its enantiomer.

In smaller comparison trials, levobupivacaine was shown to be as efficacious as bupivacaine for major extradural anaesthesia for cesarean delivery [109], epidural analgesia during labor [110], and major orthopedic surgery [111]. In a more recent study [112], levobupivacaine (7.5 mg) was compared with bupivacaine as spinal anesthetics for transurethral surgery. Less motor block and shorter motor block duration were observed with the single enantiomer treatment. Longer sensory block duration and prolonged intervals until requested supplemental analgesia were also associated with the single enantiomer dose group. In a double-blind comparison study, patients undergoing lower abdominal procedures were provided levobupivacaine, 50% enriched (S)-bupivacaine, and bupivacaine [113]. The most common procedures in the study were hysterectomy (75%) followed by tubal ligation (15%). All patients were provided

TABLE 10.11. Comparison of Marcaine® and Its Chiral Switch Successor Chirocaine®

	Marcaine®	Chirocaine®
Stereochemistry	(R/S)	(S)
API	Bupivacaine	Levobupivacaine
FDA approval[a]	1978	1999
Originator	AstraZeneca/Sanofi	UCB Celltech
Expected patent expiration[b]	Generic	2009
Peak global sales (year)[c]	N/A	N/A
Therapeutic class	Local and regional anesthetics	
Key advantages		
• Pharmacology	• Animal and receptor binding studies have confirmed that the (R)-bupivacaine is more closely related to the cardiac toxicity observed in the racemate.	
• Clinical data	• Less motor block and shorter motor block duration were observed with the single enantiomer over racemate.	

[a] Drugs@FDA.
[b] Based on FDA Orange Book data for longest possible coverage.
[c] Sales figures obtained from Thomson Reuters Integrity[SM] database.

epidural anesthesia 1 hour prior to surgery. Motor and sensory block profiles were evaluated in addition to monitoring of pulse, blood pressure, and heart rate. Motor block was evaluated according to the Bromage scale for 30 minutes prior to surgery and 30 minutes during surgery. No statistical differences were observed among patient groups with regard to cardiovascular parameters. Although similar levels of sensory block were observed in all patients, the levobupivacaine group did demonstrate the least amount of motor block compared with the two other patient groups (Table 10.11).

10.3.8. Conclusion

The preceding case studies are provided as examples of successful execution of the chiral switch strategy, which has been utilized across a variety of therapeutic classes and indications. The success of chiral switch drugs has been made possible by significant advances in enantioselective synthesis as well as through further understanding of the chiral nature of biological systems. Although the strategy has been scrutinized for merely being a tool for patent life cycle management, the clinical data suggest that there is often a demonstrable advantage of the single enantiomer over a racemic mixture. Although single enantiomer drugs have overtaken mixtures and achiral entities, the chiral switch approach may continue to provide new and improved therapeutics based on older, racemic agents.

10.4. SITE-SELECTIVE DEUTERATION APPROACH

10.4.1. Introduction

Deuterated compounds have been widely used in nonclinical settings as metabolic or PK probes both *in vitro* and *in vivo* [114, 115]. Depending on the route of metabolism and the location of the deuterium, deuteration can be metabolically silent, allowing use as a PK tracer, or it can alter the compound's metabolism, enabling use as a mechanistic probe. In spite of the potential to alter a compound's metabolism, deuterium-containing compounds have rarely been clinically explored as new therapeutic agents, and no deuterated compound has advanced beyond Phase II clinical evaluation [116–118]. This section will provide a brief review of the use of site-selective deuteration as a strategy to alter the metabolic properties of clinically validated agents and will discuss past and current approaches to the development of deuterium-containing drugs. While not all of the case studies detailed below are formally repurposing efforts in terms of developing a deuterated drug for a new indication, the reader will appreciate that improvements to the PK profiles of existing agents may make them more amenable to repositioning strategies.

10.4.2. Primary Deuterium Isotope Effect

Deuterium is a naturally occurring, stable, nonradioactive isotope of hydrogen discovered in 1932 [119]. Hydrogen consists of one electron and one proton and has a mass of 1.008 atomic mass units (AMU), whereas deuterium also contains a neutron, which results in a mass of 2.014 AMU. Due to this mass difference, deuterium–carbon bonds have a lower vibrational frequency and therefore a lower zero-point energy than a corresponding hydrogen–carbon bond [120]. The lower zero-point energy results in a higher activation energy for C–D bond cleavage and a slower reaction rate (k). This reaction rate effect is known as the primary deuterium isotope effect (DIE) and is expressed as k_H/k_D, the ratio of the reaction rate of C–H versus C–D bond cleavage with a theoretical limit of about 9 at 37°C in the absence of tunneling effects [121, 122].

A very large number of studies have appeared in the literature over the years reporting DIEs for enzyme-catalyzed reactions. The DIE has the potential to affect the biological fate of many drugs metabolized by pathways involving hydrogen–carbon bond scission. k_H/k_D is the intrinsic deuterium isotope effect and is the full isotope effect observed in reactions where the C–H bond cleavage is rate limiting. However, the observed isotope effect, $(k_H/k_D)_{obs}$, for an enzymatic/metabolic reaction is often much smaller than the intrinsic isotope effect [123, 124]. This reduction, or masking of the isotope effect, results from the complexity of biological systems and the number of competing effects. For example, if the C–H bond breaking is only partially rate limiting, a reduced DIE will be observed. Likewise, if another enzymatic step is rate limiting (e.g., product release), then no isotope effect would be observed.

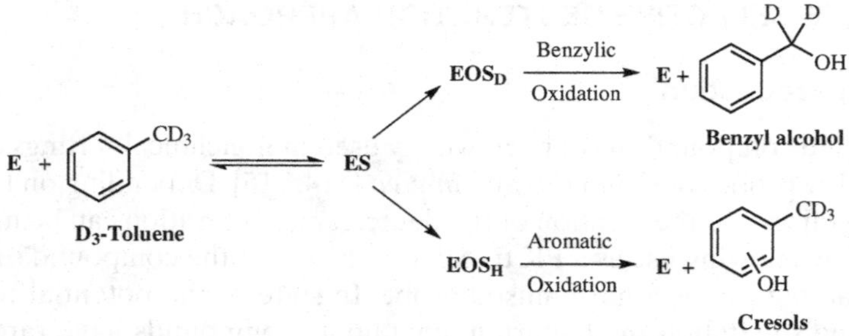

Scheme 10.3. Metabolic shunting for D_3-toluene. **E** represents free enzyme; **ES** is the enzyme–substrate (D_3-toluene) complex; **EOS$_D$** is the active oxygenating species for C–D bond oxidation to yield benzyl alcohol; **EOS$_H$** is the active oxygenating enzyme species for C–H (aromatic) oxidation to yield cresols.

Masking of the isotope effect also results from metabolic switching, which is a change from one site of metabolism to another on the molecule [121, 122, 125, 126]. When metabolic switching occurs, one can observe no change in the rate of substrate metabolism but will observe a change in the ratios of products formed [127]. There is at least one example in the literature in which an increased rate of metabolic turnover is attributed to metabolic switching [128]. In this study with D_3-toluene (Scheme 10.3), metabolic switching occurs away from benzylic oxidation, producing benzyl alcohol, to aromatic oxidation, producing cresols. The authors propose that the increase in turnover results from the more rapid product release for cresols than benzyl alcohol, thereby accelerating catalytic turnover. In spite of the ability of deuterium to alter metabolism patterns, the authors are not aware of any reports of deuteration resulting in the formation of unique metabolites that were not also observed for the all-hydrogen analog.

The complexity of biological systems and the number of competing effects in enzyme-catalyzed reactions that can mask the DIE have made the application of deuterium to drug discovery highly unpredictable and challenging [122]. The most important enzymes in drug metabolism are the cytochrome P450s (CYPs), which are responsible for the Phase I metabolism of a majority of drugs. The structures and mechanisms of CYPs have been reviewed in addition to the application of DIEs to the study of CYP-catalyzed reactions [121, 129].

In spite of the complexities surrounding the expression of a DIE, the incorporation of deuterium into pharmacologically active agents offers potential benefits such as improved exposure profiles and switching metabolic pathways away from the production of toxic metabolites [117, 130], thereby offering possible improvements in efficacy, tolerability, or safety. As noted in a recent review [131], there has been a resurgence of interest in the application of deuterium in medicinal chemistry as evidenced by the emergence of several new companies largely or solely focused on this technology.

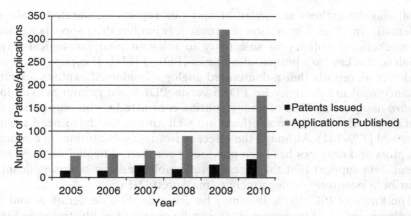

FIGURE 10.4. Issued patents and published applications containing "deuterium" or "deuterated" in the claims and "pharmaceutical" in any field for 2005–2010.

The increased level of interest in deuterated drugs by the pharmaceutical industry is also reflected by the number of published patent applications and issued patents over the last five years. A search of the USPTO database covering the years 2005 to 2010 for the terms "deuterium" or "deuterated" in the claims and "pharmaceutical" in all fields of published U.S. patent applications and issued U.S. patents resulted in 761 and 142 hits, respectively. For all years prior to 2005, the total hits were less than 80. Figure 10.4 shows the annual breakdown. There has been a large overall increase in published U.S. applications for 2008 through 2010 with a smaller but steady increase for issued patents over the same period, which shows the continuing patentability of deuterated drugs. The patentability of these new molecular entities is based on a showing of unexpected differences between the deuterated analogs and the prior art all-hydrogen compounds [132]. As more companies explore the potential of deuterated drugs and applications enter prosecution at the USPTO, it will be of great interest to see if the number of issued patents continues to grow.

10.4.3. Deuterium Effects upon Pharmacology, Metabolism, and Pharmacokinetics

When deuterium is substituted into molecules in place of hydrogen, in most respects the deuterated compound is quite similar to the all-hydrogen compound. Since the electron clouds of the atoms define the shape of a molecule, deuterated compounds have shapes and sizes that are very similar to their all-hydrogen analogs [133]. Small physical property changes have been detected in partially or fully deuterated compounds, including reduced hydrophobicity [134, 135], decreased acidity of carboxylic acids and phenols [136], and increased basicity of amines [137]. These differences tend to be quite small and the authors are aware of only one report—deuterated analogs of sildenafil—in which deuteration of a reversibly binding drug appears to change its biochemical potency or selectivity to relevant pharmacological targets, which in this case are phophodiesterases (PDEs) [138]. This paper by F. Schneider et al. reports that a deuterated analog of sildenafil exhibits a twofold enhancement in selectivity for PDE5 versus PDE6 and greater activity in an *in vitro* assay (relaxation of phenylephrine contracted rabbit corpus cavernosum strips). Binding isotope effects are well known and have been recently reviewed [139–141]. Although the effect of isotopic substitution on binding to receptors and enzymes has been previously considered negligible, these more recent data support that they are unpredictable, and can be insignificant, or contribute positively or negatively to measured DIEs.

The kinds of PK effects that may be achieved with deuteration, and that have been observed in certain cases, can be classified as illustrated in Figure 10.5. Panel 5 of Figure 10.5 illustrates the case where the major effect of deuteration, as shown by the theoretical solid line for the deuterated compound versus the theoretical dashed line for the all-hydrogen compound, is to reduce the rate of systemic clearance, which results in an increase of the biological half-life of the compound. Potential drug benefits could include a reduction in dosage and the ability to maintain similar systemic exposures with decreased peak levels (C_{max}) and enhanced trough levels (C_{min}). This could result in a lower incidence of C_{max}-associated side effects and enhanced efficacy, depending on the particular drug's PK–PD relationship. D_{15}-atazanavir shown in Figure 10.7a is an example of this effect that will be discussed in greater detail as a case study. There are also two other examples in the recent literature

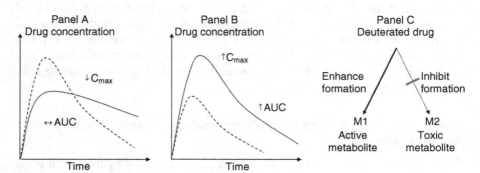

FIGURE 10.5. Panel A: Theoretical PK curves for reduced systemic clearance resulting in increased half-life for a deuterated compound (solid line) versus an all-hydrogen compound (dashed line). Panel B: Theoretical PK curves for decreased presystemic metabolism resulting in higher bioavailability of unmetabolized drug for a deuterated compound (solid line) versus an all-hydrogen compound (dashed line). Panel C: Deuterium mediated metabolic shunting resulting in reduced exposure to an undesired metabolite (M2) and increased exposure to a desired active metabolite (M1).

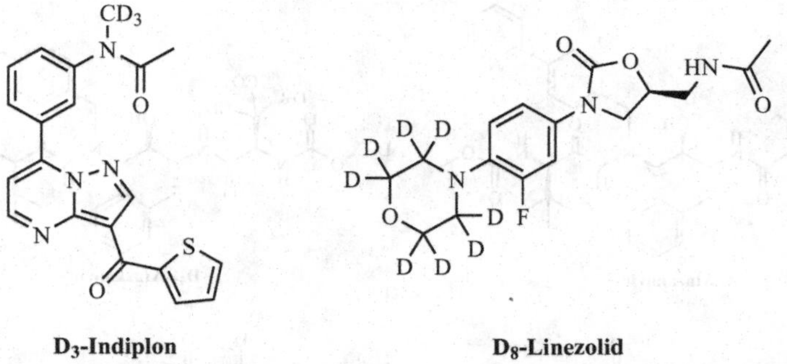

D₃-Indiplon   **D₈-Linezolid**

FIGURE 10.6. Structures of D_3-indiplon and D_8-linezolid.

shown in Figure 10.6, D_3-indiplon [142] and D_8-linezolid [143], in which deuterium substitution results in a longer half-life *in vivo*. Indiplon is a GABA$_A$ receptor agonist that was in development for the treatment of insomnia. The D_3-indiplon compound showed an approximate twofold increase in half-life when orally dosed to rats. Linezolid (Zyvox®) is the only oxazolidinone antibiotic approved for the both intravenous (IV) and oral treatment of susceptible and resistant Gram-positive pathogens, particularly methicillin-resistant *Staphylococcus aureus* (MRSA) and vancomycin-resistant enterococci (VRE). The recommended dosage regimen for linezolid is 600 mg twice per day. The D_8-linezolid compound showed a 43% increase in half-life versus linezolid following IV dosing in primates. In both cases, the increase in half-life could have potential clinical value. D_3-indiplon may have a longer duration of action and improved sleep maintenance in humans, whereas D_8-linezolid may have prolonged exposure enabling a once-daily dosing regimen. These two examples are not presented as case studies since only preclinical data have been reported.

Figure 10.5, Panel B illustrates a largely presystemic (or first-pass) effect of deuteration. In this case, reduced rates of oxidative metabolism in the gut wall and/or liver results in a larger percentage of unmetabolized deuterated drug (shown by the solid line) versus the all-hydrogen drug (shown by the dashed line) reaching systemic circulation while the overall rate of systemic clearance remains unchanged. Deuterated drugs showing this effect may have reduced dosing requirements and produce lower metabolite loads. Since, in many instances, gastrointestinal irritation has been shown to be a dose-dependent rather than a plasma concentration-dependent phenomenon, this effect could allow for enhanced tolerability and/or the ability to achieve a higher maximum tolerated dose. Figure 10.5, Panel C illustrates metabolic shunting in which a drug is metabolized to form both active (M1) and toxic metabolite (M2) species. In such a case, deuteration could result in the reduced formation of M2, the toxic or reactive metabolite, as well as the increased formation of the desirable active metabolite M1.

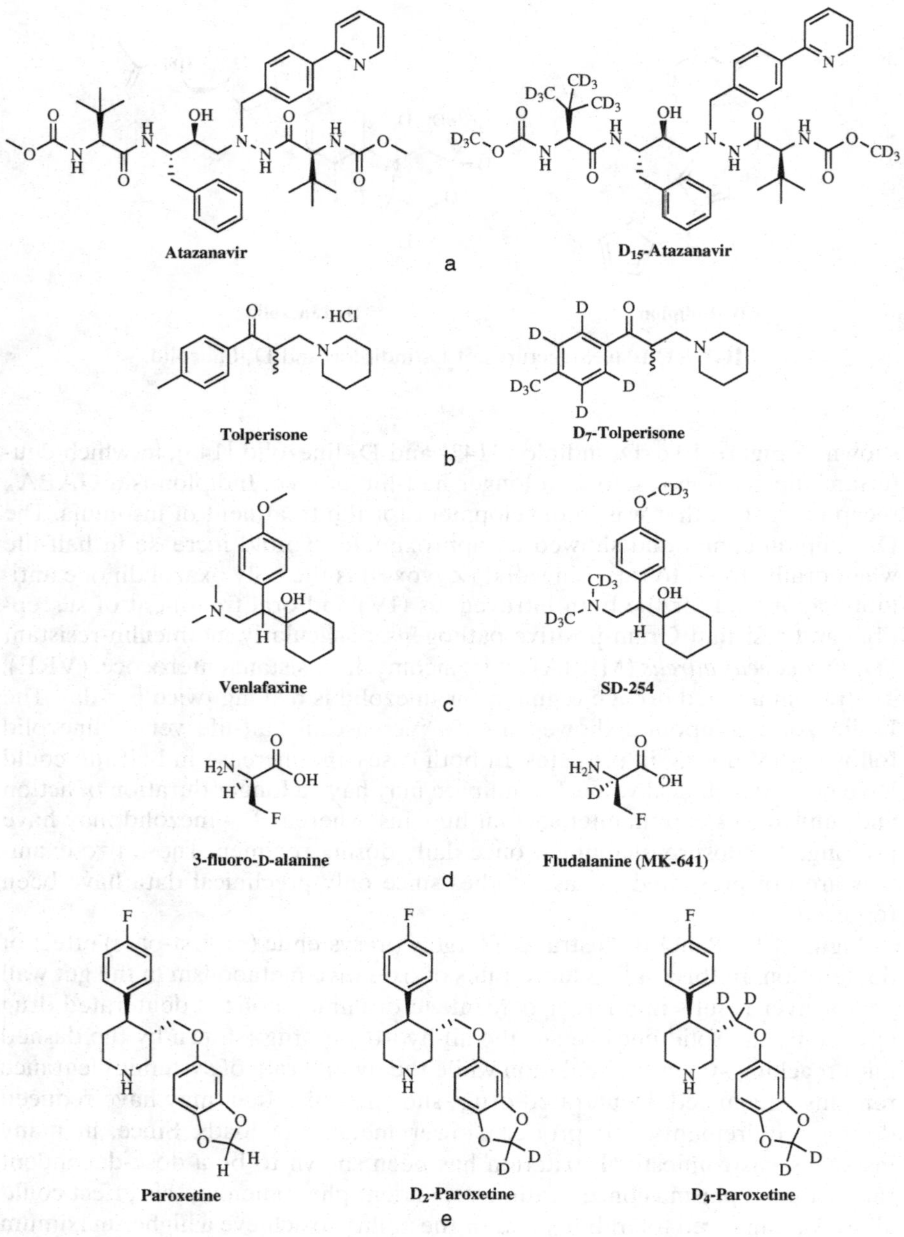

FIGURE 10.7. Structures of the site-selective deuterium modification case studies: (a) atazanavir, (b) tolperisone, (c) venlafaxine, (d) fludalanine, (e) paroxetine.

The case studies that follow are deuterated compounds exemplifying the PK effects represented in Figure 10.5. Each of these examples is a deuterated molecule that has been advanced to clinical studies in humans. However, only fludalanine progressed to clinical studies in patients; the other examples appear to have not advanced beyond Phase I studies in healthy volunteers. Deuterated atazanavir (Figure 10.7a) represents a deuterium effect to increase half-life as illustrated in Figure 10.5, Panel A. Deuterated tolperisone (Figure 10.7b) and deuterated venlafaxine (Figure 10.7c) show an increase in exposure resulting from decreased presystemic metabolism as represented in Figure 10.5, Panel B. The final two examples, fludalanine (Figure 10.7d) and deuterated paroxetine (Figure 10.7e), exhibit a deuterium effect, which produces metabolic switching away from an undesired metabolite to produce a safer or better tolerated drug (Figure 10.5, Panel C). The published data for each of these case studies will be reviewed.

10.4.4. CTP-518, Deuterated Atazanavir

Atazanavir (Reyataz®) (Figure 10.7a) is an HIV protease inhibitor (PI) launched in the United States in 2003 by Bristol-Myers Squibb and is labeled for the oral treatment of HIV-1 infection in combination with other antiretroviral agents [144]. The recommended dosage in HIV-1 positive treatment-naïve patients is either 300 mg with 100 mg ritonavir (Norvir®, a PK booster) once daily or 400 mg once daily if unable to tolerate ritonavir. For HIV-1 positive, treatment-experienced patients, the recommended dose is 300 mg with 100 mg ritonavir once daily.

Atazanavir is extensively metabolized in humans and *in vitro* studies suggest that metabolism is primarily via CYP3A4/CYP3A5 isozymes [145]. Ritonavir is an approved HIV-PI that is also a strong inhibitor of CYP3A isozymes; therefore, it can increase plasma concentrations of agents that are primarily metabolized by CYP3A [146]. Studies have shown that ritonavir increases the exposure (AUC), C_{max}, C_{min}, and half-life of atazanavir in a 300/100 once-daily regimen [145, 147]. A ritonavir-boosted atazanavir regimen is associated with greater virologic control due to greater exposure and higher C_{min} levels [148, 149]. Ritonavir, however, is associated with adverse events such as hyperlipidemia, hyperglycemia, and gastrointestinal intolerance [150]. Therefore, a once-daily, unboosted PI regimen for HIV-1 patients remains a significant unmet need.

CTP-518 is a deuterated version of the atazanavir (Figure 10.7a) that has entered Phase 1 clinical studies [131]. Selective deuteration is directed towards developing a drug that retains the anti-viral potency of atazanavir without the need for ritonavir or another PK boosting agent [151]. The structure of CTP-518 has not been published; however, D_{15}-atazanavir (Figure 10.7a) has been disclosed in a patent [152] with data showing increased human liver microsome (HLM) stability versus atazanavir. The half-life in HLM for D_{15}-atazanavir was increased 51% versus atazanavir. The increased stability in HLM translated to an *in vivo* setting. Following an IV codose of D_{15}-atazanavir and atazanavir (1:1) in primates, an average 52% increase in half-life for D_{15}-atazanavir versus atazanavir was reported. Atazanavir and D_{15}-atazanavir exhibit similar HIV anti-viral activity in an *in vitro* viral assay. No clinical data for CTP-518 have been published; however, if deuterium substitution results in a longer half-life and more closely matches the exposure and C_{min} for boosted atazanavir, then viral replication could be effectively suppressed by unboosted CTP-518.

10.4.5. BDD-10103, Deuterated Tolperisone

Tolperisone-HCl (Figure 10.7b), was introduced into Hungary in 1959 by Gedeon Richter and is used for the treatment of various spastic paralyses [153]. Tolperisone possesses several desirable characteristics including a low adverse event profile, a lack of sedation and no interaction with alcohol as well as no potential for tolerance and addiction. However, tolperisone still has several pharmacological limitations, the most notable of which is a high first-pass effect in various species that requires high daily doses [154]. The metabolism of tolperisone is highly dependent on the genetic background of the patients and thus subject to considerable inter-individual PK variation. The major metabolic path for tolperisone is hydroxylation of the aryl methyl, predominantly via CYP2D6 with some contribution from CYP2C19 [155]. CYP2D6 is a genetically polymorphic enzyme and this polymorphism can be used to separate subjects into phenotypes: poor and extensive metabolizers, which results in significant individual differences in the ability to metabolize certain drugs [156]. A clinical study in 15 healthy male Korean volunteers reported highly variable pharmacokinetics upon oral dosing of tolperisone [157]. The volunteers were given a single oral 450 mg dose of tolperisone HCL (3 × 150 mg Mydocalm® tablets) and plasma drug levels were monitored over an 8 hours period. The AUC values ranged from 125.9 to 1241.3 ng/mL-h and the Cmax values ranged from 64.2 to 784.9 ng/mL. These data emphasize the large inter-individual PK variability of tolperisone.

BDD-10103 is a deuterated analog of tolperisone that emerged from Berolina innovative Research and Development Services (BiRDS) Pharma GmbH using their Atomic Substitution Technology platform. The compound reportedly addresses current drawbacks of tolperisone while maintaining its advantageous features. The structure of BDD-10103 has yet to be reported and the intellectual property rights to the compound have recently been transferred to D4Pharma [158]. The company reports [159] that various animal models have shown oral doses of BDD-10103 to be more efficacious than the corresponding doses of tolperisone both in selected preclinical rodent and non-rodent animal models; BDD-10103 and tolperisone inhibited the monosynaptic ventral root reflex roughly to the same extent. BDD-10103 reportedly showed superiority in the tremorine test in mice after oral administration. Metabolic degradation of BDD-10103 and tolperisone was assessed in hepatic liver microsomes. The results suggested that a longer elimination half-life could be expected for BDD-10103 in humans than that reported for tolperisone. However, the corporate website reports that in a single dose (300 mg) study of BDD-10103 in man, an increase in bioavailability was observed but no mention of an increase in half-life [159]. Although the structure of BDD-10103 has not been disclosed, D_7-tolperisone has been disclosed [160] and is reported to show a 10-fold decrease in aryl methyl hydroxylation versus tolperisone by both CYP2D6 and CYP2C19. If deuterium substitution suppresses both the first-pass metabolism by CYP2D6 and interpatient variability resulting from CYP2D6 polymorphism, then BDD-10103 could be clinically superior to tolperisone. The company reports that pharmaceutical development includes the evaluation of an improved oral formulation to enhance the bioavailability of BDD-10103 in the human body, but the current clinical status of BDD-10103 is unclear.

10.4.6. SD-254, Deuterated Venlafaxine

Venlafaxine (Effexor®, Effexor XR®) is a centrally acting serotonin-norepinephrine reuptake inhibitor (SNRI) launched in the US in 1994 by Wyeth Pharmaceuticals for the treatment of MDD, generalized anxiety disorder, social anxiety disorder and panic disorder with or without agoraphobia [161]. Venlafaxine (Figure 10.7c) has also been studied clinically for the treatment of hot flashes [162, 163] and neuropathic pain [164, 165]. Venlafaxine is orally absorbed and extensively metabolized in the liver by CYP2D6 to produce its major active metabolite O-desmethylvenlafaxine (ODV) [166, 167]. ODV or desvenlafaxine (Pristiq®) was launched in the US in 2008 for the treatment of MDD [168]. Since venlafaxine is metabolized by CYP2D6, plasma levels are higher in poor metabolizers than extensive metabolizers. However, since the metabolite, ODV, is also active and the total exposure for venlafaxine plus ODV are similar in poor and extensive metabolizers, there is no recommended dose adjustment for venlafaxine in these two groups [161].

SD-254 (Figure 10.7c) is a selectively deuterated analog of venlafaxine that has advanced into clinical development. Limited clinical data are available; however, the compound has been dosed in a Phase I healthy volunteer study to evaluate the effect of deuteration on drug behavior [169]. As illustrated in Figure 10.8, site-selective deuteration of venlafaxine resulted in enhanced exposure of SD-254 while reducing the levels of the major metabolite (ODV, or O-desmethyl venlafaxine). The left panel of Figure 10.8 shows the blood plasma levels for SD-254 versus venlafaxine, represented as their time versus concentration PK profiles. The right panel shows the time versus concentration PK profile observed in healthy volunteers for the deuterated versus all-hydrogen versions of the major metabolite, ODV. The data in Figure 10.8 show that when human subjects are dosed with the SD-254, they experience higher blood concentrations of the parent drug relative to venlafaxine. The SD-254 treated subjects also exhibit lower plasma concentrations of the major

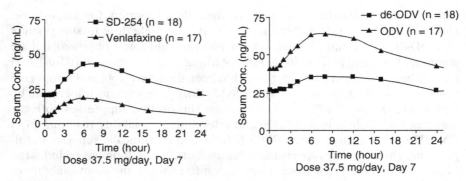

FIGURE 10.8. Left Panel: Time versus concentration PK profiles of deuterated ven-lafaxine (SD-254) and venlafaxine in healthy volunteers after 7 days of dosing. Right Panel: Time versus concentration PK profiles of the metabolites: d6-O-desmethyl ven-lafaxine and O-desmethyl venlafaxine (ODV) in healthy volunteers after 7 days of dosing. Reproduced from [169] with permission, Auspex Pharmaceuticals.

metabolite (ODV). Development in neuropathic pain is reportedly planned for SD-254 [131, 151].

10.4.7. Fludalanine (MK-641)

Fludalanine (Figure 10.7d) appears to be the earliest deuterated drug candidate to have entered clinical trials; however, very little data have been reported. Fludalanine, combined with cycloserine, displays broad and potent antibacterial activity [170]. The all-hydrogen analog 3-fluoro-D-alanine (Figure 10.7d) is a highly effective antibacterial agent that acts against bacterial cell wall synthesis [171]. However, preclinical studies reportedly showed that it was metabolized to 3-fluorolactate (Scheme 10.4), a toxin that caused brain vacuolization [172]. A recent letter reported that deuteration reduced 3-fluorolactate production to what were deemed acceptable levels in healthy volunteers [118]. However, higher 3-fluorolactate levels were observed in patients, which may have resulted from metabolic differences between healthy volunteers and patients. Studies on fludalanine were discontinued at Phase 2b.

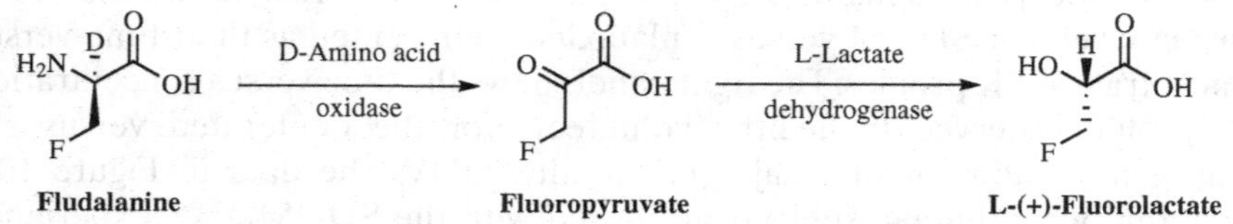

Scheme 10.4. Proposed metabolic pathway for the conversion of fludalanine to L-(+)-fluorolactate.

10.4.8. CTP-347, Deuterated Paroxetine

Paroxetine (Paxil®, Paxil CR®), shown in Figure 10.7e, is a centrally acting, SSRI launched in the United States in 1991 by GlaxoSmithKline and is labeled for the treatment of MDD, panic disorder, social anxiety disorder, and premenstrual dysphoric disorder [173]. As with venlafaxine, paroxetine has also been studied clinically for the treatment of hot flashes and neuropathic pain [163, 165]. Paroxetine is orally absorbed and extensively metabolized in the liver to produce a number of more polar and conjugated metabolites, which are readily cleared. The major metabolites have significantly less SSRI activity than paroxetine. Paroxetine is metabolized by CYP2D6; however, this enzyme is significantly inhibited by paroxetine. Therefore, co-administration of paroxetine with other drugs metabolized by CYP2D6 is contraindicated.

CTP-347 is a deuterated analog of paroxetine for the treatment of hot flashes that has completed Phase I clinical evaluation [174]. Low-dose paroxetine reportedly has good efficacy in treating hot flashes [175]. However, in patients potentially benefiting from such therapy, such as postmenopausal women and cancer patients receiving endocrine disrupting agents, paroxetine use can be complicated or contraindicated as it causes extensive drug–drug interactions (DDIs) with other drugs. The cause of these DDIs is believed to be predominantly irreversible inactivation of the hepatic enzyme CYP2D6. While CTP-347 shows similar pharmacology to paroxetine with respect to inhibition of serotonin and norepinephrine reuptake [176], CTP-347 is reported to be the first example of the use of deuterium to mitigate CYP2D6 inactivation versus paroxetine in a clinical setting [177]. The structure of CTP-347 has not been reported; however, D_2-paroxetine and D_4-paroxetine (Figure 10.7e) have been disclosed in the patent literature [178].

Increased metabolism for D_2- and D_4-paroxetines versus paroxetine in human liver microsomes is reported in the patent. The greater stability of paroxetine results from irreversible inhibition of CYP2D6 whereas the decreased stability of D_2- and D_4-paroxetines results from reduced CYP2D6 inhibition. Metabolism experiments in human liver microsomes confirmed that paroxetine was a mechanism-based inactivator of CYP2D6 (K_{inact} = 0.08 minute^{-1}); however, CTP-347 showed little or no CYP2D6 inactivation [179], possibly due to metabolic shunting that prevents the formation of a reactive metabolite that forms an irreversible complex at the active site of CYP2D6 (Scheme 10.5) [180].

A Phase I study was conducted to assess the effect of CTP-347 on mechanism-based inhibition of CYP2D6 in healthy women [176]. CTP-347 was administered (9/dose group) at doses of 10, 20, and 40 mg qd and 10 mg bid for 14 days. A 30 mg dose of dextromethorphan was administered orally on days 1 and 14. Dextromethorphan acts as a selective probe for CYP2D6 activity by measuring the urinary levels of dextrorphan, the metabolite formed by CYP2D6. Urine was collected for 8 hours and the amounts of dextromethorphan and dextrorphan were measured by liquid chromatography–tandem

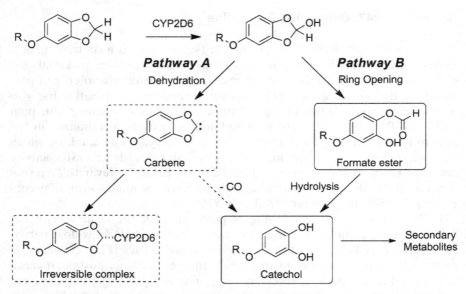

Scheme 10.5. Proposed inactivation pathway for CYP2D6 by a paroxetine metabolite. Pathway A produces a putative reactive metabolite and resultant inactivated enzyme (structures in dashed-line boxes). Pathway B produces polar metabolites via formate ester hydrolysis to the catechol (structures in solid-line boxes) that are rapidly cleared as secondary metabolites. Some of the carbene metabolite may also form the catechol via decarbonylation.

mass spectrometry (LC-MS/MS). Subjects dosed with CTP-347 retained substantially greater ability to metabolize dextromethorphan than has been reported previously for paroxetine [181, 182], correlating well with *in vitro* data (see Figure 10.9). Minor CYP2D6 inhibition was observed at higher CTP-347 doses, which is consistent with the reversible, competitive inhibition seen *in vitro.*

The five case studies presented in this section serve as clinical examples of the potential benefits of deuterium substitution. Only fludalanine has progressed to clinical trials in patients; however, the PK data for the other four examples show the potential for tangible clinical benefits. Although no human data have been reported for CTP-518, the published PK data for D_{15}-atazanavir in primates show an increase in half-life and an improved exposure profile as schematized in Figure 10.5, Panel A. The reported PK for the deuterated versions of venlafaxine and tolperisone supports a deuterium effect that reduces first-pass metabolism and increases exposure without changing half-life according to Figure 10.5, Panel B. The last two case studies, fludalanine and deuterated paroxetine, are examples of a deuterium effect that results in metabolic shunting as shown in Figure 10.5, Panel C. In both cases, deuterium substitution reduced deleterious metabolic side effects: 3-fluorolactate production from fludalanine and CYP2D6 inactivation by CTP-347. These case

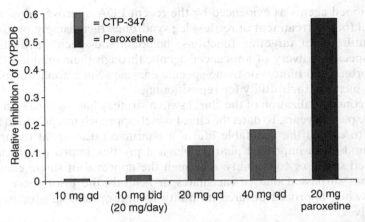

FIGURE 10.9. Drug–drug interaction between CTP-347 and dextromethorphan from Phase Ib study. [1]y-Axis shows the relative inhibition of CYP2D6 as the ratio of urinary levels of excreted dextromethorphan versus the CYP2D6 metabolite dextrorphan at four doses shown on the x-axis. The 20 mg qd paroxetine data shown are historical data from Reference [181].

studies support the ability of deuterium substitution to provide clinical agents with improved PK resulting in better efficacy, tolerability, and/or safety versus the corresponding all-hydrogen compound.

10.5. CONCLUSION

After a half century of drug discovery and development, the pharmaceutical/biotechnology industries have evolved to recognize the importance of drug repositioning as a new paradigm shift. Serendipitous discoveries, as well as concerted efforts, have led to strategies that capitalize on the advantages of repositioned drugs. The repositioning approach provides an attractive method for accelerating and concurrently de-risking drug development since these agents require less investment and time to develop and have a lower risk for late stage clinical failure. As such, repurposing offers an attractive risk-versus-reward profile in comparison with other drug development approaches and offers the potential to substantially improve performance metrics. As might be expected, there are a number of distinct challenges associated with any given repositioning strategy, which drives the development of creative approaches on the part of repositioning companies. The three strategies presented in this chapter highlight the continued progression of chemical platforms that may be utilized to facilitate these drug repositioning efforts.

The prodrug strategy has proven to be highly effective for solving many of the solubility, stability, permeability, and targeting problems necessary for certain repositioning strategies. This approach continues to yield successfully repositioned agents as evidenced by the recent FDA approval of gabapentin encarbil for the treatment of restless leg syndrome. Increasingly, prodrugs are being utilized for targeting functions, including site-specific activation and tissue-specific delivery of anticancer agents, through their unique effects on transporters, and tumor- or tissue-specific enzymes. Such applications should further increase their utility for repositioning.

The conceptualization of the chiral switch strategy has evolved significantly over the past 20 years. To date, the chiral switch approach has provided a useful option to extend the profitable life of a pharmaceutical agent by providing compounds with improved pharmacological profiles, improved efficacy, and improved safety or tolerability. Although the approval of single enantiomer drugs has surpassed that of racemates or achirals, the prior success of the chiral switch approach ensures its utility as appropriate substrates present themselves.

Finally, the site-selective deuteration strategy has recently emerged as a platform with the potential to impact positively the absorption, distribution, metabolism, and excretion (ADME) profile of clinically validated compounds, thereby possibly conferring improvements in the efficacy, tolerability, and/or safety of the deuterated entity. The examples presented in this chapter demonstrate that, in some cases, the deuterated agents possess distinct clinical benefits over the corresponding all hydrogen analogs. With more of these deuterium-containing compounds progressing into clinical evaluations, the viability of this strategy as a repositioning approach should become more evident. As such, site-selective deuteration is poised to become a standard strategic approach for both drug repositioning and discovery.

REFERENCES

1. Pammolli, F., Magazzini, L., Riccaboni, M. (2011). The productivity crisis in pharmaceutical R&D. *Nat. Rev. Drug Discov.*, *10*, 428–438.
2. Ashburn, T., Thor, K.B. (2004). Drug repositioning: Identifying and developing new uses for existing drugs. *Nat. Rev. Drug Discov.*, *3*, 673–683.
3. Rautio, J., Kumpulainen, H., Heimbach, T., Oliyai, R., Oh, D., Jarvinen, T., Savolainen, J. (2008). Prodrugs: Design and clinical applications. *Nat. Rev. Drug Discov.*, *7*, 255–270.
4. (a) Five-Year Exclusivity for Approved Prodrug Not Precluded by Prior FDA Approval of Metabolite Where Prodrug Is Not a Salt, Ester, or Other Non-Covalent Derivative of Previously-Approved Metabolite. http://ratnerprestia. com/lib/sitefiles/ANDANwsltr/Jan2011/Five-Year_Exclusivity_for_Approved_ Prodrug_Not_Precluded_by_Prior_FDA_Approval....pdf; (b) Note FDA classification of the drug Vyvanse® as a new chemical entity (NCE). http://www. accessdata.fda.gov/scripts/cder/ob/docs/patexclnew.cfm?Appl_No=021977& Product_No=001&table1=OB_Rx; (c) Note FDA classification of the drug Invega® Sustenna® as a new dosage form (NDF). http://www.accessdata.fda.gov/scripts/

cder/ob/docs/patexclnew.cfm?Appl_No=022264&Product_No=001&table1=
OB_Rx

5. Guidance for Industry: Applications Covered by Section 505(b)(2). http://
www.fda.gov/downloads/Drugs/GuidanceComplianceRegulatoryInformation/
Guidances/ucm079345.pdf

6. Murata, M. (2006). Pharmacokinetics of L-Dopa. *J. Neurol.*, *253*, iii47–iii52.

7. Antiretroviral Drugs Used in the Treatment of HIV Infection. http://www.fda.gov/
ForConsumers/ByAudience/ForPatientAdvocates/HIVandAIDSActivities/
ucm118915.htm

8. Pokorna, J., Machala, L., Rezacova, P., Konvalinka, J. (2009). Current and novel
inhibitors of HIV protease. *Viruses*, *1*, 1209–1239.

9. Noble, S., Goa, K.L. (2000). Amprenavir—A review of its clinical potential in
patients with HIV infection. *Drugs*, *60*, 1383–1410.

10. Furfine, E.S., Baker, C.D., Hale, M.H., Reynolds, D.J., Salisbury, J.A., Searle, A.D.,
Studenberg, S.D., Todd, D., Tung, R.D., Spaltenstein, A. (2004). Preclinical pharmacology and pharmacokinetics of GW433908, a water-soluble prodrug of the
human immunodeficiency virus protease inhibitor amprenavir. *Antimicrob. Agents
Chemother.*, *48*, 791–798.

11. Prescribing Information for Agenerase®. http://www.accessdata.fda.gov/
drugsatfda_docs/label/2005/021007s017lbl.pdf

12. (a) Bangsberg, D.R., Hecht, F.M., Charlebois, E.D., Zolopa, A.R., Holodniy, M.,
Sheiner, L., Bamberger, J.D., Chesney, M.A., Moss, A. (2000). Adherence to protease inhibitors, HIV-1 viral load, and development of drug resistance in an
indigent population. *AIDS*, *14*, 357–366.; (b) Stone, V.E. (2001). Strategies for
optimizing adherence to highly active anti-retroviral therapy; lessons from
research and clinical practice. *Clin. Infect. Dis.*, *33*, 865–872.

13. (a) Tung, R.D., Hale, M.R., Baker, C.T., Furfine, E.S., Kaldor, I., Kazmierski, W.W.,
Spaltenstein, A. (1999). Patent Application WO 9933815-A1.; (b) Baker, C.T.,
Chaturvedi, P.R., Hale, M.R., Bridson, G., Heiser, A., Furfine, E.S., Spaltenstein,
A., Tung, R.D. (1999). Discovery of VX-175/GW433908, A Novel, Water-Soluble
Prodrug of Amprenavir. Abstract 916. *The 39th Interscience Conference on Anti-
microbial Agents and Chemotherapy*. San Francisco, CA.

14. Wire, M.B., Shelton, M.J., Studenberg, S. (2006). Fosamprenavir: Clinical pharmacokinetics and drug interactions of the amprenavir analog. *Clin. Pharmacokinet.*,
45, 137–168.

15. Highlights of Prescribing Information (Lexiva®). http://www.accessdata.fda.gov/
drugsatfda_docs/label/2011/021548s026,022116s010lbl.pdf

16. Re: Discontinuation of AGENERASE® (amprenavir) Oral Solution and 50 mg
Capsules in the US. http://www.fda.gov/downloads/Drugs/DrugSafety/
DrugShortages/ucm086035.pdf

17. (a) U.S. Food and Drug Administration. Search results from the "OB_Disc" table
for query on "021007". http://www.accessdata.fda.gov/scripts/cder/ob/docs/obdetail.
cfm?Appl_No=021007&TABLE1=OB_Disc.; (b) U.S. Food and Drug Administration. Search results from the "OB_Rx" table for query on "022116". http://
www.accessdata.fda.gov/scripts/cder/ob/docs/obdetail.cfm?Appl_No=022116&
TABLE1=OB_Rx.

18. Financial Data for Lexiva® (Fosamprenavir Calcium). Includes revenues for Agenerase (amprenavir; EN:205414) until 2009. https://integrity.thomson-pharma.com/integrity/xmlxsl/pk_com_list.showProductSalesResults?p_entryNumber=285394

19. What Is ADHD or ADD? http://www.help4adhd.org/en/about/what

20. Voeller, K.K. (2004). Attention-deficit hyperactivity disorder (ADHD). *J. Child Neurol.*, *19*, 798–814.

21. Prous Science (2007). Lisdexamfetamine mesilate: Treatment of attention deficit hyperactivity disorder. *Drugs Future*, *32*, 223–227.

22. Mickle, T., Krishnan, S., Moncrief, J.S., Lauderback, C. (2005). Patent Application WO 2005032474-A2.

23. Mattingly, G. (2010). Lisdexamfetamine dimesylate: A prodrug stimulant for the treatment of ADHD in children and adults. *CNS Spectr.*, *15*, 315–325.

24. Boyle, L., Moncrief, S., Krishnan, S. (2006). Abstract II-3. *The 46th Annual New Clinical Drug Evaluation Unit (NCDEU) Meeting*. Boca Raton, FL.

25. FDA Approval History of Vyvanse®. Applied search using the term "vyvanse" on January 13, 2012. http://www.accessdata.fda.gov/scripts/cder/drugsatfda/index.cfm

26. Foley, S. (2006-08-16). Shire in deal with Barr to delay launch of rival to its ADHD drug. *London: The Independent*: http://www.independent.co.uk/news/business/news/shire-in-deal-with-barr-to-delay-launch-of-rival-to-its-adhd-drug-412102.html

27. Sandoz looks to market generic Vyvanse®. http://www.drugstorenews.com/article/sandoz-looks-market-generic-vyvanse

28. Thomson Reuters. https://integrity.thomson-pharma.com/integrity/xmlxsl/pk_com_list.showProductSalesResults?p_entryNumber=377425. Copyright 2012, Prous Science.

29. Campion, M.E., Gan, T.J. (2009). Fospropofol disodium for sedation. *Drugs Today*, *45*, 567–576.

30. (a) Gan, T.J. (2006). Pharmacokinetic and pharmacodynamic characteristics of medications used for moderate sedation. *Clin. Pharmacokinet.*, *45*, 855–869.; (b) Skues, M.A., Prys-Roberts, C. (1989). The pharmacology of propofol. *J. Clin. Anesth.*, *1*, 387–400.

31. Trapani, G., Altomare, C., Sanna, E., Biggio, G., Liso, G. (2000). Propofol in anesthesia. Mechanism of action, structure-activity relationships, and drug delivery. *Curr. Med. Chem.*, *7*, 249–271.

32. Fowler, C.J. (2004). Possible involvement of the endocannabinoid system in the actions of three clinically used drugs. *Trends Pharmacol. Sci.*, *25*, 59–61.

33. Haeseler, G., Leuwer, M. (2003). High-affinity block of voltage-operated rat IIA neuronal sodium channels by 2,6 di-tert-butylphenol, a propofol analogue. *Eur. J. Anaesthesiol.*, *20*, 220–224.

34. Lubarsky, D.A., Candiotti, K., Harris, E. (2007). Understanding modes of moderate sedation during gastrointestinal procedures: A current review of the literature. *J. Clin. Anesth.*, *19*, 397–404.

35. Rex, D.K. (2004). The science and politics of propofol. *Am. J. Gastroenterol.*, *99*, 2080–2083.

36. Fechner, J., Schwilden, H., Schuttler, J. (2008). Pharmacokinetics and pharmaco-dynamics of GPI 15715 or fospropofol (Aquavan injection)—A water soluble propofol prodrug. *Handb. Exp. Pharmacol.*, *182*, 253–266.

37. Propofol Update. http://www.trends-in-medicine.com/April2003/Propofol043p.pdf

38. Yavas, S., Lizdas, D., Gravenstein, N., Lampotang, S. (2008). Interactive web simulation for propofol and fospropofol, a new prodrug. *Anesth. Analg.*, *106*, 880–883.

39. Valerie Jensen, V., Rappaport, B.A. (2010). The reality of drug shortages—The case of the injectable agent propofol. *N. Engl. J. Med.*, *363*, 806–807.

40. U.S. Food and Drug Administration. Search results from the "OB_Rx" table for query on "022244". http://www.accessdata.fda.gov/scripts/cder/ob/docs/obdetail. cfm?Appl_No=022244&TABLE1=OB_Rx.

41. Owen, R.T. (2010). Paliperidone palmitate injection: Its efficacy, safety and toler-ability in schizophrenia. *Drugs Today*, *46*, 463–471.

42. Boom, S., Talluri, K., Janssens, L., Remmerie, B., De Meulder, M., Rossenu, S., van Osselaer, N., Eerdekens, M., Cleton, A. (2009). Single- and multiple-dose pharma-cokinetics and dose proportionality of the psychotropic agent paliperidone extended release. *J. Clin. Pharmacol.*, *49*, 1318–1330.

43. Nasrallah, H. (2007). The case for long-acting antipsychotics in the post CATIE era. *Acta Psychiatr. Scand.*, *115*, 260–267.

44. Pandina, G., Lane, R., Gopal, S., Gassman-Mayer, C., Hough, D., Remmerie, B., Simpson, G. (2009). Abstract 202. *The 48th Annual Meeting of the American College of Neuropsycopharmacology*. Hollywood, FL.

45. Highlights for Prescribing Information (Invega® Sustenna®). http://www. accessdata.fda.gov/drugsatfda_docs/label/2011/022264s002lbl.pdf

46. Merlino, G., Serafini, A., Lorenzut, S., Sommaro, M., Gigli, G.L., Valente, M. (2010). Gabapentin enacarbil in restless leg syndrome. *Drugs Today*, *46*, 3–11.

47. (a) Eroglu, Ç., Allen, N.J., Susman, M.W., O'Rourke, N.A., Park, C.Y., Özkan, E., Chakraborty, C., Mulinyawe, S.B., Annis, D.S., Huberman, A.D., Green, E.M., Lawler, J., Dolmetsch, R., Garcia, K.C., Smith, S.J., Luo, Z.D., Rosenthal, A., Mosher, D.F., Barres, B.A. (2009). Gabapentin receptor $\alpha 2\delta$-1 is a neuronal throm-bospondin receptor responsible for excitatory CNS synaptogenesis. *Cell*, *139*, 380–392.; (b) Hendrich, J., Minh, A.T.V., Heblich, F., Nieto-Rostro, M., Watschinger, K., Striessnig, J., Wratten, J., Davies, A., Dolphin, A.C. (2008). Pharmacological disruption of calcium channel trafficking by the alpha2delta ligand gabapentin. *Proc. Natl. Acad. Sci. U.S.A.*, *105*, 3628–3633.; (c) Davies, A., Hendrich, J., Minh, A.T.V., Wratten, J., Douglas, L., Dolphin, A.C. (2007). Func-tional biology of the alpha(2)delta subunits of voltage-gated calcium channels. *Trends Pharmacol. Sci.*, *28*, 220–228.

48. Cundy, K.C., Branch, R., Chernov-Rogan, T., Dias, T., Estrada, T., Hold, K., Koller, K., Liu, X., Man, A., Panuwat, M., Raillard, S.P., Upadhyay, S., Wu, Q.Q., Xiang, J.-N., Yan, H., Zerangue, N., Zhou, C.X., Barrett, R.W., Gallop, M.A. (2004). XP13512 [(+/-)-1-([a-isobutanoyloxyethoxy)carbonyl]aminomethyl)-1-cyclohexane acetic acid], a novel gabapentin prodrug: I. Design, synthesis, enzy-matic conversion to gabapentin, and transport by intestinal solute transporters. *J. Pharmacol. Exp. Ther.*, *311*, 315–323.

49. Cundy, K.C., Sastry, S., Luo, W., Zou, J., Moors, T.L., Canafax, D.M. (2008). Clinical pharmacokinetics of XP13512, a novel transported prodrug of gabapentin. *J. Clin. Pharmacol.*, *48*, 1378–1388.

50. Highlights for Prescribing Information (Horizant®). http://www.accessdata.fda.gov/drugsatfda_docs/label/2011/022399s000lbl.pdf

51. Núñez, M.C., García-Rubiño, E., Conejo-García, A., Cruz-López, O., Kimatrai, M., Gallo, M.A., Espinosa, A., Campos, J.M. (2009). Homochiral drugs: A demanding tendency of the pharmaceutical industry. *Curr. Med. Chem.*, *16*, 2064–2074.

52. Hutt, A.J., Valentova, J. (2003). The chiral switch: Development of single enantiomer drugs from racemates. *Acta Facultatis Pharmaceuticae Universitatis Comenianae* 7–23.

53. Strong, M. (1999). FDA policy and regulation of stereoisomers: Paradigm shift and the future of safer more effective drugs. *Food Drug Law J.*, *54*, 463–487.

54. U.S. Food and Drug Administration. FDA's policy statement for the development of new stereoisomeric drugs. http://www.fda.gov/Drugs/GuidanceComplianceRegulatoryInformation/Guidances/ucm122883.htm. U.S. Food and Drug Administration [online] (cited Jun 15. 2011).

55. Agranat, I., Caner, H., Caldwell, J. (2002). Putting chirality to work: The strategy of chiral switches. *Nat. Rev. Drug Discov.*, *1*, 753–768.

56. Hirschowitz, B.I. (1994). Medical management of esophageal reflux. *Yale J. Biol. Med.*, *67*, 223–231.

57. Olbe, L., Carlsson, E., Lindberg, P. (2003). A proton-pump inhibitor expedition: The case histories of omeprazole and esomeprazole. *Nat. Rev. Drug Discov.*, *2*, 132–139.

58. Abelö, A., Andersson, T.B., Antonsson, M., Naudot, A.K., Skånberg, I., Weidolf, L. (2000). Stereoselective metabolism of omeprazole by human cytochrome P450 enzymes. *Drug Metab. Dispos.*, *28*, 966–972.

59. Andersson, T., Röhss, K., Bredberg, E., Hassan-Alin, M. (2001). Pharmacokinetics and pharmacodynamics of esomeprazole the S-isomer of omeprazole. *Aliment. Pharmacol. Ther.*, *15*, 1563–1569.

60. Tybring, G., Böttiger, Y., Widén, J., Bertilsson, L. (1997). Enantioselective hydroxylation of omeprazole catalyzed by CYP2C19 in Swedish white subjects. *Clin. Pharmacol. Ther.*, *62*, 129–137.

61. Röhss, K., Hasselgren, G., Hedenström, H. (2002). Effect of esomeprazole 40 mg versus omeprazole 40 mg on 24-hour intragastric pH in patients with symptoms of gastroesophageal reflux disease. *Dig. Dis. Sci.*, *47*, 954–958.

62. Prous Science (2001). Esomeprazole Magnesium Nexium®. *Drugs Future*, *26*, 1108–1112.

63. Thomson Reuters. https://integrity.thomson-pharma.com/integrity/xmlxsl/pk_com_list.showProductSalesResults?p_entryNumber=272598. Copyright 2012, Prous Science.

64. Schmitt, C., Lightdale, C.J., Hwang, C. (2006). A multicenter, randomized, double-blind, 8-week comparative trial of standard doses of esomeprazole (40 mg) and omeprazole (20 mg) for the treatment of erosive esophagitis. *Dig. Dis. Sci.*, *51*, 844–850.

65. Kuipers, E.J. (1997). Helicobacter pylori and the risk and management of associated diseases: Gastritis, gastric ulcer, atrophic gastritis and gastric cancer. *Aliment. Pharmacol. Ther.*, *11*(Suppl), 71–88.

66. Huang, J.-Q., Sridhar, S., Hunt, R.H. (2002). Role of *Helicobacter pylori* infection and non-steroidal anti-inflammatory drugs in peptic-ulcer disease: A meta-analysis. *Lancet, 359*, 14–22.

67. Anagnostopoulos, G.K., Tsiakos, S., Margantinis, G., Kostopoulos, P., Arvaitidis, D. (2004). Esomeprazole versus omeprazole for the eradication of *Helicobacter pylori* infection. *J. Clin. Gastroenterol., 38*, 503–506.

68. Subei, I.M., Cardona, H.J., Bachelet, E., Useche, E., Arigbabu, A., Hammour, A.A., Miller, T. (2006). One week of esomeprazole triple therapy versus 1 week of omeprazole triple therapy plus 3 weeks of omeprazole for uodenal ulcer healing in *Helicobacter pylori*-positive patients. *Dig. Dis. Sci., 52*, 1505–1512.

69. Gladwell, M. (2004). High prices: How to hink about prescription drugs. *The New Yorker*, http://www.newyorker.com/archive/2004/10/25/041025crat_atlarge?currentPage=all, retrieved July 15, 2011

70. National Institute of Neurological Disorders and Stroke Information page on Attention Deficit-Hyperactivity Disorder http://www.ninds.nih.gov/disorders/adhd/adhd.htm

71. Volkow, N.D., Wang, G.J., Kollins, S.H., Wigal, T.L., Newcorn, J.H., Telang, F., Fowler, J.S., Zhu, W., Logan, J., Ma, Y., Pradhan, K., Wong, C., Swanson, J.M. (2009). Evaluating dopamine reward pathway in ADHD. *JAMA, 302*, 1084–1091.

72. Panizzon, L. (1944). La preparazione di piridil- e piperidil-arilacetonitrili e di alcuni prodotti di trasformazione (Parte Ia). *Helv. Chim. Acta, 27*, 1748–1756.

73. Meier, R., Gross, F., Tripod, J. (1954). Ritalin, a new synthetic compound with specific analeptic components. *Klin. Wochenschr., 32*, 445–450.

74. International Narcotics Control Board (2003) Green List: Annex to the Annual Statistical Report on Psychotropic Substances (form P). International Narcotics Board, Vienna International Centre.

75. Volkow, N.D., Wang, G.J., Fowler, J.S., Ding, Y.S. (2005). Imaging the effects of methylphenidate on brain dopamine: New model on its therapeutic actions for attention-deficit/hyperactivity disorder. *Biol. Psychiatry, 57*, 1410–1415.

76. Axton, J.M., Ivy, R., Krim, L., Winkler, J.D. (1999). Enantioselective synthesis of D-threo-Methylphenidate. *J. Am. Chem. Soc., 121*, 6511–6512.

77. Markowitz, J.S., Patrick, K.S. (2008). Differential pharmacokinetics and pharmacodynamics of methylphenidate enantiomers. Does chirality matter? *J. Clin. Psychopharmacol., 28*(3, Suppl 2), S54–S61.

78. Ding, Y.S., Fowler, J.S., Volkow, N.D., Dewey, S.L. (1997). Chiral drugs: Comparison of the pharmacokinetics of [11C]-d-threo and [11C]-l-threo-methylphenidate in the human and baboon brain. *Psychopharmacology, 131*, 71–78.

79. Ding, Y.-S., Gatley, S.J., Thanos, P.K., Shea, C., Garza, V., Xu, Y., Carter, P., King, P., Warner, D., Taintor, N.B., Park, D.J., Pyatt, B., Fowler, J.S., Volkow, N.D. (2004). Brian kinetics of methylphenidate (Ritalin) enantiomers after oral adminstration. *Synapse, 53*, 168–175.

80. Quinn, D. (2008). Does chirality matter? Pharmacodynamics of enantiomers of methylphenidate in patients with attention-deficit/hyperactivity disorder. *J. Clin. Psychopharmacol., 28*(3, Suppl 2), S62–S66.

81. Weiss, M., Wasdell, M., Patin, J. (2004). A post hoc analysis of d-threo-methylphenidate hydrochloride (Focalin) versus d,l-threo-methylphenidate hydrochloride (Ritalin). *J. Am. Acad. Child Adolesc. Psychiatry, 43*, 1145–1421.

82. World Health Organization Site http://www.who.int/mental_health/management/ depression/definition/en/

83. Hirschfeld, R.M.A. (2000). Antidepressants in long-term therapy: A review of tricyclic antidepressants and selective serotonin reuptake inhibitors. *Acta Psychiatr. Scand.*, *101*(Suppl 403), 35–38.

84. Nutt, D.J. (2008). Relationship of neurotransmitters to the symptoms of major depressive disorder. *J. Clin. Psychiatry*, *69*(Suppl E1), 4–7.

85. Maletic, V., Robinson, M., Oakes, T., Iyengar, S., Ball, S.G., Russell, J. (2007). Neurobiology of depression: An integrated view of key findings. *Int. J. Clin. Pract.*, *61*, 2030–2040.

86. Vaidya, V.A., Duman, R.S. (2001). Depresson—Emerging insights from neurobiology. *Br. Med. Bull.*, *57*, 61–79.

87. Tang, S.W., Helmeste, D.M., Leonard, B.E. (2010). Antidepressant compounds: A critical review. *Mod. Trends Pharmacopsychiatry*, *27*, 1–19.

88. Prous Science (2001). Escitalopram oxalate. *Drugs Future*, *26*, 115–120.

89. Chen, F., Larsen, M.B., Sanchez, C., Wiborg, O. (2005). The (S)-enantiomer of R,S-citalopram, increases inhibitor binding to the human serotonin transporter by an allosteric mechanism. Comparison with other serotonin transporter inhibitors. *Eur. Neuropsychopharmacol.*, *15*, 193–198.

90. Mansari, M.E., Wiberg, O., Mnie-Filali, O., Benturquia, N., Sanchez, C., Haddjeri, N. (2007). Allosteric modulation of the effect of escitalopram, paroxetine and fluoxetine: In-vitro and in-vivo studies. *Int. J. Neuropsychopharmacol.*, *10*, 31–40.

91. Kennedy, S.H., Andersen, H.F., Thase, M.E. (2009). Escitalopram in the treatment of major depressive disorder: A metaanalysis. *Curr. Med. Res. Opin.*, *25*, 161–175.

92. Yevtushenko, V.Y., Belous, A.I., Yevtushenko, Y.G., Gusinin, S.E., Buzik, O.J., Agibalova, T.V. (2007). Efficacy and tolerability of escitalopram versus citalopram in major depressive disorder: A 6-week multicenter, prospective, randomized, double-blind, active-controllwed study in adult outpatients. *Clin. Ther.*, *29*, 2319–2332.

93. Dykewicz, M.S., Hamilos, D.L. (2010). Rhinitis and sinusitis. *J. Allergy Clin. Immunol.*, *125*(2 Suppl 2), S103–S115.

94. Criado, P.R., Criado, R.F., Maruta, C.W., Machado, F.C. (2010). Histamine, histamine receptors and antihistamines: New concepts. *An. Bras. Dermatol.*, *85*, 195–210.

95. Day, J.H., Ellis, A.K., Rafeiro, E. (2004). Levocetirizine—A new and selective H1 receptor antagonist for use in allergic disorders. *Drugs Today*, *40*, 415–421.

96. Wang, D.Y., Hanotte, F., De Vos, C., Clement, P. (2001). Effect of cetirizine, levocetirizine, and dextrocetirizine on histamine-induced nasal response in healthy adult volunteers. *Allergy*, *56*, 339–343.

97. Devalia, J.L., De Vos, C., Hanotte, F., Baltes, E. (2001). A randomized, double-blind, crossover comparison among cetirizine, levocetirizine, and ucb-28557 on histamine-induced cutaneous responses in healthy adult volunteers. *Allergy*, *56*, 50–57.

98. Hunter, J.M. (1995). New neuromuscular blocking drugs. *N. Engl. J. Med.*, *332*, 1691–1699.

99. Zhang, M.-Q. (2003). Drug-specific cyclodextrins: The future of rapid neuromuscular block reversal? *Drugs Future*, *28*, 347–354.

100. Hughes, R. (1986). Atracurium: An overview. *Br. J. Anaesth.*, *58*(6 Suppl 1), 2S–5S.

101. Stenlake, J.B., Waigh, R.D., Urwin, J., Dewar, G.H., Coker, G.G. (1983). Atracurium: Conception and inception. *Br. J. Anaesth.*, *55*(Suppl 1), 3S–10S.

102. Basta, S.J., Ali, H.H., Savarese, J.J., Sunder, N., Gionfriddo, M., Cloutier, G., Lineberry, C., Cato, A.E. (1982). Clinical pharmacology of atracurium besylate (BW 33A): A new non-depolarizing muscle relaxant. *Anesth. Analg.*, *61*, 723–729.

103. Stenlake, J.B., Waigh, R.D., Dewar, G.H., Dhar, N.C., Hughes, R., Chapple, D.J., Lindon, J.C., Ferrige, A.G. (1984). Biodegradable neuromuscular blocking agents. Part 6. Stereochemical studies on atracurium and related polyalkylene di-esters. *Eur. J. Med. Chem.*, *19*, 441–450.

104. Bryson, H.M., Faulds, D. (1997). Cisatracurium besilate. A review of its pharmacology and clinical potential in anaesthetic practice. *Drugs*, *53*, 848–866.

105. Schramm, W.M., Papousek, A., Michalek-Sauberer, A., Czech, T., Illievich, U. (1998). The cerebral and cardiovascular effects of cisatracurium and atracurium in neurosurgical patients. *Anesth. Analg.*, *86*, 123–127.

106. Sorbera, L.A., Graul, A., Castañer, J. (1998). Levobupivacaine. *Drugs Future*, *23*, 838–842.

107. Vanhoutte, F., Vereecke, J., Verbeke, N., Carmeliet, E. (1991). Stereoselective effects of the enantiomers of bupivacaine on the electrophysiological properties of guinea-pig papillary muscle. *Br. J. Pharmacol.*, *103*, 1275–1281.

108. Denson, D.D., Behbehani, M.M., Gregg, R.V. (1992). Enantiomer specific effects of an intravenously administered arrhythmogenic dose of bupivacaine on neurons of the nucleus tractus solitaries and cardiovascular system in the anesthized rat. *Reg. Anesth.*, *17*, 311–316.

109. Ngamprasertwong, P., Udomtecha, D., Charuluxananan, S., Rodanant, O., Srihatajati, C., Baogham, S. (2005). Levobupivacaine versus racemic bupivacaine for extradural anesthesia for cesarean delivery. *J. Med. Assoc. Thai.*, *88*, 1563–1568.

110. Li-Zhong, W., Xiang-Yang, C., Xia, L., Xiao-Xia, H., Bei-Lei, T. (2010). Comparison of bupivacaine, ropivacaine, levobupivacaine with sufentanil for patient-controlled epidural analgesia during labor: A randomized clinical trial. *Chin. Med. J.*, *123*, 178–183.

111. Fattorini, F., Ricci, Z., Rocco, A., Romano, R., Pascarella, M.A., Pinto, G. (2006). Levobupivacaine versus racemic bupivacaine for spinal anaesthesia in orthopaedic major surgery. *Minerva Anestesiol.*, *72*, 637–644.

112. Erbay, R.H., Ennumcu, O., Hanci, V., Atalay, H. (2010). A comparison of spinal anesthesia with low dose hyperbaric levobupivacaine and hyperbaric bupivacaine for transurethral surgery: A randomized controlled trial. *Minerva Anestesiol.*, *76*, 992–1001.

113. Tanaka, P.P., Ogleari, M., Valmorbida, P., Tanaka, M.A. (2005). Levobupivacaine 0.5%, 50% enantiomeric excess bupivacaine, and racemic bupivacaine in epidural anesthesia for lower abdominal procedures. Comparative study. *Rev. Bras. Anestesiol.*, *55*, 597–605.

114. Schoenheimerand, R., Rittenberg, D. (1940). The study of intermediary metabolism of animals with the aid of isotopes. *Physiol. Rev.*, *20*, 218–248.

115. Baillie, T.A. (1981). The use of stable isotopes in pharmacological research. *Pharmacol. Rev.*, *33*, 81–132.

116. Blake, M.I., Crespi, H.L., Katz, J.J. (1975). Studies with deuterated drugs. *J. Pharm. Sci.*, *64*, 367–391.

117. Foster, A.B. (1985). Deuterium isotope effects in the metabolism of drugs and xenobiotics: Implications for drug design. *Adv. Drug Res.*, *14*, 1–40.

118. Kahan, F.M. (2009). A deuterated drug that almost succeeded. *Chem. Eng. News*, *87*, 4.

119. Urey, H.C., Brickwedde, F.C., Murphy, G.M. (1932). A hydrogen isotope of mass 2. *Phys. Rev.*, *39*, 164–165.

120. Wiberg, K.B. (1955). The deuterium isotope effect. *Chem. Rev.*, *55*, 713–743.

121. Nelson, S.D., Trager, W.F. (2003). The use of deuterium isotope effects to probe the active site properties, mechanism of cytochrome P450-catalyzed reactions, and mechanisms of metabolically dependent toxicity. *Drug Metab. Dispos.*, *31*, 1481–1498.

122. Fisher, M.B., Henne, K.R., Boer, J. (2006). The complexities inherent in attempts to decrease drug clearance by blocking sites of CYP-mediated metabolism. *Curr. Opin. Drug Discov. Devel.*, *9*, 101–109.

123. Jenks, W.P. (1987). *Catalysis in Chemistry and Enzymology*. Mineola, NY: Dover Publications Inc.; 243–279.

124. Northrop, D.B. (1975). Steady-state analysis of kinetic isotope effects in enzymic reactions. *Biochemistry*, *14*, 2644–2651.

125. Bell, R.P. (1974). Liversidge lecture. Recent advances in the study of kinetic hydrogen isotope effects. *Chem. Soc. Rev.*, *3*, 513–544.

126. Krauser, J.A., Guengerich, F.P. (2005). Cytochrome P450 3A4-catalyzed testosterone 6beta-hydroxylation stereochemistry, kinetic deuterium isotope effects, and rate-limiting steps. *J. Biol. Chem.*, *280*, 19496–19506.

127. Mutlib, A.E., Gerson, R.J., Meunier, P.C., Haley, P.J., Chen, H., Gan, L.S., Davies, M.H., Gemzik, B., Christ, D.D., Krahn, D.F., Markwalder, J.A., Seitz, S.P., Robertson, R.T., Miwa, G.T. (2000). The species-dependent metabolism of efavirenz produces a nephrotoxic glutathione conjugate in rats. *Toxicol. Appl. Pharmacol.*, *169*, 102–113.

128. Ling, K.J., Hanzlik, R.P. (1989). Deuterium isotope effects on toluene metabolism. Product release as a rate-limiting step in cytochrome P-450 catalysis. *Biochem. Biophys. Res. Commun.*, *169*, 844.

129. Meunier, B., de Visser, S.P., Shaik, S. (2004). Mechanism of oxidation reactions catalyzed by cytochrome P450 enzymes. *Chem. Rev.*, *104*, 3947–3980.

130. Kushner, D.J., Baker, A., Dunstall, T.G. (1999). Pharmacological use and perspectives of heavy water and deuterated compounds. *Can. J. Physiol. Pharmacol.*, *77*, 79–88.

131. Shao, L., Hewitt, M.C. (2010). The kinetic isotope effect in the search for deuterated drugs. *Drug News Perspect.*, *23*, 398–404.

132. Buteau, K.C. (2009). Deuterated drugs: Unexpectedly nonobvious? *J. High Tech. L.*, *10*, 22–72.

133. Di Costanzo, L., Moulin, M., Haertlein, M., Meilleur, F., Christianson, D.W. (2007). Expression, purification, assay, and crystal structure of perdeuterated human arginase I. *Arch. Biochem. Biophys.*, *465*, 82–89.

134. Tayar, N.E., Waterbeemd, H.V.D., Gryllaki, M., Testa, B., Trager, W.F. (1984). The lipophilicity of deuterium atoms. A comparison of shake-flask and HPLC methods. *Int. J. Pharm.*, *19*, 271–281.

135. Turowski, M., Yamakawa, N., Metier, J., Kimata, K., Ikegami, T., Hosoya, K., Tanaka, N., Thornton, E.R. (2003). Deuterium isotope effects on hydrophobic interactions: The importance of dispersion interactions in the hydrophobic phase. *J. Am. Chem. Soc.*, *125*, 13836–13849.

136. Perrin, C.L., Dong, Y. (2007). Secondary deuterium isotope effects on acidity of carboxylic acids and phenols. *J. Am. Chem. Soc.*, *129*, 4490–4497.

137. Perrin, C.L., Ohta, B.K., Liberman, J., Erdelyi, M. (2005). Stereochemistry of beta-deuterium isotope effects on amine basicity. *J. Am. Chem. Soc.*, *127*, 9641–9647.

138. Schneider, F., Mattern-Dogru, E., Hillgenberg, M., Alken, R.-G. (2007). Changed phosphodiesterase selectivity and enhanced in vitro efficacy by selective deuteration of sildenafil. *Arzneim. Forsch., Drug. Res.*, *57*, 293–298.

139. Ruszczycky, M.W., Anderson, V.E. (2006). Interpretation of V/K isotope effects for enzymatic reactions exhibiting multiple isotopically sensitive steps. *J. Theor. Biol.*, *243*, 328.

140. Lewis, B.E., Schramm, V.L. (2006). *Isotope Effects in Chemistry and Biology*, eds. Kohen, A., Limbach, H.-H., Boca Raton, FL: CRC Taylor & Francis; 1019.

141. Schramm, V.L. (2007). Binding isotope effects: Boon and bane. *Curr. Opin. Chem. Biol.*, *11*, 529.

142. Morales, A.J., Gallegos, R., Uttamsingh, V., Cheng, C., Harbeson, S., Zelle, R., Tung, R., Wells, D. (2008). Increased in vitro metabolic stability and in vivo exposure in rats of presicion-deuterated indiplon. Abstract 285. *The 15th North American Meeting of the International Society of Xenobiotics*. San Diego, CA.

143. Morales, A., Wells, D., Tung, R., Zelle, R., Cheng, C., Harbeson, S. (2008). Pharmacokinetic characterization of a deuterated oxazolidinone in chimpanzees. Abstract A-990. *48th Annual Interscience Conference on Antimicrobial Agents and Chemotherapy (ICAAC) and the 46th Annual Meeting of the Infectious Diseases Society of America (IDSA)*. Washington, DC.

144. Reyataz [package insert] Bristol-Myers Squibb Company, Princeton, NJ; February 2011 http://www.accessdata.fda.gov/drugsatfda_docs/label/2011/021567s025lbl.pdf

145. Colombo, S., Buclin, T., Cavassini, M., Decosterd, L.A., Telenti, A., Biollaz, J., Csajka, C. (2006). Population pharmacokinetics of atazanavir in patients with human immunodeficiency virus infection. *Antimicrob. Agents Chemother.*, *50*, 3801–3808.

146. Norvir [package insert] Abbott Laboratories, North Chicago, IL; April 2010 http://www.accessdata.fda.gov/drugsatfda_docs/label/2010/020659s050,022417s001lbl.pdf

147. Anderson, P.L., Aquilante, C.L., Gardner, E.M., Predhomme, J., McDaneld, P., Bushman, L.R., Zheng, J.-H., Ray, M., Mawhinney, S. (2009). Atazanavir pharmacokindetics in genetically determined CYP3A5 expressors versus non-expressors. *J. Antimicrob. Chemother.*, *64*, 1071–1079.

148. Horberg, M., Klein, D., Hurley, L., Silverberg, M., Towner, W., Antoniskis, D., Kovach, D., Mogyoros, M., Blake, W., Dobrinich, R., Dodge, W. (2008). Efficacy and safety of ritonavir-boosted and unboosted atazanavir among antiretroviral-naïve patients. *HIV Clin. Trials*, *9*, 367–374.

149. Gonzalez De Requena, D., Bonora, S., Canta, F., Avolio, A.D., Sciandra, M., Milia, M., DiGarbo, A., Sinicco, A., DiPerri, G. (2005). Atazanavir Ctrough is

associated with efficacy and safety: Definition of therapeutic range. *12th Conference on Retroviruses and Opportunistic Infections 2005*, poster 645.

150. Shafran, S.D., Mashinter, L.D., Roberts, S.E. (2005). The effect of low-dose ritonavir monotherapy on fasting serum lipid concentrations. *HIV Med.*, *6*, 421–425.

151. Yarnell, A. (2009). Heavy-hydrogen drugs turn heads, again. *Chem. Eng. News*, *87*, 36–39.

152. Harbeson, S.L., Tung, R.D. (2009). *Patent Application US* 2009/0036357-A1.

153. Yokohama, T., Fukuda, K.-I., Mori, S., Ogawa, M., Nagasawa, K. (1992). Determination of tolperisome enantiomers in plasma and their disposition in rats. *Chem. Pharm. Bull.*, *40*, 272–274.

154. Quasthoff, S., Mockel, C., Zieglgansberger, W., Schreibmayer, W. (2008). Tolperisone: A typical representative of a class of centrally acting muscle relaxants with less sedative side effects. *CNS Neurosci. Ther.*, *14*, 107–119.

155. Dalmadi, B., Leibinger, J., Szeberenyi, S., Borbas, T., Farkas, S., Szombathelyi, Z., Tihanyi, K. (2003). Identification of metabolic pathways involved in the biotransformation of tolperisone by human microsomal enzymes. *Drug Metab. Dispos.*, *31*, 631–636.

156. Wojtczak, A., Rychlik-Sych, M., Krochmalska-Ulacha, E., Skretkowicz, J. (2007). CYP2D6 phenotyping with dextromethorphan. *Pharmacol. Rep.*, *59*, 734–738.

157. Bae, J.W., Kim, M.J., Park, Y.S., Myung, C.S., Jang, C.G., Lee, S.Y. (2007). Considerable interindividual variation in the pharmacokinetics of tolperisone HCl. *Int. J. Clin. Pharmacol. Ther.*, *45*, 110–113.

158. http://www.d4pharma.com

159. http://www.birdspharma.com/projects/bdd_10103

160. Aiken, R.-G. (2004). *Patent Application US* 2004/0186136-A1.

161. Effexor XR [package insert] Wyeth Pharmaceuticals, Inc., Philadelphia, PA; June 2009. http://www.accessdata.fda.gov/drugsatfda_docs/label/2010/020699s090lbl.pdf

162. Kaplan, M., Mahon, S., Cope, D., Keating, E., Hill, S., Jacobson, M. (2011). Putting evidence into practice: Evidence-based interventions for hot flashes resulting from cancer therapies. *Clin. J. Oncol. Nurs.*, *15*, 149–157.

163. Pachman, D.R., Jones, J.M., Loprinzi, C.L. (2010). Management of menopause-associated vasomotor symptoms: Current treatment options, challenges and future directions. *Int. J. Womens Health*, *2*, 123–135.

164. Eardley, W., Toth, C. (2010). An open-label, non-randomized comparison of venlafaxine and gabapentin as monotherapy or adjuvant therapy in the management of neuropathic pain in patients with peripheral neuropathy. *J. Pain Res.*, *3*, 33–49.

165. Lee, Y.-C., Chen, P.-P. (2010). A review of SSRIs and SNRIs in neuropathic pain. *Expert Opin. Pharmacother.*, *11*, 2813–2825.

166. Otton, S.V., Ball, S.E., Cheung, S.W., Inaba, T., Rudolph, R.L., Sellers, E.M. (1996). Venlafaxine oxidation in vitro is catalysed by CYP2D6. *Br. J. Clin. Pharmacol.*, *41*, 149–156.

167. Fukuda, T., Yamamoto, I., Nishida, Y., Zhou, Q., Ohno, M., Takada, K., Azuma, J. (1999). Effect of CYP2D6*10 genotype on venlafaxine pharmacokinetics in healthy adult volunteers. *J. Clin. Pharmacol.*, *47*, 450–453.

168. Pristiq [Package insert] Wyeth Pharmaceuticals, Inc., Philadelphia, PA; April 2011. http://www.accessdata.fda.gov/drugsatfda_docs/label/2011/021992s022lbl.pdf

169. http://www.auspexpharma.com/auspex_SD254.html

170. Wise, R., Andrews, J.M. (1984). In vitro activity of fludalanine combined with pentizidone compared with those of other agents. *Antimicrob. Agents Chemother.*, 25, 612–617.

171. Kollonitsch, J., Barash, L. (1976). Organofluorine synthesis via photofluorination: 3-fluoro-D-alanine and 2-deuterio analogue, antibacterials related to the bacterial cell wall. *J. Am. Chem. Soc.*, 98, 5591–5593.

172. Darland, G.K., Hajdu, R., Kropp, H., Kahan, F.M., Walker, R.W., Vandenheuvel, W.J. (1986). Oxidative and defluorinative metabolism of fludalanine, 2-2H-3-fluoro-D-alanine. *Drug Metab. Dispos.*, 14, 668–673.

173. Paxil CR [Package insert] GlaxoSmithKline, Research Triangle Park, NC; July 2011. http://www.accessdata.fda.gov/drugsatfda_docs/label/2011/020936s034s044lbl.pdf

174. Uttamsingh, V., Wells, D., Soergel, D., Zelle, R. (2009). Abstract 11552. *The 38th American College of Clinical Pharmacology*. San Antonio, TX.

175. Stearns, V., Slack, R., Greep, N., Henry-Tilman, R., Osbourne, M., Bunnell, C., Ulmer, L., Gallagher, A., Cullen, J., Gehan, E., Hayes, D.F., Issacs, C. (2005). Paroxetine is an effective treatment for hot flashes: Results from a prospective randomized clinical trial. *J. Clin. Oncol.*, 23, 6919–6930.

176. Wells, D.S., Gallegos, R., Uttamsingh, V., Cheng, C., Bridson, G., Masse, C., Harbeson, S.L., Graham, P.B., Zelle, R., Tung, R., Morales, A.J. (2008). Abstract P-4. *19th Annual Meeting of the North American Menopause Society (NAMS)*. Orlando, FL.

177. Wells, D., Soergel, D., Zelle, R. (2009). Abstract 164. *The 38th American College of Clinical Pharmacology*. San Antonio, TX.

178. Tung, R. (2010). *US Patent 7,687,914.*

179. Gallegos, R., Uttamsingh, V., Morales, A., Cheng, C., Bridson, G., Liu, J.F., Tung, R., Zelle, R., Harbeson, S., Wells, D.S. (2009). Abstract 188. *The 16th North American Meeting of the International Society of Xenobiotics*. Baltimore, MD.

180. Murray, M. (2000). Mechanisms of inhibitory and regulatory effects of methylenedioxyphenyl compounds on cytochrome P450-dependent drug oxidation. *Curr. Drug Metab.*, 1, 67–84.

181. Liston, H.L., DeVane, C.L., Boulton, D.W., Risch, S.C., Markowitz, J.S., Goldman, J. (2002). Differential time course of cytochrome P450 2D6 enzyme inhibition by fluoxetine, sertraline, and paroxetine in healthy volunteers. *J. Clin. Psychopharmacol.*, 22, 169–173.

182. Alfaro, C.L., Lam, Y.M., Simpson, J., Ereshefsky, L. (2000). CYP2D6 inhibition by fluoxetine, paroxetine, sertraline, and venlafaxine in a crossover study: Intraindividual variability and plasma concentration correlations. *J. Clin. Pharmacol.*, 40, 58–66.

ACADEMIC AND NONPROFIT INITIATIVES AND THE ROLE OF ALLIANCES IN THE DRUG REPOSITIONING INDUSTRY

■■■■ CHAPTER 11

Repurposing Drugs for Tropical Diseases: Case Studies and Open-Source Screening Initiatives

CURTIS R. CHONG

11.1. INTRODUCTION

The discovery of new drugs is time-consuming and expensive, factors that bias development against tropical diseases. Independent studies estimate the cost of new drug development to be $800 million [1, 2], a price that increases annually by 7.4% over inflation. As DiMasi's original study was performed in 2001 using data from the previous 25 years, the present cost of drug development is estimated at $1.9 billion per new drug [3]. Even with advances in high-throughput screening and genome-based target identification, the average time from discovery to approval has doubled since 1964, from 6.5 to 14.8 years. Only 0.1% of drug candidates that enter preclinical animal testing proceed to Phase I trials and only 21.5% of drugs that begin Phase II human trials make it to the market [4–6].

Most of the drugs currently used to treat tropical diseases[1] were developed during the colonial era in Africa [7]. With an average per capita health expenditure of less than $20 per year, developing countries do not comprise a large enough market to attract the pharmaceutical industry's interest

---

[1] Tropical diseases defined as parasitic diseases (malaria, African trypanosomiasis, Chagas' disease, schistosomiasis, leishmaniasis, lymphatic filariasis, onchocerciasis, intestinal nematode infections), leprosy, dengue, Japanese encephalitis, trachoma, infectious diarrheal diseases, and tuberculosis.

Drug Repositioning: Bringing New Life to Shelved Assets and Existing Drugs, First Edition.
Edited by Michael J. Barratt and Donald E. Frail.
© 2012 John Wiley & Sons, Inc. Published 2012 by John Wiley & Sons, Inc.

and resources [8]. Only 10% of pharmaceutical global research and development resources are targeted to diseases comprising 90% of the global health burden [9]. There is also almost no pharmaceutical research on an estimated 5000 rare diseases that account for 10% of the global illness burden [10].

For tropical diseases or diseases with small patient populations, pharmaceutical companies are often unwilling to invest in new drug development because a return on investment is unlikely [11]. Of the 1393 new, marketed drugs introduced between 1975 and 1999, only 13 were specifically developed for tropical diseases, which account for 11.4% of the global disease burden, and three for tuberculosis (TB) [8]. Of these 13 drugs, five came from veterinary research, two from military research, and two were new formulations of old products [12]. Only one of these thirteen drugs is widely used due to pricing issues [13]. In contrast, 390 out of the 1393 drugs (28%) developed during this period were for cardiovascular or central nervous system (CNS) diseases, and these drugs account for 35% of worldwide pharmaceutical sales [8].

Beginning in 2000, greater awareness of tropical diseases led to increased funding, which reached $2.5 billion per year in 2007 [14]. Between 2000 and 2009, 26 new products for tropical diseases were approved, of which 10 were for HIV/AIDS and 11 were for malaria [15]. Although this represents a 250% increase for malaria over the number of new approvals from 1975 to 1999, no new drugs for TB, dengue fever, trachoma, or rheumatic/typhoid/paratyphoid fevers have been approved in the past decade [15]. The future outlook is more promising with 19 tropical disease drugs and 74 vaccines in current development [15]. In addition to direct support from government and philanthropic agencies, incentives such as U.S. Food and Drug Administration (FDA) priority vouchers have been launched to encourage pharmaceutical industry research on tropical diseases [16].

Even for diseases of high interest to pharmaceutical companies, the success rate of Phase I–III clinical trials is also on the decline [3]. Despite an over 30-fold increase to $50 billion in research and development from 1977 to 2008, the number of new drugs approved by the FDA remains relatively flat at 15–30 per year [17]. Indeed, at the current rate of drug discovery it will take 380 years for the number of drugs in the world to double.

11.2. DRUG DEVELOPMENT FOR NEGLECTED DISEASES

Public–private partnerships (PPP) involving collaboration between for-profit pharmaceutical companies and nonprofit organizations and academia are one proposed strategy to accelerate drug discovery for tropical diseases. The first PPP established was the United Nations Development Program/ World Bank/World Health Organization Special Programme for Research and Training in Tropical Disease in 1975 [9]. Examples of drugs introduced through PPPs include praziquantel for schistosomiasis in 1980 with Bayer, ivermectin for onchoceriasis in 1987 with Merck, eflornithine for African trypanosomiasis in 1991 with Dow, miltefosine for visceral leishmaniasis in 2002 with Zentaris, artesunate and amodiaquine for malaria with Sanofi-Aventis in 2006, and chloroproguanil-dapsone for malaria in 2003 with Glaxo-SmithKline [9, 18].

In 2005 there were an estimated 92 PPPs with a combined budget of over $1 billion [13]. The majority of funding for most PPPs comes from one or two foundations [19]. These partnerships represent part of a $35 billion increase in spending to fight tropical diseases [20]. Current PPP projects focus on improving the efficacy and toxicity of established drugs, screening chemical and natural product libraries for activity against established targets or parasites directly, and identifying novel targets for drug discovery [21]. Typically, PPPs maintain a portfolio of drug development candidates that is overseen by an external review board of experts [9].

Of the 63 tropical disease projects underway at PPPs at end of 2004, 18 new products were in clinical trials, including 9 in Phase III [22]. Reflecting a reliance on industry collaboration, an estimated two-thirds of all PPP funding goes to drug companies [22]. Although the drug development costs and timelines for PPPs are significantly better than industry benchmarks, drug development through these mechanisms remain expensive and lengthy. Specifically, the cost for each new antimalarial is estimated at $100–300 million [21]. In addition, the PPPs suffer from high pipeline failure rates that are similar to industry attrition rates. For example, the Medicines for Malaria Venture has an attrition rate of more than 90% [23].

One strategy to address the critical barrier posed by the cost and lengthiness of new drug development is to identify existing drugs that act against diseases where there is a need for new drugs [24–27]. Historically, many antiparasitic drugs were first developed for other indications [21]. Folate antagonists, tetracycline antibiotics, and iron chelators were all developed to treat different diseases but are undergoing development for malaria [28].

Several recent reports have uncovered novel and unexpected properties of established drugs that make them useful in treating new diseases (Table 11.1). For example, the anticancer properties of the antiamebic drug fumagillin were serendipitously discovered after this compound was isolated as the inhibitory factor secreted by fungi contaminating an endothelial cell culture [29]. Clioquinol, another antiamebic, underwent Phase II clinical trials for the treatment of Alzheimer's disease after it was found to dissociate zinc-containing amyloid plaques [30]. Quinacrine, an antimalarial, inhibits prion formation and was selected for screening based on its ability to cross the blood–brain barrier [31]. The antimalarial properties of fosmidomycin, an inhibitor of bacterial isoprenoid synthesis originally developed to treat urinary tract infections, were identified based on the presence of homologous biosynthetic enzymes in the *Plasmodium falciparum* genome. Arsenic, one of the oldest drugs in the world, and retinoic acid, which is also used to treat acne, were found to be highly effective facilitators of apoptosis and differentiation of acute promyelocytic leukemia (PML) [32]. In each example, researchers found new uses for existing drugs based on the chemical properties of the compound, genomic approaches, or luck.

TABLE 11.1. Examples of Existing Drugs Used to Treat New Diseases

Drug	Original Disease	New Disease
Amphotericin	Antifungal *Interferes with fungal membranes by binding to cell membrane sterols*	Leishmaniasis
Arsenic	"Oldest drug in the world [32]" *Used in early 20th century to treat tuberculosis and syphilis*	Acute promyelocytic leukemia (PML) [32] *Degrades PML–retinoic acid receptor (RAR) fusion protein*
Ceftriaxone	Antibiotic *β-lactam inhibits bacterial cell wall synthesis*	Amyotrophic lateral sclerosis [192] *Increases glutamate transporter expression*
Dapsone	Leprosy [64] *Inhibits folic acid synthesis*	Malaria *Combined with chlorproguanil in LapDap; approved by UK for treatment of malaria [43]*
DB289	Pneumocystis [79]	Malaria and early stage African trypanosomiasis [79].
Eflornithine	Cancer *Suicide inhibitor of ornithine decarboxylase, blocking polyamine biosynthesis. Failed in clinical trials [260]*	African trypanosomes *Inhibits protozoan ornithine decarboxylase [260]*
Fosmidomycin	Urinary tract infections *Inhibits isoprenoid synthesis [261]*	Antimalarial *Nonmevalonate pathway of isoprenoid biosynthesis identified in P. falciparum using genomic techniques [64]. Currently in clinical trials alone and in combination with clindamycin [66, 262]*
Fumagillin	Antiamebic *Unknown mechanism.*	Anticancer angiogenesis inhibitor *Blocks endothelial cell growth by inhibiting type II methionine aminopeptidase [263]. TNP-470, a fumagillin analog, underwent Phase III clinical trials for brain, breast, cervical, and prostate cancer [264].*
Miltefosine	Cancer *May induce apoptosis by inhibiting lipid biosynthesis [265].*	Visceral leishmania *Registered for use in India in 2002 [102].*
Minocycline	Antibiotic *Blocks entry of the aminoacyl tRNA into the ribosome.*	Amyotrophic lateral sclerosis *Inhibits cytochrome C release from mitochondria. Delays disease onset and extends survival of ALS mice [209].*

TABLE 11.1. (*Continued*)

Drug	Original Disease	New Disease
Nonsteroidal anti-inflammatory	Anti-inflammatory *Cyclooxygenase inhibitor*	Alzheimer's disease *Reduce brain Aβ levels and amyloid plaque burden [216]*
Paromomycin	Amebicide [266] *Oligosaccharide antibiotic*	Visceral leishmaniasis [9] *Administered by injection*
Quinacrine	Antimalarial *Interferes with heme crystallization [222]*	Prion diseases *Potently inhibits prion formation [31]. Anecdotal reports of improvement in patients with Creutzfeldt-Jakob disease [267].*
Retinoic acid	Acne	Acute promyelocytic leukemia *Activates transcription of genes involved in differentiation [268]*
Serotonin receptor antagonists	Antipsychotic	Progressive multifocal leukoencephalopathy *Inhibit human polyomavirus (JCV) infection of glial cells [208]*
Thalidomide	Sedative *Potent teratogen*	Cancer [269] *Inhibits angiogenesis*

In addition to discovering new activity against a disease pathogen, screening a library of clinical compounds in combination with existing treatments can identify drugs that act synergistically or reverse resistance. The creation of new combination therapies will extend the lifespan of existing treatments and reduce the frequency of treatment failure. For example, chloroquine resistance in malaria is reversed by the antihypertensive drug verapamil and by antihistamines like chlorpheniramine [33–35]. Atovaquone and proguanil combined as the antimalarial Malarone are synergistic [36]. The combination of β-lactamase inhibitors such as sulbactam and tazobactam with piperacillin and ampicillin, respectively, creates a synergistic effect that expands the therapeutic spectrum to include β-lactamase-producing bacteria [37].

Existing drugs that have comprehensive safety packages can be particularly attractive candidates for repositioning studies. It is almost impossible to perform Phase IV studies to monitor post-marketing safety in the developing world. Costs for these studies, which are estimated to be $150 million per new drug in developed countries, will likely be even higher in countries that lack an established communications and healthcare infrastructure [1]. However, studies of existing drugs may also detect new properties that may contribute to toxicity or safety problems. For example, the hepatitis B drug entecavir was thought to be a poor inhibitor of HIV replication [38]; however, re-examination using a newer, whole cell infectivity assay revealed inhibition

1000-fold more potent [39]. This contributed to the observation that entecavir monotherapy in patients co-infected with HIV and hepatitis B led to accumulation of lamivudine-resistant HIV virus [39]. As a result of this study, entecavir is no longer recommended for use in co-infected patients [40]. The discovery of unexpected toxicities during clinical development of existing drugs for tropical diseases may create hesitation in industry to support such efforts [41].

The above caveats notwithstanding, drug repurposing offers a more cost-effective and rapid means to develop new treatments for tropical diseases. This chapter highlights a number of case studies of drugs repurposed for tropical diseases including amphotericin, miltefosine, and paromomycin for leishmaniasis, dapsone, fosmidomycin, and pafuramidine (DB289) for malaria, and eflornithine for trypanosomiasis. In addition, an overview is provided of efforts being led by academia in open-source screening of drug libraries for the purpose of drug repositioning, with emphasis on tropical diseases.

11.3. DRUG REPURPOSING IN MALARIA

11.3.1. Dapsone

The development and subsequent failure of the antileprosy drug dapsone as a novel treatment for uncomplicated malaria highlights how known side effects can derail a drug repurposing effort. In order to ensure safety, clinical trials need to be powered to detect rare, albeit significant known complications of existing drugs. This is especially true in the developing world, where Phase IV post-marketing surveillance studies are nearly impossible to conduct due to a lack of infrastructure.

Dapsone was first synthesized in Germany in 1908 as a dye and was tested in the 1930s as an antimicrobial due to similarities to sulfa antibiotics [42]. Dapsone is currently used to treat leprosy and is an antifolate that inhibits dihydropteroate synthetase [43]. The antimalarial properties of dapsone were noted in the 1940s but were eclipsed by the efficacy of quinine that was already in use [42, 44, 45]. A decade later, D. L. Leiker noted the absence of malaria in leprosy patients treated with dapsone in New Guinea [42]. During the Vietnam War the U.S. Army revived research on dapsone in malaria, including studies on subjects who were infected with chloroquine-resistant malaria [42, 46].

Dapsone was developed in combination with chlorproguanil (Lapdap) or chlorproguanil/artesunate by a PPP between GlaxoSmithline, the University of Liverpool, the World Health Organization (WHO), and the British Government [47]. This collaboration aimed to create a first-line treatment that was less expensive than artemesinin-related compounds and to replace sulfadoxine-pyrimethamine, which parasites are increasingly resistant to. The PPP aimed to price dapsone at less than $1 per tablet [48, 49]. Clinical trials in African children demonstrated dapsone/chlorproguanil was more effective than sulfadoxine-pyrimethamine [50]. Dapsone was also studied in combination with chlorproguanil/artesunate in Phase III trials on *P. falciparum* [51–53] and in combination with chlorproguanil on *Plasmodium vivax* [54].

One major complication to emerge from several of these trials was the development of anemia in glucose-6-phosphate dehydrogenase (G6PD) deficient patients, which has been attributed to hemolysis due to dapsone [55]. Dapsone is known to cause hemolytic anemia in up to 20% of patients being treated for leprosy [56], in a dose-dependent fashion, and this side effect in G6PD patients has been known since 1966 [57]. The N-hydroxy metabolite of dapsone is thought to contribute to lipid peroxidation and generation of reactive oxygen species [58]. Patients with G6PD deficiency are more susceptible to such oxidative stress because they have lower levels of the antioxidant glutathione, which is recycled from glutathione disulfide using nicotinamide adenine dinucleotide phosphate (NADPH) produced by the action of G6PD on glucose-6-phosphate [59]. G6PD deficiency is thought to play a protective role against malaria and its prevalence ranges between 4% and 28% in Africa [59]. Although some of the studies were not sufficiently powered to detect adverse outcomes in G6PD deficient patients [50], the frequency of this side effect in multiple trials led to withdrawal of chlorproguanil/dapsone by Glaxo-SmithKline in 2008 [55].

11.3.2. Fosmidomycin

Fosmidomycin is an antibiotic first isolated from *Streptomyces lavendulae* in the 1970s and was later found to inhibit 1-deoxy-D-xylulose 5-phosphate (DOXP) reductoisomerase, which is a metalloenzyme involved in the DOXP isoprenoid synthesis pathway [60–62]. In animals the mevalonate pathway is used to synthesize isoprenoids, whereas in algae, eubacteria, and plants the DOXP pathway is predominant. Fosmidomycin was originally developed by Fujisawa Pharmaceuticals as an antibiotic for urinary tract infections, but clinical translation was hampered by a half-life of approximately 2 hours after oral and intravenous dosing [63].

A genomic screen identified DOXP reductoisomerase in *P. falciparum* [64]. Jomaa and colleagues showed that this protein localizes to the apicoplast, an organelle essential to parasite survival that was acquired through endosymbiosis of algae [64]. Fosmidomycin inhibits *P. falciparum* DOXP reductoisomerase with an IC_{50} of approximately 50 nM, inhibits chloroquine-sensitive and chloroquine-resistant parasites with an IC_{50} of approximately 300 nM, and cures mice of malaria [64]. The peak plasma level of approximately 190 µM is over 600-fold above the parasite IC_{50} [63]. Components of the mevalonate isoprenoid synthesis pathway used in humans are apparently absent in malaria, which helps explain the specificity of fosmidomycin [61].

Phase II clinical trials of fosmidomycin as a single agent demonstrated rapid clearance of parasitemia, but were hampered by high recrudescence rates

[65, 66]. Combination of fosmidomycin with clindamycin or artesunate led to rapid clearance of parasitemia without recrudescence in partially immune children (ages 7–14 years) [67–69]. There was less efficacy of the fosmidomycin–clindamycin combination in younger children (ages 1–2 years) who lack immunity and suffer the highest mortality from malaria [70]. In addition, both combinations were associated with neutropenia and anemia [68, 70]. The failure of fosmidomycin as a single agent illustrates how pharmacokinetic factors such as half-life can impair repurposing of a drug. Specifically, a sustained half-life is likely necessary to prevent resistance and achieve maximal parasite killing effects. Further development of fosmidomycin combinations and analogs that overcome the short half-life and side effects are ongoing.

11.3.3. Pafuramidine (DB289)

The case of pafuramidine (DB289) in malaria and other tropical diseases illustrates how medicinal chemistry is used to improve the efficacy of an existing drug against a new target. In the 1930s aromatic diamidines such as pentamidine were found to have activity against trypanosomes [71] and were tested against other protozoan infections, including simian and avian malaria in the 1940s [72, 73]. Pentamidine inhibits chloroquine-sensitive and chloroquine-resistant malaria with IC_{50} values of approximately 100 nM and, like chloroquine, concentrates in parasite-infected erythrocytes [74]. Cardiac and renal toxicity limit the use of pentamidine [75]. Since pentamidine must be administered parenterally, it is not an attractive therapy for tropical diseases, and so a search was launched to identify an orally bioavailable analog [76]. These efforts focused on modification of the charged amidine groups, which limit oral bioavailability, and attention focused on diamidoxime and methoxime analogs [77].

Pafuramidine is an orally available prodrug of the pentamidine analog DB75, which was originally developed to treat *Pneumocystis* infections and was later found to have activity against other protozoan infections, especially trypanosomes [77]. Like pentamidine, pafuramidine is thought to bind to AT-rich DNA in the minor groove and interfere with replication, and was also shown to inhibit mitochondrial oxidative phosphorylation [78] and heme crystallization in *P. falciparum* [74]. In malaria, the activated form of pafuramidine, DB75, has an IC_{50} against *P. falciparum* of 20 nM [79]. Immtech Pharmaceuticals, which holds the patent for pafuramidine, received $22.6 million from the Bill and Melinda Gates Foundation to support further development [79]. Phase II clinical trials demonstrated the efficacy of pafuramidine in the treatment of *P. falciparum* and *P. vivax* malaria [80]. Pafuramidine showed no synergy with existing antimalarials but is effective *in vitro* against *P. falciparum* and *P. vivax* [81–83]. There is no prophylactic activity of pafuramidine against malaria infection and the drug was discontinued from further development for trypanosomiasis and *Pneumocystis* by Immtech Pharmaceuticals due to liver and renal toxicity [84]. Other analogs of pafuramidine are currently under investigation as antimalarials [77].

11.4. DRUG REPURPOSING IN LEISHMANIA

11.4.1. Miltefosine

Each year 1.5–2 million people develop symptomatic leishmaniasis and approximately 70,000 people die from the disease, which is prevalent in 88 countries [85]. Leishmania infection has a diverse clinical presentation including skin ulceration, mucosal lesions, and visceral infection (kala azar) characterized by fever, weight loss, pancytopenias, and hepatosplenomegaly due to infection of the spleen, liver, and bone marrow [85]. Scottish pathologist Sir William Leishman first described the disease in 1903 after performing autopsies on British soldiers stationed near Calcutta [86]. The disease is spread through sandfly bites and parasites replicate in macrophages [85]. Sodium antimonyl gluconate, the mainstay treatment for leishmaniasis, requires a 3- to 4-week hospital stay, is expensive, has many side effects, and is becoming less effective due to parasite resistance [87].

Miltefosine is a stable analog of lecithin similar in structure to platelet aggregation factor and has the phosphorylcholine moiety attached by a lipase-resistant ether rather than an ester bond [88]. In cancer cells miltefosine is incorporated into the plasma membrane, where it interferes with lipid metabolism and affects enzymes such as protein kinase C, leading to apoptosis [88]. In Phase II clinical trials miltefosine failed to show activity against colorectal cancer [89], and its use in oncology was limited to topical treatment of skin metastases in breast cancer [90].

The antileishmanial activity of miltefosine was first described in 1987 by researchers examining existing drugs for new activity [91, 92]. Of the 17 disease-causing species of Leishmania, Croft and colleagues tested six and found miltefosine active at concentrations of between 0.12 and 37 μM [93]. Leishmania parasites treated with miltefosine exhibit apoptosis-like cell death [94], and the drug may also have immunodulatory activity that contributes to its efficacy [95].

Miltefosine is the first effective oral treatment for leishmaniasis and has shown efficacy equivalent or greater than existing treatments for cutaneous leishmaniasis [96–99] and visceral leishmaniasis in India in Phase II [100, 101] and III [102] trials. A collaborative effort between the Indian government and the WHO led to approval of miltefosine as a treatment for visceral leishmaniasis in several developing countries [103]. Due to its teratogenic potential, miltefosine must be used with contraception in women of childbearing age [104]. Vomiting and diarrhea, the principal toxicities observed in cancer trials, are less severe in patients undergoing miltefosine treatment for leishmania, and the reason is unclear [103, 105]. The antileishmanial properties of miltefosine are particularly welcome given its efficacy in patients with resistance to first-line antimonial treatments [106].

The pricing of miltefosine at $145 for a 28-day course is a major obstacle to implementation, especially in rural India where patients may make only $1/day [107]. Patients may only purchase enough medication to feel better and then relapse, which breeds resistance. To circumvent these issues, there are calls for directly observed therapy, similar to TB, and for government subsidies to lower drug cost [107]. Strains of leishmania resistant to miltefosine are thought to overexpress the P-glycoprotein *MDR1* and to undergo changes in lipid membrane composition [108, 109].

11.4.2. Amphotericin

The case of amphotericin in the treatment of leishmania infection illustrates the benefits and pitfalls of drug repurposing using a newer, on-patent version of an existing drug. Liposomal or colloidal reformulation of amphotericin reduced toxicity, yet the cost of the patented drug blocks access to patients in the developing world. The high costs of liposomal/colloidal amphotericin are a major obstacle to eradication of leishmania in India [110].

Amphotericin is a polyene antifungal drug first isolated in 1955 from *Streptomyces nostra* found growing in a soil sample from the Orinoco River in Venezuela [111]. The mechanism of amphotericin in both leishmania and fungal infections is thought to involve disruption of plasma membrane integrity through binding sterols and forming pores in the lipid membrane [112]. Amphotericin binds the 24-substituted sterols (i.e., ergosterol) found in fungal and leishmanial cells more avidly than the cholesterol found on the plasma membrane of mammalian cells, explaining its selectivity [113].

The activity of amphotericin against leishmania was first discovered in 1960 [114, 115]. The rise of antimony-resistant visceral leishmaniasis prompted clinical reinvestigation of amphotericin in India and the Sudan in the early 1990s [116, 117]. Amphotericin was found to be as effective as antimony in the treatment of visceral leishmania infection [118]. Although amphotericin is better for patients than antimony, it is associated with nephrotoxicity and hypokalemia, which limits the dose given and requires hospitalization for up to 5 weeks [119]. Lengthy hospitalization is expensive for patients who lose wages, and it places an increased burden on healthcare systems that are already overwhelmed [120].

Liposomal and lipid formulations of amphotericin were tested on patients with visceral leishmaniasis to avoid the toxicity and prolonged hospitalization necessary for the older formulation [121, 122]. Liposomal, lipid, and colloidal formulations of amphotericin were similar in efficacy to regular amphotericin [85]. Shorter courses (5–10 days) of liposomal amphotericin at lower doses are equivalent in efficacy to the 20- to 30-day treatment required for the deoxycholate formulation, and even a single dose cured 92% of patients [123–125].

Liposomal formulation reduces complications during treatment of leishmania as the macrophages that clear lipid particles from the bloodstream are the host for parasites [126].

Although shorter stays reduced 80% of the cost of hospitalization, savings were still not enough to compensate for the increased price of liposomal amphotericin [120]. Cost is a major obstacle for either formulation as liposomal amphotericin costs $390 versus $60 for amphotericin deoxycholate [127]. Even single-dose liposomal amphotericin is more costly than a 30-day course of regular amphotericin, including the cost of prolonged hospitalization [128]. In an effort to create a "homegrown" lipid formulation of amphotericin, investigators in India mixed amphotericin deoxycholate with a commercial fat emulsion. This novel formulation was similar in efficacy to liposomal amphotericin, but the majority of patients had infusion-related side effects [129].

Based on trials showing the efficacy of liposomal amphotericin in the treatment of visceral leishmania, the drug was approved for this use by the FDA in 1997 [130]. Significantly, historical controls were used as a comparator for the clinical trials, given liposomal amphotericin was the first drug approved in the United States for visceral leishmaniasis [130]. Approval of liposomal amphotericin was aided by the accumulation of Phase IV safety data from its use as an antifungal in the developed world [131]. The FDA also granted liposomal amphotericin orphan drug status, which provides market exclusivity for this indication for the originator for 7 years [131].

The WHO was able to secure a 90% discount on liposomal amphotericin, which expanded availability of the drug for treating visceral leishmaniasis [110]. With lower pricing, the goal is to eliminate leishmania from Southeast Asia by 2015 [110]. Improved pricing will also make combination treatment available to prevent development of resistance. The ideal situation will be to treat patients with a single dose of liposomal amphotericin as an outpatient and then closely follow them in the community to ensure adequate treatment [110].

The case of amphotericin in leishmania highlights the benefits and challenges of drug repurposing for tropical disease. Fortunately, the composition of the leishmania plasma membrane was similar to fungi, allowing amphotericin to be effective. Widespread use in leishmania and FDA approval of liposomal amphotericin were helped by the large body of safety data accumulated during treatment for fungal infections. Cost remains a substantial issue but is helped by partnerships between industry and government.

11.4.3. Paromomycin

Paromomycin, also called aminosidine, is an aminoglycoside antibiotic isolated from *Streptomyces rimous* and originally developed for bacterial infections but later repurposed to treat leishmania infection [111]. Popular in the 1980s, paromomycin fell out of favor as an antibiotic after it was eclipsed by cephalosporin and quinolone antibiotics [132]. Its activity against leishmania was first discovered in 1963, and it is more potent than other aminoglycosides [133]. Paromomycin was also identified in a screen of 400 existing drugs against leishmania in 1988 [134]. In bacteria, paromomycin binds to 30S ribosomes and interferes with mRNA reading and protein translation, and a similar mechanism is thought to exist in leishmania parasites [113, 135, 136].

Similar in efficacy to first-line antimonials, paromomycin must be given parenterally, via intramuscular injection, and initial use was hampered by poor oral bioavailability [111]. Reformulation allowed for clinical trials on cutaneous and visceral leismaniasis in the 1980s [137]. In particular, paromomycin was used by Médecins Sans Frontières in combination with antimonials during an outbreak of visceral leishmaniasis in the Sudan [132]. Development of paromomycin was almost side-tracked by lack of funds and the rise of miltefosine until 1999 when the Institute for OneWorld Health, with funding from the Gates Foundation, spearheaded clinical trials required for registration in India [132]. These Phase III trials established paromomycin as a safe treatment for visceral leishmaniasis with efficacy similar to amphotericin. Based on these data, the Indian government approved paromomycin in August 2006 as part of a national campaign to end visceral leishmaniasis [138]. Since humans are the main vector for leishmania in India, the goal of this campaign is to eradicate the disease [139]. Higher doses of paromomycin were necessary in trials on visceral leishmaniasis in Sudan [140, 141]. This may be due to variations in susceptibility of leishmania parasites to paromomycin, a situation also encountered with miltefosine [142].

Compared with miltefosine and amphotericin, paromomycin has several advantages. Patients treated with amphotericin must be hospitalized for weeks due to nephrotoxicity, fevers, and vomiting [143]. Liposomal amphotericin requires a 5-day treatment course but is 30-fold more expensive ($2500–3000) [87, 138]. Miltefosine is likewise expensive, can cause abortions, and is teratogenic [87]. Paromomycin is currently in Phase IV clinical trials sponsored by the Institute for OneWorld Health in India [132]. Currently paromomycin is the cheapest treatment for leishmania, with a 21-day course costing approximately $5 [132]. Combinations with other antileishmania drugs may shorten the duration of treatment and prevent the emergence of resistance.

11.5. DRUG REPURPOSING IN AFRICAN TRYPANOSOMIASIS (SLEEPING SICKNESS)

11.5.1. Eflornithine

Human African trypanosomiasis (sleeping sickness) affects up to 70,000 patients a year with 60 million susceptible to infection in 36 sub-Saharan African countries [144]. The disease is spread by the tsetse fly and is caused by *Trypanosoma brucei gambiense* in 90% of cases [145]. Infection with *T.b. gambiense* follows a chronic course of approximately 3 years, while the less common *T.b. rhodesiense* leads to death in weeks to months due to cardiac complications [146]. After inoculation parasites proliferate in the bloodstream and later invade the cerebrospinal fluid (CSF) and brain parenchyma [147]. Patients with trypanosomiasis show fever, headaches, pruritus, and lymphadenopathy in the first, hemolymphatic stage of infection, and then neuropsychiatric symptoms in a second, meningoencephalic stage [148]. The disease derives its name "sleeping sickness" due to daytime somnolence and nocturnal insomnia in late stage disease [146]. Trypanosomes can express up to 2000 variant surface glycoprotein genes, allowing evasion of the host immune response and complicating vaccine development [149].

First developed as a potential anticancer agent, eflornithine is a suicide inhibitor of ornithine decarboxylase, which is involved in the synthesis of polyamines such as spermidine and putrescine, which are essential for the stability of nucleic acids [147]. Eflornithine acts by covalently modifying a cysteine residue in ornithine decarboxylase [150]. Although preclinical data in cell lines and animal models showed eflornithine had promising antineoplastic activity, when tested in 500 patients with various cancers the results were disappointing [151].

The use of eflornithine in trypanosomiasis was pioneered in 1980 by Cyrus Bacchi, who showed it cured mice of infection and blocked putrescine synthesis in trypanosome extracts [152]. Subsequent biochemical work demonstrated inhibition of parasite ornithine decarboxylase, with the X-ray crystal structure of enzyme bound to eflornithine showing covalent modification of an active-site cysteine [153]. Eflornithine became known as the "resurrection drug" after it reversed coma related to African trypanosomiasis in a woman in Antwerp in less than three days [154]:

Patient 1. A 55-year old Zairian woman admitted to Saint-Pierre University in a comatose state. The patient had been living in the Bandundu area of Zaire, an endemic region for trypanosomiasis until October 1979, when she immigrated to Belgium to join her children. In November 1982 she presented to another hospital with a one-year history of visual disturbances and a one-month history of weight loss, generalized itching, intermittent fever, and enlarged lymph nodes...On admission in December 1982 [she had a] stage I coma...finally in January 1983 with the patient still comatose trypanosomes were detected in a bone marrow smear and also in the peripheral blood...eflornithine was administered...The clinical course of this patient was dramatic: on day 3 of treatment she awoke, on day 5 tremor became less intense; by day 7 she was fully conscious and shaking hands; on day 9 she answered questions; on day 11 she walked with assistance; on day 13 she spoke spontaneously; on day 16 she walked unassisted; on day 19 she washed and dressed herself; on day 24 she was discharged from the hospital.

Eflornithine halts proliferation of trypanosomes without any killing, which is why an intact immune system is needed for efficacy [155]. It is selective against trypanosomes due to the higher turnover of ornithine decarboxylase in mammalian cells [155]. Ornithine decarboxylase from *T.b. gambiense* lacks a C-terminal peptide sequence associated with higher turnover in mammals [156]. *T.b. rhodesiense*, which is not inhibited by eflornithine, likewise has a higher enzyme turnover and a greater specific activity of ornithine decarboxylase, explaining why the drug is not useful in infection caused by this parasite [157]. Consequentially, eflornithine treatment in *T.b. gambiense* leads to prolonged enzyme inhibition, whereas in mammalian and *T.b. rhodesiense*, ornithine decarboxylase is rapidly regenerated [158].

Eflornithine was approved by the FDA in 1990 with orphan status for the treatment of disease caused by *T.b. gambiense* after a PPP between Marion Merrell Dow and the United Nations Development Programme (UNDP)/WHO/World Bank, and is the only new drug for African trypanosomiasis in 50 years [145]. Merrell Dow subsequently ceased to exist and offered the eflornithine license to the WHO, which failed to produce the drug [159]. ILEX Oncology then inherited development rights for eflornithine in cancer and agreed to produce the drug for the WHO, but costs were prohibitive [160]. Aventis, which acquired Merrell Dow, abandoned eflornithine in 1995 for African trypanosomiasis due to market considerations and then resumed production in 2001 after outcry from the WHO and Médecins Sans Frontières [161, 162]. Discovery that eflornithine was useful for facial hair removal in women and subsequent rebranding as Vaniqa by Bristol-Myers Squibb led to resumption of manufacturing for the drug in trypanosomiasis [163, 164]. Sanofi-Aventis now provides eflonithine kits [165]. Repurposing of eflornithine as a "lifestyle drug" for women's facial hair essentially preserved its use for trypanosomiasis [166].

Treatment of African trypanosomiasis with eflornithine began in 1985 and consists of infusions every 6 hours for 14 days and patients experience chemotherapy-type side effects including vomiting, diarrhea, bone marrow suppression, and alopecia [167–172]. Clinical trials in the treatment of African trypanosomiasis are complicated by the civil wars and political instability in regions where the disease is endemic. Due to its CNS penetration, eflornithine is used primarily to treat the second, neurologic stage of *T.b. gambiense* infection whereas pentamidine is used mainly to treat the bloodstream stage of the illness [173]. A shorter 7-day course of eflornithine monotherapy failed to show efficacy in new cases of African trypanosomiasis but was efficacious in treating relapses [174]. Despite the toxicity of eflornithine, it is safer than melarsoprol, the existing treatment that is associated with up to a 10% fatality rate due to acute reactive encephalopathy [171]. There is also increasing resistance to melarsoprol, leading to use of eflornithine as a first-line treatment [175, 176]. Prompted by the expense of eflornithine ($200 for 7 days) and difficulty in administering it to patients who often live in war-torn areas of Africa, attempts have been made to find an abbreviated treatment. Despite the expense, eflornithine treatment costs approximately $560 per life saved, which is more cost effective than meningitis vaccination or antiretroviral treatment for HIV [177].

Shorter courses of eflornithine with melarsoprol, an existing treatment for African trypanosomiasis, also show efficacy [178]. Concerns about emergence of resistance to eflornithine monotherapy prompted efforts to find a two-drug regimen. Resistant parasites have been generated using *in vitro* selection and were found to have impaired eflornithine accumulation, possibly due to deficiency in the *TbAAT6* amino acid transporter [179, 180]. Nifurtimox, which is used to treat American trypanosomiasis (Chagas' disease), caused by *Trypanosoma cruzi*, shows low efficacy against African trypanosomiasis as a primary treatment but augments the efficacy of eflornithine when used in combination [181]. Nifurtimox is thought to exert its trypanocidal effects by increasing oxidative stress [182]. The nifurtimox–eflornithine combination was noninferior to eflornithine monotherapy and allowed for a shorter, less frequent eflornithine regimen (q12 hours × 7 days) in a Phase III trial [183].

The story of eflornithine in African trypanosomiasis highlights how economic pressures shape drug repurposing for tropical diseases. After eflornithine was abandoned as a cancer treatment, its new use in African trypanosomiasis became tenuous due to supply issues. Discovery that eflornithine was a cosmetic treatment for facial hair facilitated manufacturing for one of the developing world's most neglected diseases.

11.6. OPEN-SOURCE SCREENING INITIATIVES—A SYSTEMATIC APPROACH TO IDENTIFYING NEW USES FOR EXISTING DRUGS

The legendary pharmacologist Sir James Black famously said, "The most fruitful basis for the discovery of a new drug is to start with an old drug." Drug repurposing efforts in academia have typically focused on hypothesis-driven research or fortuitous discoveries. Recently high-throughput screens of libraries of existing drugs emerged as an exciting way for academics to launch drug discovery efforts. One of the first screens of existing drug libraries was done by Neal and Allen in the mid-1980s and involved testing of 400 drugs in current clinical use [134]. Efforts at screening existing drug libraries accelerated in the early-2000s through an initiative launched by the National Institutes for Neurological Disorders and Stroke (NINDS), which sponsored a screen of approximately 1000 drugs by 29 labs for activity against amyotrophic lateral sclerosis, damage due to stroke, and Huntington's and Alzheimer's diseases [24, 184–191]. One of the major findings of the NINDS effort was the discovery that the antibiotic ceftriaxone stimulates expression of the GLT1 glutamate transporter, protecting neurons from glutamate toxicity [192]. In a mouse model of amyotrophic lateral sclerosis (ALS), animals treated with ceftriaxone survived longer [192]. The use of ceftriaxone in ALS is currently being studied in a multicenter Phase III clinical trial involving 600 patients, with an expected completion date in June 2012 (NCT00349622). The library created by NINDS and MicroSource Discovery represented one of the first publicly available collections of existing drugs, and it was screened by other investigators for effects on leukemia differentiation [193], hearing loss [194], inflammation [195, 196], angiogenesis [197], TB [198, 199], giardia [200], pseudomonas [201], melanoma [202], apoptosis [203], telomerase [204], legionella [205], fungi [206], and Gaucher disease [207], among others. The NINDS library became standard in many academic high-throughput screening facilities.

Drug repurposing is seen as a promising way for academia to engage in drug discovery [25]. The small size of collections of existing drugs allows for rapid, cost-effective screening in academic labs, compared with libraries of hundreds of thousands of compounds. Many investigators in academia have high-throughput models for diseases but lack the resources necessary to take promising leads to the clinic. Academic institutions such as the National Institutes of Health, Hopkins, Rockefeller, the Harvard/MIT Broad Institute, and Kansas University have established core facilities that include collections of existing drugs [25]. The discovery of ceftriaxone as a neuroprotective agent is one example of a successful academic repurposing effort. Other examples include the identification of antipsychotic drugs that can prevent infection of glial cells by the human polyoma JC virus, which leads to progressive multifocal leukoencephalopathy in the immunosuppressed [208].

11.7. HIGH-THROUGHPUT SCREENING OF EXISTING DRUGS FOR TROPICAL DISEASES: THE JOHNS HOPKINS CLINICAL COMPOUND SCREENING INITIATIVE

The identification of new uses for known drugs in recent years presents a compelling case to collect and screen every drug known to medicine for activity against tropical diseases. Although several reports revealed unexpected properties of established drugs that make them useful in treating new diseases [29, 64, 209] only recently has a systematic high-throughput approach been undertaken to screen existing drugs for novel activities, primarily for diseases other than those most prevalent in the developing world [185, 192, 193].

Prior to establishment of the Johns Hopkins Clinical Compound Library (JHCCL) in 2003 the largest collection of existing drugs contained less than a quarter of the 3400 drugs approved by the FDA from 1938 to 2003 and less than 10% of the approximately 11,500 drugs ever used in medicine. To construct the JHCCL, drugs were identified using the Therapeutic Index of the Merck Index [210], the 2004 Physician's Desk Reference [211], the USP dictionary [212], and a list of 32,000 FDA approvals from 1938 to present purchased from FOI Services and distilled to 3464 unique drug approvals. Chemicals were purchased from a variety of commercial vendors identified using the ChemACX search program, and also from The Johns Hopkins Hospital Pharmacy, USP Reference Standard Collection, and CVS Pharma-Care pharmacy.

The JHCCL became the largest collection of existing drugs available yet only spans 22% of existing drugs [213]. Completing the library, which will entail chemical synthesis of drugs no longer in production, will likely cost tens of millions of dollars. Although in principle this existing drug library should be freely available, the need to replenish drug stocks necessitates a $5000 charge, which is still much less expensive than competitor collections [213]. To date, the JHCCL has been shared with over 45 investigators worldwide for screening on a number of diseases. The scale of the JHCCL (~24 96-well plates) allows screening in an academic lab without sophisticated high-throughput machinery. A growing array of open-source bioinformatic resources such as PubChem and DrugBank provide data on existing drugs [214]. Further development of clinical compound libraries will require the large-scale support of government or philanthropic agencies.

11.8. IDENTIFICATION OF ASTEMIZOLE AS AN ANTIMALARIAL AGENT BY SCREENING A CLINICAL COMPOUND LIBRARY

Malaria parasites are thought to infect one billion people at any time and cause between 700,000 and 3 million deaths annually, mostly in African children [215, 216]. The widespread resistance of *P. falciparum* to commonly used drugs like chloroquine and sulfadoxine–pyrimethamine directly contributes to treatment failure and increased mortality, especially in children [217]. In an effort to accelerate antimalarial drug development, we created and screened the JHCCL against *P. falciparum*. We identified the nonsedating antihistamine astemizole as a potent inhibitor of chloroquine-sensitive and multidrug-resistant *P. falciparum*. The experience with astemizole highlights several of the benefits and pitfalls of drug repurposing for tropical diseases. Specifically, although astemizole demonstrated potent inhibition of malaria parasites and is used in the developing world, its withdrawal from the U.S. market for safety concerns [218] complicated efforts to undertake clinical trials as an antimalarial treatment in the developing world.

Astemizole is one of 190 existing drugs that demonstrate more than 50% inhibition of *P. falciparum* proliferation as measured by $[^3H]$-hypoxanthine uptake at 10 μM (Figure 11.1) [219]. The known properties of drugs identified as inhibitors eliminated classes that are either too toxic or do not reach high enough plasma levels to be clinically relevant, and IC_{50} values were determined for the 87 compounds remaining. A separate screen performed by different investigators using different methodologies identified overlapping hits [220]. Compared with other antihistamines, astemizole was uniquely potent and inhibited *P. falciparum* at submicromolar concentrations, and desmethyl-astemizole, its main metabolite, was effective at 100 nM concentrations. Astemizole and desmethylastemizole are active in three mouse models of malaria, including in mice infected with chloroquine-resistant parasites at doses below that used in humans to treat allergic rhinitis (Figure 11.2).

During intraerythrocytic infection *P. falciparum* parasites crystallize heme released during hemoglobin catabolism within the food vacuole, and this crystallization reaction is inhibited by quinolines like chloroquine [221]. Astemizole and desmethylastemizole inhibit heme crystallization with

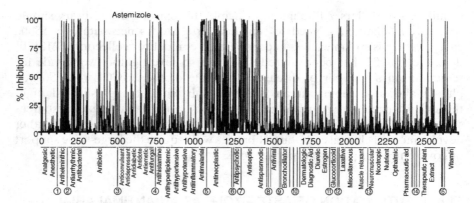

FIGURE 11.1. Identification of astemizole as an antimalarial agent by screening a library of existing drugs. Screening results for 2687 existing drugs in the JHCCL organized by therapeutic indication as indicated in the Merck Index. Drugs were incubated at 10 μM final concentration with 3D7 *P. falciparum* for 96 hours. 1: Antacid; 2: Antianginal; 3: Anticoagulant; 4: Antiglaucoma; 5: Antimigraine; 6: Antiparkinsonian, antiprotozoal, respectively; 7: Antirheumatic; 8: Antithrombotic, antitussive, antiulcerative, respectively; 9: Anxiolytic, bone resorption inhibitor, respectively; 10: Cardiotonic, choleretic, cholinergic, decongestant, respectively; 11: Expectorant; 12: Hemostatic, immunosuppressant, respectively; 13: Mydriatic; 14: Pituitary, plasma volume expander, progestogen, sedative, steroid, respectively; 15: Thyroid, tocolytic, vasodilator, respectively. The miscellaneous category includes abortifacient, alcohol deterrent, anorexic, antiamebic, anticholelithogenic, antidiarrheal, antiflatulent, antimethemoglobinemic, antiobesity, antiurolithic, capillary protectant, contraceptive, ectoparasiticide, erectile dysfunction, gastroprokinetic, hemantic, hepatic protectant, immunomodulator, insecticide, mucolytic, oxytocic, prostaglandin, respiratory stimulant, sialagogue, surfactant, uricosuric, urologic, and vaccine, respectively. *Reproduced in modified form from [219] with permission of Nature Publishing Group.*

similar potency (Figure 11.3a). Like chloroquine, this inhibition is reversible (Figure 11.3b).

The concentration of astemizole required to inhibit heme crystallization is high compared with the concentration necessary to inhibit parasite growth. The same is true for chloroquine, which accumulates at high concentrations in the acidic food vacuole of *P. falciparum* [222]. We therefore tested whether [³H]-astemizole accumulates within the acidic food vacuole of *P. falciparum*. Astemizole concentrates by 941- and 1195-fold with hemozoin co-purified from the *P. falciparum* food vacuole in chloroquine-sensitive and chloroquine-resistant parasites, respectively (Figure 11.3).

Astemizole displays potent activity against malaria both *in vitro* and in mouse models. Nwaka et al. have proposed criteria to determine which candidates should be advanced for further study based on potency, selectivity, toxicity, and animal data, among other factors [223]. Existing drugs fulfill many

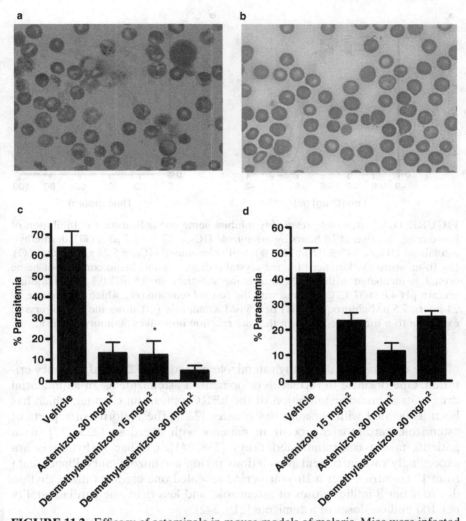

FIGURE 11.2. Efficacy of astemizole in mouse models of malaria. Mice were infected with *P. vinckei*, treated for 4 days with daily intraperitoneal (i.p.) injections of test drug, and parasitemias were counted on day 5 in a blinded fashion. Representative smears from mice treated with vehicle (a) or desmethylastemizole 15 mg/m^2/day i.p. (b) are shown. Astemizole and desmethylastemizole reduce parasitemias of mice infected with chloroquine-sensitive *Plasmodium vinckei* (c) (control $n = 9$; astemizole $n = 9$, $P = 0.000, 12$; desmethylastemizole $n = 10$, $P = 0.000,11$ (*), $P = 4.8 \times 10^{-5}$). Astemizole also reduced parasitemias in mice infected with chloroquine-resistant *Plasmodium yoelii* (d) (control $n = 9$; astemizole 15 mg/m^2 $n = 10$, $P = 0.085$; astemizole 30 mg/m^2 $n = 9$, $P = 0.017$; desmethylastemizole 15 mg/m^2 $n = 8$, $P = 0.0002$). *Reproduced in modified form from [219] with permission of Nature Publishing Group.*

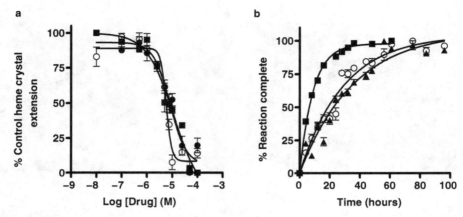

FIGURE 11.3. Astemizole reversibly inhibits heme crystallization. (a) Inhibition of heme crystallization at 16 hours by astemizole (IC_{50} = 12.3 ± 1.7 µM) (■), desmethyl-astemizole (IC_{50} = 8.13 ± 0.84 µM) (●), and chloroquine (IC_{50} = 5.74 ± 0.23 µM) (○). (b) To measure the kinetics of heme crystallization, 5 nmol (heme content) of heme crystal is incubated with 50 µM free heme substrate in 0.5 mL 0.1 M ammonium acetate, pH 4.8 at 37°C. Compared with the control reaction (■), which is complete by 24 hours, 7.5 µM chloroquine (▲) or 7.5 µM astemizole (○) slows the rate of crystal extension to a similar degree such that the reaction now takes 60 hours to finish.

of these criteria, and desmethylastemizole passed the 0.2 µg/mL potency criterion. One obstacle to further development of astemizole as an antimalarial drug is its nanomolar inhibition of the hERG potassium channel, which has been associated with torsades des pointes [224]. The majority of reports of astemizole cardiotoxicity occur in patients with overdose [225–237] or in patients taking contraindicated drugs [238–241]. Cardiac arrhythmias are exceedingly rare in patient populations taking astemizole. Surveillance data from 17 countries over a 10-year period revealed one cardiac rate or rhythm disorder per 8 million doses of astemizole, and less than one cardiac fatality per 100 million doses of astemizole [219, 242].

Astemizole was introduced in 1983 under the brand name Hismanal as a nonsedating selective H_1-histamine receptor antagonist for the treatment of allergic rhinitis that was sold in prescription strength in 106 countries and was also available over the counter [243]. Although astemizole was voluntarily withdrawn in 1999 from the United States and Europe after decreased sales due to warnings about its safety and also the much greater availability of antihistamines with fewer side effects [218], it is currently produced for sale in generic form as an antihistamine in over 30 countries, including Cambodia, Thailand, and Vietnam, which are malaria endemic (Figure 11.4) [219].

The potent human *ether-à-go-go*-related gene (hERG) channel inhibition and withdrawal of astemizole from Western markets created an obstacle to a possible clinical trial of astemizole in malaria. Specifically, even though

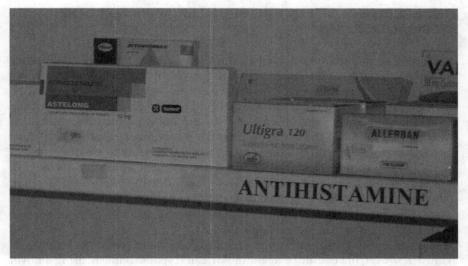

FIGURE 11.4. Astemizole sold as an antihistamine in a rural pharmacy in Livingstone, Zambia for 5000 Kwacha (US$1).

astemizole is still widely used, repurposing it as an antimalarial could imply that different safety standards exist for developing and developed countries. This argument highlights a conundrum applicable to the repurposing of any drug that has fallen out of use for safety reasons. The counterargument to this is that malaria is a serious disease for which few affordable treatments exist. The risk of further developing astemizole as an antimalarial must be balanced against the consequences of the disease. In contrast to the extensive Phase IV safety data on astemizole, no such surveillance has been done for most antimalarials, which are administered in countries where mechanisms and funding for Phase IV studies do not exist. It seems ironic to disparage the Phase IV safety of any existing drug when comparison data on other emerging antimalarials is largely incomplete or unavailable.

Even if astemizole cannot immediately enter human clinical trials for malaria, its structure represents a novel antimalarial pharmacophore. Structural modification of astemizole or its metabolites may enhance its antimalarial activity while reducing interactions with the hERG potassium channel. Such derivatization would defeat many of the cost and time savings in finding a new use for an existing drug, but illustrate how novel activities identified in a clinical compound screen can reveal new pharmacophores. This approach was used by Musonda and colleagues, who synthesized chloroquine–astemizole hybrids and demonstrated inhibition of chloroquine-resistant malaria parasites that was 3- to 10-fold more potent than chloroquine alone [244]. These hybrids demonstrated activity in a mouse malaria model, although the potency did not approach that of chloroquine [244].

11.9. SCREENING OF EXISTING DRUG LIBRARIES FOR OTHER TROPICAL DISEASES

In addition to the identification of astemizole discussed above [219], libraries of existing drugs have also been screened for activity against schistosomiasis [245], African trypanosomias [246], American trypanosomiasis (Chagas' disease) [247], TB, and onchoceriasis [248] (Table 11.2). Existing drugs have also been screened *in silico* for binding to the known structures of *P. falciparum* proteins [249]. These screens identified a number of promising leads for further development, although more work will need to be done before clinical trials are undertaken. Regardless, the authors were able to reach a further point in drug development in less time and with fewer resources than if they had embarked on a *de novo* drug discovery effort. The high-throughput assays developed for the clinical compound screens will be useful once expanded drug libraries are available.

Mackey and colleagues screened a clinical compound collection for activity against *T. brucei*, the causative agent of African trypanosomiasis, using a novel ATP-bioluminescence assay [246]. The majority of existing drugs with novel antitrypanocidal activity identified in this screen were antineoplastics, which are generally cytotoxic, or detergents/antiseptics. Orlistat, an antiobesity drug that inhibits pancreatic lipase, had a submicromolar IC_{50}; however, this drug has poor systemic absorption and a bioavailability of less than 1% [250]. This is problematic given the lymphatic, bloodstream, and CSF as sites of trypanosomal infection [144].

Trypanosoma cruzi, the causative agent of Chagas' disease, which affects millions in Latin America, was the target of a clinical drug screen by Engel and colleagues [247]. These authors created a novel image-based assay to screen a library of 909 clinical compounds [247]. Seventeen existing drugs were identified that were at least fivefold selective against *T. cruzi* over host cells [247]. Azelastine, a second-generation antihistamine, showed inhibition at 1 μM, which appears promising. Azelastine is not typically orally administered as it is approved as a nasal spray and eye drop. Extensive human oral bioavailability data exist, however, that show a peak plasma level of only 33 nM [251]. This 30-fold difference between peak plasma level and IC_{50} illustrates how the pharmacologic properties of an existing drug may eliminate it from further clinical evaluation in a tropical disease. Another exciting and potent hit identified was terconazole, a triazole antifungal used topically to treat vaginal candidiasis [252]. Early work demonstrated "moderate oral broad-spectrum activity," and it is unclear how far terconazole progressed as an oral treatment and if this data was submitted for regulatory approval [253]. The presence of such human data, however, lays the groundwork for further investigation and places terconazole ahead of drug candidates developed *de novo*.

Abdulla and colleagues tested a library of 821 existing drugs in an assay against schistosomiasis, capable of screening 640 compounds per month [245].

TABLE 11.2. Identification of New Activity against Neglected Diseases by Screening Libraries of Existing Drugs

Disease	Library	Assay	Results	Reference
African trypanosomiasis	MicroSource Spectrum	ATP bioluminescence of viable parasites	33 hits: Antiseptic (acriflavinium, alexidine, dequalinium, gentian violet, pararosaniline pamoate, phenylmercuric acetate, thimerosal) Antibiotic (aclacinomycin A1, actinomycin D, aklavine, bleomycin, gramicidin, mitomycin C, mitoxantrone, monensin, nigericin, rutilantin, rutilantinone) Antitumor (paclitaxel, anthothecol, dimethyl gambogic acid, 2,3,29-Triacetoxy-24-Nor-1,3,5,7-Friedelatetraenea, gambogic acid, patulin, pristimerin), Miscellaneous (7,8-dihydroxyflavone, digitonin, orlistat, pyrvinium pamoate) Protein synthesis inhibitor (anisomycin, emetine, lycorine, puromycin)	[246]
Chagas' disease	Iconix	Parasite-infected smooth muscle cells with 4',6-diamidino-2-phenylindole staining of DNA	55 hits with six submicromolar: furazolidone (antibiotic), cycloheximide (antineoplastic), terconazole (antifungal), docetaxel (antineoplastic), amiodarone (antiarrhythmic), azelastine (antiallergic).	[247]

(Continued)

369

TABLE 11.2. (Continued)

Disease	Library	Assay	Results	Reference
Leishmania	MicroSource NINDS Custom Collection II	Luciferase-transfected parasites	69 hits with novel antileishmanial activity, including known drugs maprotiline, tilorone, sertraline, thiourea, disulfiram, nortriptyline, and digitonin.	[255]
Malaria	JHCCL	Direct inhibition of *P. falciparum* proliferation	190 compounds with >50% inhibition at 10 μM, 87 IC_{50}s determined. Astemizole and its principal metabolite are potent inhibitors of drug-sensitive and drug-resistant malaria with activity in mouse models.	[219]
Onchocerciasis	JHCCL	Chitinase enzyme activity with confirmation on molting of *Onchocerciasis volvulus* larvae	Closantel, a veterinary anthelminthic, inhibited chitinase enzyme with micromolar potency but showed limited activity against the parasite.	[248]
Schistosomiasis	MicroSource Spectrum	Phenotypic screen of schistosomular stage parasites	5 hits tested in mice: Anisomycin (protein synthesis inhibitor), gambogic acid (natural product), lasalocid (antibiotic), diffractaic acid (natural product), niclosamide (anthelminthic).	[245]
Tuberculosis	MicroSource NINDS	Screen of growing and dormant TB using resazurin reduction	41 hits including known TB drugs (rifaximin, rifampin, moxifloxacin), fluoroquinolones, antiseptics, vancomycin, disulfiram, pentamidine, orlistat	[198]

This represents a major advance in high-throughput screening given the complexity of the schistosome life cycle, the requirement for a mammalian host, and the phenotypic nature of screening [245]. The protein synthesis inhibitor anisomycin, which is not in clinical use, and the veterinary coccidostat lasalocid were identified as having activity both *in vitro* and in a murine model [245]. The authors identified the salicylanilide class of helminthicides as promising leads in a murine model of schistosomiasis [245].

Onchoceriasis, or river blindness, affects over 37 million people in developing countries and is one of the leading causes of blindness worldwide [254]. To tackle this problem Gloeckner and colleagues screened the JHCCL for inhibitors of chitinase from the pathogenic agent *Onchocerca volvulus* [248]. Closantel, a veterinary anthelmintic, inhibits chitinase with micromolar potency and displayed activity against *O. volvulus* larvae [248]. The chemical backbone of closantel was used as a starting point for further structure–activity relationships. Future research on onchocerciasis could test existing drugs directly on the parasite, in a manner similar to the work of Abdulla and colleagues on schistosoma [245].

An existing drug library was screened for activity against leishmania. High-throughput screening of parasites is complicated by intracellular infection of macrophages and so Osorio and colleagues developed a splenic explant assay [255]. In this assay parasites transfected with luciferase were used to infect hamsters, and macrophages harvested from the spleens of infected animals were used to screen a library of existing drugs. A number of existing drugs were identified with novel activity but were not as potent as current therapies. Of note, the screen failed to detect the known antileishmania drugs fluconazole, miltefosine, and pentamidine. The most likely explanation for this is that these drugs degraded during the repetitive freeze–thaw cycles used to distribute the library. Indeed, when new stocks of these three drugs were tested the IC_{50} values were up to 50-fold more potent for freshly prepared solutions. Compound degradation in high-throughput libraries is a major problem that hampers screening, and libraries of existing drugs are not exempt. To avoid this problem, compounds in screening libraries must be freshly prepared, but this is not economical in an academic setting given the price and labor involved in plating fresh libraries.

The NINDs library was screened for activity against replicating and dormant *Mycobacterium tuberculosis* by Sala and colleagues [198]. A strain of *M. tuberculosis* that relies on streptomycin for growth was used to compare dormant versus actively proliferating cells along with a colorimetric assay for metabolic activity. These experiments identified 41 compounds active against *M. tuberculosis*, including known anti-TB drugs and fluoroquinolones, validating the assay design. New findings included the anti-TB activity of vancomycin, disulfiram, and gramicidin. One limitation of this work was that IC_{50} values were not reported. The drug screening model used will be valuable for future high-throughput screening.

11.10. CONCLUSIONS AND FUTURE DIRECTIONS

Spurred by financial support from charitable organizations such as the Gates Foundation, discovery of new uses for existing drugs in tropical diseases is taking off. Eflornithine, miltefosine, paromomycin, and amphotericin are excellent examples of repurposing efforts that have a major impact on patient care in the developing world. Economic constraints in the case of eflornithine are overcome by PPPs and the coupling of a profitable market like cosmetic hair removal to production of a drug for tropical disease.

The challenges of drug repurposing are highlighted by the failure of dapsone and the ongoing development of fosmidomycin, both of which were repurposed for malaria. A known side effect—hemolytic anemia—derailed repositioning of dapsone in malaria, and earlier mindfulness of this side effect could have saved an enormous amount of funding, and reduced potential harm to patients. Likewise, repositioning of fosmidomycin was hampered by the short half-life of the drug, which was known for over a decade before its antimalarial activity was appreciated.

The promise of finding new uses for existing drugs captivates an ever growing community of researchers. New services offered by industry and the government support these efforts. The Pharmaceutical Assets Portal (ctsapharmaportal.org) is an NIH-sponsored exchange for compounds held by the pharmaceutical industry and academics [256]. To date, Pfizer, Merck, GlaxoSmithKline, Novartis, Genentech, Abbott, AstraZeneca, and Eli Lilly have provided information on how to access proprietary compounds. The Discontinued Clinical Compound Consortium aims to acquire compounds that have been abandoned by the pharmaceutical industry for testing in academia. Meetings dedicated to drug repurposing are sponsored by the NIH and industry. Charitable organizations such as Partnership for Cures (4cures.org) provide funding for projects in drug repurposing. Signaling a new era in academic–industry collaborations, Pfizer provided access to information on 500 pharmaceutical candidates to Washington University scientists in a 5-year $22.5 million agreement [186]. Companies such as Montreal-based generic pharmaceutical company Pharmascience (pharmascience.com) are sponsoring partnership projects to support collaborations in drug repurposing.

A number of new open-source databases are available to researchers interested in drug repurposing. The European Molecular Biology Laboratory supported by the Wellcome Trust has created a database of 500,000 bioactive compounds, including pharmacologic properties (ebi.ac.uk/chembldb/index.php/target). DrugBank (drugbank.ca) is an annotated database containing pharmacologic and target data on existing drugs that has been referenced more than 400 times and has 4 million page visits per year [257]. The Therapeutic Target Database likewise correlates known drugs with their targets [258]. Many known drugs are also found in open-access databases such as PubChem and on websites like Wikipedia. Computational approaches to find off-label targets identified new drug actions that were confirmed experimentally [259]. For example, the selective serotonin reuptake inhibitors fluoxetine and paroxetine were found to bind β-adrenergic receptors, which may explain why they cause erectile dysfunction [259].

While the JHCCL remains the largest collection of existing drugs, an expanding array of libraries are available to investigators interested in drug repurposing. The NIH is distributing the Clinical Compound Collection, a library of 446 existing drugs, at cost ($805) (nihclinicalcollection.com). To date, the JHCCL has been distributed to over 45 investigators pursuing drug development for a panoply of diseases.

Drug repurposing efforts for tropical diseases have resulted in numerous success stories that benefit patients across the world. Increases in philanthropic support and sharing of existing drugs through PPPs will undoubtedly accelerate the pace of success. In a hundred years, historians may look back at this as a time when we came to realize the solutions to our most vexing and unmet medical needs were already in our therapeutic arsenal.

REFERENCES

1. DiMasi, J.A., Hansen, R.W., Grabowski, H.G. (2003). The price of innovation: New estimates of drug development costs. *Journal of Health Economics*, *22*, 151–185.
2. Tolman, P., Guy, P., Altshulter, J., Flanagan, A., Steiner, M. (2001). *A Revolution in R&D: How Genomics and Genetics are Transforming the Biopharmaceutical Industry*. Boston: Boston Consulting Group.
3. Mervis, J. (2005). Productivity counts—But the definition is key. *Science*, *309*, 726.
4. Frank, R.G. (2003). New estimates of drug development costs. *Journal of Health Economics*, *22*, 325–330.
5. Miller, H.I. (1998). Rising costs hold up drug discovery. *Nature*, *395*, 835.
6. Kraljevic, S., Stambrook, P.J., Pavelic, K. (2004). Accelerating drug discovery. *EMBO Reports*, *5*, 837–842.
7. Janssens, P.G., Kivits, M., Vuylsteke, J. (1992). *Medecine et hygiene en Afrique centrale de 1885 a nos jours*. Brussels: Fondation Roi Baudoin.
8. Trouiller, P., Olliaro, P., Torreele, E., et al. (2002). Drug development for neglected diseases: A deficient market and a public-health policy failure. *Lancet*, *359*, 2188–2194.
9. Nwaka, S., Ridley, R.G. (2003). Virtual drug discovery and development for neglected diseases through public-private partnerships. *Nature Reviews Drug Discovery*, *2*, 919–928.
10. Garattini, S. (1997). Financial interests constrain drug development. *Science*, *275*, 287.
11. Trouiller, P., Torreele, E., Olliaro, P., et al. (2001). Drugs for neglected diseases: A failure of the market and a public health failure? *Tropical Medicine and International Health*, *6*, 945–951.
12. Pecoul, B., Chirac, P., Trouiller, P., et al. (1999). Access to essential drugs in poor countries: A lost battle? *Journal of the American Medical Association*, *281*, 361–367.

13. Cohen, J. (2006). Global health. Public-private partnerships proliferate. *Science, 311*, 167.

14. Moran, M., Guzman, J., Ropars, A.L., et al. (2009). Neglected disease research and development: How much are we really spending? *PLoS Medicine, 6*, e30.

15. Cohen, J., Dibner, M.S., Wilson, A. (2010). Development of and access to products for neglected diseases. *PLoS ONE, 5*, e10610.

16. Waltz, E. (2008). FDA launches priority vouchers for neglected-disease drugs. *Nature Biotechnology, 26*, 1315–1316.

17. Kaitin, K.I. (2010). Deconstructing the drug development process: The new face of innovation. *Clinical Pharmacology and Therapeutics, 87*, 356–361.

18. Das, P. (2005). New combination drug to treat malaria. *The Lancet Infectious Diseases, 5*, 267.

19. Croft, S.L. (2005). Public-private partnership: From there to here. *Transactions of the Royal Society of Tropical Medicine and Hygiene, 99*(Suppl 1), S9–S14.

20. Cohen, J. (2006). Global health. The new world of global health. *Science, 311*, 162–167.

21. Pink, R., Hudson, A., Mouries, M.A., et al. (2005). Opportunities and challenges in antiparasitic drug discovery. *Nature Reviews Drug Discovery, 4*, 727–740.

22. Moran, M. (2005). A breakthrough in R&D for neglected diseases: New ways to get the drugs we need. *PLoS Medicine, 2*, e302.

23. Biagini, G.A., O'Neill, P.M., Bray, P.G., et al. (2005). Current drug development portfolio for antimalarial therapies. *Current Opinion in Pharmacology, 5*, 473–478.

24. Abbott, A. (2002). Neurologists strike gold in drug screen effort. *Nature, 417*, 109.

25. O'Connor, K.A., Roth, B.L. (2005). Finding new tricks for old drugs: An efficient route for public-sector drug discovery. *Nature Reviews. Drug Discovery, 4*, 1005–1014.

26. Heemskerk, J. (2005). Screening existing drugs for neurodegeneration: The National Institute of Neurologic Disorders and Stroke (NINDS) model. *Retina, 25*, S56–S57.

27. Heemskerk, J., Tobin, A.J., Bain, L.J. (2002). Teaching old drugs new tricks. Meeting of the Neurodegeneration Drug Screening Consortium, 7–8 April 2002, Washington, DC, USA. *Trends in Neurosciences, 25*, 494–496.

28. Rosenthal, P.J. (2003). Antimalarial drug discovery: Old and new approaches. *The Journal of Experimental Biology, 206*, 3735–3744.

29. Ingber, D., Fujita, T., Kishimoto, S., et al. (1990). Synthetic analogues of fumagillin that inhibit angiogenesis and suppress tumour growth. *Nature, 348*, 555–557.

30. Cherny, R.A., Atwood, C.S., Xilinas, M.E., et al. (2001). Treatment with a copper-zinc chelator markedly and rapidly inhibits beta-amyloid accumulation in Alzheimer's disease transgenic mice. *Neuron, 30*, 665–676.

31. Korth, C., May, B.C., Cohen, F.E., et al. (2001). Acridine and phenothiazine derivatives as pharmacotherapeutics for prion disease. *Proceedings of the National Academy of Sciences of the United States of America, 98*, 9836–9841.

32. Zhu, J., Chen, Z., Lallemand-Breitenbach, V., et al. (2002). How acute promyelocytic leukaemia revived arsenic. *Nature Reviews. Cancer, 2*, 705–713.

33. Martin, S.K., Oduola, A.M., Milhous, W.K. (1987). Reversal of chloroquine resistance in *Plasmodium falciparum* by verapamil. *Science*, *235*, 899–901.

34. Bagla, P. (1997). Malaria fighters gather at site of early victory. *Science*, *277*, 1437–1438.

35. Sowunmi, A., Oduola, A.M., Ogundahunsi, O.A., et al. (1997). Enhanced efficacy of chloroquine-chlorpheniramine combination in acute uncomplicated falciparum malaria in children. *Transactions of the Royal Society of Tropical Medicine and Hygiene*, *91*, 63–67.

36. Looareesuwan, S., Chulay, J.D., Canfield, C.J., et al. (1999). Malarone (atovaquone and proguanil hydrochloride): A review of its clinical development for treatment of malaria. Malarone Clinical Trials Study Group. *The American Journal of Tropical Medicine and Hygiene*, *60*, 533–541.

37. Livermore, D.M. (1993). Determinants of the activity of beta-lactamase inhibitor combinations. *The Journal of Antimicrobial Chemotherapy*, *31*(Suppl A), 9–21.

38. Innaimo, S.F., Seifer, M., Bisacchi, G.S., et al. (1997). Identification of BMS-200475 as a potent and selective inhibitor of hepatitis B virus. *Antimicrobial Agents and Chemotherapy*, *41*, 1444–1448.

39. McMahon, M.A., Jilek, B.L., Brennan, T.P., et al. (2007). The HBV drug entecavir—Effects on HIV-1 replication and resistance. *New England Journal of Medicine*, *356*, 2614–2621.

40. Hirsch, M.S. (2007). Entecavir surprise. *New England Journal of Medicine*, *356*, 2641–2643.

41. Nwaka, S., Hudson, A. (2006). Innovative lead discovery strategies for tropical diseases. *Nature Reviews Drug Discovery*, *5*, 941–955.

42. Barr, J. (2010). A short history of dapsone, or an alternative model of drug development. *Journal of the History of Medicine and Allied Sciences*, *66*, 425–467.

43. Lang, T., Greenwood, B. (2003). The development of Lapdap, an affordable new treatment for malaria. *The Lancet Infectious Diseases*, *3*, 162–168.

44. Ramakrishnan, S.P., Basu, P.C., Singh, H., et al. (1962). Studies on the toxicity and action of diaminodiphenyl-sulfone (DDS) in avian and simian malaria. *Bulletin of the World Health Organization*, *27*, 213–221.

45. Coggeshall, L.T., Maier, J., Best, C.A. (1941). The effectiveness of two new types of chemotherapeutic agents in malaria. *Journal of the American Medical Association*, *117*, 1077–1081.

46. Degowin, R.L., Eppes, R.B., Carson, P.E., et al. (1966). The effects of diaphenylsulfone (DDS) against chloroquine-resistant *Plasmodium falciparum*. *Bulletin of the World Health Organization*, *34*, 671–681.

47. Winstanley, P. (2001). Chlorproguanil-dapsone (LAPDAP) for uncomplicated falciparum malaria. *Tropical Medicine and International Health*, *6*, 952–954.

48. Kenyon, G. (2001). GSK renews malaria efforts. GlaxoSmithKline Biologicals. *Nature Medicine*, *7*, 389.

49. Pincock, S. (2003). Drug company to offer new malaria drug cheaply in Africa. *British Medical Journal*, *327*, 360.

50. Alloueche, A., Bailey, W., Barton, S., et al. (2004). Comparison of chlorproguanil-dapsone with sulfadoxine-pyrimethamine for the treatment of uncomplicated

falciparum malaria in young African children: Double-blind randomised controlled trial. *Lancet, 363,* 1843–1848.

51. Fanello, C.I., Karema, C., Ngamije, D., et al. (2008). A randomised trial to assess the efficacy and safety of chlorproguanil/dapsone + artesunate for the treatment of uncomplicated *Plasmodium falciparum* malaria. *Transactions of the Royal Society of Tropical Medicine and Hygiene, 102,* 412–420.

52. Premji, Z., Umeh, R.E., Owusu-Agyei, S., et al. (2009). Chlorproguanil-dapsone-artesunate versus artemether-lumefantrine: A randomized, double-blind phase III trial in African children and adolescents with uncomplicated *Plasmodium falciparum* malaria. *PLoS ONE, 4,* e6682.

53. Tiono, A.B., Dicko, A., Ndububa, D.A., et al. (2009). Chlorproguanil-dapsone-artesunate versus chlorproguanil-dapsone: A randomized, double-blind, phase III trial in African children, adolescents, and adults with uncomplicated *Plasmodium falciparum* malaria. *The American Journal of Tropical Medicine and Hygiene, 81,* 969–978.

54. Leslie, T., Mayan, M.I., Hasan, M.A., et al. (2007). Sulfadoxine-pyrimethamine, chlorproguanil-dapsone, or chloroquine for the treatment of Plasmodium vivax malaria in Afghanistan and Pakistan: A randomized controlled trial. *Journal of the American Medical Association, 297,* 2201–2209.

55. Luzzatto, L. (2010). The rise and fall of the antimalarial Lapdap: A lesson in pharmacogenetics. *Lancet, 376,* 739–741.

56. Puavilai, S., Chutha, S., Polnikorn, N., et al. (1984). Incidence of anemia in leprosy patients treated with dapsone. *Journal of the Medical Association of Thailand, 67,* 404–407.

57. Degowin, R.L., Eppes, R.B., Powell, R.D., et al. (1966). The haemolytic effects of diaphenylsulfone (DDS) in normal subjects and in those with glucose-6-phosphate-dehydrogenase deficiency. *Bulletin of the World Health Organization, 35,* 165–179.

58. Jollow, D.J., Bradshaw, T.P., McMillan, D.C. (1995). Dapsone-induced hemolytic anemia. *Drug Metabolism Reviews, 27,* 107–124.

59. Beutler, E., Duparc, S. (2007). Glucose-6-phosphate dehydrogenase deficiency and antimalarial drug development. *The American Journal of Tropical Medicine and Hygiene, 77,* 779–789.

60. Okuhara, M., Kuroda, Y., Goto, T., et al. (1980). Studies on new phosphonic acid antibiotics. I. FR-900098, isolation and characterization. *The Journal of Antibiotics, 33,* 13–17.

61. Wiesner, J., Borrmann, S., Jomaa, H. (2003). Fosmidomycin for the treatment of malaria. *Parasitology Research, 90*(Suppl 2), S71–S76.

62. Ridley, R.G. (1999). Planting the seeds of new antimalarial drugs. *Science, 285,* 1502–1503.

63. Kuemmerle, H.P., Murakawa, T., Soneoka, K., et al. (1985). Fosmidomycin: A new phosphonic acid antibiotic. Part I: Phase I tolerance studies. *International Journal of Clinical Pharmacology, Therapy, and Toxicology, 23,* 515–520.

64. Jomaa, H., Wiesner, J., Sanderbrand, S., et al. (1999). Inhibitors of the nonmevalonate pathway of isoprenoid biosynthesis as antimalarial drugs. *Science, 285,* 1573–1576.

65. Lell, B., Ruangweerayut, R., Wiesner, J., et al. (2003). Fosmidomycin, a novel chemotherapeutic agent for malaria. *Antimicrobial Agents and Chemotherapy, 47,* 735–738.

66. Missinou, M.A., Borrmann, S., Schindler, A., et al. (2002). Fosmidomycin for malaria. *Lancet, 360,* 1941–1942.

67. Borrmann, S., Issifou, S., Esser, G., et al. (2004). Fosmidomycin-clindamycin for the treatment of *Plasmodium falciparum* malaria. *The Journal of Infectious Diseases, 190,* 1534–1540.

68. Borrmann, S., Adegnika, A.A., Moussavou, F., et al. (2005). Short-course regimens of artesunate-fosmidomycin in treatment of uncomplicated *Plasmodium falciparum* malaria. *Antimicrobial Agents and Chemotherapy, 49,* 3749–3754.

69. Oyakhirome, S., Issifou, S., Pongratz, P., et al. (2007). Randomized controlled trial of fosmidomycin-clindamycin versus sulfadoxine-pyrimethamine in the treatment of *Plasmodium falciparum* malaria. *Antimicrobial Agents and Chemotherapy, 51,* 1869–1871.

70. Borrmann, S., Lundgren, I., Oyakhirome, S., et al. (2006). Fosmidomycin plus clindamycin for treatment of pediatric patients aged 1 to 14 years with *Plasmodium falciparum* malaria. *Antimicrobial Agents and Chemotherapy, 50,* 2713–2718.

71. Lourie, E.M., Yorke, W. (1939). Studies in chemotherapy XXI. The trypanocidal action of certain aromatic diamidines. *Annals of Tropical Medicine and Parasitology, 33,* 289–304.

72. Das Gupta, B.M., Siddons, L.B. (1944). Treatment of simian malaria (P knowlesi) with stilbamidine. *Indian Medical Gazette, 79,* 527.

73. Fulton, J.D. (1940). The course of *Plasmodium relictum* infection in canaries and the treatment of bird and monkey malaria with synthetic bases. *Annals of Tropical Medicine and Parasitology, 34,* 53–66.

74. Stead, A.M., Bray, P.G., Edwards, I.G., et al. (2001). Diamidine compounds: Selective uptake and targeting in *Plasmodium falciparum. Molecular Pharmacology, 59,* 1298–1306.

75. Purfield, A.E., Tidwell, R.R., Meshnick, S.R. (2009). The diamidine DB75 targets the nucleus of *Plasmodium falciparum. Malaria Journal, 8,* 104.

76. Midgley, I., Fitzpatrick, K., Taylor, L.M., et al. (2007). Pharmacokinetics and metabolism of the prodrug DB289 (2,5-bis[4-(N-methoxyamidino)phenyl]furan monomaleate) in rat and monkey and its conversion to the antiprotozoal/antifungal drug DB75 (2,5-bis(4-guanylphenyl)furan dihydrochloride. *Drug Metabolism and Disposition, 35,* 955–967.

77. Werbovetz, K. (2006). Diamidines as antitrypanosomal, antileishmanial and antimalarial agents. *Current Opinion in Investigational Drugs, 7,* 147–157.

78. Lanteri, C.A., Trumpower, B.L., Tidwell, R.R., et al. (2004). DB75, a novel trypanocidal agent, disrupts mitochondrial function in *Saccharomyces cerevisiae. Antimicrobial Agents and Chemotherapy, 48,* 3968–3974.

79. Yeates, C. (2003). DB-289 Immtech International. *IDrugs, 6,* 1086–1093.

80. Yeramian, P., Meshnick, S.R., Krudsood, S., et al. (2005). Efficacy of DB289 in Thai patients with *Plasmodium vivax* or acute, uncomplicated *Plasmodium falciparum* infections. *The Journal of Infectious Diseases, 192,* 319–322.

81. Bell, C.A., Hall, J.E., Kyle, D.E., et al. (1990). Structure-activity relationships of analogs of pentamidine against *Plasmodium falciparum* and *Leishmania mexicana amazonensis*. *Antimicrobial Agents and Chemotherapy, 34*, 1381–1386.

82. Kocken, C.H., van der Wel, A., Arbe-Barnes, S., et al. (2006). *Plasmodium vivax*: In vitro susceptibility of blood stages to synthetic trioxolane compounds and the diamidine DB75. *Experimental Parasitology, 113*, 197–200.

83. Purfield, A.E., Tidwell, R.R., Meshnick, S.R. (2008). Interactions of DB75, a novel antimalarial agent, with other antimalarial drugs in vitro. *Antimicrobial Agents and Chemotherapy, 52*, 2253–2255.

84. Nyunt, M.M., Hendrix, C.W., Bakshi, R.P., et al. (2009). Phase I/II evaluation of the prophylactic antimalarial activity of pafuramidine in healthy volunteers challenged with *Plasmodium falciparum* sporozoites. *The American Journal of Tropical Medicine and Hygiene, 80*, 528–535.

85. Murray, H.W., Berman, J.D., Davies, C.R., et al. (2005). Advances in leishmaniasis. *Lancet, 366*, 1561–1577.

86. Leishman, W. (1903). On the possibility of the occurrence of trypanosomiasis in India. *British Medical Journal, 1*, 1252.

87. Guerin, P.J., Olliaro, P., Sundar, S., et al. (2002). Visceral leishmaniasis: Current status of control, diagnosis, and treatment, and a proposed research and development agenda. *The Lancet Infectious Diseases, 2*, 494–501.

88. Barratt, G., Saint-Pierre-Chazalet, M., Loiseau, P.M. (2009). Cellular transport and lipid interactions of miltefosine. *Current Drug Metabolism, 10*, 247–255.

89. Planting, A.S., Stoter, G., Verweij, J. (1993). Phase II study of daily oral miltefosine (hexadecylphosphocholine) in advanced colorectal cancer. *European Journal of Cancer, 29A*, 518–519.

90. Smorenburg, C.H., Seynaeve, C., Bontenbal, M., et al. (2000). Phase II study of miltefosine 6% solution as topical treatment of skin metastases in breast cancer patients. *Anti-Cancer Drugs, 11*, 825–828.

91. Croft, S.L., Neal, R.A., Pendergast, W., et al. (1987). The activity of alkyl phosphorylcholines and related derivatives against *Leishmania donovani*. *Biochemical Pharmacology, 36*, 2633–2636.

92. Achterberg, V., Gercken, G. (1987). Cytotoxicity of ester and ether lysophospholipids on *Leishmania donovani* promastigotes. *Molecular and Biochemical Parasitology, 23*, 117–122.

93. Escobar, P., Matu, S., Marques, C., et al. (2002). Sensitivities of Leishmania species to hexadecylphosphocholine (miltefosine), ET-18-OCH(3) (edelfosine) and amphotericin B. *Acta Tropica, 81*, 151–157.

94. Paris, C., Loiseau, P.M., Bories, C., et al. (2004). Miltefosine induces apoptosis-like death in *Leishmania donovani* promastigotes. *Antimicrobial Agents and Chemotherapy, 48*, 852–859.

95. Wadhone, P., Maiti, M., Agarwal, R., et al. (2009). Miltefosine promotes IFN-gamma-dominated anti-leishmanial immune response. *Journal of Immunology, 182*, 7146–7154.

96. Soto, J., Arana, B.A., Toledo, J., et al. (2004). Miltefosine for new world cutaneous leishmaniasis. *Clinical Infectious Diseases, 38*, 1266–1272.

97. Killingley, B., Lamb, L.E., Davidson, R.N. (2009). Miltefosine to treat cutaneous leishmaniasis caused by *Leishmania tropica*. *Annals of Tropical Medicine and Parasitology*, *103*, 171–175.

98. Machado, P.R., Ampuero, J., Guimaraes, L.H., et al. (2010). Miltefosine in the treatment of cutaneous leishmaniasis caused by *Leishmania braziliensis* in Brazil: A randomized and controlled trial. *PLoS Neglected Tropical Diseases*, *4*, e912.

99. Chrusciak-Talhari, A., Dietze, R., Chrusciak Talhari, C., et al. (2011). Randomized controlled clinical trial to access efficacy and safety of miltefosine in the treatment of cutaneous leishmaniasis caused by *Leishmania* (Viannia) *guyanensis* in Manaus, Brazil. *The American Journal of Tropical Medicine and Hygiene*, *84*, 255–260.

100. Jha, T.K., Sundar, S., Thakur, C.P., et al. (1999). Miltefosine, an oral agent, for the treatment of Indian visceral leishmaniasis. *New England Journal of Medicine*, *341*, 1795–1800.

101. Sundar, S., Rosenkaimer, F., Makharia, M.K., et al. (1998). Trial of oral miltefosine for visceral leishmaniasis. *Lancet*, *352*, 1821–1823.

102. Sundar, S., Jha, T.K., Thakur, C.P., et al. (2002). Oral miltefosine for Indian visceral leishmaniasis. *New England Journal of Medicine*, *347*, 1739–1746.

103. Croft, S.L., Engel, J. (2006). Miltefosine—Discovery of the antileishmanial activity of phospholipid derivatives. *Transactions of the Royal Society of Tropical Medicine and Hygiene*, *100*(Suppl 1), S4–S8.

104. Desjeux, P. (2004). Leishmaniasis. *Nature Reviews Microbiology*, *2*, 692.

105. Sundar, S., Chatterjee, M. (2006). Visceral leishmaniasis—Current therapeutic modalities. *The Indian Journal of Medical Research*, *123*, 345–352.

106. Croft, S.L., Seifert, K., Yardley, V. (2006). Current scenario of drug development for leishmaniasis. *The Indian Journal of Medical Research*, *123*, 399–410.

107. Sundar, S., Murray, H.W. (2005). Availability of miltefosine for the treatment of kala-azar in India. *Bulletin of the World Health Organization*, *83*, 394–395.

108. Perez-Victoria, J.M., Perez-Victoria, F.J., Parodi-Talice, A., et al. (2001). Alkyl-lysophospholipid resistance in multidrug-resistant *Leishmania tropica* and chemo-sensitization by a novel P-glycoprotein-like transporter modulator. *Antimicrobial Agents and Chemotherapy*, *45*, 2468–2474.

109. Rakotomanga, M., Saint-Pierre-Chazalet, M., Loiseau, P.M. (2005). Alteration of fatty acid and sterol metabolism in miltefosine-resistant *Leishmania donovani* promastigotes and consequences for drug-membrane interactions. *Antimicrobial Agents and Chemotherapy*, *49*, 2677–2686.

110. Matlashewski, G., Arana, B., Kroeger, A., et al. (2011). Visceral leishmaniasis: Elimination with existing interventions. *The Lancet Infectious Diseases*, *11*, 322–325.

111. Mishra, J., Saxena, A., Singh, S. (2007). Chemotherapy of leishmaniasis: Past, present and future. *Current Medicinal Chemistry*, *14*, 1153–1169.

112. Hartsel, S., Bolard, J. (1996). Amphotericin B: New life for an old drug. *Trends in Pharmacological Sciences*, *17*, 445–449.

113. Croft, S.L., Yardley, V. (2002). Chemotherapy of leishmaniasis. *Current Pharmaceutical Design*, *8*, 319–342.

114. Furtado, T.A., Cisalpino, E.O., Santos, U.M. (1960). In vitro studies of the effect of amphotericin B on *Leishmania brasiliensis*. *Antibiotics and Chemotherapy*, *10*, 692–693.

115. Sampaio, S.A., Godoy, J.T., Paiva, L., et al. (1960). The treatment of American (mucocutaneous) leishmaniasis with amphotericin B. *Archives of Dermatology*, *82*, 627–635.

116. Mishra, M., Biswas, U.K., Jha, D.N., et al. (1992). Amphotericin versus pentamidine in antimony-unresponsive kala-azar. *Lancet*, *340*, 1256–1257.

117. Seaman, J., Boer, C., Wilkinson, R., et al. (1995). Liposomal amphotericin B (AmBisome) in the treatment of complicated kala-azar under field conditions. *Clinical Infectious Diseases*, *21*, 188–193.

118. Thakur, C.P., Narayan, S. (2004). A comparative evaluation of amphotericin B and sodium antimony gluconate, as first-line drugs in the treatment of Indian visceral leishmaniasis. *Annals of Tropical Medicine and Parasitology*, *98*, 129–138.

119. Sundar, S., Mehta, H., Chhabra, A., et al. (2006). Amphotericin B colloidal dispersion for the treatment of Indian visceral leishmaniasis. *Clinical Infectious Diseases*, *42*, 608–613.

120. Sundar, S., Mehta, H., Suresh, A.V., et al. (2004). Amphotericin B treatment for Indian visceral leishmaniasis: Conventional versus lipid formulations. *Clinical Infectious Diseases*, *38*, 377–383.

121. Davidson, R.N., Croft, S.L., Scott, A., et al. (1991). Liposomal amphotericin B in drug-resistant visceral leishmaniasis. *Lancet*, *337*, 1061–1062.

122. Croft, S.L., Davidson, R.N., Thornton, E.A. (1991). Liposomal amphotericin B in the treatment of visceral leishmaniasis. *The Journal of Antimicrobial Chemotherapy*, *28*(Suppl B), 111–118.

123. Davidson, R.N., Di Martino, L., Gradoni, L., et al. (1996). Short-course treatment of visceral leishmaniasis with liposomal amphotericin B (AmBisome). *Clinical Infectious Diseases*, *22*, 938–943.

124. Sundar, S., Jha, T.K., Thakur, C.P., et al. (2002). Low-dose liposomal amphotericin B in refractory Indian visceral leishmaniasis: A multicenter study. *The American Journal of Tropical Medicine and Hygiene*, *66*, 143–146.

125. Sundar, S., Agrawal, G., Rai, M., et al. (2001). Treatment of Indian visceral leishmaniasis with single or daily infusions of low dose liposomal amphotericin B: Randomised trial. *British Medical Journal*, *323*, 419–422.

126. Berman, J.D., Ksionski, G., Chapman, W.L., et al. (1992). Activity of amphotericin B cholesterol dispersion (Amphocil) in experimental visceral leishmaniasis. *Antimicrobial Agents and Chemotherapy*, *36*, 1978–1980.

127. Sundar, S., Rai, M. (2002). Advances in the treatment of leishmaniasis. *Current Opinion in Infectious Diseases*, *15*, 593–598.

128. Murray, H.W. (2000). Treatment of visceral leishmaniasis (kala-azar): A decade of progress and future approaches. *International Journal of Infectious Diseases*, *4*, 158–177.

129. Sundar, S., Gupta, L.B., Rastogi, V., et al. (2000). Short-course, cost-effective treatment with amphotericin B-fat emulsion cures visceral leishmaniasis. *Transactions of the Royal Society of Tropical Medicine and Hygiene*, *94*, 200–204.

130. Meyerhoff, A. (1999). U.S. Food and Drug Administration approval of AmBisome (liposomal amphotericin B) for treatment of visceral leishmaniasis. *Clinical Infectious Diseases, 28*, 42–48; discussion 49–51.

131. Berman, J.D. (1999). U.S. Food and Drug Administration approval of AmBisome (liposomal amphotericin B) for treatment of visceral leishmaniasis. *Clinical Infectious Diseases, 28*, 49–51.

132. Davidson, R.N., den Boer, M., Ritmeijer, K. (2009). Paromomycin. *Transactions of the Royal Society of Tropical Medicine and Hygiene, 103*, 653–660.

133. Kellina, O.I. (1963). Investigations of the chemotherapeutic activity of monomycin in experimental cutaneous leishmaniasis in mice. *Meditsinskaia Parazitologiia i Parazitarnye Bolezni, 32*, 572–575.

134. Neal, R.A., Allen, S. (1988). In vitro anti-Leishmanial activity of compounds in current clinical use for unrelated diseases. *Drugs under Experimental and Clinical Research, 14*, 621–628.

135. Maarouf, M., Lawrence, F., Brown, S., et al. (1997). Biochemical alterations in paromomycin-treated *Leishmania donovani* promastigotes. *Parasitology Research, 83*, 198–202.

136. Maarouf, M., Lawrence, F., Croft, S.L., et al. (1995). Ribosomes of *Leishmania* are a target for the aminoglycosides. *Parasitology Research, 81*, 421–425.

137. Berman, J.D. (1997). Human leishmaniasis: Clinical, diagnostic, and chemotherapeutic developments in the last 10 years. *Clinical Infectious Diseases, 24*, 684–703.

138. Sundar, S., Jha, T.K., Thakur, C.P., et al. (2007). Injectable paromomycin for visceral leishmaniasis in India. *New England Journal of Medicine, 356*, 2571–2581.

139. Klempner, M.S., Unnasch, T.R., Hu, L.T. (2007). Taking a bite out of vector-transmitted infectious diseases. *New England Journal of Medicine, 356*, 2567–2569.

140. Hailu, A., Musa, A., Wasunna, M., et al. (2010). Geographical variation in the response of visceral leishmaniasis to paromomycin in East Africa: A multicentre, open-label, randomized trial. *PLoS Neglected Tropical Diseases, 4*, e709.

141. Musa, A.M., Younis, B., Fadlalla, A., et al. (2010). Paromomycin for the treatment of visceral leishmaniasis in Sudan: A randomized, open-label, dose-finding study. *PLoS Neglected Tropical Diseases, 4*, e855.

142. Neal, R.A., Allen, S., McCoy, N., et al. (1995). The sensitivity of *Leishmania* species to aminosidine. *The Journal of Antimicrobial Chemotherapy, 35*, 577–584.

143. Wilson, M.E. (2008). Alternative drug treatments for visceral leishmaniasis: Paromomycin. *Current Infectious Disease Reports, 10*, 40–41.

144. Brun, R., Blum, J., Chappuis, F., et al. (2010). Human African trypanosomiasis. *Lancet, 375*, 148–159.

145. Kuzoe, F.A. (1993). Current situation of African trypanosomiasis. *Acta Tropica, 54*, 153–162.

146. Barrett, M.P., Burchmore, R.J., Stich, A., et al. (2003). The trypanosomiases. *Lancet, 362*, 1469–1480.

147. Burchmore, R.J., Ogbunude, P.O., Enanga, B., et al. (2002). Chemotherapy of human African trypanosomiasis. *Current Pharmaceutical Design, 8*, 256–267.

148. Murray, H.W., Pepin, J., Nutman, T.B., et al. (2000). Tropical medicine. *British Medical Journal, 320*, 490–494.

149. Kennedy, P.G. (2008). The continuing problem of human African trypanosomiasis (sleeping sickness). *Annals of Neurology, 64*, 116–126.

150. Wang, C.C. (1995). Molecular mechanisms and therapeutic approaches to the treatment of African trypanosomiasis. *Annual Review of Pharmacology and Toxicology, 35*, 93–127.

151. McCann, P.P., Pegg, A.E. (1992). Ornithine decarboxylase as an enzyme target for therapy. *Pharmacology and Therapeutics, 54*, 195–215.

152. Bacchi, C.J., Nathan, H.C., Hutner, S.H., et al. (1980). Polyamine metabolism: A potential therapeutic target in trypanosomes. *Science, 210*, 332–334.

153. Grishin, N.V., Osterman, A.L., Brooks, H.B., et al. (1999). X-ray structure of ornithine decarboxylase from *Trypanosoma brucei*: The native structure and the structure in complex with alpha-difluoromethylornithine. *Biochemistry, 38*, 15174–15184.

154. Taelman, H., Schechter, P.J., Marcelis, L., et al. (1987). Difluoromethylornithine, an effective new treatment of Gambian trypanosomiasis. Results in five patients. *The American Journal of Medicine, 82*, 607–614.

155. Docampo, R., Moreno, S.N. (2003). Current chemotherapy of human African trypanosomiasis. *Parasitology Research, 90*(1), S10–S13.

156. Phillips, M.A., Coffino, P., Wang, C.C. (1987). Cloning and sequencing of the ornithine decarboxylase gene from *Trypanosoma brucei*. Implications for enzyme turnover and selective difluoromethylornithine inhibition. *The Journal of Biological Chemistry, 262*, 8721–8727.

157. Iten, M., Mett, H., Evans, A., et al. (1997). Alterations in ornithine decarboxylase characteristics account for tolerance of *Trypanosoma brucei* rhodesiense to D,L-alpha-difluoromethylornithine. *Antimicrobial Agents and Chemotherapy, 41*, 1922–1925.

158. Denise, H., Barrett, M.P. (2001). Uptake and mode of action of drugs used against sleeping sickness. *Biochemical Pharmacology, 61*, 1–5.

159. Sjoerdsma, A., Schechter, P.J. (1999). Eflornithine for African sleeping sickness. *Lancet, 354*, 254.

160. Barrett, M.P. (1999). The fall and rise of sleeping sickness. *Lancet, 353*, 1113–1114.

161. Checchi, F., Barrett, M.P. (2008). African sleeping sickness. *British Medical Journal, 336*, 679–680.

162. Pecoul, B., Gastellu, M. (1999). Production of sleeping-sickness treatment. *Lancet, 354*, 955–956.

163. Wickware, P. (2002). Resurrecting the resurrection drug. *Nature Medicine, 8*, 908–909.

164. Barrett, M.P. (2006). The rise and fall of sleeping sickness. *Lancet, 367*, 1377–1378.

165. Burri, C. (2010). Chemotherapy against human African trypanosomiasis: Is there a road to success? *Parasitology, 137*, 1987–1994.

166. Coyne, P.E., Jr (2001). The eflornithine story. *Journal of the American Academy of Dermatology, 45*, 784–786.

167. Van Nieuwenhove, S., Schechter, P.J., Declercq, J., et al. (1985). Treatment of gambiense sleeping sickness in the Sudan with oral DFMO (DL-alpha-

difluoromethylornithine), an inhibitor of ornithine decarboxylase; first field trial. *Transactions of the Royal Society of Tropical Medicine and Hygiene*, *79*, 692–698.

168. Balasegaram, M., Young, H., Chappuis, F., et al. (2009). Effectiveness of melarsoprol and eflornithine as first-line regimens for gambiense sleeping sickness in nine Medecins Sans Frontieres programmes. *Transactions of the Royal Society of Tropical Medicine and Hygiene*, *103*, 280–290.

169. Khonde, N., Pepin, J., Mpia, B. (1997). A seven days course of eflornithine for relapsing *Trypanosoma brucei* gambiense sleeping sickness. *Transactions of the Royal Society of Tropical Medicine and Hygiene*, *91*, 212–213.

170. Burri, C., Brun, R. (2003). Eflornithine for the treatment of human African trypanosomiasis. *Parasitology Research*, *90*(Suppl 1), S49–S52.

171. Chappuis, F., Udayraj, N., Stietenroth, K., et al. (2005). Eflornithine is safer than melarsoprol for the treatment of second-stage *Trypanosoma brucei gambiense* human African trypanosomiasis. *Clinical Infectious Diseases*, *41*, 748–751.

172. Milord, F., Pepin, J., Loko, L., et al. (1992). Efficacy and toxicity of eflornithine for treatment of *Trypanosoma brucei gambiense* sleeping sickness. *Lancet*, *340*, 652–655.

173. Chappuis, F. (2007). Melarsoprol-free drug combinations for second-stage Gambian sleeping sickness: The way to go. *Clinical Infectious Diseases*, *45*, 1443–1445.

174. Pepin, J., Khonde, N., Maiso, F., et al. (2000). Short-course eflornithine in Gambian trypanosomiasis: A multicentre randomized controlled trial. *Bulletin of the World Health Organization*, *78*, 1284–1295.

175. Priotto, G., Pinoges, L., Fursa, I.B., et al. (2008). Safety and effectiveness of first line eflornithine for *Trypanosoma brucei gambiense* sleeping sickness in Sudan: Cohort study. *British Medical Journal*, *336*, 705–708.

176. Balasegaram, M., Harris, S., Checchi, F., et al. (2006). Melarsoprol versus eflornithine for treating late-stage Gambian trypanosomiasis in the Republic of the Congo. *Bulletin of the World Health Organization*, *84*, 783–791.

177. Robays, J., Raguenaud, M.E., Josenando, T., et al. (2008). Eflornithine is a cost-effective alternative to melarsoprol for the treatment of second-stage human West African trypanosomiasis in Caxito, Angola. *Tropical Medicine and International Health*, *13*, 265–271.

178. Mpia, B., Pepin, J. (2002). Combination of eflornithine and melarsoprol for melarsoprol-resistant Gambian trypanosomiasis. *Tropical Medicine and International Health*, *7*, 775–779.

179. Vincent, I.M., Creek, D., Watson, D.G., et al. (2010). A molecular mechanism for eflornithine resistance in African trypanosomes. *PLoS Pathogens*, *6*, e1001204.

180. Wang, C.C. (1991). A novel suicide inhibitor strategy for antiparasitic drug development. *Journal of Cellular Biochemistry*, *45*, 49–53.

181. Checchi, F., Piola, P., Ayikoru, H., et al. (2007). Nifurtimox plus eflornithine for late-stage sleeping sickness in Uganda: A case series. *PLoS Neglected Tropical Diseases*, *1*, e64.

182. Fairlamb, A.H., Henderson, G.B., Bacchi, C.J., et al. (1987). In vivo effects of difluoromethylornithine on trypanothione and polyamine levels in bloodstream forms of *Trypanosoma brucei*. *Molecular and Biochemical Parasitology*, *24*, 185–191.

183. Priotto, G., Kasparian, S., Mutombo, W., et al. (2009). Nifurtimox-eflornithine combination therapy for second-stage African *Trypanosoma brucei gambiense* trypanosomiasis: A multicentre, randomised, phase III, non-inferiority trial. *Lancet*, *374*, 56–64.

184. Heemskerk, J. (2004). High throughput drug screening. *Amyotrophic Lateral Sclerosis and Other Motor Neuron Disorders*, *5*(Suppl 1), 19–21.

185. Pollitt, S.K., Pallos, J., Shao, J., et al. (2003). A rapid cellular FRET assay of polyglutamine aggregation identifies a novel inhibitor. *Neuron*, *40*, 685–694.

186. Wang, W., Duan, W., Igarashi, S., et al. (2005). Compounds blocking mutant huntingtin toxicity identified using a Huntington's disease neuronal cell model. *Neurobiology of Disease*, *20*, 500–508.

187. LeVine, H., 3rd, Ding, Q., Walker, J.A., et al. (2009). Clioquinol and other hydroxyquinoline derivatives inhibit Abeta(1-42) oligomer assembly. *Neuroscience Letters*, *465*, 99–103.

188. Desai, U.A., Pallos, J., Ma, A.A., et al. (2006). Biologically active molecules that reduce polyglutamine aggregation and toxicity. *Human Molecular Genetics*, *15*, 2114–2124.

189. Barber, S.C., Higginbottom, A., Mead, R.J., et al. (2009). An in vitro screening cascade to identify neuroprotective antioxidants in ALS. *Free Radical Biology and Medicine*, *46*, 1127–1138.

190. Wang, X., Zhu, S., Pei, Z., et al. (2008). Inhibitors of cytochrome c release with therapeutic potential for Huntington's disease. *Journal of Neuroscience*, *28*, 9473–9485.

191. Stavrovskaya, I.G., Narayanan, M.V., Zhang, W., et al. (2004). Clinically approved heterocyclics act on a mitochondrial target and reduce stroke-induced pathology. *The Journal of Experimental Medicine*, *200*, 211–222.

192. Rothstein, J.D., Patel, S., Regan, M.R., et al. (2005). Beta-lactam antibiotics offer neuroprotection by increasing glutamate transporter expression. *Nature*, *433*, 73–77.

193. Stegmaier, K., Ross, K.N., Colavito, S.A., et al. (2004). Gene expression-based high-throughput screening(GE-HTS) and application to leukemia differentiation. *Nature Genetics*, *36*, 257–263.

194. Ou, H.C., Santos, F., Raible, D.W., et al. (2010). Drug screening for hearing loss: Using the zebrafish lateral line to screen for drugs that prevent and cause hearing loss. *Drug Discovery Today*, *15*, 265–271.

195. Kim, J.Y., Lee, W.K., Yu, Y.G., et al. (2010). Blockade of LTB4-induced chemotaxis by bioactive molecules interfering with the BLT2-Galphai interaction. *Biochemical Pharmacology*, *79*, 1506–1515.

196. Ouertatani-Sakouhi, H., El-Turk, F., Fauvet, B., et al. (2010). Identification and characterization of novel classes of macrophage migration inhibitory factor (MIF) inhibitors with distinct mechanisms of action. *The Journal of Biological Chemistry*, *285*, 26581–26598.

197. Cho, H., Lee, H.Y., Ahn, D.R., et al. (2008). Baicalein induces functional hypoxia-inducible factor-1alpha and angiogenesis. *Molecular Pharmacology*, *74*, 70–81.

198. Sala, C., Dhar, N., Hartkoorn, R.C., et al. (2010). Simple model for testing drugs against nonreplicating *Mycobacterium tuberculosis*. *Antimicrobial Agents and Chemotherapy*, *54*, 4150–4158.

199. Anthony, K.G., Strych, U., Yeung, K.R., et al. (2011). New Classes of alanine racemase inhibitors identified by high-throughput screening show antimicrobial activity against *Mycobacterium tuberculosis*. *PLoS ONE*, *6*, e20374.

200. Bonilla-Santiago, R., Wu, Z., Zhang, L., et al. (2008). Identification of growth inhibiting compounds in a *Giardia lamblia* high-throughput screen. *Molecular and Biochemical Parasitology*, *162*, 149–154.

201. Junker, L.M., Clardy, J. (2007). High-throughput screens for small-molecule inhibitors of *Pseudomonas aeruginosa* biofilm development. *Antimicrobial Agents and Chemotherapy*, *51*, 3582–3590.

202. Saunders, L.P., Ouellette, A., Bandle, R., et al. (2008). Identification of small-molecule inhibitors of autotaxin that inhibit melanoma cell migration and invasion. *Molecular Cancer Therapeutics*, *7*, 3352–3362.

203. Boon-Unge, K., Yu, Q., Zou, T., et al. (2007). Emetine regulates the alternative splicing of Bcl-x through a protein phosphatase 1-dependent mechanism. *Chemistry and Biology*, *14*, 1386–1392.

204. Cristofari, G., Reichenbach, P., Regamey, P.O., et al. (2007). Low- to high-throughput analysis of telomerase modulators with Telospot. *Nature Methods*, *4*, 851–853.

205. Charpentier, X., Gabay, J.E., Reyes, M., et al. (2009). Chemical genetics reveals bacterial and host cell functions critical for type IV effector translocation by Legionella pneumophila. *PLoS Pathogens*, *5*, e1000501.

206. Breger, J., Fuchs, B.B., Aperis, G., et al. (2007). Antifungal chemical compounds identified using a *C. elegans* pathogenicity assay. *PLoS Pathogens*, *3*, e18.

207. Maegawa, G.H., Tropak, M.B., Buttner, J.D., et al. (2009). Identification and characterization of ambroxol as an enzyme enhancement agent for Gaucher disease. *The Journal of Biological Chemistry*, *284*, 23502–23516.

208. Elphick, G.F., Querbes, W., Jordan, J.A., et al. (2004). The human polyomavirus, JCV, uses serotonin receptors to infect cells. *Science*, *306*, 1380–1383.

209. Zhu, S., Stavrovskaya, I.G., Drozda, M., et al. (2002). Minocycline inhibits cytochrome c release and delays progression of amyotrophic lateral sclerosis in mice. *Nature*, *417*, 74–78.

210. O'Neill, M.J. (2001). *The Merck index: An encyclopedia of chemicals, drugs, and biologicals*. Merck; Harcourt Whitehouse Station, N.J. London.

211. PDR (2004). *Physicians' Desk Reference: PDR*. Oradell, NJ: Medical Economics Co.

212. *USP Dictionary of USAN and International Drug Names, 2002*. Rockville, MD: U.S. Pharmacopeia, 2002.

213. Chong, C.R., Sullivan, D.J., Jr (2007). New uses for old drugs. *Nature*, *448*, 645–646.

214. Wishart, D.S., Knox, C., Guo, A.C., et al. (2006). DrugBank: A comprehensive resource for in silico drug discovery and exploration. *Nucleic Acids Research*, *34*, D668–D672.

215. Breman, J.G., Egan, A., Keusch, G.T. (2001). The intolerable burden of malaria: A new look at the numbers. *The American Journal of Tropical Medicine and Hygiene*, *64*, iv–vii.

216. Guerin, P.J., Olliaro, P., Nosten, F., et al. (2002). Malaria: Current status of control, diagnosis, treatment, and a proposed agenda for research and development. *The Lancet Infectious Diseases*, *2*, 564–573.

217. Attaran, A. (2004). Where did it all go wrong? *Nature, 430,* 932–933.
218. Gottlieb, S. (1999). Antihistamine drug withdrawn by manufacturer. *British Medical Journal, 319,* 7.
219. Chong, C.R., Chen, X., Shi, L., et al. (2006). A clinical drug library screen identifies astemizole as an antimalarial agent. *Nature Chemical Biology, 2,* 415–416.
220. Weisman, J.L., Liou, A.P., Shelat, A.A., et al. (2006). Searching for new antimalarial therapeutics amongst known drugs. *Chemical Biology and Drug Design, 67,* 409–416.
221. Slater, A.F., Cerami, A. (1992). Inhibition by chloroquine of a novel haem polymerase enzyme activity in malaria trophozoites. *Nature, 355,* 167–169.
222. Chong, C.R., Sullivan, D.J., Jr (2003). Inhibition of heme crystal growth by antimalarials and other compounds: Implications for drug discovery. *Biochemical Pharmacology, 66,* 2201–2212.
223. Nwaka, S., Ramirez, B., Brun, R., et al. (2009). Advancing drug innovation for neglected diseases-criteria for lead progression. *PLoS Neglected Tropical Diseases, 3,* e440.
224. Cavalli, A., Poluzzi, E., De Ponti, F., et al. (2002). Toward a pharmacophore for drugs inducing the long QT syndrome: Insights from a CoMFA study of HERG K(+) channel blockers. *Journal of Medicinal Chemistry, 45,* 3844–3853.
225. Heidemann, S.M., Sarnaik, A.P. (1996). Arrhythmias after astemizole overdose. *Pediatric Emergency Care, 12,* 102–104.
226. Hoppu, K., Tikanoja, T., Tapanainen, P., et al. (1991). Accidental astemizole overdose in young children. *Lancet, 338,* 538–540.
227. Saviuc, P., Danel, V., Dixmerias, F. (1993). Prolonged QT interval and torsade de pointes following astemizole overdose. *Journal of Toxicology. Clinical Toxicology, 31,* 121–125.
228. Honig, P.K., Sevka, M.J. (1993). Comment: Ventricular fibrillation and anoxic encephalopathy secondary to astemizole overdose. *The Annals of Pharmacotherapy, 27,* 1407.
229. Clark, A., Love, H. (1991). Astemizole-induced ventricular arrhythmias: An unexpected cause of convulsions. *International Journal of Cardiology, 33,* 165–167.
230. Bishop, R.O., Gaudry, P.L. (1989). Prolonged Q-T interval following astemizole overdose. *Archives of Emergency Medicine, 6,* 63–65.
231. Craft, T.M. (1986). Torsade de pointes after astemizole overdose. *British Medical Journal (Clinical Research Edition), 292,* 660.
232. Hasan, R.A., Zureikat, G.Y., Nolan, B.M. (1993). Torsade de pointes associated with Astemizole overdose treated with magnesium sulfate. *Pediatric Emergency Care, 9,* 23–25.
233. Burke, T.G., Mutnick, A.H. (1993). Ventricular fibrillation and anoxic encephalopathy secondary to astemizole overdose. *The Annals of Pharmacotherapy, 27,* 239–241.
234. Wiley, J.F., 2nd, Gelber, M.L., Henretig, F.M., et al. (1992). Cardiotoxic effects of astemizole overdose in children. *The Journal of Pediatrics, 120,* 799–802.
235. Tobin, J.R., Doyle, T.P., Ackerman, A.D., et al. (1991). Astemizole-induced cardiac conduction disturbances in a child. *Journal of the American Medical Association, 266,* 2737–2740.

236. Leor, J., Harman, M., Rabinowitz, B., et al. (1991). Giant U waves and associated ventricular tachycardia complicating astemizole overdose: Successful therapy with intravenous magnesium. *The American Journal of Medicine*, *91*, 94–97.

237. Rao, K.A., Adlakha, A., Verma-Ansil, B., et al. (1994). Torsades de pointes ventricular tachycardia associated with overdose of astemizole. *Mayo Clinic Proceedings. Mayo Clinic*, *69*, 589–593.

238. Tsai, W.C., Tsai, L.M., Chen, J.H. (1997). Combined use of astemizole and ketoconazole resulting in torsade de pointes. *Journal of the Formosan Medical Association*, *96*, 144–146.

239. Hsieh, M.H., Chen, S.A., Chiang, C.E., et al. (1996). Drug-induced torsades de pointes in one patient with congenital long QT syndrome. *International Journal of Cardiology*, *54*, 85–88.

240. Goss, J.E., Ramo, B.W., Blake, K. (1993). Torsades de pointes associated with astemizole (Hismanal) therapy. *Archives of Internal Medicine*, *153*, 2705.

241. Kulkarni, S.M., Agarwal, H.K., Shaikh, A.A. (1994). Torsade de pointes complicating treatment with astemizol. *Indian Heart Journal*, *46*, 179–180.

242. Lindquist, M., Edwards, I.R. (1997). Risks of non-sedating antihistamines. *Lancet*, *349*, 1322.

243. Janssens, M.M. (1993). Astemizole. A nonsedating antihistamine with fast and sustained activity. *Clinical Reviews in Allergy*, *11*, 35–63.

244. Musonda, C.C., Whitlock, G.A., Witty, M.J., et al. (2009). Chloroquine-astemizole hybrids with potent in vitro and in vivo antiplasmodial activity. *Bioorganic and Medicinal Chemistry Letters*, *19*, 481–484.

245. Abdulla, M.H., Ruelas, D.S., Wolff, B., et al. (2009). Drug discovery for schistosomiasis: Hit and lead compounds identified in a library of known drugs by medium-throughput phenotypic screening. *PLoS Neglected Tropical Diseases*, *3*, e478.

246. Mackey, Z.B., Baca, A.M., Mallari, J.P., et al. (2006). Discovery of trypanocidal compounds by whole cell HTS of Trypanosoma brucei. *Chemical Biology and Drug Design*, *67*, 355–363.

247. Engel, J.C., Ang, K.K., Chen, S., et al. (2010). Image-based high-throughput drug screening targeting the intracellular stage of *Trypanosoma cruzi*, the agent of Chagas' disease. *Antimicrobial Agents and Chemotherapy*, *54*, 3326–3334.

248. Gloeckner, C., Garner, A.L., Mersha, F., et al. (2010). Repositioning of an existing drug for the neglected tropical disease onchocerciasis. *Proceedings of the National Academy of Sciences of the United States of America*, *107*, 3424–3429.

249. Jenwitheesuk, E., Samudrala, R. (2005). Identification of potential multitarget antimalarial drugs. *Journal of the American Medical Association*, *294*, 1490–1491.

250. Padwal, R.S., Majumdar, S.R. (2007). Drug treatments for obesity: Orlistat, sibutramine, and rimonabant. *Lancet*, *369*, 71–77.

251. Riethmuller-Winzen, H., Peter, G., Buker, K.M., et al. (1994). Tolerability, pharmacokinetics and dose linearity of azelastine hydrochloride in healthy subjects. *Arzneimittel-Forschung*, *44*, 1136–1140.

252. Weisberg, M. (1989). Terconazole—A new antifungal agent for vulvovaginal candidiasis. *Clinical Therapeutics*, *11*, 659–668.

253. Van Cutsem, J., Van Gerven, F., Zaman, R., et al. (1983). Terconazole—A new broad-spectrum antifungal. *Chemotherapy*, *29*, 322–331.

254. Taylor, M.J., Hoerauf, A., Bockarie, M. (2010). Lymphatic filariasis and onchocerciasis. *Lancet*, *376*, 1175–1185.

255. Osorio, Y., Travi, B.L., Renslo, A.R., et al. (2011). Identification of small molecule lead compounds for visceral leishmaniasis using a novel ex vivo splenic explant model system. *PLoS Neglected Tropical Diseases*, *5*, e962.

256. Schubert, C. (2010). Matchmaking service links up researchers to wallflower drugs. *Nature Medicine*, *16*, 7.

257. Knox, C., Law, V., Jewison, T., et al. (2011). DrugBank 3.0: A comprehensive resource for "omics" research on drugs. *Nucleic Acids Research*, *39*, D1035–D1041.

258. Zhu, F., Han, B., Kumar, P., et al. (2010). Update of TTD: Therapeutic target database. *Nucleic Acids Research*, *38*, D787–D791.

259. Keiser, M.J., Setola, V., Irwin, J.J., et al. (2009). Predicting new molecular targets for known drugs. *Nature*, *462*, 175–181.

260. Marton, L.J., Pegg, A.E. (1995). Polyamines as targets for therapeutic intervention. *Annual Review of Pharmacology and Toxicology*, *35*, 55–91.

261. Shigi, Y. (1989). Inhibition of bacterial isoprenoid synthesis by fosmidomycin, a phosphonic acid-containing antibiotic. *The Journal of Antimicrobial Chemotherapy*, *24*, 131–145.

262. Borrmann, S., Adegnika, A.A., Matsiegui, P.B., et al. (2004). Fosmidomycin-clindamycin for *Plasmodium falciparum* infections in African children. *The Journal of Infectious Diseases*, *189*, 901–908.

263. Griffith, E.C., Su, Z., Turk, B.E., et al. (1997). Methionine aminopeptidase (type 2) is the common target for angiogenesis inhibitors AGM-1470 and ovalicin. *Chemistry and Biology*, *4*, 461–471.

264. Kruger, E.A., Figg, W.D. (2000). TNP-470: An angiogenesis inhibitor in clinical development for cancer. *Expert Opinion on Investigational Drugs*, *9*, 1383–1396.

265. Croft, S.L., Seifert, K., Duchene, M. (2003). Antiprotozoal activities of phospholipid analogues. *Molecular and Biochemical Parasitology*, *126*, 165–172.

266. Botero, D. (1978). Chemotherapy of human intestinal parasitic diseases. *Annual Review of Pharmacology and Toxicology*, *18*, 1–15.

267. Nakajima, M., Yamada, T., Kusuhara, T., et al. (2004). Results of quinacrine administration to patients with Creutzfeldt-Jakob disease. *Dementia and Geriatric Cognitive Disorders*, *17*, 158–163.

268. Fang, J., Chen, S.J., Tong, J.H., et al. (2002). Treatment of acute promyelocytic leukemia with ATRA and As2O3: A model of molecular target-based cancer therapy. *Cancer Biology and Therapy*, *1*, 614–620.

269. D'Amato, R.J., Loughnan, M.S., Flynn, E., et al. (1994). Thalidomide is an inhibitor of angiogenesis. *Proceedings of the National Academy of Sciences of the United States of America*, *91*, 4082–4085.

CHAPTER 12

Drug Repositioning Efforts by Nonprofit Foundations

12.1. INTRODUCTION

DONALD E. FRAIL

Nonprofit foundations have played a major role in the advancement of break-throughs in basic research over the years. Historically, the primary research role assumed by the foundations was to allocate funds raised through donations through investigator-initiated grant proposals and peer review. More recently, a number of existing foundations and their supporters (e.g., the Fast Forward arm of the Multiple Sclerosis Society, and the three highlighted within this chapter), as well as a new breed of "philanthropic entrepreneurs" (e.g., The Myelin Repair Foundation and the Spinal Muscular Atrophy Association), have been frustrated by the pace at which these enormous basic research discoveries have been translated to new medicines for patients and have therefore established programs or organizations specifically directed toward the clinical translation of these discoveries and the development of new medicines. The development of a new medicine is an expensive proposition with high risks for the most experienced pharmaceutical company. For these very reasons, diseases with a low potential return on investment, higher risk, or unprecedented and long development paths are often underserved by the traditional pharmaceutical or biotechnology industry. Certain foundations therefore seek to fill or supplement the translation of basic discoveries to testing potential new medicines in humans and have embraced drug repositioning as one important strategy due to the potential lower costs involved and quicker timelines to success.

In this chapter the clinical translation models of three different nonprofit foundations, the Leukemia & Lymphoma Society, the Michael J. Fox Foundation, and the Polycystic Kidney Disease Foundation, are highlighted and each includes drug repositioning as a key strategy. These three examples are by no

Drug Repositioning: Bringing New Life to Shelved Assets and Existing Drugs, First Edition.
Edited by Michael J. Barratt and Donald E. Frail.
© 2012 John Wiley & Sons, Inc. Published 2012 by John Wiley & Sons, Inc.

means exclusive, but collectively they highlight the key opportunities and challenges involved. Common themes include:

- The establishment of specific programs targeted toward these efforts, separate from their existing basic research efforts.
- The use of their network of academic experts to identify advancing basic research opportunities and potential therapeutic targets for intervention.
- The inclusion and often proactive engagement of pharmaceutical and biotechnology companies, which can include funding. While this may seem counterintuitive—a nonprofit providing funding to a for-profit entity—it is often necessary for the company to engage. This is particularly true for drug repositioning since the company may have a compound of high interest to the foundation but the specific disease may not be within the strategy of the company. The interest by a foundation in obtaining a return on investment if the funding leads to a marketed medicine varies across foundations.
- Unlike a basic research grant, the continued funding by a foundation is often based on the achievement of predetermined milestones in the near term (a year or less) and is done in collaboration with the foundation.

A common challenge also emerges from these experiences. Intellectual property issues can create barriers to advancing a successful molecule to the market, as discussed elsewhere in this book (for example, see Chapter 2). This is a double-edged sword. On the one hand, if a company has intellectual property on a certain molecule, then the repositioning effort is dependent on the endorsement of the company. On the other hand, if there is no intellectual property remaining on the molecule, then the ability to gain a return on the significant investment needed to advance through Phase III development and to the market does not exist. This latter situation is more often the case since many shelved development and marketed compounds have little or no remaining patent life. While the potential new use of the molecule may be patentable, it must be entirely novel and not disclosed previously, and even then may suffer from off-labeling prescribing of a generic substitute. Finally, theoretically, data exclusivity (see Chapters 2 and 4) can provide a sufficient incentive, but more often than not, the risk-adjusted costs of the development and marketing activities cannot be recovered within the current standard data exclusivity period.

Foundations are playing an increasingly important role in the initial translation of basic discoveries to the clinic and drug repositioning is a key strategy. They are well positioned to bridge the basic science of the experts they fund within academic centers, networks of investigators, pharmaceutical and biotech companies, and government. In this chapter, we profile three such efforts, each highlighting their drug repositioning model, their opportunities, and their challenges.

12.2. REPOSITIONING OF DRUGS FOR HEMATOLOGICAL MALIGNANCIES: PERSPECTIVE FROM THE LEUKEMIA & LYMPHOMA SOCIETY

LOUIS DEGENNARO, AARON SCHIMMER, JAMES KASPER, and RICHARD WINNEKER

12.2.1. Introduction

This section highlights a collaborative effort between a not-for-profit voluntary health agency, academic institutions, and the private sector to successfully discover, drive the development of, and initiate human clinical testing of an off-patent topical antifungal with previously under-recognized activity in hematological malignancies. This case history serves as an example of how parties that serve different stakeholders with varying goals and outcome metrics have cooperated to enable a mutually desirable and beneficial goal, namely the rapid acceleration of a potential novel acute leukemia agent into human clinical testing. As an introduction to the process, we discuss the history of the not-for-profit agency and the programs and resources utilized in this effort before reviewing the details of the repositioned drug project.

12.2.2. The Hematological Malignancies

The hematological malignancies are cancers that originate in the cells of the blood system. While the most familiar forms of these diseases are leukemia, lymphoma, and myeloma, a recent World Health Organization (WHO) classification lists over 140 diseases in the full spectrum of hematological malignancies, including numerous subtypes of leukemia, lymphoma, and myeloma and a host of rare myelodysplastic and myeloproliferative disorders [1]. The hematological malignancies are among the most well-understood cancers and significant progress has been made in their treatment. Cancer chemotherapy, stem cell transplant technology, and cancer therapies targeting specific molecular pathways were each developed initially through the study of blood cancers. Notable successes include a chemotherapy regimen that yields an 85% cure rate in young children diagnosed with acute lymphoblastic leukemia (ALL), Gleevec® for the treatment of chronic myelogenous leukemia (CML), where 90% of newly diagnosed patients in chronic phase achieve complete remission, and the thalidomide-based drugs extending average survival of myeloma patients to 10 years post-diagnosis. Nearly half of all cancer therapies approved by the FDA in the past decade (2001–2010) were approved initially for a blood cancer indication. Nonetheless, the hematological malignancies remain a significant unmet medical need. In 2011, approximately 130,000 newly diagnosed cases are expected to occur in North America alone (~40,000 leukemia diagnoses, ~70, 000 lymphoma diagnoses, and ~15,000 myeloma diagnoses) and approximately 60,000 patients will succumb to their disease.

Altogether, approximately 1 million North Americans are currently living with the consequences of a blood cancer diagnosis. Even with the therapeutic advances cited above, 50% of newly diagnosed patients do not live beyond 5 years post-diagnosis and the majority of patients who do survive beyond 5 years are at high risk for relapse or the occurrence of a secondary cancer, post-treatment. Thus, a significant opportunity and, indeed, need exists for the development of new therapies to treat these diseases.

12.2.3. The Leukemia & Lymphoma Society (LLS)

The LLS is the world's largest voluntary health organization dedicated to finding cures for hematological malignancies. LLS was founded as the de Villiers Foundation in 1949 and has awarded more than $800 million in research funding with total research spending in fiscal year 2010 alone totaling over $71 million. LLS-funded research programs include traditional grant-based funding to academic researchers as well as a recently developed funding model that focuses on drug discovery and development. For over 60 years, LLS has vetted and financed the most innovative and state-of-the-art blood cancer research in the world. Indeed, LLS-funded research directly influenced many advances in blood cancer therapy including bone marrow transplant techniques and novel medicines including pivotal work on drugs such as Gleevec®, Velcade®, and Rituxan®, among others. In 1949, a blood cancer diagnosis was almost surely fatal but today, thanks to innovative research funded partly through LLS, the survival rates for certain blood cancers have doubled or even tripled in some cases.

12.2.4. The Therapy Acceleration Program (TAP) of the LLS

TAP is the LLS's recently developed initiative designed to speed the development of blood cancer treatments and supportive diagnostics. The program was conceived to: (1) capitalize on research advances made by academic investigators funded through the LLS research grant programs, (2) catalyze interest in the development of blood cancer therapies by biotechnology and pharmaceutical companies; and (3) seek opportunities to lower the regulatory and clinical development hurdles faced by new treatments. The program complements the grant programs at LLS by assisting potential therapies from discovery through clinical development, stages of development notorious for extremely high failure rates and frequently referred to as "the valley of death." TAP was established in June 2007 and is composed of three divisions: Biotechnology Accelerator (BA), Clinical Trials (CT) and Academic Concierge (AC).

12.2.5. Biotechnology Accelerator (BA) Division

The BA division seeks to support biotechnology and small pharmaceutical companies that have potential blood cancer therapies but lack expertise and/

or resources to develop the therapy for a blood cancer indication. Through corporate alliances (not grants), the BA invests in specific projects to assist companies with gaining proof-of-concept data to demonstrate the therapeutic efficacy for blood cancer patients. Potential partnership projects are vetted through a multistep due diligence process that involves the LLS Research Department staff and a panel of biotechnology, pharmaceutical, business, and intellectual property volunteer experts. Partnerships are governed by contracts with timelines, milestones, and deliverables tied to LLS funding as well as diligence stipulations and a return on investment for LLS should a product move to the market. The BA is most likely to fund projects that will result in key results or milestones that enable a company to partner or raise additional funds; therefore, projects in late preclinical or early clinical development best fit the goals of this division. Examples of current partners include Avila Therapeutics for a Phase I trial of a Bruton's tyrosine kinase inhibitor to treat leukemia and lymphoma; Shape Pharmaceuticals for preclinical and Phase I testing of a novel, topical histone deacetylase (HDAC) inhibitor to treat cutaneous T-cell lymphoma; Celator Pharmaceuticals for Phase II testing of a novel liposomal formulation of chemotherapeutic agents to treat acute myeloid leukemia; and Onconova Therapeutics for a Phase III, pivotal, registration trial of a multikinase inhibitor for the treatment of high risk myelodysplastic syndrome.

12.2.6. Clinical Trials (CT) Division

The CT division seeks to develop a network of Phase I and Phase II clinical trial sites that use new strategies to reach underrepresented patient populations with the goals of increasing clinical trial enrollment and bringing the most recent therapies into communities distant from major cancer centers. Following this "take the trial to the patient" strategy, the CT division established its first partnership through the creation of The Clinical Trial Center for Hematologic Malignancies, jointly with the Cleveland Clinic, to facilitate the implementation of Phase I and Phase II clinical trials in a community-based setting. TAP provides funds to support some of the personnel (study nurses, protocol monitors, data managers) required to conduct clinical trials in six community-based hospitals affiliated with The Clinic. Clinical trials conducted at the Center are drawn from LLS-funded academic and private sector projects and can be proposed by The Clinic medical staff as well. Active trials testing various therapies currently are open and accruing at Cleveland Clinic-affiliated community centers across Northern Ohio.

12.2.7. Academic Concierge (AC) Division

The most novel division of TAP is the AC division that leverages LLS's 60-year history of vetting and funding top quality research at academic centers around the world. This program identifies active projects within the LLS grant

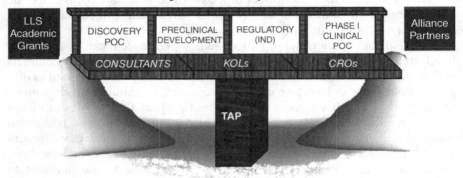

THERAPY ACCELERATION PROGRAM (TAP)
Academic Concierge
A Bridge across the Valley of Death

FIGURE 12.1. Schematic representation of the Academic Concierge (AC) division of LLS's Therapy Acceleration Program (TAP). The AC program's goal is to identify and chaperone key project/assets from LLS's portfolio of academic research grants to enable them to complete the necessary studies to bridge the gap to advanced clinical trials, key commercialization partnerships, and eventual access to patients. KOL, key opinion leaders.

portfolio (~400 projects representing a $56 million annual investment in fiscal year 2010) that may have therapy potential and could benefit from additional resources (Figure 12.1). LLS grantees submit annual progress reports and promising projects are identified when these reports are reviewed by LLS Research Department staff that has industry drug development experience. Typically, approximately 10% of grant-funded projects reviewed each year fall into the development space and are considered candidates for additional support. The LLS staff also actively reaches out to academic investigators with promising projects to stay informed of the latest data. Once a project is identified, the TAP staff uses internal expertise as well as contract research organizations (CROs) and volunteer experts in hematology, drug discovery, regulatory affairs, business development, and intellectual property to vet the project and establish a path forward for investigational new drug (IND) enabling studies and clinical development. Accelerating progress toward potential therapies is enabled by the investment of additional financial support and LLS staff-directed guidance through the process of drug development.

The AC division is especially relevant regarding drug repositioning as these types of studies are often conducted in an academic institution due to lack of large pharmaceutical interest—driven primarily by intellectual property concerns or apparent lack of commercialization potential. However, recent initiatives announced by many of the larger pharmaceutical companies indicate a renewed interest in drug repositioning as one means of searching for novel indications and uses for existing drugs.

12.2.8. Partnering to Reposition a Drug to Treat Hematological Malignancies—A Case Study of Ciclopirox Olamine (CPX)

Drug repositioning is a strategy to rapidly advance new therapeutic options for drugs that have been shown previously to have clinical safety and/or efficacy. The repositioning of thalidomide as a therapeutic agent for the treatment of multiple myeloma and myelodysplasia is one of the best-known examples of this strategy and there are other examples. However, to date, the identification of old drugs with unrecognized anticancer activity has been largely serendipitous. For example, the antifungal ketoconazole was discovered to inhibit the production of androgens from the testes and adrenals in rat models [2]. Given this finding, ketoconazole was rapidly advanced into clinical trials for patients with prostate cancer where it displayed clinical efficacy in early studies [3, 4]. By contrast, the partnership described here between the LLS, Dr. Aaron Schimmer at Princess Margaret Hospital in Toronto, the University of Kansas Medical Center (UKMC), and Beckloff Associates took a systematic approach to the identification and development of previously well-characterized compounds for the treatment of acute leukemias.

12.2.8.1. Compound Screening Commercially available and in-house libraries of on-patent and off-patent drugs from the Canadian and U.S. drug formularies were compiled by Dr. Schimmer, an LLS grantee, and used in two parallel screens to identify novel anticancer agents. These screens led to the identification of the topical anti-fungal agent CPX (Figure 12.2A) [5].

The first screen sought to identify compounds that were potentially cytotoxic to leukemia stem cells. Specifically, a chemical screen was conducted to identify drugs that reduced the viability of TEX and M9-ENL1 cells. TEX and M9-ENL1 cells, derived from lineage-depleted human cord blood cells (Lin-CB) transduced with TLS-ERG or MLL-ENL oncogenes, respectively,

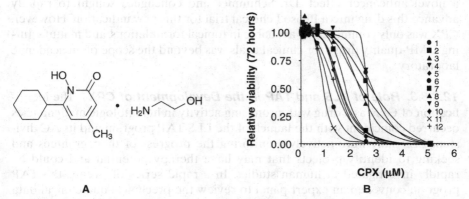

FIGURE 12.2. (A) The chemical structure of ciclopirox olamine (CPX). (B) Growth inhibitory effects of CPX on primary cells in culture derived from patients with acute myeloblastic leukemia. Individual symbols represent individual patient samples.

display properties similar to leukemia stem cells such as a hierarchal differentiation and marrow repopulation [6, 7]. In this screen, TEX and M9-ENL1 cells were treated with aliquots of known drug libraries and cell viability was measured. This screen identified 76 compounds, including CPX, which reduced the viability of TEX and M9-ENL1. A second screen was also conducted in parallel that sought to identify drugs that inhibited survivin transactivation. Survivin, a regulator of cell cycle and apoptosis, is preferentially expressed in malignant cells when compared with normal adult cells [8–10]. Dr. Schimmer hypothesized that compounds capable of directly or indirectly inhibiting survivin expression might possess anticancer activity. This screen also identified CPX. In secondary studies, CPX induced cell death in leukemia and myeloma cell lines and primary acute myeloblastic leukemia (AML) patient samples (Figure 12.2B) preferentially over normal hematopoietic cells at concentrations that appeared pharmacologically achievable. Moreover, CPX was preferentially cytotoxic to leukemia stem cells over normal hematopoietic stem cells. In mouse models of leukemia, CPX delayed tumor growth without evidence of toxicity. Mechanistically, CPX's anticancer effects appeared related to its ability to bind intracellular iron and inhibit iron-dependent enzymes such as ribonucleotide reductase.

12.2.8.2. The Compound CPX is an alpha-hydroxypyridone that is approved for the treatment of cutaneous fungal infection [11]. Although not previously administered systemically to humans for therapeutic use, its safety after oral and intravenous administration had been extensively tested in animals. Importantly, repeat dose toxicology studies following oral and intravenous administration in rats and dogs indicated a sufficient therapeutic safety margin to propose a Phase I clinical study. Given the existence of prior toxicology and pharmacology studies of CPX, its prior approval as a topical antifungal based on those studies, and the strong preclinical data demonstrating a novel anticancer effect, Dr. Schimmer and colleagues sought to rapidly advance this drug into a Phase I clinical trial for this new indication. However, CPX was only commercially available in topical formulations, and manufacturing GMP-quality drugs for clinical trials was beyond the scope of an academic laboratory.

12.2.8.3. Role of LLS and TAP in the Development of CPX The identification of CPX as a drug with promising activity in hematologic malignancies occurred coincident with the launch of the LLS TAP program and its AC division. LLS staff were actively monitoring the progress of their grantees and seeking to identify projects that may have therapy potential and could be rapidly investigated in human studies. In a rapid series of events, the TAP program convened an expert panel to review the preclinical and clinical data surrounding CPX. In addition, opinions were sought regarding the status of the intellectual property and the potential for commercial development. After the appropriate due diligence on the part of LLS, a partnership was established to advance CPX into the clinic for patients with relapsed and refractory hematologic malignancy, with LLS providing funding for the project. The partnership included LLS, Dr. Schimmer, UKMC, and the regulatory group Beckloff Associates. This partnership established a team from a voluntary health organization, two academic institutions, and the private sector to individually add expertise that when combined would facilitate and accelerate the investigation of this drug in a previously unrecognized indication.

12.2.8.4. Intellectual Property Considerations
As a charitable organization, intellectual property considerations are given less weight in LLS's decision to adopt a project into its AC program. Although a stronger intellectual property position than the off-patent status of CPX would have been preferable, the mandate of LLS is to find cures for blood cancers. Thus, LLS was willing to support a promising therapy despite concerns around intellectual property. It was also recognized that as a drug for the treatment of AML or myeloma, CPX would qualify for orphan drug status and thus offer a route for commercial development and market exclusivity (see Chapters 2 and 4 for more details on exclusivity protection). Moreover, the clinical data obtained with CPX would support the development of analogs that would potentially be more potent and have a stronger future intellectual property position.

12.2.8.5. Drug Reformulation and Chemistry, Manufacturing, and Controls
The drug development unit at the University of Kansas was charged with developing an oral formulation of CPX suitable for use in a clinical trial. While a number of formulations were considered and tested, the joint team decided to initiate the clinical trial with a simple oral formulation of CPX dissolved in Ora-Sweet®. Although this formulation was felt to offer the greatest dose flexibility in the Phase I study, it was recognized that it would likely not be the formulation that would advance into later stage clinical trials.

Beckloff Associates coordinated the manufacturing and stability testing of CPX for the Phase I study. CPX drug substance is obtained from PCAS in France. The drug product, "Ciclopirox Olamine Powder for Oral Suspension," is manufactured under cGMP conditions at KP Pharmaceutical Technology in Indiana. The manufacturing consists of quality control testing and weighing and filling bulk supplies into smaller containers. For use in the proposed clinical trial, 1 g is provided in 120-mL amber polyethylene bottles, to be reconstituted with a commercially available suspending agent (Ora-Sweet®) to a final concentration of 10 mg/mL. The pH of the final product once suspended is approximately 7 to 8. Drug stability studies of the reconstituted suspension indicated that it can be stored at 4°C for up to 2 weeks.

12.2.8.6. Regulatory Approval and Phase I Clinical Trial
The repositioning of an approved drug for a new indication offers the significant advantage of existing IND-enabling safety studies that can be submitted in the process of seeking regulatory approval for a clinical trial. In the case of CPX, the team

did not perform GLP toxicology studies but relied on data that were publicly available from studies performed in support of the original approval of the topical products (included in the approved labeling and summarized in the published literature). The studies performed identified potential target organs of toxicity and were judged to be adequate to support clinical trials of CPX in patients with advanced cancer. Median lethal doses (LD_{50}) in adult rodents exceeded 1700 to 2500 mg/kg administered orally, consistent with the lower oral bioavailability; intravenous LD_{50} was 20-fold lower. Repeated oral dose toxicity studies of up to 13 weeks were performed in rats and dogs. Similar to the mouse, CPX is rapidly converted to the glucuronide in these species and oral bioavailability in the dog is reported to be approximately 20–30%. In both species, the no-adverse effect-level (NOAEL) was determined to be 10 mg/kg/day. A standard battery of reproductive toxicity studies had been performed by oral and subcutaneous routes of administration of CPX (studies were also performed with the free acid). There was no evidence of adverse effects on fertility or of teratogenesis or developmental effects using doses that appear to be the highest achievable on the basis of the toxicology results. Neither CPX nor ciclopirox (free acid) was genotoxic in standard *in vitro* and *in vivo* assays.

Beckloff Associates provided an analysis of the prior pharmacology and toxicology studies related to CPX as well as the existing Drug Master File. This comprehensive analysis identified a German-language publication that described a study in which healthy volunteers received a single 10 mg dose of radiolabeled CPX. This study was the only reported series of systemic administration of CPX to humans. Compiling the existing regulatory data available for CPX, together with Dr. Schimmer's data on the antileukemic activity of the compound, the team created a data dossier for presentation to Health Canada in a Clinical Trial Application seeking approval for a Phase I safety study in acute leukemia patients. The team received a "No Objections" letter from Health Canada 28 days after submitting the application, allowing a Phase I study to commence.

Through collaboration and the combination of the individual skills of the team partners, the project had moved through IND-enabling studies into a Phase I clinical trial approved by Health Canada (NCT00990587) in less than 12 months from the time Dr. Schimmer's LLS progress report was read by the LLS staff. The trial opened, initially, at Princess Margaret Hospital and, in order to speed accrual, the British Columbia Cancer Center in Vancouver, British Columbia, Canada, was added to the trial as a second site. The trial is an ascending dose Phase I study in patients with relapsed or refractory hematologic malignancies (AML, ALL, chronic lymphocytic leukemia [CLL]) high risk myelodysplasia, CML blast crisis, multiple myeloma, non-Hodgkin's lymphoma, or Hodgkin's lymphoma for which all potentially curative therapy options have been exhausted). Single and multiple dose pharmacokinetics are being characterized. The study was initiated at a CPX oral dose of 10 mg/day, given as an aqueous suspension once daily in a fasting state for 5 days (one cycle); the dose corresponds to approximately 5 mg/m²/day in a patient with a body surface area of 2 m². Pharmacodynamic studies are also being conducted to demonstrate proof of mechanism in leukemic blasts isolated from the peripheral blood of patients on study.

12.2.8.7. Handoff to Industry LLS undertook the CPX project with the ultimate goal of delivering a new therapy to blood cancer patients. Nonetheless, LLS recognized that later stages of drug development (Phase II and III trials) and commercialization were beyond its resources and expertise. Thus, LLS sought a private sector partner with expertise in drug repositioning to carry the program beyond the Phase I trial. BioTheryX, a biotechnology company with such expertise, has been added to the partnership through an equity investment in the company by LLS. BioTheryX will seek regulatory approval to open a trial of the parent compound in the United States and will engage in prodrug and analog programs to improve on the pharmacokinetic and pharmacody-namic properties of CPX, as well as to secure the intellectual property neces-sary to warrant further development and investment in the project.

12.2.9. Summary and Lessons Learned

The CPX project illustrates how an existing drug can be rapidly repositioned and entered into human clinical studies for a new indication by combining the expertise of a voluntary health organization, academic institutions and the private sector. A systematic approach, building upon strong laboratory studies that suggested an unexpected anti-neoplastic activity in CPX and the existing preclinical and clinical experience with this approved compound, allowed rapid advancement into the clinic. Keys to the success of this collaboration were clearly defined roles and responsibilities for all collaborators and a project management team spearheaded by LLS who coordinated these activi-ties. It is critical to work with people/organizations that have the appropriate expertise and experience to move quickly and find or generate the data needed for a successful registration document and development strategy. This collabo-ration between multiple partners around a specific goal, driven by "industry-quality" metrics and reporting, has yielded significant progress over a compressed time frame. Only future clinical studies will confirm the utility of CPX, or derivatives of the compound, in the treatment of hematological malig-nancies. LLS, and its partners are committed to carrying out those studies.

12.3. REPOSITIONING DRUGS FOR PARKINSON'S DISEASE: PERSPECTIVE FROM THE MICHAEL J. FOX FOUNDATION

TODD B. SHERER, ALISON URKOWITZ, and KULDIP D. DAVE

12.3.1. Parkinson's Disease: Research Challenges and Opportunities

Parkinson's disease (PD) is the second most common neurodegenerative disease, affecting 1% of individuals over the age of 60 years of age. PD is marked by progressive degeneration of select populations of brain cells and predominantly characterized by motor symptoms. The cardinal motor symptoms of PD include bradykinesia (slowness of movement), rigidity, tremor, and postural instability. Recently, it has become increasingly appreciated that PD patients suffer from a host of symptoms beyond the widely recognized motor dysfunction. These nonmotor symptoms include mood disorders, cognitive dysfunction, sleep problems as well as autonomic dysfunction including cardiac, bladder, and dysfunction of other physiological systems [12].

Pathologically, PD is marked by selective degeneration of the dopaminergic neurons of the substantia nigra as well as neuronal loss in other brain regions including the locus coerulus, among others. Lewy bodies and Lewy neurites, protein aggregates, are also seen in widespread regions of brains of PD patients and are used as a final clinico-pathological marker for PD diagnosis. In addition to being found in the brains of PD patients, these protein aggregates are seen in many areas of the peripheral nervous system [13].

In most cases, the cause of PD remains largely unknown and is widely attributed to an interaction between environmental and genetic factors. On one extreme, in certain rare familial PD cases, the cause of PD can be specifically linked to genetic mutations in genes such as LRRK2, alpha-synuclein, glucocerebrosidase, PINK1, parkin, and DJ-1 [14–22]. Recent genome-wide association studies in idiopathic PD cases have also pointed to genetic contributions to PD in genes such as alpha-synuclein and tau [23]. On the other extreme, also in rare instances, there is evidence for a direct environmental cause for PD. In the 1980s, it was found that accidental exposure to the chemical, 1-methyl-4-phenyl-1,2,3,6-tetrahydropyridine (MPTP) by drug users in Northern California resulted in acute, onset of parkinsonism in these individuals [24]. More commonly, evidence suggests that exposure to pesticides, rural living, or well water increases risk for developing PD, while smoking and exposure to ibuprofen may decrease PD risk [25–27].

Current pharmacological treatments for PD predominately focus on dopamine replacement strategies in order to improve function of the basal ganglia system responsible for controlling movement. The gold standard for PD treatment remains levodopa therapy, with the goal of increasing production of dopamine in the brain. Additional therapies include dopamine receptor agonists, inhibitors of dopamine metabolism, and a combination of all these approaches. Dopamine-based PD therapies can be effective for a period of time in treating a subset of motor symptoms of the disease. However, their effectiveness wanes over time and is marked by significant side effects including motor fluctuations and dyskinesia, uncontrollable abnormal movements [28]. Additionally, dopamine-based therapies are ineffective at treating the array of nonmotor symptoms seen in PD. In fact, most of these nonmotor symptoms remain poorly managed in PD patients despite attempts to treat using available therapies (approved antidepressants, sleep treatment, etc.) for PD patients. Surgical approaches such as deep brain stimulation may be used in later stage PD patients and seem to impact a similar symptomology as with dopamine-based therapies. However, surgical approaches are also marked by potential side effects of brain surgery as well as specific treatment-based side effects that may impact cognition, speech, or other symptoms [29].

As described above, there are some available treatments for a subset of motor symptoms of PD. However, there is currently no proven disease-modifying therapy for PD. That is, there has been no therapy definitely demonstrated to slow or reverse the underlying progressive disease process. With increasing knowledge of PD etiology and pathophysiology, there are an increasing number of targets to explore as potential disease-modifying therapies.

In the face of the existing challenges for treatment of PD patients, there are a number of clear needs and opportunities for developing improved treatments. Developing improved symptomatic treatments for PD patients that leverage the success of dopamine-based treatments but without the side effects of dyskinesia would have a profound impact on the lives of patients. Currently, patients are forced to decide between optimal symptomatic benefit in the face of these side effects. Additionally, there are clear needs to develop treatments for the currently untreated symptoms of PD, including cognitive dysfunction and postural/gait disturbances. Current symptomatic drug development programs are focusing on nondopamine-based approaches with the aim of targeting other neurotransmitter systems such as adenosine or glutamate that also function to control movement [30, 31]. Finally, the impact of a successful, disease-modifying therapy that slows or even reverses the progression of PD would dramatically change the landscape of PD treatment and greatly improve prognosis for patients following a PD diagnosis.

12.3.2. The Michael J. Fox Foundation for Parkinson's Research

In late 2000, The Michael J. Fox Foundation for Parkinson's Research (MJFF) was founded by actor Michael J. Fox after his diagnosis with PD. MJFF was founded with the clear mission of developing an aggressive scientific research agenda with the goal of developing improved treatments and ultimately a cure for PD. To achieve this ambitious goal, MJFF has developed a proactive research strategy to engage with other stakeholders (government, academia, biotech, and pharmaceutical) to prioritize research opportunities and to de-risk PD research for wide-scale investment. By focusing on validating promising targets, promoting research at key translational decision points, developing and sharing critical research tools, and partnering with invested members of the medical research community, MJFF works to accelerate the translation of PD research into potential novel therapeutics. In addition to direct research funding, MJFF also plays an important role in promoting problem solving around ongoing PD research challenges by serving as a neutral convener of experts across the sector.

The MJFF research funding strategy involves two main avenues of activity (Figure 12.3). The Foundation's Pipeline Programs (Figure 12.4) provide open, investigator-initiated funding opportunities at various stages of the drug

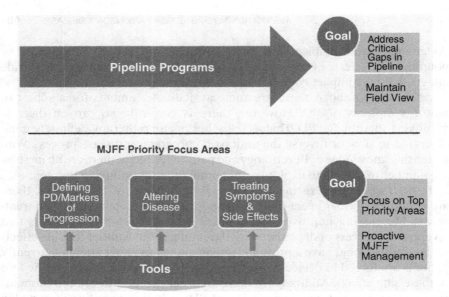

FIGURE 12.3. MJFF's research funding strategy involves two main avenues of activity: Pipeline Programs and MJFF Priority Focus Areas. The Pipeline Programs present MJFF with the opportunity to fund a wide-range of academia and industry investigator-initiated science covering various stages of drug development. MJFF-driven Priority Areas, in contrast, are specific research topics that have been identified by staff, in consultation with the Foundation's Scientific Advisory Board, and are the targets of a more proactive approach by the research team.

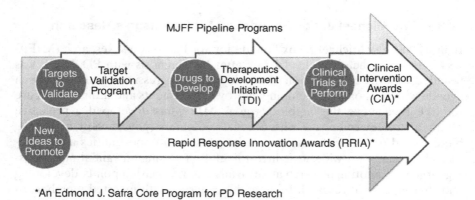

*An Edmond J. Safra Core Program for PD Research

FIGURE 12.4. MJFF's Pipeline Programs are annual funding opportunities that present the Foundation with the opportunity to fund a wide-range of investigator-initiated science covering various stages of drug development. In 2011, these included the Therapeutics Development Initiative, a funding mechanism to support and stimulate preclinical PD research led by companies, and the Edmond J. Safra Core Programs for PD Research: Rapid Response Innovation Awards, supporting high-risk, high-reward projects; Target Validation, supporting work demonstrating whether modulation of a novel biological target has impact in a PD-relevant animal model; Clinical Intervention Awards, funding clinical testing of promising PD therapies.

development pipeline. Applications are encouraged from both academic and industry researchers. Rapid Response Innovation Awards (RRIA), an Edmond J. Safra Core Program for PD Research, is a 1-year program that seeks to support new, innovative PD hypotheses, through $75,000 awards. Target Validation, an Edmond J. Safra Core Program for PD Research, supports proposals to provide the first initial validation of novel therapeutic targets in relevant PD animal models. The Therapeutics Development Initiative (TDI) supports preclinical development of novel therapies exclusively in biotechnology or pharmaceutical companies. The MJFF LEAPS program (Linked Efforts to Accelerate Parkinson's Solutions) provide multimillion dollar awards to all-star teams focused on moving a therapy from preclinical development into and including early clinical testing. Finally, the Clinical Intervention Award (CIA), an Edmond J. Safra Core Program for PD Research, provides support for testing of novel therapies in the clinic, whether to evaluate safety, dosing, or efficacy. Through these Pipeline Programs, MJFF seeks to solicit the best hypotheses from the PD research community and provide rapid funding to move these ideas further down the drug development pipeline. In 2010, MJFF supported roughly $12 million of research through its Pipeline Programs.

MJFF supplements its Pipeline Programs with more focused efforts through its Priority Area efforts. To specifically address critical challenges in PD research and to proactively move research in targets of high priority toward the clinic, MJFF has identified specific research areas of high potential impact. In these Priority Areas, MJFF develops specific roadmaps of activities and develops proactive strategies to implement these initiatives. The Priority Area topics are developed, in consultation with the Foundation's Scientific Advisory Board, based on the needs of PD patients and the existing scientific opportunities and roadblocks. Currently, MJFF's priority topics focus on the following specific areas (Figure 12.5): (1) develop markers of PD progression—including an emphasis on biomarkers, (2) develop disease-modifying therapies focused on the high priority targets based on PD genetics (alpha-synuclein, Lrrk2) and neurorestorative potential (i.e., neurotrophic factors), (3) develop improved symptomatic PD treatments by developing treatments for levodopa-induced dyskinesia and targeting untreated symptoms such as cognition and posture/gait disorders, and (4) develop and make widely available critical research tools such as animal models, antibodies, and assays to broadly accelerate PD research.

12.3.3. MJFF's Work in Drug Repositioning

As part of this aggressive research agenda, MJFF is always looking for ways to accelerate the timeline for developing novel PD therapies. On average, it is estimated that a new therapy can take over a decade to develop and well over $1.0 billion including research and time costs [32]. Due to these significant challenges facing central nervous system (CNS) drug development in general and PD development in particular, innovative approaches must be considered

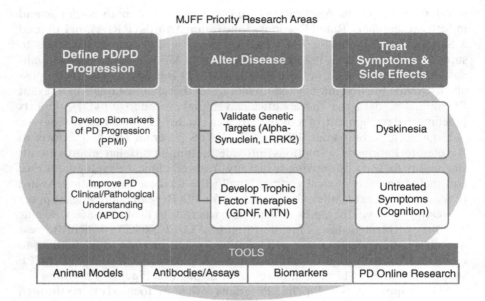

FIGURE 12.5. MJFF's Priority Focus Areas are specific research topics that have been identified by staff and are the targets of a more proactive approach by the research team. In 2011, these included: Defining PD/Markers of Progression, Altering Disease, Treating Symptoms and Side Effects, and Tools. PPMI, Parkinson's Progression Marker's Initiative; APDC, Arizona Parkinson's Disease Consortium; GDNF, glial-derived neurotrophic factor; NTN, neurturin.

in an attempt to accelerate this timeframe and reduce expenses. One approach that MJFF has used focuses on drug repositioning, with a specific goal of identifying clinically available compounds/therapies that may influence the activity of PD targets identified as high priority. MJFF has taken two main approaches to drug repositioning. The first approach includes an opportunistic strategy where a clinically available compound is identified that may influence a newly validated PD target. This opportunistic strategy has been supplemented with a specific funding program developed in 2010–2011 to proactively solicit research proposals that seek to repurpose existing, clinically available therapies for PD. In both of these cases, focus is particularly paid to therapeutic approaches with the potential to overcome the limitations of currently available PD therapies by addressing either untreated symptoms, side effects of existing medications, or ideally a disease-modifying treatment.

In assessing and prioritizing opportunities for repositioning drugs for PD, some specific PD-related issues must be taken into consideration. Therapies for PD and other CNS diseases must have sufficient permeability to cross the blood–brain barrier in order to interact with targets within the CNS. Many clinically available drugs developed for other non-CNS indications were not developed or selected for based on blood–brain barrier permeability and thus may not be suitable for testing in PD. In some cases, the brain bioavailability data may not be known and must be generated as part of the PD repositioning development plan. Investment in this work may not be of immediate interest to the drug owner. However, additional data generated with Foundation support may provide greater incentive for further company investment and application to PD. Finally, as most PD patients are elderly and PD is a chronic disorder, attention must be paid to potential safety and toxiciological issues when repurposing drugs for PD, especially if the drug was originally developed either for an acute treatment or for use in younger patient populations.

Included in the section below are specific case studies describing MJFF's attempts to support research to reposition drugs for use in PD. The following is described for each case: the scientific rationale for the target, the preclinical data supporting the approach for the repurposed drug, the current state of development, MJFF's role in accelerating the research and any specific challenges and lessons learned. Additionally, details have been included describing the specific 2011 MJFF Drug Repositioning Program to highlight issues in soliciting and evaluating opportunities for drug repositioning for PD.

12.3.4. Repositioning Drugs for PD: Disease-Modifying Therapy Case Studies

A major goal of PD research is to develop therapies that slow, stop, or even reverse the progression of the disease—a so-called disease-modifying therapy. Currently, there are no treatments that have been definitively shown to be disease-modifying for PD. Developing a disease-modifying treatment comes with many challenges, including, but not limited to, lengthy timelines and very large expenses and resources required for preclinical and clinical development as well as significant risk due to the lack of a clear regulatory path for approval. For these reasons, in addition to working to develop novel disease-modifying therapies using the standard drug development approach—from target to lead compound to preclinical and clinical development—MJFF has also supported opportunities to reposition treatments as disease-modifying therapies.

12.3.4.1. Case Study #1—Isradipine as a Disease-Modifying Therapy for PD

Drug   Isradipine is FDA-approved for hypertension (brand name—Dynacirc®).

Researchers Involved   D. James Surmeier, PhD, and Tanya Simuni, MD, at Northwestern University.

Scientific Rationale   The scientific basis for exploring isradipine as a disease-modifying treatment for PD comes from both laboratory and epidemiological evidence. The selective vulnerability of the dopaminergic neurons of the substantia nigra in PD may derive from the unique electrophysiological properties of these neurons. In fact, work from the laboratory of D. James

Surmeier at Northwestern University suggests that these cells rely on a specific calcium channel, L-type Ca_v 1.3, to regulate neuronal excitability [33]. Studies in relevant *in vitro* and *in vivo* PD models have indicated that exposure to isradipine, a dihydropyridine calcium channel antagonist, protects nigrostriatal dopaminergic neurons [33]. In addition to this laboratory evidence, recent epidemiological studies have demonstrated that long-term use of calcium channel blockers may reduce risk for a PD diagnosis. This effect was specific to calcium channel blockers when compared to other antihypertensive therapies [34].

MJFF Role in Development of Isradipine for PD   MJFF moved quickly to work with Drs. Surmeier and Simuni soon after the initial publication of the discovery of the protective role for isradipine in animal models of PD. As isradipine was not initially developed as a therapy for a CNS indication, detailed dosing and pharmacokinetic data were needed in order to quickly translate the animal data into a clinical application. Through an Edmond J. Safra Core Program for PD Research RRIA grant, Dr. Surmeier conducted critical dose-finding and pharmacokinetic studies in PD animal models to determine whether the effective doses for neuroprotection observed in the rodent models fell within the feasible range for human exposure based on the history of human use of isradipine. The results of the MJFF-funded preclinical study provided critical dosing and confirmed previous bioavailability data [35] that informed the design of an ongoing MJFF-funded clinical study testing isradipine in PD patients.

Based on the scientific rationale described above and results from the additional preclinical studies, Dr. Simuni conducted an initial open-label safety and tolerability study of isradipine in normotensive PD patients. One concern with using isradipine in PD patients is that many PD patients suffer from hypotension [36] so there is a potential risk of exposing this population to an additional antihypertensive drug. The results of this study suggested that isradipine, at the exposures deemed effective in the animal studies, was well tolerated in PD patients independent of the presence of hypertension in the subjects. The main adverse events reported were leg edema and dizziness that required reducing dose exposure [37]. This small clinical study set the stage for a larger clinical evaluation focused on dose selection that is now being conducted in early idiopathic PD patients by Dr. Simuni and supported by MJFF.

Challenges and Lessons Learned   The isradipine project highlights some specific examples of the opportunities and challenges of repositioning drugs for PD. As is the case with many repositioning opportunities, isradipine was not originally developed for use in the CNS, and therefore, specific attention and care had to be taken to analyze data around blood–brain barrier permeability. In this case, researchers were fortunate to identify a calcium channel blocker with brain permeability. Frequently, animal studies may provide evidence for efficacy but do not specifically confirm that the activity of the drug is occurring centrally. Additionally, specific dose–response studies should be conducted in animal models to confirm that the effective dose is in the range of possibility for safe human exposure prior to proceeding into the clinical studies. Finally, specific characteristics of the patient population must be taken into consideration prior to proceeding into clinical studies—in the case of PD and isradipine, for example, researchers needed to consider the potential interaction between an antihypertensive drug and hypotension in the patient population.

An important, nonscientific challenge that also remains to be addressed relates to the future development of isradipine for PD. Due to intellectual property considerations, that is, a lack of intellectual property protection and therefore a limited return on investment, there is currently no industrial partner to help move isradipine forward for PD. MJFF and Dr. Simuni are working to determine mechanisms for potential partnering with governmental agencies on future development, but even if government support is obtained, the path forward to market remains unclear given the large costs involved in Phase III studies, product manufacturing, and distribution.

12.3.4.2. Case Study #2—Pioglitazone as a Disease-Modifying Therapy for PD

Drug   Pioglitazone is FDA-approved for diabetes (Brand name—Actos®).

Researchers Involved   Marina E. Emborg, PhD, Jeffrey A. Johnson, PhD, Joseph Kemnitz, PhD, University of Wisconsin-Madison; Tanya Simuni, MD, Northwestern University; and David K. Simon, MD, PhD, Harvard University.

Scientific Rationale   Increased oxidative stress due to increased reactive oxygen species (ROS) production is associated with neuronal cell death in PD [38]. One of the ways that cells respond to oxidative insults is by activation of the antioxidant-responsive element (ARE) through activation of the nuclear factor erythroid 2-related factor (Nrf2) [39]. The ARE–Nrf2 system regulates expression of antioxidant genes and detoxification enzymes, which promote neuroprotection via increased glutathione synthesis, nicotinamide adenine dinucleotide phosphate (NADPH) production, and ROS scavenging. Thiazolidinediones, such as pioglitazone, a brain-penetrable FDA-approved antidiabetic drug, have been shown to possess anti-inflammatory properties via activation of the peroxisome proliferators-activated receptor gamma (PPARγ) [40] and enhance mitochondrial biogenesis by activating the Nrf system [41], making it an attractive compound to repurpose for PD. Indeed, pioglitazone was demonstrated to prevent dopaminergic cell death in the MPTP mouse PD models [42, 43]. Dr. Emborg proposed to test pioglitazone (given orally) in a nonhuman primate model (macaque monkey) to assess for neuroprotection in PD.

MJFF Role in Development of Pioglitazone for PD   MJFF funded the efficacy study in nonhuman primates through its Pipeline Program. This study showed that, at a dose equivalent to the one used in the clinic to treat diabetic patients, pioglitazone treatment induced moderate but significant functional (motor) and neuroprotective (anatomical) effects in monkeys. Subsequently, MJFF provided supplemental funding to Dr. Emborg to assess levels of pioglitazone in the cerebrospinal fluid (CSF) of normal monkeys using three different doses, to understand brain availability and pharmacokinetic/pharmacodynamic relationship with regard to its efficacy. The results of these studies confirmed that pioglitazone, given orally at doses shown to be efficacious in monkeys, does indeed penetrate the brain. Following these positive results, MJFF brokered collaboration between Dr. Emborg and a group of PD clinicians, leading a consortium charged with evaluating disease-modifying therapies in early PD patients. As a result of this collaboration, pioglitazone is now being tested in humans (for early PD) as part of the NET-PD (Neuroprotection Exploratory Trials in PD) studies sponsored by the National Institute of Neurological Disorders and Stroke (NINDS). To supplement this clinical efficacy testing, MJFF has provided funding to add biomarker analysis to the clinical study (through a grant to David K. Simon, MD, PhD, at Harvard University) to complement clinical outcome measures and provide increased data to evaluate the effectiveness of pioglitazone.

Challenges and Lessons Learned   Many of the challenges described above in the isradipine example directly apply to the work on repositioning pioglitazone for PD. Careful attention to drug dosing and CNS exposure levels in deciding whether to move the project forward into the clinic was critical. In the case of pioglitazone, the partnership with NINDS provided the funding required to initiate the clinical trial. A collaborative effort among scientists with different areas of expertise (animal models, PD mechanistic science, clinical researchers, and biomarkers) was critical in prioritizing and designing appropriate studies.

The business challenge remains. Without a clear industrial partner, funding support for the full clinical program remains unclear. Additionally, issues such as drug supply and formulations need to be fully addressed in order to allow for continued therapeutic development of pioglitazone through the stages of clinical development.

12.3.4.3. Case Study #3—Nicotine as a Disease-Modifying Therapy for PD

Drug   Nicotine patches are approved as an aid in nicotine replacement therapy for smokers

Researchers Involved   Wolfgang H. Oertel, MD, and Marcus M. Unger, MD, Philipps-University Marburg; Karl Kieburtz, MD, MPH, University of Rochester Medical Center

Scientific Rationale The scientific rationale for testing nicotine in PD comes from numerous epidemiological studies that have consistently shown an inverse relationship between tobacco consumption and susceptibility in PD. A clinical study of 144 PD patients and 464 control subjects showed that smokers had a lower risk of developing PD than nonsmokers [25], and the incidence of PD was inversely correlated with the dose of cigarette smoking [44], providing evidence that nicotine may be neuroprotective in PD. Nicotine has been shown to up-regulate antiapoptotic proteins [45], induce enzymes of cytochrome P450 [46], and stimulate trophic factors [47], and these effects may underlie nicotine's protective effects. In nonhuman primates, nicotine exposure prior to MPTP lesion was demonstrated to protect against toxin-induced nigrostriatal neurodegeneration and significantly normalized evoked dopamine release, dopamine turnover, synaptic plasticity, long-term depression, vesicular monoamine transporter levels, and striatal tyrosine hydroxylase (TH) expression [48].

MJFF Role in Development of Nicotine for PD Dr. Oertel proposed a clinical trial to assess, for the first time, the disease-modifying potential of transdermal nicotine in very early stage drug-naïve PD patients over a treatment period of 12 months. MJFF funded, through its Clinical Intervention Awards, an Edmond J. Safra Core Program for PD Research, the randomized, placebo-controlled, double-blind multicenter trial (called NIC-PD), the first investigator-initiated transatlantic collaboration between PD networks in Germany and the United States.

Challenges and Lessons Learned An important aspect of repositioning nicotine for PD was dose selection for the transdermal patch. For NIC-PD, a slow up-titration (over 12 weeks) dose progression will be employed to enhance tolerability of nicotine, minimize side effects, and preserve blinding of the study. Additionally, a washout design approach will be used to assess primary endpoint clinical motor scores and minimize any confounding direct or enduring symptomatic effects of chronic nicotine treatment.

Other challenges facing the study are obtaining transdermal nicotine and placebo patches from the manufacturer, as well as coordinating contractual agreements for multiple clinical sites in two different countries. While the study is still in the planning phases, positive results from this trial would be of great value, as this approach could easily be translated in routine care due to the wide availability of nicotine patches.

12.3.5. Repositioning Drugs for PD: Symptomatic Treatments for PD

In parallel with working to develop disease-modifying therapies for PD, researchers are focused on developing treatments that improve the current symptomatic treatment of the disease and could result in significant improvement of quality of life for PD patients. This section will discuss efforts to reposition therapies to treat dyskinesia and compulsions, two debilitating side effects of current dopamine-based PD therapies. Following chronic exposure to Sinemet® (levodopa/carbidopa), the current gold standard treatment for a subset of the motor symptoms of PD, nearly all PD patients will develop dyskinesia, uncontrollable abnormal movements, over time. As a result, PD patients are faced with the difficult choice between receiving the optimal therapeutic benefit of Sinemet® and suffering a difficult side effect, or receiving a reduced dose of Sinemet® (thus lessening the therapeutic benefit) and avoiding the side effect. This difficult balancing act makes treating the motor symptoms of PD extremely difficult.

Because the side effects of Sinemet® are difficult to manage, many clinicians and patients prefer to use dopamine agonists for symptomatic treatment, especially early in the disease. However, these treatments are also marked by potentially damaging side effects including debilitating behavioral side effects with dramatic effects on patient quality of life including impulse control disorders [49].

12.3.5.1. Case Study #1—Eltoprazine as an Antidyskinetic Therapy

Drug Eltoprazine—being developed for CNS indications by the biotechnology firm PsychoGenics—shown to be safe in over 500 human subjects to date.

Researchers Involved Anders Björklund, MD, PhD, Lund University, in collaboration with PsychoGenics, Inc.

Scientific Rationale Dr. Anders Björklund, Lund University, and colleagues have generated extensive data suggesting that serotonin (5-HT) neurons in the brain take up levodopa to produce and release dopamine as a "false transmitter," contributing to the development and maintenance of levodopa-induced dyskinesia in PD. Using both selective lesion and pharmacological approaches in animal models of levodopa induced dyskinesia, Dr. Björklund validated 5-HT_{1a} and 5-HT_{1b} receptors as therapeutic targets for dyskinesia [50–53]. Specifically, he showed that agonists at both of these receptors are needed to suppress dyskinesia so a drug with these dual effects could be a potential antidyskinesia treatment. After a patent and literature search for potential compounds, Dr. Björklund identified eltoprazine, a partial agonist combining activity at both 5-HT_{1a} and 5-HT_{1b} receptors.

MJFF Role in Development of Eltoprazine for PD In addition to supporting Dr. Björklund's preclinical studies to determine the efficacy of eltoprazine (described above), MJFF is funding an initial dose selection clinical study being conducted in Sweden in collaboration with PsychoGenics, Inc. This initial study in PD patients suffering from dyskinesia seeks to identify an effective dose for use in a future, large clinical efficacy study as well as to confirm information on the pharmacokinetics of eltoprazine in PD patients. Additionally, the researchers will evaluate whether eltoprazine has any adverse interactions with Sinemet® that would limit its utility in PD patients. MJFF has played an important role in coordinating and aiding the new collaboration between Dr. Björklund and researchers at PsychoGenics, Inc.

Challenges and Lessons Learned   The eltoprazine project highlights some unique lessons in repositioning drugs for PD. Again, a major challenge in this project was the identification and selection of a compound with the appropriate receptor selectivity (in this case 5-HT1$_a$/5-HT1$_b$ agonism) to move forward. Many drugs that target serotonin receptors in various stages of development exist, and a combination of drug profile and accessibility was required for the selection of eltoprazine to move forward. As eltoprazine was already under development for CNS indications, much of the data regarding its CNS exposure and dosing was already available, and through partnering with Psycho-Genics, Inc., Dr. Björklund was able to leverage this existing information.

Some unique challenges that arose, however, were in the planning and development of the clinical trial. Even though eltoprazine has been tested in hundreds of individuals, a distinct development package needed to be developed and submitted to the Swedish regulatory authorities for approval to conduct the trial in PD. Again, in this case, the collaboration with PsychoGenics was helpful given their development knowledge and work with the compound.

12.3.5.2. Case Study #2: Simvastatin as an Antidyskinetic Treatment for PD

Drug   Simvastatin—FDA-approved to treat high cholesterol (Brand name— Zocor®)

Researchers Involved   Erwan Bezard, PhD, Francois Tison, MD, PhD, University Hospital of Bordeaux; Olivier Rascol, MD, PhD, Toulouse University Hospital.

Scientific Rationale   Evidence suggests that alterations in the Ras-ERK signaling cascade in the striatum of levodopa-treated dopamine-depleted animals contribute to the development and maintenance of dyskinesia. As a result, inhibitors of the MAP kinase cascade have been proposed as potential antidyskinetic treatments [54]. Additional studies have validated ERK signaling as a promising therapeutic target for antidyskinetic treatments by using pharmacological gene therapy and other genetic approaches [55, 56]. However, most inhibitors of this signaling pathway are not very specific and use of them as an antidyskinetic treatment would result in unacceptable side effects. The widely used statins inhibit RAS activity and ERK 1/2 phosphorylation [57] and were shown to reduce levodopa-induced dyskinesia in animal models [58]. Additionally, epidemiological data suggest that statin use is associated with lower risk of both PD and PD dementia [59]. Along with these data and the fact that statins have been widely used in humans for decades, Dr. Bezard and his colleagues proposed to conduct a small pilot clinical study of statins on PD patients suffering from dyskinesia.

MJFF Role in Development of Simvastatin for PD   Through its Clinical Intervention Award (CIA) program, an Edmond J. Safra Core Program for PD Research, MJFF worked with Dr. Bezard to support a small crossover study examining the effectiveness of statins in treating dyskinesia in PD patients. Simvastatin was selected for the study as it was known to have adequate brain penetration when compared to other statins. In this study, an $n = 1$ crossover design was used in which each patient serves as their own control following drug washout periods. Simvastatin was used at 40 mg/day and the primary outcome was improvement in dyskinesia without worsening drug wearing-off effects. The results of the study were reported in the fall of 2010 and demonstrated that simvastatin failed to show positive effects on treating dyskinesia [60].

Challenges and Lessons Learned   As discussed in the previous case studies, an important issue that requires specific attention when repositioning drugs for PD is brain bioavailability and dose selection of the molecule being tested. As many of these "repositioned" drugs were not designed for CNS indications, they have not been optimized for blood–brain barrier permeability or for dosing to the CNS. Additionally, clinical studies should include some type of marker, so that the biological activity of the tested compound can be observed and the study results can be interpreted more fully. As part of the statin study, Dr. Bezard included an informative biomarker read-out, examining ERK phosphorylation in peripheral blood cells. At the dose selected in the study, there was only a weak effect observed on this biomarker read-out suggesting that a higher dose of drug may have been required to generate the intended biological effect [60]. However, concerns regarding potential side effects at higher doses limited the interest to test higher doses.

While the study demonstrated that simvastatin was not effective as an antidyskinetic treatment at a dose the effectively treats dyslipidemia, the Ras-ERK hypothesis remains untested due to limitations of the compound. Dose selection is a critical variable in moving forward with clinical studies in drug repositioning and although animal studies can be informative, it is important to carefully consider whether an effective dose can be used in human subjects. Finally, inclusion of biological/biomarker read-outs in these clinical studies can also provide critical information to help interpret a negative result.

12.3.5.3. Case Study #3—Naltrexone for Impulse Control Disorders (ICDs) in PD

Researchers Involved   Daniel Weintraub, MD, University of Pennsylvania.

Scientific Rationale   The common use of dopamine agonists for the treatment of PD has given rise to ICDs associated with compulsive gambling, buying, eating, and sexual behavior. More recently, a large international cross-sectional study showed that 17% of dopamine agonist-treated PD patients experience at least one ICD at any given time and that 36% of those with an ICD have multiple ICDs [49]. ICDs can represent a significant clinical problem in PD due to impairments in psychosocial functioning, interpersonal relationships, and quality of life issues such as gambling and at-risk sexual behavior. Stimulation of dopamine function in mesocorticolimbic pathways, areas involved in reward and reinforcement behaviors, may underlie the pathophysiology of ICDs [61]. Endogenous opioids modulate mesolimbic dopamine pathways [62] and opioid antagonism has been proposed to block opioid receptors in the dopamine reward areas, thus providing efficacy in dependency/addiction states. A long-acting nonselective opioid receptor antagonist, naltrexone, is approved by the FDA for treatment of alcohol addiction [63] and is shown to be clinically efficacious against opioid dependence [64] and pathological gambling [65]. Thus, naltrexone may decrease ICDs correlated with dopamine agonist treatment in PD. Although naltrexone alone has been shown to be ineffective as anti-parkinsonian [66] or antidyskinetic [67] therapeutic, it was well tolerated in the PD population and had no worsening effects on motor or dyskinesia symptoms.

MJFF Role in Development of Naltrexone for ICDs in PD   Dr. Weintraub proposed an 8-week study in which 48 PD patients diagnosed with one or more ICDs that developed during PD and in the context of DA agonist treatment would receive either naltrexone or placebo treatment. Through CIA, an Edmond J. Safra Core Program for PD Research, MJFF funded the randomized, stratified, double-blind, placebo-controlled trial to test the efficacy and tolerability of naltrexone for the treatment of ICDs in PD.

Challenges and Lessons Learned   One of the most important challenges in this trial has been identifying and recruiting PD ICD patients. Dr. Weintraub has tremendous experience with clinical management of PD patients suffering from ICDs such as compulsive gambling, buying, sex behavior, and eating. Additionally, Dr. Weintraub developed and validated a new self-administered questionnaire for ICDs called the Questionnaire for Impulse-Compulsive Disorders in Parkinson's disease (QUIP) [49], which will be used as the screening agent for potential subjects. While the study is still ongoing, positive results from this trial would permit treatment of ICDs with little impact on motor symptoms and allow continued use of dopamine agonists by PD patients.

12.3.6. An Open, Investigator-Initiated Solicitation: Repositioning Drugs for PD 2011

As described above, MJFF has supported a number of projects focused on drug repositioning for PD. However, MJFF had neither proactively looked for these types of investments nor developed a mechanism to compare different opportunities until 2010. Similarly, it is not clear how many researchers were mining their compound libraries to reposition compounds to PD. Therefore, in September 2010, MJFF launched a funding initiative to attract both academic and industry researchers testing drug compounds for indications outside of PD that could have potential utility for PD. The funding announcement was posted in various online publications in order to attract as many non-PD researchers as possible, including the *Nature* online publication. Announced with $3 million worth of funding available, *Repositioning Drugs for PD*, challenged investigators to reposition compounds proven safe in the clinic, or through regulatory approval, to PD research. Applicants were encouraged to identify promising compounds and propose ways these might target PD pathways. Through the initiative, MJFF was prepared to fund both preclinical and clinical studies depending on the available rationale for testing in PD.

Researchers were required to submit to two application phases: a pre-proposal phase and an application phase. Those who passed the review during the initial phase were invited to submit a full proposal for funding. The difference between the two phases was that the full proposals included more details about the proposed experiments, whereas the initial phase included more information about why the therapeutic should be tested for PD.

Over 60 applicants submitted pre-proposals to the program, with 31% of these coming from the for-profit sector. With the help of the expanded advertising, over 16% of the researchers that submitted proposals to the program had never before applied to MJFF for funding. Applicants proposed repositioning drugs to PD from clinical research in epilepsy, Alzheimer's disease, malaria, organ transplantation, autism, and depression among others, with the goals of developing disease-modifying, antidyskinetic, or nonmotor symptomatic treatments for PD.

During the initial phase, researchers were required to complete a "Therapeutic Scorecard" (Figure 12.6) detailing prior preclinical and clinical results. To be eligible for funding consideration, proposed therapeutics needed to be proven safe in a clinical setting. Some applicants had also completed preclinical testing on their compounds in order to inform the dosing, duration, or formulation to be used when testing in PD models or in PD subjects. All of this information, combined with details on the proposed experiments to be carried out under the MJFF initiative, was reviewed by MJFF internal scientific staff and several external advisors.

This review committee evaluated the clarity of safety data presented for the therapeutic, the rationale for testing in PD, and the nature of the scientific experiments proposed for MJFF funding. When evaluating the rationale, the committee considered the targets each proposed therapeutic would hit. MJFF looked for targets with strong rationale for PD when considering if the proposed therapeutic would be worthy of moving forward. About half of those who submitted pre-proposals for funding were invited to expand their proposals for the second stage of review. Full proposals were due to the Foundation in March 2011.

The Michael J. Fox Foundation for Parkinson's Research
Repositioning Drugs for PD 2011 - THERAPEUTIC SCORECARD

Principal Investigator, Institution/Company, Project Title:

SECTION 1: General Information/Rationale
Provide a brief description of the therapeutic, its intended target and mechanism of action through which therapeutic is hypothesized to improve a PD-relevant symptom/feature. Please also explain the rationale for developing therapeutic, including how proposed therapeutic may address needs not currently met by existing treatments or therapies in later stage clinical development.

SECTION 2: Prior Clinical Testing
Please provide a brief summary of the prior clinical development of the proposed therapeutic. Include the indication in which it was tested, the farthest clinical phase reached and any reasons for failure in the clinic.

SECTION 3: Therapeutic Data
Please complete the following table by shading/highlighting the appropriate box that best represents the level of supporting data you have for your therapeutic. You may include clarification points within the 'notes' field at the bottom of each section, although please do not include extensive data or descriptions.

Therapeutic Name	The current name/designation for the therapeutic				
Patent/License Holder	Who owns the license/patent for the therapeutic being developed				
DRUG-TARGET RELATIONSHIP					
Selectivity	Untested/ Unknown	Non-Selective; "hits" many targets	Non- Selective; "Hits" targets within general class	Selective for Target Family/isoforms	Selective for Target
Potency	Untested/ Unknown	Micromolar	Nanomolar (>100 nM)	Nanomolar (>10 nM)	Nanomolar (<10 nM)
Note:					
THERAPEUTIC CHARACTERISTICS					
ADME/PK	Untested/ Unknown	ICV dosing in animal models	IP dosing in animal models	SC dosing in animal models	Oral dosing in animal models
BBB Penetrability in Target Region	Untested/ Unknown	Does Not Cross BBB	Limited (<10% systemic exposure)	Moderate (<50% systemic exposure)	Good (<100% systemic exposure)
Target Engagement	Untested/ Unknown	Not Possible to Determine	Suggested by PK	Confirmed; No Dose Relationship Established	Confirmed; Dose Dependent
Note:					
EFFICACY IN PRECLINICAL MODELS					
Experience in Parkinson's Disease Model: INDICATE MODEL	Untested/ Unknown	Negative	Positive, but high exposure required	Relevant Rodent Model	Relevant Primate Model
Experience in Other CNS Disease Model: INDICATE MODEL	Untested/ Unknown	Negative	Positive, but high exposure required	Relevant Rodent Model	Relevant Primate Model

FIGURE 12.6. "Therapeutic Scorecard" developed and used by the Michael J. Fox Foundation that required researchers to submit as part of the investigator initiated solicitation of repositioned drugs for Parkinson's disease for 2011. The "scorecard" asked applicants to summarize essential information about the proposed therapeutic, and was used during the review process to determine whether the proposed therapeutic was based on strong preliminary rationale and sufficient preclinical data to justify testing in animal models of PD or for moving into human testing.

Experience in Other Non-CNS Disease Model: **INDICATE MODEL**	Untested/ Unknown	**Negative**	**Positive, but high** exposure required	Relevant Rodent Model	Relevant Primate Model
Note:					
IND ENABLING STUDIES					
Safety Pharmacology	Untested/ Unknown	NOAEL known SR < 1	NOAEL known SR < 10	NOAEL known SR < 50	
Toxicological Studies	Untested/ Unknown	Single Species	**Multiple Species**	IND Enabling Studies Completed	
Formulation	Untested/ Unknown	**Initial Clinical Formulation** Developed	Bridging Clinical Formulation Developed	**Final Clinical Formulation Developed**	
ADME/PK	Untested/ Unknown	Support IV dosing	Support SC dosing	Support BID/TID oral dosing	Support QD oral dosing
Note:					
CLINICAL EXPERIENCE WITH THERAPEUTIC					
Phase 1: Dosing	Untested/ Unknown	Currently Being Tested	Completed	Dose Selected	
Phase 1: Safety And Tolerability	Untested/ Unknown	**Dose limiting safety/tolerability identified**	MTD not yet **Identified** – further studies needed	**MTD Identified**	No MTD **Identified** - no further studies needed
Pharmacodynamic Outcome	Untested/ Unknown	Not Possible to Determine	Suggested by PK	Confirmed, No Dose Relationship Established	Confirmed and Dose Dependent
Phase 2: Dosing	Untested/ Unknown	IV dosing for efficacy studies	SC dosing for efficacy studies	BID/TID oral dosing for efficacy studies	QD oral dosing for efficacy studies
Phase 2: Safety And Tolerability	Untested/ Unknown	**Dose limiting safety/tolerability identified**	Safety/Tolerability of significant concern	Safety/Tolerability of minor concern	Supports advancement to Phase 3
Phase 2: Efficacy	Untested/ Unknown	Not established			Supports advancement to Phase 3
Experience in Humans: NON-PD (INDICATE DISEASE)	Untested	Tested; Safety Liability	Tested; Safe in Phase I Studies	Tested; **Effective/Safe** in Pivotal Phase 2/3 trials	FDA Approved
Experience in Humans: PD	Untested	Tested in Humans – Safety Liability	Tested in Humans – Safe in Phase I Studies	Tested in Humans- **Effective/Safe** in Pivotal Phase 2/3 trials	
Note:					

SECTION 4: Proposed Experiments

Please briefly describe the proposed experiments you wish to perform. If preclinical experiments, please include any animal models to be tested as well as the outcome measures you will test. If a clinical trial, please include the basic trial design/phase, targeted subject population and primary outcome measures you will test. Please note that investigators invited to submit a full proposal will be able to expand on details of their proposed experiments.

FIGURE 12.6. (*Continued*)

For the evaluation of full proposals during the second phase, MJFF organized a formal review meeting where the applications were assessed for scientific rationale for repositioning the proposed drug for PD, potential impact of developing treatments for PD patients, design of the proposed preclinical or clinical experiments, expertise of project team, budget and timeline rationale, fit within MJFF portfolio, and intellectual property/drug development plan. This last point is especially important to understand the commercial landscape and anticipate potential hurdles for licensing or further development as a PD therapeutic. Applicants were asked to explain their plan for development after the MJFF award, and if any potential intellectual property challenges stand in the way.

Once projects were recommended for funding, MJFF staff worked with the Principal Investigators to incorporate any reviewer recommendations or feedback. In some cases, collaborations with PD experts could be recommended for researchers new to PD to ensure their projects are set up for success from the beginning. MJFF worked with each awardee to outline clear milestones and deliverables that were included in the contract letter sent to each project team. These are used as a guide throughout the project for both the researchers and the MJFF staff, and are discussed during progress assessment conversations every 6 months.

MJFF will look for projects most deserving of funding under the Repositioning Drugs for PD initiative. Although $3 million has been allocated to the program for the first call for proposals, MJFF will only fund the projects testing candidates with the most promise for development into a PD therapeutic. If only $2 million worth of projects fit these criteria, then MJFF will invest the remaining money elsewhere. If projects representing more than $3 million deserve funding, MJFF will look through its budget to potentially supplement further funding. Breadth of awardees, along with progress made over the first year will be key factors when deciding whether MJFF should launch the program in the future.

12.3.7. Conclusions from MJFF Drug Repositioning Efforts for PD

Despite some available treatments, clear unmet medical needs for PD patients still exist. Developing novel therapeutics for PD can be a high risk, lengthy, and expensive process. For this reason, multiple approaches need to be advanced in parallel. In addition to focusing on developing a rich, novel drug development pipeline, opportunities to jumpstart this process through drug repositioning are also worthy of investment. In PD, drug repositioning should focus on validated hypotheses that could benefit from leveraging clinically safe and available compounds. Specific focus needs to be paid to issues related to drug dosing, selectivity, blood–brain barrier permeability (as PD is a CNS disease) and unique aspects of PD patient populations. Promoting collaborations between PD experts and drug development experts can help to address some of these scientific issues, but generation of additional data will often be required to plan for a clinical trial with the repositioned compound. These studies should be held to the same scientific standards as those testing novel therapeutics in terms of the preclinical packages and data required to justify clinical investigation.

An additional challenge associated with drug repositioning may result from the intellectual property position of different therapies. Drugs "off patent," but safe in humans, may provide a promising opportunity for repositioning, but funding for late stage clinical development may be difficult to obtain.

Given the difficulty in bringing new molecules through the rigorous preclinical development pipeline, drug repositioning plays an important role in a portfolio approach to accelerating development of new treatments for PD patients.

12.4. REPOSITIONING DRUGS FOR POLYCYSTIC KIDNEY DISEASE: PERSPECTIVES FROM THE POLYCYSTIC KIDNEY DISEASE FOUNDATION

JILL PANETTA and JOHN MCCALL

12.4.1. Introduction: Accelerating Treatments for Patients (ATP) Program

Dr. Jared Grantham, MD, co-founder of the Polycystic Kidney Disease (PKD) Foundation, remembers a time when the genes for PKD had not yet been identified, when there was only a handful of researchers working in PKD science and when the promise for therapies was a distant dream. Since the organization's founding in 1982, the PKD Foundation has invested over $30 million around the world in critical PKD basic science and clinical research projects that have led to the identification of potential targets for drug discovery and many important clinical trials. The Foundation's significant and productive investments in basic research created a robust field of PKD science that is now ripe for drug therapy development. In fact, the progress has been so great in such a relatively short amount of time that Dr. Grantham admits he often reminds himself that the first treatments for PKD appear to be within sight. The PKD Foundation is reacting to these advances with newly implemented strategic initiatives that seek to realize this vision.

12.4.2. PKD

Autosomal dominant polycystic kidney disease (ADPKD) is a hereditary systemic disorder that most notably affects the kidneys, causing bilateral renal cysts and loss of renal function. ADPKD is a progressive disease that leads to renal failure in about half of patients by their mid-50s. The incidence of ADPKD is high with a frequency of more than one in 1000 and a patient population of about 600,000 in the United States alone. ADPKD is the fourth most common cause of renal failure; it is more common than sickle cell disease, Huntington's, and cystic fibrosis combined. Direct medical costs for ADPKD exceed $1.5 billion per year [68].

PKD is relentlessly progressive. As the disease develops, cysts appear on both kidneys and the kidneys themselves enlarge, often up to five times their normal size. Hypertension and pain are common. Patients usually become symptomatic after the age of 30 to 40 when the latent disease begins to show itself. As the kidneys begin to fail, patients suffer life-threatening cardiovascular disease, including aneurysms, strokes, and heart attacks. For the half of PKD victims that develop kidney failure, dialysis, and transplantation are the only available treatments.

ADPKD is a multifactorial disease. Cysts, which often become necrotic, result from cell proliferation, fluid secretion, and the development of abnormal basement membranes. Predictably, the disease has a significant inflammatory component. The progressive nature of PKD can lead to different therapeutic strategies that address both the proliferation and inflammation.

But what is the root cause? Over 90% of the PKD cases are inherited as an autosomal dominant trait. PKD results from mutation in either the PKD-1 or PKD-2 genes with about 85% of cases due to mutations in the PKD-1 gene on chromosome 16. The PKD-1 and PKD-2 genes direct the synthesis of proteins called polycystins. PKD-1 produces polycystin-1, which is believed to act as a G-protein coupled receptor. PKD-2 produces the protein polycystin-2, which acts as an ion channel for calcium and other ions (reviewed in Reference [69]).

With so much at stake for the 12.5 million people around the world with polycystic kidney disease, the PKD Foundation has initiated its Accelerating Treatment to Patients (ATP) program. The primary goal of the ATP program is the translation of PKD research discoveries made over the past three decades into the first treatments ever available for PKD patients. The hope of the ATP program is to foster the discovery and development of new therapies for PKD and to build a robust clinical trial pipeline. Ultimately, these efforts will lead to the clinical testing of more potential new treatments, thereby increasing the likelihood of new medicines for patients.

Historically, the PKD Foundation has supported important basic research that has made it possible to move in this new direction. In 2010, the Foundation decided to expand its preclinical focus to include more translational work that has as its ultimate goal the registration of new therapies. This translational program focuses the resources and experience of the Foundation on work that directly impacts the movement of new therapies to the clinic. This strategic decision is important in that it recognizes the importance of moving drugs into clinical trials for PKD as quickly and effectively as possible.

The PKD Foundation recognizes that translational research proceeds through a set of well-recognized and gated milestone steps. The path to registration for any drug is notoriously long, arduous, and expensive, and patients are left waiting. This traditional path is well understood. Pharmaceutical companies follow it as they discover and develop new therapies. Controllable risk is minimized as much as possible by including a variety of assays, or test systems, at all states of the drug discovery and development process. A holistic approach that eliminates compounds early that may not be appropriate for the target disease and identifies potential winners is the key to translational work.

12.4.3. Drug Repurposing: De-Risking and Expediting the Drug Discovery and Development Process

Researchers and clinicians studying PKD now understand many of the disease pathways and mechanisms involved in the onset and progression of PKD. As mentioned previously, PKD is a disease of cell proliferation (cell growth, fluid secretion, and inflammation). Cysts appear on the kidneys prenatally and then multiply and also grow on the kidneys. Through discovery biology, we have learned that many of the disease mechanisms described in PKD are also implicated in cancer and inflammation. This is where the strongest opportunities for drug treatments present themselves. With this knowledge in hand, experts in the field of PKD believe the time has come to move to the next level in discovering treatments for the disease.

The most cost-effective, least risky and most expedient way of accomplishing the goal of finding new therapies is to implement a drug repurposing strategy. This is at the heart of the ATP program. We define drug repurposing as the process of developing new uses for existing drugs or candidate compounds. It takes advantage of work that has been done for a different therapeutic use, thereby decreasing development costs and time to launch. The PKD Foundation strategy is to assist biotechnology and pharmaceutical organizations, or other research organizations, in evaluating whether their drug candidates have potential as therapeutic agents for PKD.

The three advantages of repurposing are reduced risk, shorter time lines, and lower cost. If a drug under development is at or near candidate stage, much is known about how it can be delivered, what its pharmacokinetic properties are, what doses hit the intended target reliably, what safety issues exist, and how the candidate can be prepared and formulated. This saves time and removes risk that others have already evaluated. In addition, by the time that a compound reaches candidate stage, a pharmaceutical company will typically have spent between $10 million and $30 million. By repurposing at the candidate stage, we avoid these early costs and save years of research time. In its simplest terms, this is the translational research model that we have embraced.

PKD is a genetic disease, and although we cannot yet cure the genetics involved in the disease onset, we can have a positive impact on progression of the disease. We need only look to the example of aspirin, first used to treat pain and now used for treatment of cardiovascular disease, in order to illustrate this primary prevention model. The PKD Foundation intends to find the first treatments that slow down or even reverse the process of cyst formation in patients with PKD. If we can accomplish this, we can delay or even prevent patients with PKD from going into renal failure.

We have identified over 20 drug compounds that work on mechanisms at different points in the onset and progression of PKD. We also have animal models of cystic kidney disease that took years to develop and that help us better understand how the disease ultimately affects the human body.

12.4.4. The PKD Foundation Methodology

To begin this journey into translational research, the new position of Chief Scientific Officer (CSO) was established at the PKD Foundation, and a small (<10 scientists) Drug Development Advisory Board was recruited. This latter group includes experts in drug discovery and development and project management. Members of this board are retired or active senior leaders in the pharmaceutical industry and are committed to applying their skills and experience in the efforts of the Foundation.

We kicked off the PKDF translational program with a scientific conference in April 2010. This conference was pivotally important. Members of the PKD Scientific Advisory Committee (SAC) who are leading experts in the PKD field (clinical work and basic science), members of pharmaceutical and biotechnology companies who were developing compounds that had potential in PKD, and representatives from the FDA and National Institutes of Health all attended the meeting. For the PKD Foundation, this conference was a dramatic declaration of our intent to launch the new ATP initiative, as well as an effort to educate pharmaceutical companies on the basic and clinical science and market potential of PKD. The meeting format was designed to mix PKD researchers and pharmaceutical/biotechnology researchers, to build new alliances, and to build interest in moving drugs forward for PKD patients.

We very intentionally defined the value proposition of the effort and articulated the reasons that a pharmaceutical company should be interested in PKD. We were aware that simple altruism on the part of the company is neither a sufficient nor realistic motivation for launching a drug development program in PKD. Clinical trials can be difficult, and a faster path to registration is still being debated. During the conference, we argued that we now understand much of the etiology of the disease and have good ideas on how PKD can be treated. With the emerging science that may lead to faster registration trials and a reasonable probability of success, the inherent commercial value to pharmaceutical companies of a PKD program swings in a very positive direction. PKD is not an orphan disease. It is very common with a worldwide population of 12.5 million people. The market potential in the United States alone is large, with a population of over 600,000 and projected revenues well over $500 million. Because the need for detailing or marketing cost is low given this patient population, the margins in PKD should be excellent. We believe that, in time, through the work of the Foundation's PKD Outcomes Consortium that registration of a compound using renal enlargement (total kidney volume) as an endpoint will become possible, thus favorably changing the risk, time, and cost factors involved significantly. So altruism aside, there is good reason to view PKD as a strategically important indication for a pharmaceutical company. Pharmaceutical and biotechnology companies are now recognizing this and showing significant interest in the potential of PKD.

Returning to repurposing and the methodology used, members of the Scientific Advisory Committee and a team of PKD scientist clinicians teamed up to assemble a list of drug targets/mechanisms/pathways that are implicated in the pathogenesis of PKD. The Drug Development Advisory Board took this list and generated a virtual portfolio of compounds from public sources that are in various stages of discovery and development at various pharmaceutical and biotechnology companies and that have mechanisms of action that we think might be important in the successful treatment of PKD. The virtual portfolio helped us better understand the possibilities that lay before us. The numbers of compounds that are in development and that have the potential in PKD are large. A few examples from our virtual portfolio are shown in Table 12.1.

As part of the ATP program, the PKD Foundation is entering into collaborative agreements for drug repurposing opportunities with biotechnology or pharmaceutical sponsors. The overarching goals are to determine if inhibition of specific mechanisms will serve as an effective treatment for PKD and to generate a drug efficacy package which, when combined with appropriate safety assessment data, forms the basis to advance a drug candidate into clinical development. In exchange for the compounds that are being tested, industry partners are benefiting from this collaboration model by receiving high quality preclinical testing data that would enhance the rationale for moving to clinical testing.

We seek to work to the rigorous standards used within the industry, which includes a standardized testing scheme that provides consistent and comparable results to aid in prioritization and decision making. Academic laboratories that do basic and translational research are not typically equipped or motivated to fulfill the role of a testing organization. Therefore, in order to guarantee a consistent evaluation of opportunities, we decided to establish a single laboratory that would run potential candidate compounds on behalf of the PKD Foundation rodent models of cystic disease.

The PKD Foundation is engaging Contract Research Organizations (CROs)—service organizations that provide support to the pharmaceutical and biotechnology industries—to develop a complete preclinical efficacy packages. These packages can then be used to support and encourage an IND application. After the efficacy package is complete, we will deliver the package back to the biotechnology or pharmaceutical organization. A schematic of our working business model and the various partners that are needed to make this work is shown in Figure 12.7.

The PKD Foundation has engaged PreClinOmics in Indianapolis as our CRO for the assessment of efficacy. PreClinOmics is providing preclinical research services in connection with drug efficacy testing for the treatment of human PKD and drug exposures are being assessed by PharmOptima. Professor Vincent Gattone (Indiana School of Medicine, a member of our PKD Scientific Advisory Committee and an expert in animal models of PKD) is serving as an advisor to PreClinOmics. Dr. Gattone is evaluating the kidneys in the cystic rodent model drug trials.

TABLE 12.1. Examples from the PKD Foundation "Virtual Portfolio"

Mechanism of Action	Compound	Company	Comments
Antioxidant inflammation modulators (AIMs)	Bardoxolone methyl—RTA 402	Reata	Phase II
avB6 integrin antibody	STX100	Stromedix	Being investigated for chronic allograft nephropathy
Calcimimetrics	Cinacalcet	Amgen	
Cdk4	PD 0332991	Pfizer	Selective. From Parke Davis/Onyx
GlcCer synthase inhibition	Genz-123346 and Genz-112638		Pharmacologic support in PKD exists for this class of compounds. Genz-112638 in P2/3 for Gaucher's Syndrome. Tested in preclinical models. Positive
20 HETE	Eis Avner compounds		Dropped in development
MEK	98059	Parke Davis/Pfizer	Preclinical
mTORC1/2	Non-rapalog inhibitors	Intellikine, S*Bio	
NF-kB inhibitor	VBP15	Validus Biopharm	Developed for Duchenne, preclinical
TGF Beta 1 inhibitor	GC1008, fresolimumab	Genzyme, AZ	Fresolimumab is being developed for idiopathic pulmonary fibrosis. It is a growth factor that acts by transforming tumor growth factor (TGFBR1) and induces oncogenic transformation in kidney fibroblasts
TGF Beta 1 inhibitor	P17 (Peptide)	Digna Biotech	Aerosol for lung fibrosis
TGF Beta1 inhibitor	Ang1122.	Angion Biomedical Corp	Inhibits signaling and causes differentiation of fibroblasts into fibrogenic myofibroblasts. Developed for lung fibrosis
V2 Vasopressin antagonism	SR 121463	Sanofi	
Pioglitazone analog, non-PPAR		Metabolic Solutions	Phase II, metabolic syndrome
P70 S6K1 inhibition	PF-4708671	Pfizer	A novel and highly specific inhibitor of p70 ribosomal S6 kinase (S6K1)
Read through, frame shift	PTC124 (Ataluren)	PTC Therapeutics	Needs to be targeted/tailored by genotyping to the ~30% of PKD1 patients with nonsense mutations. Phase II/III for cystic fibrosis and Duchenne muscular dystrophy
PI3K inhibitor, delta selective	Cal101	Calistoga	

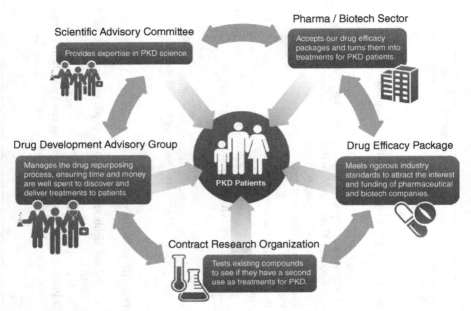

FIGURE 12.7. PKD Foundation drug repurposing model and the various partners that are needed to make this work.

Animal models are critical in supporting studies of disease pathogenesis and in testing potential new therapies. They are instrumental in the drug development process. Ideally, the perfect animal model should mirror the human condition completely. In the case of PKD, the model should carry a mutation in a gene orthologous to the human disease-carrying gene. The development of the disease in such an orthologous model should have the same course, severity, segmental origin of cysts, and extrarenal manifestations as seen in the human condition. Unfortunately, at this time, there is no ideal model. Therefore, in our drug repurposing and development program it is wise to test a potential therapy in more than one PKD model to determine its utility for clinical testing in PKD. This will give us the confidence to move a clinical candidate forward for testing in PKD patients.

PreClinOmics runs three different rodent models of PKD: two spontaneous mouse models (pcy and jck) and one rat model (pck). In the pcy mouse, cystic disease is slowly progressive with cyst formation similar to ADPKD. The jck mouse model resembles human ADPKD phenotypically despite the autosomal recessive mode of inheritance. The development of the cysts in the jck mouse is characterized by the development of cysts in multiple nephron segments. The pck rat is an inherited model of PKD and polycystic liver disease

(PLD) with a natural history and renal and hepatic histologic abnormalities that resemble human autosomal dominant PKD.

As a first step, validation of these cystic animal models has been completed at PreClinOmics using standard compounds that have already been shown to be effective in these models. In our ATP initiative, compound selection has been guided by the target candidate profile for PKD: an orally administered compound or a biologic that leads to a safe and effective therapy. All compounds are being tested in the same way so data will be comparable across different compounds and the pharmacokinetic profile of the test compound is established prior to testing.

Our collaborative arrangement with Intellikine, announced in February, 2010, is illustrative of our approach. Intellikine, a leader in the development of small molecule drugs targeting the PI3K/mTOR pathway, is collaborating to investigate novel, orally available small molecule kinase inhibitors of the TORC1 and TORC2 complexes as a potential treatment for patients with PKD. The mTOR kinase represents an important potential target for drug development in PKD. Unlike rapamycin analogs, such as sirolimus and everolimus, which have had only limited success in treating patients with PKD, TORC1/2 inhibitors block both TORC1 and TORC2, thus more potently inhibiting mTOR kinase, and may provide for greater efficacy in the treatment of PKD. Through the ATP program, Intellikine is having their compound assessed in the animal models, and they are able to engage the entire PKD community, from research and clinical experts in the field. The ATP program allows Intellikine to broaden their research and development activities in PKD beyond what the company would do on its own.

12.4.5. Lessons Learned To Date

Since inception of our ATP initiative, what have we learned? In creating our virtual portfolio, we have seen that the partnership between the PKD Foundation and the drug owners is essential and important. Both the drug and experience with that drug are provided by the drug owners. The Foundation provides access to state of the art screens and contact with the PKD scientific community. The preparation of a high quality data package that can support IND filing at minimal monetary cost is just one incentive. Second, we have concluded that a well-controlled triage assay is important for prioritizing opportunities in a way that is standardized for all compounds. This gives the foundation and our partners a sense of how competitive individual approaches will be. This desire for standardization led us to establish an exclusive relationship with PreClinOmics, our CRO. All compounds are being tested in the same way so data will be comparable across the different compounds. Third, we recognize that the preclinical work that we are doing is very expensive. We must acquire and dedicate funds in strategic and well-considered ways.

From the PKD Foundation perspective, this means we need to move more money into translational work if the effort is going to be both far-reaching and effective. Secure in the strength of the basic and translational research that we have already funded—discovery biology that has gotten us to this point—the time is now to move forward with the drug repurposing ATP initiative. Finally, we are increasingly convinced that this approach can work and that it can help move new and promising drugs into clinical evaluation for PKD. We are resolved to advance new therapies in PKD as quickly as possible.

REFERENCES

1. Swerdlow, S.H., Campo, E., Harris, N. L., Jaffe, E.S., Pileri, S.A., Stein, H., Thiele, J., Vardiman, J.W., eds. (2008). *WHO Classification of Tumours of Haematopoietic and Lymphoid Tissues*. Lyon, France: International Agency for Research on Cancer.
2. Ideyama, Y., Kudoh, M., Tanimoto, K., Susaki, Y., Nanya, T., Nakahara, T., Ishikawa, H., Yoden, T., Okada, M., Fujikura, T., Akaza, H., Shikama, H. (1998). Novel nonsteroidal inhibitor of cytochrome P450(17alpha) (17alpha-hydroxylase/C17-20 lyase), YM116, decreased prostatic weights by reducing serum concentrations of testosterone and adrenal androgens in rats. *Prostate, 37*, 10–18.
3. Sella, A., Kilbourn, R., Amato, R., Bui, C., Zukiwski, A.A., Ellerhorst, J., Logothetis, C.J. (1994). Phase II study of ketoconazole combined with weekly doxorubicin in patients with androgen-independent prostate cancer. *Journal of Clinical Oncology, 12*, 683–688.
4. Millikan, R., Thall, P.F., Lee, S.J., Jones, D., Cannon, M.W., Kuebler, J.P., Wade, J., III, Logothetis, C.J. (2003). Randomized, multicenter, phase II trial of two multicomponent regimens in androgen-independent prostate cancer. *Journal of Clinical Oncology, 21*, 878–883.
5. Eberhard, Y., McDermott, S.P., Wang, X., Gronda, M., Venugopal, A., Wood, T.E., Hurren, R., Datti, A., Batey, R.A., Wrana, J., Antholine, W.E., Dick, J.E., Schimmer, A.D. (2009). Chelation of intracellular iron with the antifungal agent ciclopirox olamine induces cell death in leukemia and myeloma cells. *Blood, 114*, 3064–3073.
6. Warner, J.K., Wang, J.C., Takenaka, K., Doulatov, S., McKenzie, J.L., Harrington, L., Dick, J.E. (2005). Direct evidence for cooperating genetic events in the leukemic transformation of normal human hematopoietic cells. *Leukemia, 19*, 1794–1805.
7. Barabe, F., Kennedy, J.A., Hope, K.J., Dick, J.E. (2007). Modeling the initiation and progression of human acute leukemia in mice. *Science, 31*, 600–604.
8. Altieri, D.C. (2008). Survivin, cancer networks and pathway-directed drug discovery. *Nature Reviews. Cancer, 8*, 61–70.
9. Fukuda, S., Pelus, L.M. (2006). Survivin, a cancer target with an emerging role in normal adult tissues. *Molecular Cancer Therapeutics, 5*, 1087–1098.
10. Altieri, D.C. (2001). The molecular basis and potential role of survivin in cancer diagnosis and therapy. *Trends in Molecular Medicine, 7*, 542–547.
11. Sehgal, V.N. (1976). Ciclopirox: A new topical pyrodonium antimycotic agent. A double-blind study in superficial dermatomycoses. *The British Journal of Dermatology, 95*, 83–88.
12. Langston, J.W. (2006). The Parkinson's complex: Parkinsonism is just the tip of the iceberg. *Annals of Neurology, 59*, 591–596.

13. Halliday, G.M., Del Tredici, K., Braak, H. (2006). Critical appraisal of brain pathology staging related to presymptomatic and symptomatic cases of sporadic Parkinson's disease. *Journal of Neural Transmission. Supplementum*, *70*, 99–103.

14. Polymeropoulos, M.H., Lavedan, C., Leroy, E., Ide, S.E., Dehejia, A., Dutra, A., Pike, B., Root, H., Rubenstein, J., Boyer, R., Stenroos, E.S., Chandrasekharappa, S., Athanassiadou, A., Papapetropoulos, T., Johnson, W.G., Lazzarini, A.M., Duvoisin, R.C., Di Iorio, G., Golbe, L.I., Nussbaum, R.L. (1997). Mutation in the alpha-synuclein gene identified in families with Parkinson's disease. *Science*, *276*, 2045–2047.

15. Hattori, N., Kitada, T., Matsumine, H., Asakawa, S., Yamamura, Y., Yoshino, H., Kobayashi, T., Yokochi, M., Wang, M., Yoritaka, A., Kondo, T., Kuzuhara, S., Nakmura, S., Shimizu, N., Mizuno, Y. (1998). Molecular genetic analysis of a novel Parkin gene in Japanese failies with autosomal recessive juvenile parkinsonism: Evidence for variable homozygous deletions in the parkins gene in affected individuals. *Annals of Neurology*, *44*, 935–941.

16. Kruger, R., Kuhn, W., Muller, T., Woitalla, D., Graeber, M., Kosel, S., Przuntek, H., Epplen, J.T., Schols, L., Reiss, O. (1998). Ala30Pro mutation in the gene encoding alpha-synuclein in Parkinson's disease. *Nature Genetics*, *18*, 106–108.

17. Bonifati, V., Rizzu, P., van Baren, M.J., Schaap, O., Breedveld, G.J., Krieger, E., Dekker, M.C., Squitieri, F., Ibanez, P., Joosse, M., van Dongen, J.W., Vanacore, J.W., van Swieten, J.C., Brice, A., Meco, G., van Duijn, C.M., Oostra, B.A., Heutink, P. (2003). Mutations in DJ-1 gene associated with autosomal recessive early-onset parkinsonism. *Science*, *299*, 256–259.

18. Singleton, A.B., Farrer, M., Johnson, J., Singleton, A., Hague, S., Kachergus, J., Hulihan, M., Peuralinna, T., Dutra, A., Nussbaum, R., Lincoln, S., Crawley, A., Hanson, M., Maraganore, D., Adler, C., Cookson, M.R., Muenter, M., Baptista, M., Miller, D., Blancato, J., Hardy, J., Gwinn-Hardy, K. (2003). Alpha-synuclein locus triplication causes Parkinson's disease. *Science*, *302*, 841.

19. Paisan-Ruiz, C., Jain, S., Evans, E.W., Gilks, W.P., Simon, J., van der Brug, M., Lopez De Munain, A., Aparicio, S., Gil, A.M., Khan, N., Johnson, J., Martinez, J.R., Nicholl, D., Carrera, I.M., Pena, A.S., de Silva, R., Lees, A., Marti-Masso, J.F., Perez-Tur, J., Wood, N.W., Singleton, A.B. (2004). Cloning of the gene containing mutations that cause PARK8-linked Parkinson's disease. *Neuron*, *44*, 595–600.

20. Valente, E.M., Abou-Sleiman, P.M., Caputo, V., Muqit, M.M., Harvey, K., Gispert, S., Ali, Z., Del Turco, D., Bentivoglio, A.R., Healy, D.G., Albanese, A., Nussbaum, R., Gonzalez-Maldonado, R., Deller, T., Salvi, S., Cortelli, P., Gilks, W.P., Latchman, D.S., Harvey, R.J., Dallapiccola, B., Auburger, G., Wood, N.W. (2004). Hereditary early-onset Parkinson's disease caused by mutations in PINK1. *Science*, *304*, 1158–1160.

21. Zimprich, A., Biskup, S., Leitner, P., Lichtner, P., Farrer, M., Lincoln, S., Kachergus, J., Hulihan, M., Uitti, R.J., Calne, D.B., Stoessl, A.J., Pfeiffer, R.F., Patenge, N., Carbajal, I.C., Vieregge, P., Asmus, F., Muller-Myhsok, B., Dickson, D.W., Meitinger, T., Strom, T.M., Wszolek, Z.K., Gasser, T. (2004). Mutations in LRRK2 cause autosomal-dominant parkinsonism with pleomorphic pathology. *Neuron*, *44*, 601–607.

22. Sidransky, E., Nalls, M.A., Aasly, J.O., Aharon-Peretz, J., Annesi, G., Barbosa, E.R., Bar-Shira, A., Berg, D., Bras, J., Brice, A., Chen, C.M., Clark, L.N., Condroyer, C., De Marco, E.V., Durr, A., Eblan, M.J., Fahn, S., Farrer, M.J., Fung, H.C., Gan-Or, Z., Gasser, T., Gershoni-Baruch, R., Giladi, N., Griffith, A., Gurevich, T.,

Januario, C., Kropp, P., Lang, A.E., Lee-Chen, G.J., Lesage, S., Marder, K., Mata, I.F., Mirelman, A., Mitsui, J., Mizuta, I., Nicoletti, G., Oliveira, C., Ottman, R., Orr-Utreger, A., Pereira, L.V., Quattrone, A., Rogaeva, E., Rolfs, A., Rosenbaum, H., Rozenberg, R., Samii, A., Samaddar, T., Schulte, C., Sharma, M., Singleton, A., Spitz, M., Tan, E.K., Tayeni, N., Toda, T., Troiano, A.R., Tsuji, S., Wittsock, M., Wolfsberg, T.G., Wu, Y.R., Zabetian, C.P., Zhao, Y., Ziegler, S.G. (2009). Multicenter analysis of glucocerebrosidase mutations in Parkinson's disease. *New England Journal of Medicine, 361,* 1651–1661.

23. Simon-Sanchez, J., Schulte, C., Bras, J.M., Sharma, M., Gibbs, J.R., Berg, D., Paisan-Ruiz, C., Lichtner, P., Scholz, S.W., Hernandez, D.G., Kruger, R., Federoff, M., Klein, C., Goate, A., Perlmutter, J., Bonin, M., Nalls, M.A., Illig, T., Gieger, C., Holden, H., Steffens, M., Okun, M., Racette, B.A., Cookson, M.R., Foote, K.D., Fernandez, H.H., Traynor, B.J., Schreiber, S., Arepalli, S., Zonozi, R., Gwinn, K., van der Brug, M., Lopez, G., Chanock, S.J., Schatzkin, A., Park, Y., Hollenbeck, A., Gao, J., Huang, X., Wood, N.W., Lorenz, D., Deuschl, G., Chen, H., Riess, O., Hardy, J.A., Singleton, A.B., Gasser, T. (2009). Genome-wide association study reveals genetic risk underlying Parkinson's disease. *Nature Genetics, 41,* 1308–1312.

24. Langston, J.W., Ballard, P., Tetrud, J.W., Irwin, I. (1983). Chronic Parkinsonism in humans due to a product of meperidine-analog synthesis. *Science, 25,* 979–980.

25. Gorell, J.M., Rybicki, B.A., Johnson, C.C., Peterson, E.L. (1999). Smoking and Parkinson's disease: A dose-response relationship. *Neurology, 52,* 115–119.

26. Petrovich, H., Ross, G.W., Abbott, R.D., Sanderson, W.T., Sharp, D.S., Tanner, C.M., Masaki, K.H., Blanchette, P.L., Popper, J.S., Foley, D., Launer, L., White, L.R. (2002). Plantation work and risk of Parkinson's disease in a population-based longitudinal study. *Archives of Neurology, 59,* 1787–1792.

27. Chen, H., Jacobs, E., Schwarzschild, M.A., McCullough, M.L., Calle, E.E., Thun, M.J., Ascherio, A. (2005). Nonsteroidal anti-inflammatory drug use and the risk of Parkinson's disease. *Annals of Neurology, 58,* 963–967.

28. Rascol, O., Payoux, P., Ory, F., Ferreira, J.J., Brefel-Courbon, C., Montastruc, J.L. (2003). Limitations of current Parkinson's disease therapy. *Annals of Neurology, 53*(Suppl 3), S3–S12.

29. Bronstein, J.M., Tagliati, M., Alterman, R.L., Lozano, A.M., Volkmann, J., Stefani, A., Horak, F.B., Okun, M.S., Foote, K.D., Krack, P., Pahwa, R., Henderson, J.M., Hariz, M.I., Bakay, R.A., Rezai, A., Marks, W.J., Jr, Moro, E., Vitek, J.L., Weaver, F.M., Gross, R.E., Delong, M.R. (2010). Deep brain stimulation for Parkinson's disease: An expert consensus and review of key issues. *Archives of Neurology, 68*(2), 165.

30. Simola, N., Morelli, M., Pinna, A. (2008). Adenosine A2A receptor antagonists and Parkinson's disease: State of the art and future directions. *Current Pharmaceutical Design, 14,* 1475–1489.

31. Johnson, K.A., Conn, P.J., Niswender, C.M. (2009). Glutamate receptors as therapeutic targets for Parkinson's disease. *CNS & Neurological Disorders Drug Targets, 8,* 475–491.

32. DiMasi, J.A., Grabowski, H.G. (2007). The cost of biopharmaceutical R and D: Is biotech different? *Managerial and Decision Economics, 28,* 469–479.

33. Chan, C.S., Guzmna, J.N., Ilijic, E., Mercer, J.N., Rick, C., Tkatch, T., Meredith, G.E., Surmeier, D.J. (2007). "Rejuventation" protects neurons in mouse models of Parkinson's disease. *Nature, 447,* 1081–1086.

34. Ritz, B., Rhodes, S.L., Qian, L., Schernhammer, E., Olsen, J.H., Friis, S. (2010). L-type calcium channels and Parkinson's disease in Denmark. *Annals of Neurology*, *67*(5), 600–606.

35. Urien, S., Pinquier, J.L., Paquette, B., Chaumet-Riffaud, P., Kiechel, J.R., Tillement, J.P. (1987). Effect of the binding of israpidine and darodipine to different plasma proteins on their transfer through the rat blood brain barrier. Drug binding to lipoproteins does not limit the transfer of drug. *The Journal of Pharmacology and Experimental Therapeutics*, *242*, 349–353.

36. Viscomi, P., Jeffrey, J. (2010). Development of clinical practice guidelines for patient management of blood pressure instability in multiple system atrophy, Parkinson's disease, and other neurological disorders. *Canadian Journal of Neuroscience Nursing*, *32*, 6–19.

37. Simuni, T., Borushko, E., Avram, M.J., Miskevics, S., Martel, A., Zadikoff, C., Videnovic, A., Weaver, F.M., Williams, K., Surmeier, D.J. (2010). Tolerability of isradipine in early Parkinson's disease: A pilot dose escalation study. *Movement Disorders*, *25*, 2863–2866.

38. Olanow, C.W. (1990). Oxidation reactions in Parkinson's disease. *Neurology*, *40*(Suppl 3), suppl 32–37, discussion 37–39.

39. Nguyen, T., Yang, C.S., Pickett, C.B. (2004). The pathways and molecular mechanisms regulating Nrf2 activation in response to chemical stress. *Free Radical Biology and Medicine*, *47*(4), 433–441.

40. Sakamoto, J., Kimura, H., Moriyama, S., Odaka, H., Momose, Y., Sugiyama, Y., Sawada, H. (2000). Activation of human peroxisome proliferator-activated receptor (PPAR) subtypes by pioglitazone. *Biochemical and Biophysical Research Communications*, *278*(3), 704–711.

41. Fujisawa, K., Nishikawa, T., Kukidome, D., Imoto, K., Yamashiro, T., Motoshima, H., Matsumura, T., Araki, E. (2009). TZDs reduce mitochondrial ROS production and enhance mitochondrial biogenesis. *Biochemical and Biophysical Research Communications*, *379*(1), 43–48.

42. Breidert, T., Callebert, J., Heneke, M.T., Landreth, G., Launay, J.M., Hirsch, E.C. (2002). Protective action of the peroxisome proliferator-activated receptor-gamma agonist pioglitazone in a mouse model of Parkinson's disease. *Journal of Neurochemistry*, *82*(3), 615–624.

43. Dehmer, T., Heneka, M.T., Sastre, M., Dichgans, J., Schulz, J.B. (2004). Protection by pioglitazone in the MPTP model of Parkinson's disease correlates with I kappa B alpha induction and block of NF kappa B and iNOS activation. *Journal of Neurochemistry*, *88*(2), 494–501.

44. Tanner, C.M., Goldman, S.M., Aston, D.A., Ottman, R., Ellenberg, J., Mayeux, R., Langston, J.W. (2002). Smoking and Parkinson's disease in twins. *Neurology*, *58*(4), 581–588.

45. Dasgupta, P., Kinkade, R., Joshi, B., Decook, C., Haura, E., Chellappan, S. (2006). Nicotine inhibits apoptosis induced by chemotherapeutic drugs by up-regulating XIAP and survivin. *Proceedings of the National Academy of Sciences of the United States of America*, *103*(16), 6332–6337.

46. Miksys, S., Tyndale, R.F. (2006). Nicotine induces brain CYP enzymes: Relevance to Parkinson's disease. *Journal of Neural Transmission. Supplementum*, *70*, 177–180.

47. Belluardo, N., Mudo, G., Blum, M., Fuxe, K. (2000). Central nicotinic receptors, neurotrophic factors and neuroprotection. *Behavioural Brain Research*, *113*(1–2), 227–245.

48. Quik, M., Parameswaran, N., McCallum, S.E., Bordia, T., Bao, S., McCormack, A., Kim, A., Tyndale, R.F., Langston, J.W., Di Monte, D.A. (2006). Chronic oral nicotine treatment protects against striatal degeneration in MPTP-treated primates. *Journal of Neurochemistry, 98*, 1866–1875.

49. Weintraub, D., Koester, J., Potenza, M.N., Siderowf, A.D., Stacy, M., Voon, V., Whetteckey, J., Wunderlich, G.R., Lang, A.E. (2010). Impulse control disorders in Parkinson's disease: A cross sectional study of 3090 patients. *Archives of Neurology, 67*(5), 589–595.

50. Carta, M., Carlsson, T., Kirik, D., Bjorklund, A. (2007). Dopamine released from 5HT terminals is the cause of L-DOPA-induced dyskinesia in parkinsonian rats. *Brain, 130*(Pt 7), 1819–1833.

51. Carlsson, T., Carta, M., Winkler, C., Bjorklund, A., Kirik, D. (2007). Serotonin neuron transplants exacerbate L-DOPA-induced dyskinesia in a rat model of Parkinson's disease. *Journal of Neuroscience, 27*(30), 8011–8022.

52. Munoz, A., Li, Q., Gardoni, F., Marcello, E., Qin, C., Carlsson, T., Kirik, D., Di Luca, M., Bjorklund, A., Bezard, E., Carta, M. (2008). Combined 5HT1A and 5HT1B receptor agonists for treatment of L-DOPA-induced dyskinesia. *Brain, 131*(Pt 12), 3380–3394.

53. Munoz, A., Carlsson, T., Tronic, E., Kirik, D., Bjorklund, A., Carta, M. (2009). Serotonin neuron-dependent and –independent reduction of dyskinesia by 5HT1A and 5HT1B receptor agonists in the rat Parkinson model. *Experimental Neurology, 219*, 298–307.

54. Gerfen, C.R., Miyachi, S., Paletzki, R., Brown, P. (2002). D1 dopamine receptor supersensitivity in the dopamine-depleted striatum results from a switch in the regulation of ERK1/2MAP kinase. *Journal of Neuroscience, 22*(12), 5042–5054.

55. Santini, E., Valjent, E., Usiello, A., Carta, M., Borgkvist, A., Girault, J.A., Herve, D., Greegard, P., Fisone, G. (2007). Critical involvement of cAMP/DARPP-32 and extracellular signal-regulated protein kinase signaling in L-DOPA-induced dyskinesia. *Journal of Neuroscience, 27*(26), 6995–7005.

56. Fasano, S., Bezard, E., D'Antoni, A., Francardo, V., Indrigo, M., Qin, L., Dovero, S., Cerovic, M., Cenci, M.A., Brambilla, R. (2010). Inhibition of Ras-guanine nucleotide-releasing factor 1(Ras-GRF1) signaling in the striatum reverts motor symptoms associated with L-dopa-induced dyskinesia. *Proceedings of the National Academy of Sciences of the United States of America, 107*(50), 21824–21829.

57. Li, W., Cui, Y., Kushner, S.A., Brown, R.A., Jentsch, J.D., Frankland, P.W., Cannon, T.D., Silva, A.J. (2005). The HMG-CoA reductase inhibitor lovastatin reverses the learning and attention deficits in a mouse model of neurofibromatosis type 1. *Current Biology, 15*(21), 1961–1967.

58. Schuster, S., Nadjar, A., Guo, J.T., Li, Q., Ittrich, C., Hengerer, B., Bezard, E. (2008). The 3-hydroxy-3-methylglutaryl-CoA reductase inhibitor lovastatin reduces severity of L-DOPA-induced abnormal involuntary movements in experimental Parkinson's disease. *Journal of Neuroscience, 28*(17), 4311–4316.

59. Wolozin, B., Wang, S.W., Li, N.C., Lee, A., Lee, T.A., Kazis, L.E. (2007). Simvastatin is associated with a reduced incidence of dementia and Parkinson's disease. *BMC Medicine, 5*, 20.

60. Bezard, E. (2010). Discussion: The Pilot Simvastatin Trial Sponsored by MJFF. [cited 2010, November 30] In: PD Online Research [internet]. New York: The

Michael J Fox Foundation for Parkinson's Research. Available from http://www. pdonlineresearch.org/news/2010-05/21/cholesterol-drug-side-effects-need-watching-study#28178

61. Carlezon, W.A., Thomas, M.J. (2009). Biological substrates of reward and aversion: A nucleus accumbens activity hypothesis. *Neuropharmacology, 56*(Suppl 1), 122–132.

62. Johnson, S.W., North, R.A. (1992). Opioids excite dopamine neurons by hyperpolarization of local interneurons. *Journal of Neuroscience, 12*(2), 483–488.

63. Ray, L.A., Chin, P.F., Miotto, K. (2010). Naltrexone for the treatment of alcoholism: Clinical findings, mechanisms of action, and pharmacogenetics. *CNS & Neurological Disorders Drug Targets, 9*(1), 13–22.

64. Hulse, G.K., Morris, N., Arnold-Reed, D., Tait, R.J. (2009). Improving clinical outcomes in treating heroin dependence: Randomized, controlled trial of oral or implant naltrexone. *Archives of General Psychiatry, 66*(10), 1108–1115.

65. Kim, S.W., Grant, J.E., Adson, D.E., Shin, Y.C. (2001). Double-blind naltrexone and placebo comparison study in the treatment of pathological gambling. *Biological Psychiatry, 49*(11), 914–921.

66. Rascol, O., Fabre, N., Blin, O., Poulik, J., Sabatini, U., Senard, J.M., Ane, M., Mostastruc, J.L., Rascol, A. (1994). Naltrexone, an opiate antagonist, fails to modify motor symptoms in patients with Parkinson's disease. *Movement Disorders, 9*(4), 437–440.

67. Manson, A.J., Katzenschlager, R., Hobart, J., Lees, A.J. (2001). High dose naltrexone for dyskinesias induced by levodopa. *Journal of Neurology, Neurosurgery, and Psychiatry, 70*(4), 554–556.

68. Torres, V.E., Harris, P.C. (2009). *Kidney International, 76*, 149–168.

69. Harris, P.C., Torres, V.E. (2009). Polycystic kidney disease. *Annual Review of Medicine, 60*, 321–337.

■■■■■■ CHAPTER 13

Business Development Strategies in the Repositioning Industry[1]

ARIS PERSIDIS and ELIZABETH T. STARK

13.1. INTRODUCTION

While the business case for drug repositioning has been articulated extensively in earlier chapters of this book, it is perhaps, not surprisingly, often viewed primarily from the perspective of the large pharmaceutical companies since they hold much of the potential substrate for reprofiling activities. However, in recent years, the drug development industry in general has become increasingly dependent on strategic alliances that spread risk and reward while bringing together complementary resources and expertise from various parties. The discipline of drug repositioning is no exception. Indeed, as will be discussed here, it can be argued that repositioning is at the forefront of innovative business development models between large pharmaceutical companies, specialty pharmaceutical companies, small biotechnology companies, academic institutions, venture capital (VC) investors, and patient advocacy groups, all of whom have differing perspectives and drivers with respect to drug repositioning (Table 13.1).

In this chapter we will discuss these drivers, some of the types of business deals that have been done and creative business development strategies being pursued to reposition existing drugs and drug candidates for new indications. To further exemplify some of the pertinent considerations for alliances in this area, the subsequent chapter in this book provides a detailed case study on Sosei, a Japanese biopharmaceutical company that pioneered a unique business platform for reprofiling previously shelved drug candidates using a sophisticated shared risk partnership model.

[1] The opinions stated in this chapter are those of the authors and not of their employers.

Drug Repositioning: Bringing New Life to Shelved Assets and Existing Drugs, First Edition.
Edited by Michael J. Barratt and Donald E. Frail.
© 2012 John Wiley & Sons, Inc. Published 2012 by John Wiley & Sons, Inc.

TABLE 13.1. Key Drivers for Drug Repositioning Business Deals per Stakeholder

Stakeholder	Drivers
Large pharmaceutical companies	• Extracting maximum value from portfolio • Sharing financial risk • Speed to market • Loss of exclusivity
Specialty pharmaceutical companies	• Franchise growth
Small biotechnology companies	• Decreasing risk of company failure
Venture capital firms	• Due diligence—explore new indications to assess additional potential value • Decreased risk
Patient advocacy groups	• Speed to clinical trial • Known safety
Academia	• Access to drugs for research use

13.2. LARGE PHARMACEUTICAL COMPANIES

13.2.1. Extracting Maximum Value from the R&D Portfolio

In this era of severe research and development (R&D) budget constraints for most large pharmaceutical companies, there is a big driver to extract maximum value from existing R&D portfolios. Large pharmaceutical companies have extensive collections of ongoing and discontinued compounds and biotherapeutics that have preclinical and clinical data packages, making them potentially ripe for repositioning initiatives. However, narrow therapeutic focus and pressure to invest in "core" diseases may result in limited internal resources and capabilities devoted to systematic reprofiling of promising candidates across the therapeutic spectrum. Nevertheless, many companies are recognizing that novel ideas for repositioning their compounds can be generated "outside their walls" by organizations with unique technology platforms, or more expertise in particular disease areas that lie outside core areas of focus for the large pharmaceutical partner, but still represent areas of high medical need. Coupled with a more open mindset toward collaboration that is driven by the high cost of failure and attrition, there is a gradual trend for large pharmaceutical companies to be more forthcoming with data they are willing to share more broadly with prospective partners—a trend that can only serve to benefit patients in need of new treatments in the long run.

For these reasons, a number of major R&D collaborations have been initiated by large pharmaceutical companies in recent years, such as the deals that AstraZeneca struck with Galderma for dermatology indications and Alcon for ophthalmic indications [1, 2]. These deals save time and money for Alcon and

Galderma by giving them access to numerous relatively mature clinical candidates for testing and repurposing in their areas of expertise, and provide AstraZeneca with the potential for new revenue streams for products in disease areas that they would likely not have built expertise in or pursued on their own. This model has some similarities to a venture—called Anaderm—which had been developed in 1996 between Pfizer, OSI Pharmaceuticals, and dermatologists at New York University to access Pfizer's drug library to search for compounds to treat various dermatological conditions—an area in which Pfizer had limited internal expertise at the time [3].

A different sort of collaboration to generate testable hypotheses for new indications is being explored by Biovista in separate deals with Novartis [4] and Pfizer's Indications Discovery Unit [5]. Biovista, Inc. is a small privately held drug development and pharmaceutical services company based in Charlottesville, Virginia, USA, and Athens, Greece (http://www.biovista.com), which has developed a proprietary bioinformatics-based drug repositioning platform called COSS™ (Clinical Outcomes Search Space). (This technology is described in more detail in Chapter 6, "Mining Scientific and Clinical Databases to Identify Novel Uses for Existing Drugs.") In these collaborations with major pharmaceutical companies, Biovista is using their COSS™ platform to identify new indications for a number of proprietary drugs or drug candidates selected by the pharmaceutical partner. Biovista received upfront payments to perform the work and, in addition, will receive milestone payments if certain success criteria are met.

In another effort to capture additional value from their portfolio of clinic-ready compounds, Pfizer in 2010 initiated an innovative 5-year R&D collaboration with Washington University in St. Louis—one of the leading U.S. academic medical centers—aimed at identifying new indications for existing Pfizer drugs and drug candidates [6]. In this collaboration, Pfizer committed funding and agreed to provide Washington University investigators with access to information on hundreds of ongoing and discontinued clinical candidates through a secure web portal, with the goal of funding research proposals that identify and develop new therapeutic uses for these biotherapeutics. A key difference between the aims of this collaboration and many other industry/academia research collaborations is the strong focus on moving drug candidates quickly into early stage clinical studies to test the proposed new indication, as opposed to spending years on basic research [7].

13.2.2. Sharing Financial Risk

Another approach that large pharmaceutical companies are taking to share financial risk and to capture more value, or at least recoup investment costs, from discontinued drug candidates is out-licensing them for new indications. Creative out-licensing deals with VC-backed startups or other small biopharmaceutical companies for early clinical stage assets can be an attractive option for a large company that wants to retain the option to bring the drug back in-house for late stage development after it has been significantly de-risked. This partnering strategy can also be used when a drug is in development for one indication at a large pharmaceutical company, but there are other potential indications to be pursued in which the pharmaceutical company is unable to invest resources or does not have sufficient expertise. However, this sort of a "split indication" deal can be quite complex and has its risks and challenges. A legitimate concern, for example, is that one company might generate toxicity data during development of its indication that would create additional regulatory work for the other company, even if the particular toxicity data are not relevant for the second company's indication or targeted patient population. (Of course, this could also happen if two indications are being pursued by the same company, but additional complexities exist with two separate development parties.) Another potential issue with split indication deals is that if both the large pharmaceutical company and the licensee launch the same compound for different indications, then each company's drug formulation or route of administration (e.g., oral vs. topical) would need to be unique enough for its approved indication that the risk of off-label use is eliminated. In addition, patent protection issues, such as which company will have the right to apply for a patent term extension for its product, must be managed.

13.2.3. Speed to Market

Many pharmaceutical companies are under enormous pressure to enhance their late stage pipelines in order to offset the drop in revenue anticipated due to recent and upcoming patent expiries for their blockbuster drugs. A number of these best-selling drugs reach the end of the period of exclusivity in the period from 2011 to 2013. In-licensing a repositioned clinical candidate that has existing Phase I (or higher) data provides the potential for a shortened development timeline and a reduced risk of failure due to safety or poor pharmacokinetic properties, although the risk of achieving the high bar for efficacy in Phase III trials remains. The Cephalon/BioAssets Development Corporation deal for repositioning Enbrel for sciatica [8] exemplifies this strategy, but it remains to be seen whether the investment made by Cephalon will pay off.

13.2.4. Loss of Exclusivity

When a drug loses exclusivity (usually provided by patent protection and/or data exclusivity), two events occur. First, a generic version of the drug produced by one or more generic drug manufacturers can immediately go on sale. Second, the market availability of the generic results in substantial revenue loss for the original developer of the drug. It is estimated that over $100 billion will be lost from branded drug sales as these transition to their generic counterparts over the period from 2011 to 2014 [9]. This is obviously beneficial to consumers and payers. But innovator companies can take steps to continue to participate in the market and encourage competition in a variety of ways, including in-licensing promising compounds in development, and implementing various initiatives to boost both the number of Phase II/III starts and, importantly, the survival and differentiation of these candidates from existing marketed therapies.

One such approach is repositioning their existing marketed drugs. If a company validates a new indication that requires a distinct route of administration or formulation, this may be patentable. Even if a patent is not granted, the company may be able to obtain a grant from the U.S. Food and Drug Administration (FDA) (under the Hatch–Waxman Act) of three years of data exclusivity in the market [10]. Of course, the repositioning of a compound previously discontinued in development will not be affected by a generic product, but it may have limited composition of matter patent life remaining. In these cases, the value of a new method-of-use patent or data exclusivity granted by the FDA can be high, particularly if the drug represents a novel mechanism of action that will not be subject to competition from compounds of the same class already on the market (see Chapter 2 for further discussion of this topic).

13.3. FRANCHISE GROWTH FOR SPECIALTY PHARMACEUTICAL COMPANIES

Specialty pharmaceutical companies can be thought of as those with a small number of drugs on the market and a smaller sized development pipeline or as a pharmaceutical company working in a narrow therapeutic space. In most cases, one or two marketed drugs account for a significant portion of their revenues. Such companies can be thought of as small pharmaceutical companies, or as companies that early stage biotechnology companies aspire to become.

In order to ensure continued revenue stability and growth and to maintain a competitive position, specialty pharmaceutical companies are under constant pressure to find the next drug with a short path to revenues. They too are active in acquisitions and in-licensing of drug candidates from other companies. They can also drive their development by repositioning drugs, as this approach offers the advantages of speed to advanced clinical trials and reduced risk of attrition for safety reasons. Smaller/specialty pharmaceutical companies also usually have lower revenue requirements for an indication than their larger counterparts and therefore are often more willing to pursue indications with smaller revenue potential (e.g., <$250 million annually).

A good example is Celgene, which collaborated with academic investigators to reposition the off-patent and banned drug thalidomide—originally introduced in Europe by German company Grunenthal in the late 1950s to treat morning sickness but withdrawn when it was tragically found to cause birth defects [11]—as Thalomid, for two new indications based on new understanding of it mechanisms of action. First, Celgene obtained approval for treatment of erythema nodosum leprosum and later they received approval for its use as a first-line treatment in multiple myeloma [12].

13.4. SMALL BIOTECHNOLOGY COMPANIES—REDUCING THE RISK OF COMPANY FAILURE

Small biotechnology companies are inherently high-risk ventures—their employees and investors bet the company's success on a very small number of drugs. They usually have small pipelines of preclinical and perhaps a few Phase I/IIa compounds. Many biotechnology companies also have a platform technology such as a novel antibody technology or screening methodology that they can make available to partner pharmaceutical companies as a service in order to generate revenue to sustain their R&D pipeline (see case studies in Part II of this book for examples). But, ultimately, most small biotechnology companies need to have one or two successful Phase I or IIa clinical trials in order to provide a financial return for their investors, typically through acquisition of the company by a larger pharmaceutical company, or less typically nowadays via an initial public offering (IPO).

Since clinical attrition and failure of drugs in trials is a very frequent occurrence, small biotechnology companies are under tremendous pressure to ensure that their few drug candidates have the maximum probability of success in the clinic. Exploration of additional and potentially non-obvious indications for their drugs that have been shown to be safe in early trials is an approach that is cost-effective and time-sensitive. This increases the chances that the single drugs may find a number of distinct markets. However, a key challenge with repositioning for biotechnology companies is the need to focus scarce resources on only a few clinical studies. This can limit their ability to invest in new indications for their own drugs, which may limit their overall chances of success, and also create a potential weakness in their patent position, especially if a competitor realizes that they can acquire new use intellectual property (IP) on these drugs.

13.4.1. Case Studies

Intellikine, a biotech focused on developing small molecule drugs targeting the PI3K/mTOR pathway, has found a way to obtain external financial support as well as access to research and clinical expertise for repurposing some of their small molecule kinase inhibitors in polycystic kidney disease (PKD). In early 2011, Intellikine announced a collaboration with the PKD Foundation for investigating their TORC1/2 inhibitors for treatment of PKD, as part of the PKD Foundation's Accelerating Treatments to Patients program [13]. This case study is described in more detail in Chapter 12, "Drug Repositioning Efforts by Nonprofit Foundations."

Melior Discovery is a small biotechnology company dedicated to repositioning existing drugs, both for its own and its partners' pipelines. At the company's core is its *thera*Trace® indications discovery platform, which includes over 40 animal models representing a broad spectrum of disease areas. The company provides research services to other companies and counts Merck, Astra Zeneca, Johnson and Johnson, and Pfizer among its collaborators [14], but also uses its platform to investigate discontinued, off-patent drugs for new potential indications on its own. In 2008, Melior entered into an agreement with Pfizer that provided access for Melior to certain data relating to a discontinued Pfizer drug candidate that had been in development for gastric ulcers. Melior was later granted a patent covering the use of this compound, MLR-1023, for the the treatment of type 2 diabetes, obesity, and metabolic syndrome [15, 16].

Zalicus, formerly CombinatoRx, is a biotechnology company with a unique approach to drug repositioning. The company seeks to identify synergistic combinations of existing drugs through screening in cell-based assays of disease to develop new products [17]. The company's lead un-partnered clinical candidate, Synavive®, is in development for treating arthritis. Synavive® is a combination of the cardiovascular drug dipyridamole and a very low dose of the corticosteroid prednisolone [18]. This case study, as well as the screening platform in which it was discovered, is described in more detail in Chapter 8.

13.5. EXPANDING THE VALUE PROPOSITION FOR VENTURE CAPITAL

A Venture Capital (VC) group spends a considerable amount if its time performing due diligence on investment opportunities. In the healthcare/biotechnology space, this often means examining drugs and pipelines of early stage investment possibilities, and also in-licensing candidates for their portfolio companies. It also means that they perform the reverse action, where they represent the drugs of their portfolio companies to other VC groups or potential pharmaceutical acquirers, as part of a co-investment proposal or acquisition exit. Within the context of these activities, understanding potential new uses for drugs can be a significant advantage for the VC companies that perform the task. Once they know potential additional indications, which may be validated by preclinical data, then the package of information around the drug of interest would have expanded value.

Interestingly, the use of repositioning insights and data may be used by VC groups in two principal ways, depending on whether the drug is being assessed for investment, or being packaged for out-licensing or acquisition by another party. In the case of due diligence for investment, repositioning insights may alter the negotiating posture or valuation discussion. The VC company may realize that the drug they are considering investing in may have further uses that the originator may not actually be aware of. This may alter how the investment may be agreed upon. In the case of out-licensing one of their portfolio company drugs, repositioning may add to the attractiveness of the asset to a potential partner.

A number of VCs are becoming attracted to establishing startup companies based on a repositioning opportunity. These opportunities can arise from various sources, including academic investigators who uncover new science that provides confidence in rationale for a new indication of an older drug, or from pharmaceutical companies who have more repositioning opportunities for relatively newer drugs (with patent life) than they can afford to pursue. Advantages of repositioning opportunities can include existing Phase I data establishing safety and known favorable pharmacokinetic properties, existing drug product available for new clinical studies, and an issued composition-of-matter patent application, thus greatly reducing the cost and risk as compared with most startup pharmaceutical opportunities. Disadvantages frequently include: limited or no patent life remaining on the compound, strings that may be attached to an asset from a large pharmaceutical company (e.g., an option for the pharmaceutical company to take the drug back), and the complications and risks of splitting the rights on indications with the large pharmaceutical company or another licensee.

Incline Therapeutics is one interesting example of a company created by VCs to develop a repositioning opportunity. Incline is developing IONSYS™ (fentanyl iontophoretic transdermal system), an investigational product candidate intended to provide patient-controlled analgesia for adult inpatients requiring opioids following surgery. The IONSYS system was approved by both the FDA and the European Medicines Agency (EMA) in 2006; however, IONSYS is not currently marketed anywhere in the world due to limitations in the technology. Frazier Healthcare Ventures led the formation of Incline to acquire the asset and obtain regulatory approval from both the FDA and EMA for new patient safety features being developed into the system [19].

13.6. SPEED AND SAFETY FOR PATIENT ADVOCACY GROUPS

Patient Advocacy Groups (PAGs) exist to help accelerate the pace of research and development of drugs for specific indications. They are active fundraisers relying on philanthropy to fund research that is proceeding too slowly or that would otherwise not be undertaken by pharmaceutical or biotechnology companies. These organizations are usually founded and driven by people with a personal stake in the particular disease who are highly motivated to find new therapies to improve the quality of life or to save the lives of loved ones.

Repositioning offers the known benefits of speed and safety, since it makes use of already existing drugs that have passed early safety trials. In the case of PAGs, this is a particularly attractive proposition, as it means that they can explore advanced clinical candidates for potential efficacy in humans, with a reduced investment in preclinical efficacy validation research. Numerous examples from three PAGs, The Leukemia and Lymphoma Society, The Michael J. Fox Foundation, and the Polycystic Kidney Disease Foundation, are highlighted in Chapter 12.

13.7. ACADEMIA—ACCESS TO DRUGS FOR RESEARCH USE

Scientists undertaking basic research often test existing drugs for potential new uses in their assays and animal models, and it is common practice for pharmaceutical and biotechnology companies to enter into material transfer agreements with academic institutions for this purpose. Also commonplace is the provision of formulated drug and funding to clinical researchers at academic medical centers for clinical studies to test existing drugs/drug candidates in new indications under an Investigator Initiated Research Agreement, in which the academic institution is responsible for the regulatory requirements and conduct of the study. In addition to the novel collaboration between Washington University in St. Louis and Pfizer for drug repositioning discussed earlier in this chapter, many other academic initiatives for drug repositioning are being explored.

One such effort has been initiated by the Center for World Health and Medicine (CWHM) at St. Louis University, in collaboration with the University of Missouri St. Louis, which is dedicated to the development of treatments for rare and neglected diseases, with a focus on diseases in the developing world. Part of CWHM's strategy is to test existing drugs and abandoned drug candidates for efficacy in models for selected rare and neglected diseases. CWHM seeks to form alliances and partnerships with pharmaceutical companies, patient advocacy groups, the World Health Organization, and others to access the specific drug candidates and funding for advancing new treatment opportunities through clinical trials [20].

13.8. FUTURE PROSPECTS FOR BUSINESS DEALS IN THE REPOSITIONING INDUSTRY

As discussed in this chapter and shown in Table 13.2, a number of unique business deals based on repositioning drugs have been entered into over the past several years. We foresee increased deal activity in this space over the next few years after some of the previous deals bear fruit and demonstrate success in the clinic and the marketplace, further demonstrating the value of drug repositioning.

As large pharmaceutical companies continue to narrow their focus in a smaller number of core therapeutic areas, they will seek more partnerships for developing their existing drugs and drug candidates in therapeutic areas outside their core expertise. As VC firms look for new investment

TABLE 13.2. Some Recent Drug Repositioning Deals

Partners	Focus	Year	Financials
Novartis–Biovista	Biovista to propose new uses for selected Novartis drugs	2011	Upfront plus milestones, not disclosed [4]
AstraZeneca–Galderma	5-year R&D collaboration providing Galderma with access to AstraZeneca compounds for developing in dermatological diseases	2011	Not disclosed [1]
Intellikine–Polycystic Kidney Disease Foundation	Collaboration to investigate Intellikine's TORC1/2 inhibitors for treating PKD	2011	Research funding (amount not disclosed) [13]
Pfizer–Washington University	Washington University investigators provided access to information on Pfizer clinical compound collection in order to propose new indications and awarded grants to pursue those of mutual interest	2010	$22.5 million over 5 years [6]
Frazier Healthcare Ventures (FHV and other VCs)—Incline Therapeutics	FHV led the startup and Series A financing of Incline to add new features to IONSYS (fentanyl iontophoretic transdermal system) to support new regulatory filings to enable successful marketing	2010	$43 million Series A equity financing [19]
Pfizer–Biovista	Biovista to propose new uses for selected Pfizer drugs	2010	Upfront plus milestones, not disclosed [5]
LPath–Pfizer	Pfizer obtains license option to ocular formulation of mAb (iSONEP) to treat wet age-related macular degeneration AMD while LPath continues clinical development of systemic formulation of the same mAb (ASONEP) for cancer	2010	$14 million upfront, shared development costs, milestones, and royalties [21]
Cephalon–BioAssets Development Corporation (BDC)	Cephalon acquisition of BDC to obtain IP on tumor necrosis factor (TNF) inhibitors for sciatica (for repositioning from rheumatoid arthritis and other autoimmune disorders)	2009–2010	$30 million option payment followed by $12.5 million stock purchase plus milestones [8]

TABLE 13.2. (*Continued*)

Partners	Focus	Year	Financials
AstraZeneca–Alcon	5-year collaborative research agreement providing Alcon with access to AstraZeneca compounds for development in ophthalmic indications	2009	Milestones and royalties to be negotiated [2]
MacuSight–Santen	Santen in-license of rights to IP from MacuSight for sirolimus (rapamycin), an immunosuppressant to prevent transplant rejection for ophthalmic diseases	2008	$50 million upfront plus milestones and royalties [22]
Medivation–Pfizer	Medivation and Pfizer agree to co-development and co-marketing deal for Dimebon, an antihistamine, developed by Medivation for Alzheimer's and Huntington's diseases	2008	$225 million upfront plus additional payments, milestones, and royalties [23]
Melior–Pfizer	License option and data license for MLR-1023— repositioning former Pfizer gastric ulcer drug candidate in type 2 diabetes	2008	Upfront payment [16]

opportunities, some will certainly be attracted to funding startups that use off-patent drugs as substrate for developing treatments in new indications—with new IP—because of the decreased risk as compared with developing new chemical lead matter, as well as the shortened development timeline. Especially attractive will be deals for drugs repositioned into diseases with a high unmet medical need and fewer competing therapies, where the efficacy bar in Phase III trials is not as high as in disease areas that are already well served by effective drugs.

REFERENCES

1. AstraZeneca. http://www.astrazeneca.com/Research/news/Article/AstraZeneca-and-Galderma-enter-into-RandD-collaboration
2. Progressive Digital Media Group Plc. http://www.pharmaceutical-business-review.com/news/alcon_signs_agreement_with_astrazeneca_on_eye_drug_development_090722
3. Farlex, Inc. http://www.thefreelibrary.com/PFIZER,+ONCOGENE+FORM+COMPANY+TO+DISCOVER+AND+DEVELOP+PRESCRIPTION..-a018216119

4. PR Newswire Association LLC. http://www.prnewswire.com/news-releases/biovista-announces-research-collaboration-with-a-major-pharmaceutical-company-120772669.html

5. PR Newswire Association LLC. http://www.prnewswire.com/news-releases/biovista-announces-a-drug-repositioning-collaboration-with-pfizer-106955943.html

6. Washington University in St. Louis. http://news.wustl.edu/news/Pages/20770.aspx

7. Jarvis, L.M. (2010). Opening the Medicine Cabinet. *Chemical & Engineering News*, *88*(45), 14–20.

8. Cephalon, Inc. http://www.exterapartners.com/pdfs/Cephalon%20_%20BDC-NewsRelease_Nov2010.pdf

9. EvaluatePharma® (2009). Evaluate Pharma Alpha World Preview 2014. Evaluate Pharma report.

10. Kesselheim, A.S., Solomon, D.H. (2010). Incentives for drug development-the curious case of colchicine. *N. Engl. J. Med.*, *362*, 2045–2047.

11. The Thalidomide Society 2006. http://www.thalidomidesociety.co.uk/publications.htm

12. Celgene Corporation. http://www.thalomid.com/

13. Intellikine. http://www.intellikine.com/pdf/Intellikine_PressRelease_Feb10_2011.pdf

14. Melior Discovery. http://www.meliordiscovery.com/about_overview.html

15. Intellectual Property Today. http://www.iptoday.com/news-article.asp?id=6003&type=tech

16. Vocus PRW Holdings, LLC. http://www.prweb.com/releases/melior/pfizer/prweb1055874.htm

17. Xconomy, Inc. http://www.xconomy.com/boston/2010/09/20/zalicus-formerly-the-bicoastal-biotech-combinatorx-seeks-new-identity-with-name-fit-for-a-warrior/

18. Zalicus. http://www.zalicus.com/product-pipeline/pipeline-overview.asp

19. Incline Therapeutics, Inc. http://inclinethera.com/?p=1

20. Saint Louis University. http://www.cwhm.org/index.php?page=alliances-and-partnerships

21. EvaluatePharma®. http://www.evaluatepharma.com/Universal/View.aspx?type=Story&id=232977

22. Santen Pharmaceutical Co., Ltd. http://www.santen.com/news/20080602-1.jsp

23. Business Wire. http://investors.medivation.com/ReleaseDetail.cfm?releaseid=331827

■■■■ **CHAPTER 14**

A Case Study in Drug Repositioning: Sosei

AKINORI MOCHIZUKI and MAKIKO AOYAMA

14.1. INTRODUCTION

Sosei is a Japanese biopharmaceutical company that pioneered a unique open innovation business platform for drug reprofiling using a sophisticated shared risk partnership model.

Initiated in 1999, its Drug Reprofiling Platform (DRP) was actively driven by a core team of five full time personnel, yielding a number of internal projects based on its systematic approach to serendipitous new indications discovery. The full extent of its success is yet to be realized; however, at the time of writing, DRP has resulted in the identification of dozens of off-target activities from a relatively small library of over 50 compounds, of which one asset, SD118, has successfully completed Phase I clinical trials under current regulations after showing significant activity in several models for its newly identified indication (neuropathic pain). These pioneering initiatives led to the acquisition of Arakis, now known as Sosei R&D with a similar business model. Its lead pipeline product, NVA237, is a drug that was already on the European Union (EU) market for the reduction of saliva secretion and has been repositioned into a potential blockbuster for the treatment of chronic obstructive pulmonary disease (COPD). NVA237 has now been licensed to Novartis along with the combination product with indacaterol, and both are in Phase III trials at the time of writing.

The initial high "hit rate" in DRP can be attributed to the unique nature of the risk sharing model that provides a relatively small library of high quality compounds for screening against a variety of platform technologies, involving minimal upfront costs for all parties involved. There is also a historical and

---

Drug Repositioning: Bringing New Life to Shelved Assets and Existing Drugs, First Edition.
Edited by Michael J. Barratt and Donald E. Frail.
© 2012 John Wiley & Sons, Inc. Published 2012 by John Wiley & Sons, Inc.

445

opportunistic perspective to the evolution of the model, made possible through Sosei's presence in Japan and through its balanced corporate pipeline strategy outside of the DRP scheme.

This chapter will first explore some environmental factors that contributed to the development of the DRP and progress to describing the business strategy in further detail, highlighting advantages of its open innovation approach together with its limitations. In doing so, the chapter will analyze ways of optimally engaging partners in a shared risk partnership model. Finally, we will discuss how the drug repositioning landscape might evolve in the future from a business development perspective.

14.2. HISTORICAL PERSPECTIVE

Sosei was established in 1990 as a technology transfer company at a time when the financial environment was especially unfavorable in Japan. Over the following few years, much restructuring activity occurred within the Japanese pharmaceutical industry involving a number of merger and acquisition (M&A) transactions and realignment of pipeline portfolios. In common with what has been observed in the rest of the world, these activities were in response to rising development costs, heightened regulatory hurdles, and fewer products successfully reaching the market. Many companies developing "me-too" or "me-better" drugs from the 1980s also faced the need to focus on certain therapeutic areas.

This movement in the 1990s resulted in the termination of many assets, often not for safety or efficacy reasons but for strategic reasons such as changes to the companies' pipeline strategy. Some such assets were licensed out for further development; however, many others remained on the shelves together with their substantial data packages.

Sosei was one of the first companies to realize and act on the potential of such terminated assets, especially those sitting on the shelves of Japanese pharmaceutical companies with confirmed safety data. More than 99% of synthesized drugs cannot be administered to humans due to toxicity or unfavorable physicochemical properties, and a further 60–80% of compounds will not pass first-in-man studies due to tolerability issues or undesirable pharmacokinetic profiles. As such, assets with confirmed safety and tolerability in humans are highly attractive for development in a new indication, as has been described elsewhere in this book.

The most important factor for capitalizing on this idea was to access information on these Japanese assets, which are almost invisible outside of Japan. Such information is not publicized, and pharmaceutical companies are traditionally reluctant to give out the exact reason of termination of their halted projects. Sosei, however, approached a number of Japanese pharmaceutical companies using established relationships it had built up during its years of activity in the technology transfer business, and managed to secure over 50 compounds that were halted in late stage clinical development for reasons other than toxicity.

In 1999, with the growth of venture capital for biotech companies in Japan, Sosei shifted its business focus from technology transfer to pharmaceutical development, launching the DRP as an initiative for discovering new indications to halted compounds collected from Japanese pharmaceutical companies.

On a corporate scale, Sosei took on two other pipeline strategies for overall risk distribution: one to in-license products already on the Western market for development in Japan (low-medium risk and low-medium return); the other to develop a new chemical entity (NCE) and a novel antibody in collaboration with academia and a biotechnology company (high risk and high return). DRP was considered medium risk and medium return.

In 2004, the company successfully achieved an initial public offering on the Mothers market of the Tokyo Stock Exchange (4565:JP), raising over $100 million. In 2005, it acquired Arakis Ltd (Cambridge, UK), a drug discovery company dedicated to repositioning existing drugs. Its lead pipeline product, NVA237, had been repositioned from a drug already on the EU market for the reduction of saliva secretion to a potential blockbuster drug for the treatment of COPD along with its combination product with indacaterol.

14.3. DRP®

The Drug Reprofiling Platform (DRP) was formed around a library of over 50 halted compounds from Japanese pharmaceutical companies, together with access to their substantial data packages including reasons for termination. These compounds were subjected to a vast array of screening platforms in order to identify off-target activities for new indications discovery. An intensive screening program was made possible by partnering up with a large number of screening companies. In essence, the DRP acted as a coordinator of a sophisticated compound screening network, managing the flow of compounds and information between Japanese originators and screening partners (Figure 14.1). The model was unique from the outset, and still remains so today.

Its feasibility could be attributed to how all parties would benefit in a win–win manner with limited risk and upfront costs involved. The Japanese originators were able to offload their terminated assets to Sosei and have their compounds tested in a variety of state-of-the-art technologies under a single agreement similar to a Material Transfer Agreement. The screening partners were able to access valuable proprietary compounds with tolerability in humans. If a "hit" was identified by a screening partner, and the new activity considered scientifically and commercially attractive, then the finding would be patented with its rights shared between the partner, originator, and Sosei. The originator may retain rights to development primarily in Japan, and the partner and Sosei may share rights to the rest of the world (Figure 14.2).

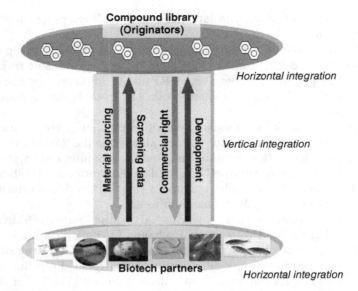

FIGURE 14.1. Sosei DRP®—An integrated reprofiling platform.

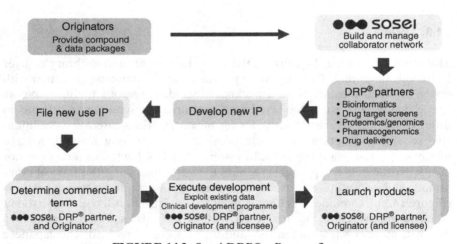

FIGURE 14.2. Sosei DRP®—Process flow.

Unlike other companies, Sosei used the term "reprofiling" instead of "repositioning," because the DRP network provided an array of new information on each compound, even if they were not significant enough on their own to indicate a new use. Each partner provided results of their assays for each of the compounds screened, including those that were negative. These include

TABLE 14.1. Strategic Considerations for Reprofiling

1 Knowledge-base or serendipitous reprofiling
  • Strong rationale/off-target discovery
2 In-house or collaboration
  • Well established technique/proprietary technology
3 High-throughput screening (*in vitro*) or animal model
  • Small quantities of compound/higher relevancy to human
4 Marketed drug or halted compound
  • Easy access to safe entity/avoid generic emergence

---

high-throughput data from *in vitro* assays as well as information-rich data from *in vivo* studies.

The DRP scheme did not rely entirely on serendipitous discovery of new activities, and Sosei conducted its own internal knowledge-base screening at the earliest stage of incorporating a new compound into the compound library. Partners with high-throughput technologies chose to screen the whole library; however this was often unattractive (and unethical) for partners with expensive assays such as animal models. Some partners chose to screen only a handful that they believed are most promising for their particular technology, target, or therapeutic focus area. Therefore, the DRP approach was not entirely serendipitous and had some direction to its screening.

There are four main strategic considerations to drug repositioning, with associated advantages and disadvantages to each approach (Table 14.1). Sosei chose to diversify on most accounts, rather than to specialize in any one category:

14.3.1. Knowledge-Base Versus Serendipitous Screening

With a strong scientific team and computational power, a knowledge-based or targeted approach is possible using information that is publicly available such as chemical structure, known pharmacology and clinical data, which can provide a strong motivation for development, being based upon on firm scientific rationale. At the same time, however, the approach is limited to available information, and the discovery of off-target pharmacology is often unpredictable. The DRP scheme has identified a number of totally unpredictable findings from serendipitous screening.

14.3.2. In-House Versus Collaboration

Since the 1990s there has been a rapid emergence of biotechnology companies with "omics"-derived technologies with good potential for new indications discovery from chemical libraries. However, almost all such companies focus on a specific pharmacology, target/pathway, or therapeutic area; therefore, subjecting a compound only to their in-house assay is limiting in terms of elucidating the full potential of a compound. Sosei therefore chose to form alliances, similar in principle to the concept of open innovation, with a number of such biotechnology companies as screening partners to maximize the chances for new indications discovery.

14.3.3. High-Throughput Screening (*In Vitro*) Versus Animal Model

The advantages of high-throughput screening platforms are of course their high-throughput capacities and the small quantities of compound that are required for each assay. Animal models, on the other hand, require considerably more of compound and are expensive to run but have higher relevance to humans and yield more informative data. Some companies utilize animals for whole body assays in a high-throughput manner, for example using nematode, drosophila, or zebrafish, involving insights into systems biology. The DRP incorporated various non-overlapping technology partners to achieve the best of both strategies.

14.3.4. Marketed Drug Versus Halted Drug

Many drug repositioning companies work on marketed drugs as their starting material as they are easy to access, have published data, and are proven safe to use at least in their existing formulation and dosage. Working on halted compounds, however, has advantages, such as avoidance of generic emergence and higher hurdles for competitors due to the difficulty in obtaining information and compound material. Data exclusivity can be significantly longer (5 years in the United States, as much as 10 years elsewhere regardless of patent life) after marketing authorization of a repositioned halted compounds because these would be classified as NCEs, whereas a repositioned marketed drug will only have 3 to 5 years of market exclusivity (see also Chapters 2 and 4 for further discussion of this topic). The DRP compound library is thus highly attractive due to its confirmed safety profile and proprietary nature.

Sosei's reprofiling activity was not, however, limited to halted compounds. The team paid much attention to drugs that are marketed only in Japan and gathered a compound library of several hundred commercially available compounds for screening. In addition, Sosei acquired a UK-based drug repositioning company, Arakis Ltd (Cambridge) in 2005, which focused on revealing hidden pharmacology of marketed drugs using a proprietary bioinformatics tool called SearchLite®. Their lead project, NVA237 (glycopyrronium bromide), is a drug already on the market to reduce saliva secretion, administered by oral or intravenous injection. Arakis predicted its activity as a long acting muscarinic antagonist, and proved its competitive bronchodialation property through inhalation in the clinic. The finding was patented and licensed out to Novartis for further clinical development for COPD. In addition to monotherapy, its combination drug with Novartis' long acting beta agonist, indacaterol, has blockbuster potential. This would be one of the most successful examples of reprofiling.

14.4. ACCESSING HALTED COMPOUNDS

The value of the DRP scheme could be attributed to its uniquely attractive compound library obtained from pharmaceutical companies in Japan. Sosei utilized its established relationships with pharmaceutical companies and successfully gained access to compounds that were halted in late stage clinical development for reasons other than toxicity.

Under an MTA-like agreement, the originators were offered development and marketing rights primarily in Japanese territory for new indications identified through the scheme. They were also entitled to reports of screening data from all screening partners on a regular basis. The DRP scheme offered them an opportunity to expose their halted assets to a wide range of screening technologies under a single agreement with minimal administrative burden on their part. Such scientific data were attractive to the originators, even if the findings were negative or of weak potency, particularly if they were developing derivatives or analogs internally.

The challenge of using halted compounds for reprofiling, however, is in obtaining their genuine reasons of development termination, which are usually held in strictest confidence. Such information is generally not publicized and is often vaguely described, if at all. The originators of the DRP scheme were willing to share this information because this was a critical factor in going about repositioning these compounds. This secrecy, however, created a high barrier for other repositioning companies to enter the arena. In addition, the halted compounds themselves are not commercially available and are difficult to obtain, unless their synthesis methods are publicized, in which case a high cost of synthesis would be involved.

The reasons of termination for the compounds Sosei took on were various, but were typically for lack of efficacy, changes to the company's therapeutic focus area, worsening of the competitive environment, introduction of additional development requirements by the regulatory authority, or termination of an existing collaborative agreement.

As for the associated data packages, Sosei gathered as much information as possible including physicochemical profiles, preclinical assays, clinical data, chemistry, manufacturing, and controls (CMC), and regulatory documents. Many of the compounds collected under the DRP scheme had already completed first-in-man trials with no safety concerns, making the library invaluable for repurposing.

The remaining period of the composition-of-matter patent for the compounds, however, was diminishing when they were incorporated into the DRP library. This was expected considering the compounds had been taken into clinical stages of development. A short period of substance patent is quite often perceived as the end of the value of a compound; however, this was less of an issue under the DRP scheme because a new use patent could be filed for the new indication or data exclusivity could be obtained. Sometimes, commercial rights of the derivatives would be secured.

Antitumor agents, especially those with cytotoxicity as their main pharmacology, were one type of compound that the DRP did not incorporate into its library. Even if such compounds had substantial patent life remaining or robust and up-to-date data packages, it was almost impossible to dissociate potential side effects because of the difficulty in obtaining acceptable therapeutic windows, and their new use would be limited to very narrow usages with local applications. It might be possible to reposition such assets to other types of cancer, but the originators or licensee candidates would often have already tested such possibilities. Moreover, repositioning of an antitumor agent to a different malignant neoplasm would most likely be insufficient for securing a use patent. Considering the risk versus benefit, these compounds were not incorporated into the DRP library.

Another type of product that was not included in the DRP was biologicals. In general, biological products are highly specific in terms of pharmacological action or target entity; thus, unexpected or off-target activity is less likely to be observed.

14.5. ESTABLISHING A STRONG SCREENING NETWORK

As the business model relies on establishing a strong, unique screening network, it is important to assess the partners well before launching into a collaborative agreement. Sosei actively approached and selected companies with sound and non-overlapping technologies to avoid duplication of screening efforts. The process of establishing such a network of screening companies outside of Sosei itself was an early adoption of the now popular concept of open innovation.

Technologies varied from *in vitro* screening to animal models of various disease states. Some companies possessed unique systemic exposure models in genetically modified *Caenorhabditis elegans*, drosophila, and zebrafish. All screening partners were located in the United States or Europe.

Partners in the DRP had a large incentive for running the compounds through their assays, as under the agreement they would have shared commercial rights to the new indication in all territories outside of Japan. Since the 1990s, platform-based biotechnology companies have been keen to possess an internal development pipeline derived from their own technology while at the same time running a fee-for-service screening business. Fundraising for clinical development was still possible and a successful proof-of-concept study provided greater exit opportunities for the investors. It was, however, often too risky and expensive for these platform technology companies to work on

NCEs and so they generally focused on screening marketed drugs for repositioning opportunities. The DRP compound library was attractive to them as they were proprietary and had associated data packages.

14.6. PATENTING

Patentability is an important aspect of drug repositioning and unpredictability/nonobviousness is an essential factor for filing new use patents. Knowledge-based repositioning is weak in this respect as the hypotheses and rationale behind the new use could be argued as an obvious step, especially if the class effect in pharmacology is already in public domain. A serendipitous approach is therefore more likely to discover off-target activities that are patentable as new use.

The data exclusivity period after marketing authorization is also another significant monopoly opportunity. The period of exclusivity differs depending on whether the compound is a new chemical entity or a marketed product, and on the status of the indication, such as for orphan diseases. Compounds repositioned by the DRP scheme are attributable as NCEs, and therefore their longest possible exclusive period is up to 10 years regardless of patent life, which is essential for recovering investment into drug development (see also Chapter 2). In comparison, repositioning of marketed compounds, sometimes through the 505(b)(2) application discussed in Chapter 4, will provide only 3 to 5 years of market exclusivity.

Examining old patents may open up repositioning opportunities, such as new crystal polymorphisms, novel synthesis pathways, and improved or new formulations. If these are patentable, repositioning under the original indication could become a commercially attractive option. Furthermore, a change in administration route to meet an unmet medical need, for example from intravenous injection to inhalation, may reveal unknown properties of the compound, opening up possibilities for a new use. If a proprietary delivery device is used for the repositioned compound, it could also prevent the emergence of generic products and potentially dominate the market.

14.7. LIMITATIONS

There are some limitations to repositioning using Sosei's DRP strategy.

14.7.1. Compound Material

The DRP scheme is attractive because of its ability to access compound material from the originator companies; however, this also renders the system dependent on the quantity available from the originators in the first instance. After multiple shipments to screening partners requiring high oral dosage in animal models, the stock will decrease quite significantly and will subsequently only be available for *in vitro* assays. Originators are usually not committed to synthesizing additional batches.

14.7.2. Dependence on Screening Partners

Much of the post-repositioning development strategy depends on the capability and experience of the screening partner, including its ability to raise funds. Even a small-scale proof-of-principle study requires substantial cash and resource; therefore, if the partner finds itself financially constrained, and many companies are, then Sosei may not be able to take on the cost and risk of development on its own.

14.7.3. Patent Ownership

Under the DRP scheme, a new use patent is filed as a joint application between the three parties. Although Sosei was fortunate enough not to see significant problems arising during its DRP activity, conceivably this could be a risk factor in the long term, such as potential disagreements arising on future development or out-licensing strategies.

14.7.4. Value Capture of Findings Outside of Therapeutic Focus

Due to its serendipitous nature, the DRP scheme sometimes identified repositioning opportunities in an unexpected therapeutic area outside of the core business interests of the screening partner and of the originator. The DRP scheme did not have an efficient way of capitalizing on such potentially interesting discoveries, as patent filing and subsequent proof-of-concept studies required significant commitment, yet were required for out-licensing to potentially interested parties. Such findings were usually not patented but remained within the internal database.

14.8. LONG-TERM PERSPECTIVE—FUTURE OF REPOSITIONING

Following the rapid emergence of numerous repositioning companies since the late 1990s, it will be interesting to see how many of them produce successful case studies.

The pharmaceutical environment is changing rapidly and existing drug repositioning strategies will need to adapt in order to be successful. Moreover, many global pharmaceutical companies are now actively profiling their assets even prior to launch. This activity may become a threat for smaller repositioning companies since the compounds will be thoroughly investigated internally, including off-target activities. Major pharmaceutical companies are also opening up their extensive compound libraries to charitable organizations such as Medicines for Malaria Venture (MMV) for discovering drug candidates in commercially less attractive indications.

Such activity is particularly evident in the development of therapeutics for rare or neglected disease. With the help of the internet, patient groups are getting together with academia and advocacy groups to making significant efforts on testing marketing drugs to treat their own conditions. One example is the patient advocacy group "PatientsLikeMe" (http://www.patientslikeme.com), a social web community for patients that started with amyotrophic lateral sclerosis (ALS or Lou Gehrig's disease) and has expanded, initially started its activity by sharing published information on the use of lithium as a potential treatment. It subsequently moved on to running a patient-driven trial to test its efficacy by establishing data-sharing partnerships with doctors, pharmaceutical companies, research organizations, and nonprofit organizations. Although such trials are likely to be less coordinated compared with traditional drug development trials, the future is all about thinking outside of the box. Such movements are starting to attract the attention of large pharmaceutical companies and may be indicating a dawn of a new paradigm of open-source reprofiling. This topic is discussed further in Chapters 12 and 13 of this book.

14.9. CONCLUSION

Since the conventional approach to drug development can no longer be solely relied upon due to its high risk, the industry has seen the blossoming of a variety of drug repositioning initiatives as a lower risk alternative. The concept is relatively easy to understand for investors and larger pharmaceutical companies have already taken up the strategy internally.

Approaches to repositioning are becoming more diversified with the progress of science and technology. As discussed in Part II of this book, advances in computerized information technology, for example, are rapidly accelerating our understanding of the biology behind many disease states by integrating and correlating enormous amounts of biological data, and as such, bioinformatics tools may provide much more accurate predictions on how a compound would behave inside a human body.

Compounds developed since the 1990s often have significantly richer clinical data than their earlier predecessors; therefore, reprofiling relatively new compounds can take completely different directions from that of DRP. It will be interesting to see how this might change the effectiveness and return from future repositioning efforts.

It has been a decade since drug repositioning gained momentum in the industry, and many repositioned candidates are now under clinical development for their new indications. The relative successes of the various strategies taken will be better understood in the years to come. From a business development perspective, the direction seems to be moving toward a collaborative partnership model between traditional pharmaceutical companies, platform technology companies, academia, and nonprofit organizations. As many pharmaceutical companies continue to shift their research strategy from relying entirely on internal resources to a framework of open innovation, this paradigm will no doubt extend beyond strategies for drug repositioning in an age of expansion of collaborative R&D.

████ **APPENDIX**

Additional Drug Repositioning Resources and Links*

MARK A. MITCHELL AND MICHAEL J. BARRATT

TABLE A.1. Drug Repositioning Databases and Miscellaneous Resources

Database/Resource	Synopsis	Reference
Ondex database	The Ondex database is an integrated dataset for *in silico* drug discovery.	1
PROMISCUOUS database	PROMISCUOUS is an exhaustive resource of protein–protein and drug–protein interactions aimed at providing a uniform dataset for a variety of purposing including drug repositioning.	2
MATADOR: Manually Annotated Targets and Drugs Online Resource	MATADOR is a resource for protein–chemical interactions and may be valuable in uncovering both direct and indirect connections between targets and drugs.	3
DrugBank	DrugBank database combines detailed drug data with drug target information. DrugBank includes information on over 1500 FDA-approved small molecule and protein-based drugs.	4
SuperTarget	SuperTarget integrates drug-related information along with their adverse effects and targets.	5

(Continued)

* While every effort has been made to ensure the accuracy of these resources/links at press time, the fast moving nature of the field that means we cannot guarantee their accuracy at the time of reading.

Drug Repositioning: Bringing New Life to Shelved Assets and Existing Drugs, First Edition.
Edited by Michael J. Barratt and Donald E. Frail.
© 2012 John Wiley & Sons, Inc. Published 2012 by John Wiley & Sons, Inc.

TABLE A.1. (*Continued*)

Database/Resource	Synopsis	Reference
TDD: Therapeutics Targets Database	The TTD is a database that provides information about the already explored drug targets and corresponding pathway information and drugs directed at each of the targets. Links to other databases are also provided.	6
Linked-In group: Drug repurposing— reprofiling— repositioning	This Linked-In group engages in online discussions about current topics of interest to people interested in drug repurposing.	7
Off-Label.com	Using Off-Label's Core Database along with their Target Library, one can connect druggable targets with potentially new clinical outcomes and identify "hidden phenotypes" to exploit.	8
Collaborative Drug Discovery (CDD)	CDD is a platform for cloud-based collaborative drug discovery. CDD hosts Public-Access Data relevant to drug discovery from a number of resources including the FDA.	9
FDA Adverse Event Reporting System (AERS)	The Adverse Event Reporting System (AERS) is a computerized information database designed to support the FDA's post-marketing safety surveillance program for all approved drug and therapeutic biologic products. Submissions to the database are voluntary as they are made from the point of care by healthcare professionals. The FDA uses AERS to monitor for new adverse events and medication errors that might occur with these marketed products. However, it can also provide the repositioning practitioner with insight into potential new uses for existing drugs based on their side effect profiles.	10

1) http://www.ondex.org/
2) http://bioinformatics.charite.de/promiscuous
3) http://matador.embl.de/
4) http://drugbank.ca/
5) http://bioinf-apache.charite.de/supertarget/
6) http://bidd.nus.edu.sg/group/cjttd/ttd.asp
7) http://www.linkedin.com/groups?home=&gid=3705627
8) http://www.off-label.com/
9) https://www.collaborativedrug.com/
10) http://www.fda.gov/Drugs/GuidanceComplianceRegulatoryInformation/Surveillance/AdverseDrugEffects/default.htm

TABLE A.2. A Selection of Companies involved in Drug Repurposing

Organization	Synopsis	Reference
Ampio Pharmaceuticals (formed from the merger of Chay Enterprises and DMI Life Sciences)	Ampio Pharmaceuticals has several repurposed drugs in its pipeline for treatment of premature ejaculation, diabetic retinopathy, diabetic macular edema, and diabetic nephropathy.	1
Anaxomics	Axanomics uses Systems Biology approaches and its bio-pathological maps technology and curated databases to reprofile existing drugs.	2
Aureus	Aureus applies its knowledge management processes to build predictive databases covering targets, pharmacology, absorption, distribution, metabolism, and excretion (ADME), drug–drug interactions, and experimental structure–activity relationship (SAR) data.	3
Biovista	Biovista uses its Clinical Outcomes Search Space platform (COSS) technology, which matches data about drug and disease mechanisms of action and adverse effects to identify drug repurposing opportunities.	4
Celentyx	Celentyx uses a platform technology that allows for rapid analysis of drug action on human immune cells to identify new uses in immune system diseases.	5
Concert Pharmaceuticals	Concert applies precision deuterium chemistry across the pharmacopeia of approved drugs and clinically validated compounds, generating numerous patentably distinct new chemical entities (NCEs). Deuteration can impact certain drugs'ADME properties, creating the potential for improved drug efficacy, safety, and tolerability.	6
Cypress Bioscience, Inc. (now acquired by Royalty Pharma)	Cypress received FDA approval for use of milnacipran HCl in the treatment of fibromyalgia. Milnacipran HCl is available in other countries for treatment of depression.	7, 8
Dualsystems Biotech	Dualsystems Biotech provides screening services specializing in drug profiling using a screening technology based on drug–protein binding.	9
Essentialis	Essentialis is developing a specific salt form of diazoxide (vasodialator for hypertension) and repurposing it as a treatment for dyslipidemia.	10

(Continued)

TABLE A.2. (*Continued*)

Organization	Synopsis	Reference
Gene Logic (Acquired by Ocimum Biosolutions)	Gene Logic is an integrated genomics company providing comprehensive genomic reference databases that can be used in genomic-driven bio-discovery programs.	11
Jenken Biosciences	Jenken Biosciences has identified two repurposed drugs as TLR4 antagonists that are capable of modulating excessive inflammatory responses.	12
Melior Discovery	Melior Discovery has pioneered a high-throughput *in vivo* pharmacology platform to identify novel indications for both preclinical and development stage drug candidates.	13
NeuroHealing Pharmaceuticals	NeuroHealing's stated mission is to repurpose neurologically active compound. Its pipeline is targeting three different indications and includes one agent formulated as a muco-adhesive thin film.	14
Numedicus	Numedicus uses a knowledge-based approach using a database combining known drug entities with mechanism and indication to identify new therapeutic switching opportunities.	15
NuMedii	NuMedii's New Indications Discovery technology is comprised of a proprietary database of genome-wide molecular profiles for more than 300 unique disease conditions and comprehensive, hierarchical knowledge bases of drug efficacy information. The technology also includes novel and proprietary integration and inference algorithms that incorporate multiple data resources to infer Signatures of Efficacy (SOE)™ as a molecular and probabilistic representation of drug efficacy.	16
Optimata	Optimata uses predictive biosimulation to build mathematical models of physiological and pathological processes. These models can be used drug repurposing projects.	17

TABLE A.2. (*Continued*)

Organization	Synopsis	Reference
Ore Pharmaceutical Holdings	As a pharmaceutical asset management company, all of Ore's in-licensed drug candidates were identified through drug repositioning collaborations with major pharmaceutical companies.	18
Pharnext	Pharnext uses underlying biological networks to identify combinations of already approved drugs to combine and repurpose as a new therapeutic treatment.	19
SOM Biotech	SOM Biotech uses an *in silico* technology developed by Intelligent Pharma to identify new applications for existing drugs candidates.	20
Sosei	Sosei's business model is primarily based on identifying drug repurposing opportunities using a drug reprofiling platform.	21
SWITCHBIOTECH	SWITCHBIOTECH employs data mining technology to match biological and compound data to predict potential drug candidates for dermatological diseases. They have established a development strategy based on systematic drug reprofiling and perhaps reformulation for topical use.	22
VervaPharmaceuticals (formerly ChemGenex and Adipogen)	Verva utilizes a Gene Expression Signature (GES) platform to identify new drug repurposing opportunities for metabolic diseases.	23
Vicus Therapeutics	Vicus product candidates are novel combinations and dosing regimens of two established generic drugs that have been selected based on published literature and expert knowledge.	24
Vivia Biotech	Vivia Biotech uses its automated flow cytometry approach to analyze the effect of drugs or combinations of drugs on *ex vivo* biological samples from many patients. This has resulted in identifying a repurposing opportunity for at least one drug.	25

(Continued)

TABLE A.2. (*Continued*)

Organization	Synopsis	Reference
XenoPort	Proprietary Transported Prodrug™ technology utilizes the body's natural mechanisms for actively transporting nutrients through cellular barriers. Suboptimal drugs are chemically modified to create a Transported Prodrug™ that utilizes transporters to gain efficient absorption into the bloodstream through active transport. Once in the blood stream, Transported Prodrugs™ are engineered to split apart, releasing the drug and natural substances that generally have well-studied, favorable safety characteristics.	26
Zalicus (formerly CombinatoRx)	Using its combination high-throughput screening technology, Zalicus has identified several unique combinations of repurposed drugs for specific indications.	27

1) http://ampiopharma.com/
2) http://www.anaxomics.com/drug-reprofiling.php
3) http://www.aureus-pharma.com
4) http://www.biovista.com/content.php?categ=10&pid=59
5) http://www.celentyx.com
6) http://www.concertpharma.com
7) http://www.cypressbio.com
8) http://www.royaltypharma.com/
9) http://www.drug-profiling.com/
10) http://www.essentialistherapeutics.com/
11) http://www.genelogic.com
12) http://www.jenkenbio.com
13) http://www.meliordiscovery.com/about_overview.html
14) http://www.neurohealing.com/
15) http://www.numedicus.co.uk
16) http://www.numedii.com/
17) http://www.optimata.com
18) http://www.orepharma.com/
19) http://www.pharnext.com/en/component/content/article/58-home/111-pharnext-news
20) http://www.sombiotech.com
21) http://www.sosei.com/
22) http://www.switch-biotech.com
23) http://www.vervapharma.com
24) http://www.vicustherapeutics.com
25) http://www.viviabiotech.com
26) http://www.xenoport.com
27) http://www.zalicus.com/

TABLE A.3. Drug Reformulation Companies

Organization	Synopsis	Reference
APT Pharmaceuticals	APT Pharmaceuticals is focused on the development of cyclosporine inhalation solution (CIS) for the prevention and treatment of chronic rejection in lung transplantation.	1
Collegium Pharmaceutical	Collegium is focused on the development of late stage, formulation-based product improvements protected by intellectual property.	2
Intarcia Therapeutics (formerly BioMedicines, Inc.)	Intarcia is focused on applying its proprietary subcutaneous delivery system along with stabilizing formulations to the delivery of drugs for the treatment of diabetes, obesity, and HCV.	3
iCeutica	iCeutica is focused on improving reformulated pharmaceutical drugs using a proprietary platform for preparing nanosized particles aimed at improving the solubility of reformulated drugs.	4
NeuroHealing Pharmaceuticals	NeuroHealing Pharmaceuticals discovers new uses for known drugs through reformulating and designing drug delivery modes suited to specific patient populations.	5
Zalicus (formed from CombinatoRx and Neuromed)	Zalicus has developed novel formulations and combinations of known drugs to achieve unique safety/efficacy profiles for specific indications.	6

1) http://www.aptbio.com/
2) http://collegiumpharma.com/
3) http://www.intarcia.com
4) http://iceutica.com/
5) http://www.neurohealing.com/
6) http://www.zalicus.com/

TABLE A.4. Academic and Publicly Funded Repositioning Initiatives

Organization/Initiative	Synopsis	Reference
University of California Davis School of Medicine—Clinical & Translational Science Awards (CTSA) Pharmaceutical Assets Portal	The UC Davis School of Medicine Clinical and Translational Science Center has coordinated the CTSA Academic Consortium and the implementation of the Pharmaceutical Assets Portal. The CTSA Pharmaceutical Assets Portal is funded as part of the National Institutes of Health Roadmap for Medical Research and has the ultimate goal of improving collaboration between industry and academia in the area of drug repositioning.	1
DTRA: Defense Department's Defense Threat Reduction Agency	DTRA awarded a contract to SRI International to lead a drug discovery and development program to identify approved drugs that could also be effective against biological threats.	2
FDA: The Rare Disease Repurposing Database (RDRD)	The RDRD includes data and cross-indexed information of already released FDA information about drugs, which offers sponsors a new tool for finding special opportunities to develop niche therapies that are already well advanced through development.	3
Johns Hopkins Clinical Compound Screening Initiative	The Johns Hopkins Clinical Compound Screening Initiative aims to collect all drugs ever used in medicine and use the collection to identify new uses for existing drugs. Currently over 3100 existing drugs make up the collection.	4
NIH Chemical Genomics Center (NCGC) Pharmaceutical Screening Collection (NPC)	NPC is a comprehensive, publicly accessible collection of approved and investigational drugs for high-throughput screening that proves a valuable resource for identifying candidates for repurposing and is being applied to neglected diseases among others, through TRND (see below).	5

TABLE A.4. (*Continued*)

Organization/Initiative	Synopsis	Reference
Sandler Center for Drug Discovery at University of California, San Francisco (UCSF)	The Sandler Center for Drug Discovery is a consortium of core laboratories at UCSF supporting development of new drugs for devastating global parasitic diseases. The Center seeks contributions of FDA-approved drugs and drugs that have successfully passed Phase I trials as these can provide a rich source of potential drugs for repurposing through their screening efforts.	6
TRND: Therapeutics for Rare and Neglected Diseases initiative (NIH)	TRND collaborative project proposals may be initiated at different stages of the drug development process. These include studies on drugs previously approved for another indication and with efficacy in an animal or cellular model of a rare or neglected disease, but in need of formulation, dose-finding disease-specific toxicology, or other studies to allow clinical testing to commence.	7

1) http://www.ctsapharmaportal.org
2) http://www.sri.com/news/releases/100407.html
3) http://www.fda.gov/ForIndustry/DevelopingProductsforRareDiseasesConditions/
   HowtoapplyforOrphanProductDesignation/ucm216147.htm
4) http://www.jhccsi.org
5) http://tripod.nih.gov/npc/
6) http://sandler.cgl.ucsf.edu/
7) http://trnd.nih.gov/

TABLE A.5. Nonprofit Organizations with Drug Repositioning Initiatives

Organization	Synopsis	Reference
BIO Ventures for Global Health	BIO Ventures for Global Health conducted an evaluation of the drug pipelines for neglected diseases in its study of the core capabilities of the entities focused on developing drugs for neglected diseases. They noted that several "quick wins" included repurposed drugs (Paromomycin and artesunate–amodiaquine).	1
Center for World Health and Medicine (CWHM) at Saint Louis University	The CWHM draws from a variety of resources for its lead identification, including redirecting marketed and advanced drug candidates toward neglected diseases.	2
The Chordoma Foundation	The Chordoma Foundation conducts a collaborative "drug repurposing" project with the NIH Chemical Genomics Center (NCGC). The NCGC is screening all approved drugs against chordoma cell lines.	3
Drugs for Neglected Diseases initiative (DNDi)	Among other strategies, the DNDi seeks new indications for existing medicines in the field of the most neglected diseases.	4
Leukemia & Lymphoma Society (LLS)	The Therapy Acceleration Program (TAP) at The Leukemia & Lymphoma Society (LLS) is a strategic initiative to speed the development of blood cancer treatments and supportive diagnostics. TAP looks to fund projects—including repositioned drugs—related to therapies that have the potential to change the standard of care for patients with blood cancer, especially in areas of high unmet medical need.	5
Michael J. Fox Foundation (MJJF) (Parkinson's disease [PD])	Awarded $2.4 million in funding in 2011 under its Repositioning Drugs for PD 2011 Request For Applications (RFA). Through this initiative, MJFF seeks to identify and reposition therapies for PD that are already clinically available for other indications in order to mitigate the time and costs involved in finding drugs that could help people living with Parkinson's.	6

TABLE A.5. (*Continued*)

Organization	Synopsis	Reference
Partnership for Cures	Partnership for Cures and its funding partners support researchers who undertake clinical trials and other "Rediscovery Research" including repurposing FDA-approved drugs and combining older drugs with newer drugs to improve new drug effectiveness.	7
The Polycystic Kidney Disease (PKD) Foundation	The PKD Foundation has launched an integrated research and development program including drug development through repurposing, targeted research grants, core grants, scientific meeting support, etc.	8
Rett Syndrome Research Trust (RSRT)	The RSRT is a start-up nonprofit organization focused on Rett Syndrome and MECP2 research. The Trust has funded the *in vivo* screening of FDA approved drugs and compounds of interest in mouse models of Rett. In addition, RSRT has initiated a collaboration with Melior Discovery to screen drug-candidates in an *in vivo* model of Rett Syndrome.	9
World Health Organization (WHO) Special Programme for Tropical Disease Research (TDR)	TDR has facilitated the partnering of industry with a network of compound assessment centers in an effort to capitalize on relevant compounds that pharmaceutical and animal healthcare companies possess that have not been previously assessed for their potential to treat tropical diseases.	10

1) http://www.bvgh.org/LinkClick.aspx?fileticket=3An6aKB2z6Y%3d&tabid=103
2) http://www.cwhm.org/index.php?page=sources-of-lead-molecules-for-drug-development
3) http://www.chordomafoundation.org/research/#Drug%20Repurposing
4) http://www.dndi.org/building-portfolio.html
5) http://www.lls.org/#/researchershealthcareprofessionals/drugdevelopment/therapyacceleration/
6) http://www.michaeljfox.org/newsEvents_mjffInTheNews_pressReleases_article.cfm?ID=486
7) http://www.4cures.org/home/funding_opportunities_for_researchers
8) http://www.pkdcure.org/Research/DrugDevelopment.aspx
9) http://www.rsrt.org/
10) http://apps.who.int/tdr/documents/TDR-business-plan-2008.pdf

TABLE A.6. U.S. and European Regulatory Agency Guidance Resources

Resource	Summary Text	Reference
FDA Regulatory Process: Guidance, Compliance, and Regulatory Information	High level FDA website for accessing information pertaining to FDA regulatory processes and other FDA-related information.	1
FDA Regulatory Process: Applications Covered by Section 505(b)(2) Draft 10/1999 Guidance	Examples of NDA applications submitted under Section 505(b)(2) include: changes in formulation, new combination products, and new indications for previously approved drugs.	2
FDA Regulatory Process: Fast Track Drug Development Programs	This guidance outlines criteria for qualifying for a Fast Track Drug Development program under Section 506(a) of the amended Federal Food, Drug, and Cosmetic Act.	3
European Medicines Agency (EMA): Preauthorization Process	This section of the EMA website provides information for companies and individuals involved in developing and marketing medicines for use in the European Union.	4
EMA: Guidance on new therapeutic indication for a well-established substance	One guiding principle for the preclinical/clinical studies under this Guidance is that the studies should have been conducted or sponsored by the applicant. However, see information pertaining to the generic/hybrid application process.	5
EMA: Pre-authorization Q&A: Generic/hybrid applications	Hybrid applications under Article 10(3) of Directive 2001/83/EC differ from generic applications in that the results of appropriate preclinical and clinical studies will be necessary in the case where there are changes in the active substance(s), therapeutic indications, strength, pharmaceutical form, or route of administration of the generic product compared with the reference medicinal product.	6

1) http://www.fda.gov/Drugs/GuidanceComplianceRegulatoryInformation/default.htm
2) http://www.fda.gov/downloads/Drugs/GuidanceComplianceRegulatoryInformation/Guidances/ucm079345.pdf
3) http://www.fda.gov/downloads/Drugs/GuidanceComplianceRegulatoryInformation/Guidances/ucm079736.pdf
4) http://www.ema.europa.eu/ema/index.jsp?curl=pages/regulation/general/general_content_000197.jsp&murl=menus/regulations/regulations.jsp&mid=WC0b01ac058002251c
5) http://ec.europa.eu/health/files/eudralex/vol-2/c/10%20_5_%20guideline_11-2007_en.pdf
6) http://www.ema.europa.eu/ema/index.jsp?curl=pages/regulation/general/general_content_000179.jsp&murl=menus/regulations/regulations.jsp&mid=WC0b01ac0580022717

Drug Repositioning: Bringing New Life to Shelved Assets and Existing Drugs, First Edition. Edited by Michael J. Barratt and Donald E. Frail. © 2012 John Wiley & Sons, Inc. Published 2012 by John Wiley & Sons, Inc.

Naltrexone, 28, 232, 412–413
National Center for Biotechnology
  Information (NCBI), 139, 143, 191
National Institutes for Neurological
  Disorders and Stroke (NINDS),
  361–362, 370–371, 408
National Institutes of Health (NIH), 168,
  362, 372–373, 421
Natural Language Processing (NLP),
  147–148, 153
neglected disease, 4, 5, 78, 169, 187, 348,
  361, 441, 455. *See also* orphan
  disease, rare disease
network analysis, 114, 116, 118–119, 124,
  127, 167, 176
neurodegenerative disease, 17, 116, 190,
  219, 263, 274, 399
Neurontin, 254, 256, 264, 278, 293,
  301–302, 332
new biologic entity (NBE), 45–47, 54.
  See also new chemical entity, new
  molecular entity
new chemical entity (NCE), 43, 45–47,
  54–55, 58–60, 63, 79, 137, 207, 229,
  282, 292, 303, 447, 450, 453. *See also*
  new biologic entity, new molecular
  entity
new drug application (NDA),11–14, 61,
  65–69, 71, 75–86, 231–292. *See also*
  505(b)(1), 505(b)(2), abbreviated
  new drug application
new indication, 26, 41–45, 55–64, 91–94,
  279–281, 433–435, 437–443, 445–447,
  449–452. *See also* additional
  indication, alternate indication,
  indications discovery, original
  indication, orphan indication,
  primary indication
new molecular entity (NME), 9–13, 18,
  20, 35, 83–85, 207, 226, 292, 304, 321.
  See also new biologic entity, new
  chemical entity
Nexium, 305–309
next-generation sequencing, 127–128,
  141
nicotine, 408–409
Nimbex, 305, 315–316
nonprofit organization, 4, 49, 348,
  389–391, 455–456

Norvir, 294–295, 325
null-effect model, 214–216

obesity, 102, 106–107, 113–115, 189, 254,
  274, 278, 364, 368, 439
off-label drug, 54, 58, 82, 83, 254–255,
  269, 279–281, 372, 390, 436.
  See also generic drug, over-the-
  counter drug
off-patent drug, 43, 391, 395, 397, 417,
  437, 439, 443. *See also* on-patent
  drug
off-target effect, 3, 35, 109, 116, 164,
  166–167, 177, 181, 183–184, 187, 191,
  193, 227, 278–279, 303, 445, 447, 449,
  452–454. *See also* on-target effect
omeprazole. *See* Prilosec
on-patent drug, 356, 395. *See also*
  off-patent drug
on-target effect, 3, 34, 109, 209, 269, 273,
  277–279, 281. *See also* off-target
  effect
onchoceriasis, 347–348, 368, 370–371
Online Mendelian Inheritance in Man
  (OMIM), 98, 100–101, 105, 146, 149,
  155
open-source database, 143–144, 363,
  372
open-source screening, 101, 142, 347, 352,
  361, 455
OpenBabel, 143–144, 156
original indication, 18, 33, 53, 226, 231,
  257, 266, 270, 279–282, 453. *See also*
  additional indication, alternate
  indication, indications discovery,
  new indication, orphan indication,
  primary indication
orphan disease, 4, 29, 44–45, 280, 421,
  453. *See also* neglected disease, rare
  disease
orphan drug, 15, 23, 28–29, 45, 79, 84–85,
  231, 357, 360, 397
  Orphan Drug Act (ODA), 29, 45
  Orphan Drug Database, 45
orphan indication, 44–46. *See also*
  additional indication, alternate
  indication, indications discovery,
  new indication, original indication,
  primary indication

Printed in the United States
by Bookmasters

Printed in the United States
By Bookmasters